PSYCHOPATHOLOGY

PSYCHOPATHOLOGY

Foundations for a Contemporary Understanding

SECOND EDITION

EDITED BY

JAMES E. MADDUX

AND

BARBARA A. WINSTEAD

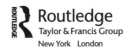

Routledge
Taylor & Francis Group
New York   London

Routledge
Taylor & Francis Group
270 Madison Avenue
New York, NY 10016

Routledge
Taylor & Francis Group
2 Park Square
Milton Park, Abingdon
Oxon OX14 4RN

© 2008 by Taylor & Francis Group, LLC
Routledge is an imprint of Taylor & Francis Group, an Informa business

Printed in the United States of America on acid-free paper
10 9 8 7 6 5 4 3 2

International Standard Book Number-13: 978-0-8058-6169-3 (Hardcover)

Library of Congress Cataloging-in-Publication Data

Psychopathology : foundations for a contemporary understanding / editors, James E. Maddux and
 Barbara A. Winstead. -- 2nd ed.
     p. cm.
 Includes bibliographical references and index.
 ISBN-13: 978-0-8058-6169-3 (alk. paper)
 ISBN-10: 0-8058-6169-6 (alk. paper)
  1. Psychology, Pathological. I. Maddux, James E. II. Winstead, Barbara A.

RC454.P786 2008
616.89--dc22   2007018747

**Visit the Taylor & Francis Web site at
http://www.taylorandfrancis.com**

**and the Routledge Web site at
http://www.routledge.com**

Contents

Contributors

Michele Boivin
University of Toronto

Annie Bollini
Emory University

Dianne L. Chambless
University of Pennsylvania

Georg H. Eifert
Chapman University

William Fals-Stewart
The Addiction and Family Research Group
RTI International

Katherine A. Fowler
Emory University

Paul J. Frick
University of New Orleans

Dolores Gallagher-Thompson
Stanford University School of Medicine

Howard N. Garb
University of Pittsburgh

Jennifer T. Gosselin
Sacred Heart University

Peter J. Guarnaccia
Rutgers, State University of New Jersey

C. Peter Herman
University of Toronto

Karen Hochman
Emory University

Rick Ingram
University of Kansas

Lisa Kestler
Emory University

Eva R. Kimonis
University of California, Irvine

Lisa M. Kinoshita
Stanford University School of Medicine

Keith Klostermann
The Addiction and Family Research Group
RTI International

Scott O. Lilienfeld
Emory University

Steven R. López
University of California, Los Angeles

Ashleigh Louis
Chapman University

Jennifer R. Lowe
University of Kentucky

James E. Maddux
George Mason University

Vijay A. Mittal
Emory University

Jack Naglieri
George Mason University

Thomas H. Ollendick
Virginia Polytechnic Institute and
  State University

Janet Polivy
University of Toronto

Johannes Rojahn
George Mason University

Claudia Salter
George Mason University

Janis Sanchez-Hucles
Old Dominion University

Janay B. Sander
University of Texas at Austin

Alison L. Shortt
University College London, England

Lucy Trenary Smith
University of Colorado

Robert F. Smith
George Mason University

Kristen H. Sorocco
University of Oklahoma Health Sciences Center

Rebecca E. Stewart
University of Pennsylvania

Elaine Walker
Emory University

Thomas A. Widiger
University of Kentucky

S. Lloyd Williams
University of Basel, Switzerland

Barbara A. Winstead
Old Dominion University

Michael J. Zvolensky
University of Vermont

Preface to the Second Edition

Since 1990, well over 30 textbooks have been published for abnormal psychology courses taught to undergraduates. This count does not include revised editions of existing books. The same period has seen the publication of numerous "handbooks" on psychopathology and psychiatry, which are conceived primarily as reference books for clinical practitioners and researchers. What has been missing is a true textbook of psychopathology for first-year graduate students in clinical psychology, counseling psychology, and related fields. Our goal in creating this book was to provide the "missing link" in the continuum. We designed the content and coverage for students in their first graduate-level course. The book also is appropriate for an advanced undergraduate course for exceptional students or those who have already taken an entry-level undergraduate course in abnormal psychology. This book was designed and written with *students* in mind. The length, organization, content, and level and style of writing reflect this intention. We, the editors, are clinical psychologists with together over 50 years of experience teaching doctoral students in clinical psychology. The chapter authors are among the most distinguished researchers in the fields of clinical psychology and psychopathology.

We are gratified that this book has been so well received that the publisher asked us to put together a second edition so soon after the first edition was published. The contributors were all eager for the opportunity to update their chapters and to provide the reader with the most current knowledge on their topics.

We had two primary goals for the book:

The first goal was to provide up-to-date information about theory and research on the etiology and treatment of the most important psychological disorders. Toward this end, we chose well-known authors who were not only familiar with the cutting-edge research in their areas of specialization but also were actively making contributions to it.

The second goal was to challenge students to think critically about psychopathology, not just memorize information. We tried to accomplish this goal in two ways. First, we encouraged authors to challenge traditional assumptions and theories about the problems they were addressing. Second, and more important, we commissioned chapters that dealt directly and in depth with such crucial and controversial issues as the definition of psychopathology; the influences of culture and gender; the validity of psychological testing; clinical judgment and decision making; the validity and utility of traditional psychiatric diagnosis; the role of biological factors in the cause of psychological problems; and (in a new chapter) psychotherapy research. We believe strongly that a sophisticated understanding of psychopathology in general and of specific psychological problems requires much more than the memorization of a list of *DSM* diagnostic criteria or the findings of numerous studies. Instead, it requires the mastery of ideas and concepts and how to use them in order to be critical users of the *DSM* and critical consumers of research.

We believe that most current books pay too little attention to these ideas, concepts, and issues. In Part I, we devote seven chapters to these issues. The major reason for placing these "issues" chapters before the "disorders" chapters is to give students a set of conceptual tools that will help them read more thoughtfully and critically the material on specific disorders.

This textbook is divided into two main parts. Part I is devoted to discussions of the ideas, concepts, and issues noted previously. Part II is devoted to the discussion of the most common problems and disorders. We asked authors to follow, to the extent possible, a common format consisting of:

1. A definition and description of the disorder or disorders.
2. A brief history of the study of the disorder.
3. Theory and research on etiology.
4. Research on empirically validated treatments.
5. A discussion of the issues covered in Part I where appropriate.

Editors always must make choices regarding what should be included in a textbook and what should not. A book that devoted a chapter to each and every disorder described in the *DSM* would be unwieldy and impossible to cover in a single semester. Our choices regarding what to include and what to exclude were guided primarily by our experiences of the kinds of psychological problems that clinical students typically encounter in their training and in their subsequent clinical careers. For these reasons, we included three chapters on the psychological and cognitive problems of children and adolescents.

We hope that both instructors and students will find our approach to psychopathology challenging and useful. We have learned much from our contributing authors in the process of editing their chapters, and we hope that students will learn much from reading what the authors have produced.

JAMES E. MADDUX
George Mason University
Fairfax, VA
BARBARA A. WINSTEAD
Old Dominion University
Norfolk, VA

I
Thinking about Psychopathology

1

Conceptions of Psychopathology

A Social Constructionist Perspective

James E. Maddux, Jennifer T. Gosselin, and
Barbara A. Winstead

A textbook about a topic should begin with a clear definition of the topic. Unfortunately, for a textbook on psychopathology, this is a difficult if not impossible task. The definitions or conceptions of *psychopathology* and such related terms as *mental disorder* have been the subject of heated debate throughout the history of psychology and psychiatry, and the debate is far from over (e.g., Gorenstein, 1984; Horwitz, 2002; Widiger, 1997). Despite its many variations, this debate has centered on a single overriding question: Are *psychopathology* and related terms such as *mental disorder* and *mental illness* scientific terms that can be defined objectively and by scientific criteria, or are they *social constructions* (Gergen, 1985) that are defined entirely by societal and cultural values? It is important to address this issue in the opening chapter because the reader's view of the rest of this book will be influenced by his or her view on this issue.

This chapter deals with *conceptions* of psychopathology. A conception of psychopathology is not a *theory* of psychopathology (Wakefield, 1992a). A conception of psychopathology attempts to define the term—to delineate which human experiences are considered psychopathological and which are not. A conception of psychopathology does not try to *explain* the psychological phenomena that are considered pathological but instead tells us which psychological phenomena are considered pathological and thus need to be explained. A *theory* of psychopathology, however, *is* an attempt to explain those psychological phenomena and experiences that have been identified by the conception as pathological. Theories and explanations for what is currently considered to be psychopathological human experience can be found in a number of other chapters, including all of those in part II.

Understanding various conceptions of psychopathology is important for a number of reasons. As medical philosopher Lawrie Reznek (1987) said, "Concepts carry consequences—classifying things one way rather than another has important implications for the way we behave towards such things" (p. 1). In speaking of the importance of the conception of *disease*, Reznek wrote:

> The classification of a condition as a disease carries many important consequences. We inform medical scientists that they should try to discover a cure for the condition. We inform benefactors that they should support such research. We direct medical care towards the

condition, making it appropriate to treat the condition by medical means such as drug therapy, surgery, and so on. We inform our courts that it is inappropriate to hold people responsible for the manifestations of the condition. We set up early warning detection services aimed at detecting the condition in its early stages when it is still amenable to successful treatment. We serve notice to health insurance companies and national health services that they are liable to pay for the treatment of such a condition. Classifying a condition as a disease is no idle matter. (p. 1)

If we substitute *psychopathology* or *mental disorder* for the word *disease* in this paragraph its message still holds true. How we conceive of psychopathology and related terms has wide-ranging implications for individuals, medical and mental health professionals, government agencies and programs, and society at large.

Conceptions of Psychopathology

A variety of conceptions of psychopathology has been offered over the years. Each has its merits and its deficiencies, but none suffices as a truly scientific definition.

Psychopathology as Statistical Deviance

A common and "commonsense" conception of psychopathology is that pathological psychological phenomena are those that are *abnormal*—statistically deviant or infrequent. Abnormal literally means "away from the norm." The word *norm* refers to what is typical or average. Thus, this conception views psychopathology as a deviation from statistical psychological normality.

One of the merits of this conception is its commonsense appeal. It makes sense to most people to use words such as *psychopathology* and *mental disorder* to refer only to behaviors or experiences that are infrequent (e.g., paranoid delusions, hearing voices) and not to those that are relatively common (e.g., shyness or sadness following the death of a loved one).

A second merit to this conception is that it lends itself to accepted methods of measurement that give it at least a semblance of scientific respectability. The first step in employing this conception scientifically is to determine what is statistically normal (typical, average). The second step is to determine how far a particular psychological phenomenon or condition deviates from statistical normality. This is often done by developing an instrument or measure that attempts to quantify the phenomenon and then assigns numbers or scores to people's experiences or manifestations of the phenomenon. Once the measure is developed, *norms* are typically established so that an individual's score can be compared to the mean or average score of some group of people. Scores that are sufficiently far from average are considered to be indicative of "abnormal" or "pathological" psychological phenomena. This process describes most tests of intelligence and cognitive ability and many commonly used measures of personality and emotion (e.g., the Minnesota Multiphasic Personality Inventory). Despite its common sense appeal and its scientific merits, this conception presents problems. It sounds relatively objective and scientific because it relies on well-established psychometric methods for developing measures of psychological phenomena and developing norms. Yet, this approach leaves much room for subjectivity.

The first point at which subjectivity comes into play is in the *conceptual definition* of the construct for which a measure is developed. A measure of any psychological construct, such as intelligence, must begin with a conceptual definition. We have to ask ourselves "What is 'intelligence'?" Of course, different people (including different psychologists) will come up with different answers to this question. How then can we scientifically and objectively determine which definition or conception is "true" or "correct"? The answer is that we cannot. Although we have tried-and-true methods for developing a reliable and valid measure (i.e., it consistently predicts what we want to predict) of a psychological construct once we have agreed on its conception or definition, we cannot use these same methods to determine which conception or definition is true or correct. The bottom line is that there is not a "true" definition of intelligence and no objective, scientific way of determining one. Intelligence is not a thing that exists inside of people and makes them behave in certain ways and that awaits our discovery of its "true" nature. Instead, it is an abstract idea that is defined by people as they use the words *intelligence* and *intelligent* to describe certain kinds of human behavior and the covert mental processes that supposedly precede or are at least concurrent with the behavior.

We usually can observe and describe patterns in the way most people use the words *intelligence* and *intelligent* to describe the behavior of themselves and others. The descriptions of the patterns then comprise the definitions of the words. If we examine the patterns of the use of *intelligence* and *intelligent*, we find that at the most basic level, they describe a variety of specific behaviors and abilities that society values and thus encourages; unintelligent behavior is a variety of behaviors that society does not value and thus discourages. The fact that the definition of *intelligence* is grounded in societal values explains the recent expansion of the concept to include good interpersonal skills (i.e., social and emotional intelligence), self-regulatory skills, artistic and musical abilities, and other abilities not measured by traditional tests of intelligence. The meaning of *intelligence* has broadened because society has come to place increasing value on these other attributes and abilities, and this change in societal values has been the result of a dialogue or discourse among the people in society, both professionals and laypersons. One measure of intelligence may prove more reliable than another and more useful than another measure in predicting what we want to predict (e.g., academic achievement, income), but what we want to predict reflects what we value, and values are not scientifically derived.

Another point for the influence of subjectivity is in the determination of *how deviant* a psychological phenomenon must be from the norm to be considered abnormal or pathological. We can use objective, scientific methods to construct a measure such as an intelligence test and develop norms for the measure, but we are still left with the question of how far from normal an individual's score must be to be considered abnormal. This question cannot be answered by the science of psychometrics because the distance from the average that a person's score must be to be considered "abnormal" is a matter of debate, not a matter of fact. It is true that we often answer this question by relying on statistical conventions such as using one or two standard deviations from the average score as the line of division between normal and abnormal. Yet the decision to use that convention is itself subjective. Why should one standard deviation from the norm designate "abnormality"? Why not two standard deviations? Why not half a standard deviation? Why not use percentages? The lines between normal and abnormal can be drawn at many different points using many different strategies. Each line of demarcation may be more or less useful for certain purposes, such as determining the criteria for eligibility for limited services and resources. Where the line is set also determines the prevalence of "abnormality" or "mental disorder" among the general population (Kutchens & Kirk, 1997), so it has great practical significance. But no such line is more or less "true" than the others even when based on statistical conventions.

We cannot use the procedures and methods of science to draw a definitive line of demarcation between normal and abnormal psychological functioning, just as we cannot use them to draw lines of demarcation between "short" and "tall" people or "hot" and "cold" on a thermometer. No such lines exist in nature awaiting our discovery.

Psychopathology as Maladaptive (Dysfunctional) Behavior

Most of us think of psychopathology as behavior and experience that are not just statistically abnormal but also maladaptive (dysfunctional). *Normal* and *abnormal* are statistical terms, but *adaptive* and *maladaptive* refer not to statistical norms and deviations but to the effectiveness or ineffectiveness of a person's behavior. If a behavior "works" for the person—if the behavior helps the person deal with challenges, cope with stress, and accomplish his or her goals—then we say the behavior is more or less adaptive. If the behavior does not help in these ways, or if the behavior makes the problem or situation worse, we say it is more or less maladaptive.

Like the statistical deviance conception, this conception has commonsense appeal and is consistent with the way most laypersons use words such as *pathology, disorder,* and *illness.* Most people would find it odd to use these words to describe statistically infrequent, high levels of intelligence, happiness, or psychological well-being. To say that someone is "pathologically intelligent" or "pathologically well-adjusted" seems contradictory because it flies in the face of the commonsense use of these words.

The major problem with the conception of psychopathology as maladaptive behavior is its inherent subjectivity. Like the distinction between normal and abnormal, the distinction between adaptive and maladaptive is fuzzy and often arbitrary. We have no objective, scientific way of making a clear distinction. Very few human behaviors are in and of themselves either adaptive or maladaptive; their adaptiveness and maladaptiveness depend on the situations in which they are enacted and on the judgment and values of the actor and the observers. Even behaviors that are statistically rare, and therefore abnormal, will be more or less adaptive under different conditions and more or less adaptive in the opinion of different observers. The extent to which a behavior or behavior pattern is viewed as more or less adaptive or maladaptive depends on a number of factors, such as the goals the person is trying to accomplish and the social norms and expectations of a given situation. What works in one situation might not work in another. What appears adaptive to one person might not appear so to another. What is usually adaptive in one culture might not be so in another (see Lopez & Guarnaccia, this volume). Even a so-called normal personality involves a good deal of occasionally maladaptive behavior, which we can find evidence for in our own lives and the lives of friends and relatives. In addition, people given official "personality disorder" diagnoses by clinical psychologists and psychiatrists often can manage their lives effectively and do not always behave in disordered ways.

Another problem with the "psychopathological equals maladaptive" conception is that determinations of adaptiveness and maladaptiveness are logically unrelated to measures of statistical deviation. Of course, often we do find a strong relationship between the statistical abnormality of a behavior and its maladaptiveness. Many of the problems described in the *Diagnostic and Statistical Manual of Mental Disorders (DSM-IV-TR;* American Psychiatric Association, 2000) and in this textbook are both maladaptive and statistically rare. There are, however, major exceptions to this relationship. First, psychological phenomena that deviate from the norm or the average are not all maladaptive. In fact, sometimes deviation from the norm is adaptive and healthy. For example, IQ scores of 130 and 70 are equally deviant from the norm, but abnormally high intelligence is much more adaptive than abnormally low intelligence. Likewise, people who consistently score abnormally low on measures of anxiety and depression are probably happier and better adjusted than people who consistently score equally abnormally high on such measures.

Second, maladaptive psychological phenomena are not all statistically infrequent and vice versa. For example, shyness is very common and therefore is statistically frequent, but shyness is almost always maladaptive to some extent, because it almost always interferes with a person's ability to accomplish what he or she wants to accomplish in life and relationships. This is not to say that shyness is "pathological" but only that it makes it difficult for some people to live full and happy lives. The same is true of many of the problems with sexual functioning that are included in the *DSM* as "mental disorders" but are relatively common (see Gosselin, this volume).

Psychopathology as Distress and Disability

Some conceptions of psychopathology invoke the notions of *subjective distress* and *disability.* Subjective distress refers to unpleasant and unwanted feelings such as anxiety, sadness, and anger. Disability refers to a restriction in ability (Ossorio, 1985). People who seek mental health treatment usually are not getting what they want out of life, and many feel that they are unable to do what they need to do to accomplish their valued goals. They may feel inhibited or restricted by their situation, their fears, or emotional turmoil, or by physical or other limitations. Individuals may lack the necessary self-efficacy beliefs (beliefs about personal abilities), physiological or biological components, self-regulatory skills, or situational opportunities to make positive changes (Bergner, 1997).

Subjective distress and disability are simply two different but related ways of thinking about adaptiveness and maladaptiveness rather than alternative conceptions of psychopathology. Although the notions of subjective distress and disability may help refine our notion of maladaptiveness, they do nothing to resolve the subjectivity problem. Different people will define personal distress and personal disability in vastly different ways, as will different mental health professionals and different cultures. Likewise, people differ in how much distress or disability they can tolerate. Thus, we are still left with the problem of how to determine normal and abnormal levels of distress and disability. As noted previously, the question "How much is too much?" cannot be answered using the objective methods of science.

Another problem is that some conditions or patterns of behavior (e.g., pedophilia, antisocial personality disorder) that are considered psychopathological (at least officially, according to the *DSM*) are *not* characterized by subjective distress, other than the temporary distress that might result from social condemnation or conflicts with the law.

Psychopathology as Social Deviance

Psychopathology has also been conceived as behavior that deviates from social or cultural norms. This conception is simply a variation of the conception of psychopathology as statistical abnormality, only in this case judgments about deviations from normality are made informally by people rather than formally by psychological tests or measures.

This conception also is consistent to some extent with common sense and common parlance. We tend to view psychopathological or mentally disordered people as thinking, feeling, and doing things that most other people do not do and that are inconsistent with socially accepted and culturally sanctioned ways of thinking, feeling, and behaving.

The problem with this conception, as with the others, is its subjectivity. Norms for socially normal or acceptable behavior are not scientifically derived but instead are based on the values, beliefs, and historical practices of the culture, which determine who is accepted or rejected by a society or culture. Cultural values develop not through the implementation of scientific methods but through numerous informal conversations and negotiations among the people and institutions of that culture. Social norms differ from one culture to another, and therefore what is psychologically abnormal in one culture may not be so in another (see Lopez & Guarnaccia, this volume). Also, norms of a given culture change over time; therefore, conceptions of psychopathology will change over time, often very dramatically, as evidenced by American society's changes over the past several decades in attitudes toward sex, race, and gender. For example, psychiatrists in the 1800s classified masturbation, especially in children and women, as a disease, and it was treated in some cases by clitoridectomy (removal of the clitoris), which Western society today would consider barbaric (Reznek, 1987). Homosexuality was an official mental disorder in the *DSM* until 1973 (see also Gosselin, this volume).

In addition, the conception of psychopathology as social norm violation is at times in conflict with the conception of psychopathology as maladaptive behavior. Sometimes violating social norms is healthy and adaptive for the individual and beneficial to society. In the 19th century, women and African Americans in the United States who sought the right to vote were trying to change well-established social norms. Their actions were uncommon and therefore "abnormal," but these people were far from psychologically unhealthy, at least not by today's standards. Earlier in the 19th century, slaves who desired to escape from their owners were said to have "drapetomania." Although still practiced in some parts of the world, slavery is almost universally viewed as socially deviant and pathological, and the desire to escape enslavement is considered to be as normal and healthy as the desire to live and breathe.

Psychopathology as Harmful Dysfunction

A more recent attempt at defining psychopathology is Wakefield's (1992a, 1992b, 1993, 1997, 1999) *harmful dysfunction* (HD) conception. Presumably grounded in evolutionary psychology (e.g., Cosmides, Tooby, & Barkow, 1992), the HD conceptionacknowledges that the conception of mental disorder is influenced strongly by social and cultural values. It also proposes, however, a supposedly scientific, factual, and objective core that is not dependent on social and cultural values. In Wakefield's (1992a) words:

> a [mental] disorder is a harmful dysfunction wherein *harmful* is a value term based on social norms, and *dysfunction* is a scientific term referring to the failure of a mental mechanism to perform a natural function for which it was designed by evolution…a disorder exists when the failure of a person's internal mechanisms to perform their function as designed by nature impinges harmfully on the person's well-being as defined by social values and meanings. (p. 373)

One of the merits of this description is that it acknowledges that the conception of mental disorders must include a reference to social norms; however, this conception also tries to ground the concept of mental disorder in a scientific theory—that is, the theory of evolution.

Wakefield (2006) recently has reiterated this definition in writing that a mental disorder "satisfies two requirements: (1) it is negative or harmful according to cultural values; and (2) it is caused by a dysfunction (i.e., by a failure of some psychological mechanism to perform a natural function for which it was evolutionarily designed)" (p. 157). He and his colleagues also write, "Problematic mismatches between designed human nature and current social desirability are not disorders…[such as] adulterous longings, taste for fat and sugar, and male aggressiveness" (Wakefield, Horwitz, & Schmitz, 2006, p. 317).

However, the claim that identifying a failure of a "designed function" is a scientific judgment and not a value judgment is open to question. Wakefield's (1992a, p. 383) claim that dysfunction can be defined in "purely factual scientific" terms rests on the assumption that the "designed functions" of human "mental mechanisms" have an objective and observable reality and, thus, that failure of the mechanism to execute its designed function can be objectively assessed. A basic problem with this notion is that although the physical inner workings of the body and brain can be observed and measured, "mental mechanisms" have no objective reality and thus cannot be observed directly—no more so than the "unconscious" forces that provide the foundation for Freudian psychoanalysis.

Evolutionary theory provides a basis for explaining human behavior in terms of its contribution to reproductive fitness. A behavior is considered more functional if it increases the survival of those who share your genes in the next generation and the next and less functional if it does not. Evolutionary psychology cannot, however, provide a catalogue of "mental mechanisms" and their natural functions. Wakefield states that "discovering what in fact is natural or dysfunctional may be extraordinarily difficult" (1992b, p. 236). The problem with this statement is that, when applied to human behavior, "natural" and "dysfunctional" are not properties that can be "discovered"; they are value judgments. The judgment that a behavior represents a dysfunction relies on the observation that the behavior is excessive or inappropriate under certain conditions. Arguing that these behaviors represent failures of evolutionarily designed "mental mechanisms" (itself an untestable hypothesis because of the occult nature of "mental mechanisms") does not relieve us of the need to make value judgments about what is excessive or inappropriate in what circumstances. These are value judgments based on social norms not scientific "facts," an issue that we will explore in greater detail later in this chapter (see also Widiger, this volume).

Another problem with the HD conception is that it is a moving target. Recently, Wakefield modified the HD conception by saying that it is concerned not with what a mental disorder *is* but only with what most scientists *think* it is. For example, he states that "My comments were intended to argue, not that PTSD [posttraumatic stress disorder] is a disorder, but that the HD analysis is capable of explaining why the symptom picture in PTSD is *commonly judged* to be a disorder" (1999, p. 390, emphasis added). Wakefield's original goal was to "define mental disorders *prescriptively*" (Sadler, 1999, p. 433, emphasis added) and to "help us decide whether someone is mentally disordered or not" (Sadler, 1999, p. 434). His more recent view, however, "avoids making any prescriptive claims, instead focusing on explaining the conventional clinical use of the disorder concept" (Sadler, 1999, p. 433). Wakefield "has abandoned his original task to be prescriptive and has now settled for being *descriptive* only, for example, telling us why a disorder is judged to be one" (Sadler, 1999, p. 434, emphasis added).

Describing how people have agreed to define a concept is not the same as defining the concept in scientific terms, even if those people are scientists. Thus, Wakefield's revised HD conception simply offers another criterion that people (clinicians, scientists, and laypersons) might use to judge whether or not something is a "mental disorder." But consensus of opinion, even among scientists, is not scientific evidence. Therefore, no matter how accurately this criterion might describe how some or most people define "mental disorder," it is no more or no less scientific than other conceptions that also are based on how some people *agree* to define "mental disorder." It is no more scientific than the conceptions involving statistical infrequency, maladaptiveness, or social norm violations (see also Widiger, this volume).

The DSM Definition of Mental Disorder

Any discussion of conceptions of psychopathology has to include a discussion of the most influential conception of all—that of the *Diagnostic and Statistical Manual of Mental Disorders (DSM)*. The *DSM* documents "what is currently understood by most scientists, theorists, researchers, and clinicians to be the predominant forms of psychopathology" (Widiger, this volume). First published in 1952 and revised and expanded five times since, the *DSM* provides the organizational structure for virtually every textbook (including this one) on abnormal psychology and psychopathology, as well as almost every professional book on the assessment and treatment of psychological problems (see Widiger, this volume, for a more detailed history of psychiatric classification and the *DSM*).

Just as a textbook on psychopathology should begin by defining its key term, so should a taxonomy of mental disorders. To their credit, the authors of the *DSM* attempted to do that. The difficulties inherent in attempting to define psychopathology and related terms are clearly illustrated by the definition of "mental disorder" found in the latest edition of the *DSM*, the *DSM-IV-TR* (American Psychiatric Association, 2000):

> ...a clinically significant behavioral or psychological syndrome or pattern that occurs in an individual and that is associated with present distress (e.g., a painful symptom) or disability (i.e., impairment in one or more important areas of functioning) or with a significantly increased risk of suffering death, pain, disability, or an important loss of freedom. In addition, this syndrome or pattern must not be merely an expectable and culturally sanctioned response to a particular event, for example, the death of a loved one. Whatever its cause, it must currently be considered a manifestation of a behavioral, psychological, or biological dysfunction in the individual. Neither deviant behavior (e.g., political, religious, or sexual) nor conflicts that are primarily between the individual and society are mental disorders unless the deviance or conflict is a symptom of a dysfunction in the individual, as described above. (p. xxxi)

All of the conceptions of psychopathology described previously can be found to some extent in this definition—statistical deviation (i.e., not "expectable"); maladaptiveness, including distress and disability; social norms violations; and some elements of the harmful dysfunction conception ("a dysfunction in the individual") although without the flavor of evolutionary theory. For this reason, it is a comprehensive, inclusive, and sophisticated conception and probably as good, if not better, than any proposed so far. Nonetheless, it falls prey to the same problems with subjectivity as other conceptions. For example, what is the meaning of "clinically significant" and how should "clinical significance" be measured? Does clinical significance refer to statistical infrequency, maladaptiveness, or both? How much distress must a person experience or how much disability must a person exhibit before he or she is said to have a mental disorder? Who gets to judge the person's degree of distress or disability? How do we determine whether or not a particular response to an event is "expectable" or "culturally sanctioned"? Who gets to determine this? How does one determine whether or not deviant behavior or conflicts "are primarily between the individual and society"? What exactly does this mean? What does it mean for a dysfunction to exist or occur "in the individual"? Certainly a biological dysfunction might be said to be literally "in the individual," but does it make sense to say the same of psychological and behavioral dysfunctions? Is it possible to say that a psychological or behavioral dysfunction can occur "in the individual" apart from the sociocultural and interpersonal milieu in which the person is acting? Clearly, the *DSM*'s conception of mental disorder raises as many questions as do the conceptions it was meant to supplant.

Dichotomies and Categories versus Dimensions The difficulty inherent in the *DSM* conception of psychopathology and other attempts to distinguish between normal and abnormal or adaptive and maladaptive is that they are *dichotomous* or *categorical models* that attempt to describe guidelines for clearly distinguishing between individuals who are normal or abnormal and for determining which specific abnormality or "disorder" a person has. An alternative model, overwhelmingly supported by research, is the *dimensional model*. In the dimensional model, normality and abnormality, as well as effective and ineffective psychological functioning, lie along a continuum; so-called psychological disorders are simply extreme variants of normal psychological phenomena and ordinary problems in living (Keyes & Lopez, 2002; Widiger, this volume). The dimensional model is concerned not with classifying people or disorders but with identifying and measuring individual differences in psychological phenomena such as emotion, mood, intelligence, and personality styles (e.g., Lubinski, 2000). Great differences among individuals on the dimensions of interest are expected, such as the differences we find on standardized tests of intelligence. As with intelligence, divisions between normality and abnormality may be demarcated for convenience or efficiency but are not to be viewed as indicative of true discontinuity among "types" of phenomena or "types" of people. Also, statistical deviation is not viewed as necessarily pathological, although extreme variants on either end of a dimension (e.g., introversion-extraversion, neuroticism, intelligence) may be maladaptive if they lead to inflexibility in functioning.

Empirical evidence for the validity of a dimensional approach to psychological adjustment is strongest in the area of personality and personality disorders (Costello, 1996; Maddux & Mundell, 1999; Coker & Widiger, this volume). Factor analytic studies of personality problems among the general population and clinical populations with "personality disorders" demonstrate striking similarity between the two groups. In addition, these factor structures are not consistent with the *DSM*'s system of classifying disorders of personality into categories (Maddux & Mundell, 1999) and support a dimensional rather than a categorical view. For example, the most recent evidence strongly suggests that psychopathic personality (or antisocial personality) and other externalizing disorders of adulthood display a dimensional structure, not a categorical structure (Edens, Marcus, Lilienfeld, & Poythress, 2006; Krueger, Markon, Patrick, & Iacono, 2005; Larsson, Andershed, & Lichtenstein,

2006). The dimensional view of personality disorders also is supported by cross-cultural research (Alarcon, Foulks, & Vakkur, 1998).

Research on other problems supports the dimensional view. Studies of the varieties of normal emotional experiences (e.g., Oatley & Jenkins, 1992) indicate that "clinical" emotional disorders are not discrete classes of emotional experience that are discontinuous from everyday emotional upsets and problems. Research on adult attachment patterns in relationships strongly suggests that dimensions are more useful descriptions of such patterns than are categories (Fraley & Waller, 1998). Research on self-defeating behaviors has shown that they are extremely common and are not by themselves signs of abnormality or symptoms of "disorders" (Baumeister & Scher, 1988). Research on children's reading problems indicates that "dyslexia" is not an all-or-none condition that children either have or do not have but occurs in degrees without a natural break between "dyslexic" and "nondyslexic" children (Shaywitz, Escobar, Shaywitz, Fletcher, & Makuch, 1992). Research on attention deficit/hyperactivity (Barkley, 1997) and posttraumatic stress disorder (Anthony, Lonigan, & Hecht, 1999) demonstrates this same dimensionality. Research on depression and schizophrenia indicates that these "disorders" are best viewed as loosely related clusters of dimensions of individual differences, not as diseaselike syndromes (Claridge, 1995; Costello, 1993a, 1993b; Persons, 1986). For example, a study on depressive symptoms among children and adolescents found a dimensional structure for all of the *DSM-IV* symptoms of major depression (Hankin, Fraley, Lahey, & Waldman, 2005). The inventor of the term *schizophrenia*, Eugene Bleuler, viewed so-called pathological conditions as continuous with so-called normal conditions and noted the occurrence of "schizophrenic" symptoms among normal individuals (Gilman, 1988). In fact, Bleuler referred to the major symptom of "schizophrenia" (thought disorder) as simply "ungewonlich," which in German means "unusual," not "bizarre," as it was translated in the first English version of Bleuler's classic monograph (Gilman, 1988). Essentially, the creation of "schizophrenia" was "an artifact of the ideologies implicit in nineteenth century European and American medical nosologies" (Gilman, 1988, p. 204). Indeed, research indicates that the hallucinations and delusions exhibited by people diagnosed with a schizophrenic disorder are continuous with experiences and behaviors among the general population (Johns & van Os, 2001; see also Walker, Bollini, Hochman, & Kestler, this volume). Finally, biological researchers continue to discover continuities between so-called normal and abnormal (or pathological) psychological conditions (Claridge, 1995; Livesley, Lang, & Vernon, 1998).

Social Constructionism and Conceptions of Psychopathology

If we cannot come up with an objective and scientific conception of psychopathology and mental disorder, then what way is left to us to understand these terms? How then are we to conceive of psychopathology? The solution to this problem is not to develop yet another definition of psychopathology. The solution, instead, is to accept the fact that the problem has no solution—at least not a solution that can be arrived at by scientific means. We have to give up the goal of developing a scientific definition and accept the idea that psychopathology and related terms are not the kind of terms that can be defined through the processes that we usually think of as scientific. We have to stop struggling to develop a scientific conception of psychopathology and attempt instead to try to understand the struggle itself—why it occurs and what it means. We need to better understand how people go about trying to conceive of and define psychopathology, what they are trying to accomplish when they do this, and how and why these conceptions are the topic of continual debate and undergo continual revision.

We start by accepting the idea that psychopathology and related concepts are abstract ideas that are not scientifically constructed but *socially* constructed. To do this is to engage in *social constructionism*, which involves "elucidating the process by which people come to describe, explain, or otherwise account for the world in which they live" (Gergen, 1985, pp. 3–4). Social constructionism is concerned with "examining ways in which people understand the world, the social and political processes that influence how people define words and explain events, and the implications of these definitions and explanations—who benefits and who loses because of how we describe and understand the world" (Muehlenhard & Kimes, 1999, p. 234). From this point of view, words and concepts such as *psychopathology* and *mental disorder* "are products of particular historical and cultural understandings rather than...universal and immutable categories of human experience" (Bohan, 1996, p. xvi). Universal or "true" definitions of concepts do not exist because these definitions depend primarily on who gets to do the defining. The people who define them are usually people with power, and so these definitions reflect and promote their interests and values (Muehlenhard & Kimes, 1999, p. 234). Therefore, "When less powerful people attempt to challenge existing power relationships and to promote social change, an initial battleground is often the words used to discuss these problems" (Muehlenhard & Kimes, 1999, p. 234). Because the interests of people and institutions are based on their values, debates over the definition of concepts often become clashes between deeply and implicitly held beliefs about the way the world works or should work and about the difference between right and wrong. Such clashes are evident in the debates over the definitions of *domestic violence* (Muehlenhard & Kimes, 1999), *child sexual abuse* (Holmes & Slapp, 1998; Rind, Tromovich, & Bauserman, 1998), and other such terms.

The social constructionist perspective can be contrasted with the *essentialist* perspective. Essentialism assumes that there are natural categories and that all members of a given category share important characteristics (Rosenblum & Travis, 1996). For example, the essentialist perspective views our categories of race, sexual orientation, and social class as objective categories that are independent of social or cultural processes. It views these categories as representing "empirically verifiable similarities among and differences between people" (Rosenblum & Travis, 1996, p. 2). In the social constructionist view, however, "reality cannot be separated from the way that a culture makes sense of it" (Rosenblum & Travis, 1996, p. 3). In social constructionism, such categories represent not what people *are* but rather the ways that people think about and attempt to make sense of differences among people. Social processes also determine what differences among people are more important than other differences (Rosenblum & Travis, 1996).

Thus, from the essentialist perspective, psychopathologies and mental disorders are natural entities whose true nature can be discovered and described. From the social constructionist perspective, however, they are but abstract ideas that are defined by people and thus reflect their values—cultural, professional, and personal. The meanings of these and other concepts are not *revealed* by the methods of science but are *negotiated* among the people and institutions of society who have an interest in their definitions. In fact, we typically refer to psychological terms as *constructs* for this very reason—that their meanings are constructed and negotiated rather that discovered or revealed. The ways in which conceptions of so basic a psychological construct as the "self" (Baumeister, 1987) and "self-esteem" (Hewitt, 2002) have changed over time and the different ways they are conceived by different cultures (e.g., Cross & Markus, 1999; Cushman, 1995; Hewitt, 2002) provide an example of this process at work. Thus "all categories of disorder, even physical disorder categories convincingly explored scientifically, are the product of human beings constructing meaningful systems for understanding their world" (Raskin & Lewandowski, 2000, p. 21). In addition, because "what it means to be a person is determined by cultural ways of talking about and conceptualizing personhood...identity and disorder are socially constructed, and there are as many disorder constructions as there are cultures" (Neimeyer & Raskin, 2000, pp. 6–7; see also Lopez and Guarnaccia, this volume). Finally, "if people cannot reach the objective truth about what disorder really is, then viable constructions of disorder must compete with one another on the basis of their use and meaningfulness in particular clinical situations" (Raskin & Lewandowski, 2000, p. 26).

From the social constructionist perspective, sociocultural, political, professional, and economic forces influence professional and lay conceptions of psychopathology. Our conceptions of psychological normality and abnormality are not facts about people but abstract ideas that are constructed through the implicit and explicit collaborations of theorists, researchers, professionals, their clients, and the culture in which all are embedded and that represent a shared view of the world and human nature. For this reason, "mental disorders" and the numerous diagnostic categories of the *DSM* were not "discovered" in the same manner that an archaeologist discovers a buried artifact or a medical researcher discovers a virus. Instead, they were invented (Raskin & Lewandowski, 2000). By saying that mental disorders are invented, however, we do not mean that they are "myths" (Szasz, 1974) or that the distress of people who are labeled as mentally disordered is not real. Instead, we mean that these disorders do not "exist" and "have properties" in the same manner that artifacts and viruses do. Therefore, a conception of psychopathology "does not simply describe and classify characteristics of groups of individuals, but...actively constructs a version of both normal and abnormal...which is then applied to individuals who end up being classified as normal or abnormal" (Parker, Georgaca, Harper, McLaughlin, & Stowell-Smith, 1995, p. 93).

Conceptions of psychopathology and the various categories of psychopathology are not mappings of psychological facts about people. Instead, they are social artifacts that serve the same sociocultural goals as do our conceptions of race, gender, social class, and sexual orientation—those of maintaining and expanding the power of certain individuals and institutions and maintaining social order, as defined by those in power (Beall, 1993; Parker et al., 1995; Rosenblum & Travis, 1996). As with other social constructions, our concepts of psychological normality and abnormality are tied ultimately to social values—in particular, the values of society's most powerful individuals, groups, and institutions—and the contextual rules for behavior derived from these values (Becker, 1963; Parker et al., 1995; Rosenblum & Travis, 1996). As McNamee and Gergen (1992) state: "The mental health profession is not politically, morally, or valuationally neutral. Their practices typically operate to sustain certain values, political arrangements, and hierarchies of privilege" (p. 2). Thus, the debate over the definition of psychopathology, the struggle over who gets to define it, and the continual revisions of the *DSM*, are not aspects of a search for "truth." Rather, they are debates over the definition of socially constructed abstractions and struggles for the personal, political, and economic power that derives from the authority to define these abstractions and thus to determine what and whom society views as normal and abnormal. As David Patrick (2005) concluded about a definition of mental disorder offered by the British government in a mental health bill, "The concept of mental disorder is of dubious scientific value but it has substantial political utility for several groups who are sane by mutual consent" (p. 435).

These debates and struggles are described in detail by Allan Horwitz (2000) in *Creating Mental Illness*. According to Horwitz,

> The emergence and persistence of an overly expansive disease model of mental illness was not accidental or arbitrary. The widespread creation of distinct mental diseases developed in specific historical circumstances and because of the interests of specific social groups.... By the time the *DSM-III* was developed in 1980, thinking of mental illnesses as discrete disease entities...offered mental health professionals many social, economic, and political advantages. In addition, applying disease frameworks to a wide variety of behaviors and to a large number of people benefited a number of specific social groups including not only clinicians but also research scientists, advocacy groups, and pharmaceutical companies, among others. The disease entities of diagnostic psychiatry arose because they were useful for the social practices of various groups, not because they provided a more accurate way of viewing mental disorders. (p. 16)

Psychiatrist Mitchell Wilson (1993) has offered a similar position. He has argued that the dimensional/continuity view of psychological wellness and illness posed a basic problem for psychiatry because it "did not demarcate clearly the well from the sick" (p. 402) and that "if conceived of psychosocially, psychiatric illness is not the province of medicine, because psychiatric problems are not truly medical but social, political, and legal" (p. 402). The purpose of *DSM-III*, according to Wilson, was to allow psychiatry a means of marking out its professional territory. Kirk and Kutchins (1992) reached the same conclusion following their thorough review of the papers, letters, and memos of the various *DSM* working groups.

The social construction of psychopathology works something like this: Someone observes a pattern of behaving, thinking, feeling, or desiring that deviates from some social norm or ideal or identifies a human weakness or imperfection that, as expected, is displayed with greater frequency or severity by some people than by others. A group with influence and power decides that control, prevention, or "treatment" of this problem is desirable or profitable. The pattern is then given a scientific-sounding name, preferably of Greek or Latin origin. The new scientific name is capitalized. Eventually, the new term may be reduced to an acronym, such as OCD (obsessive-compulsive disorder), ADHD (attention-deficit/hyperactivity disorder), and BDD (body dysmorphic disorder). The new disorder then takes on an existence all its own and becomes a diseaselike entity. As news about "it" spreads, people begin thinking they have "it;" medical and mental health professionals begin diagnosing and treating "it," and clinicians and clients begin demanding that health insurance policies cover the "treatment" of "it." Once the "disorder" has been socially constructed and defined, the methods of science can be employed to study it, but the construction itself is a social process, not a scientific one. In fact, the more "it" is studied, the more everyone becomes convinced that "it" really is "something."

Medical philosopher Lawrie Reznek (1987) has demonstrated that even our definition of physical disease is socially constructed. He writes:

> Judging that some condition is a disease is to judge that the person with that condition is less able to lead a good or worthwhile life. And since this latter judgment is a normative one, to judge that some condition is a disease is to make a normative judgment…. This normative view of the concept of disease explains why cultures holding different values disagree over what are diseases (p. 211) … Whether some condition is a disease depends on where we choose to draw the line of normality, and this is not a line that we can discover.(p. 212) … disease judgments, like moral judgments, are not factual ones.

Likewise, Sedgwick (1982) points out that human diseases are natural processes. They may harm humans, but they actually promote the "life" of other organisms. For example, a virus's reproductive strategy may include spreading from human to human. Sedgwick writes:

> There are no illnesses or diseases in nature. The fracture of a septuagenarian's femur has, within the world of nature, no more significance than the snapping of an autumn leaf from its twig; and the invasion of a human organism by cholera-germs carries with it no more the stamp of "illness" than does the souring of milk by other forms of bacteria. Out of his anthropocentric self-interest, man has chosen to consider as "illnesses" or "diseases" those natural circumstances which precipitate death (or the failure to function according to certain values). (p. 30)

If these statements are true of physical disease, they are certainly true of psychological "disease" or psychopathology. Like our conception of physical disease, our conceptions of psychopathology are social constructions that are grounded in sociocultural goals and values, particularly our assumptions about how people should live their lives and about what makes life worth living. This truth is illustrated clearly in the American Psychiatric Association's 1952 decision to include homosexuality in the first edition of the *DSM* and its 1973 decision to revoke its "disease" status (Kutchins & Kirk, 1997; Shorter, 1997). As stated by Wilson (1993), "The homosexuality controversy seemed to show that psychiatric diagnoses were clearly wrapped up in social constructions of deviance" (p. 404). This issue also was in the forefront of the debates over posttraumatic stress disorder, paraphilic rapism, and masochistic personality disorder (Kirk & Kutchins, 1997), as well as caffeine dependence, sexual compulsivity, low-intensity orgasm, sibling rivalry, self-defeating personality, jet lag, pathological spending, and impaired sleep-related painful erections, all of which were proposed for inclusion in *DSM-IV* (Widiger & Trull, 1991). Others have argued convincingly that *schizophrenia* (Gilman, 1988), *addiction* (Peele, 1995), *personality disorder* (Alarcon et al., 1998), and *dissociative identity disorder* (formerly *multiple personality disorder*) (Spanos, 1996) also are socially constructed categories rather than disease entities.

With each revision, our most powerful professional conception of psychopathology, the *DSM*, has had more and more to say about how people should live their lives. Between 1952 and 2000, the number of pages in the *DSM* increased from 86 to 943, and the number of mental disorders increased from 106 to 385. As the scope of "mental disorder" has expanded with each *DSM* revision, life has become increasingly pathologized, and the sheer number of people with diagnosable mental disorders has continued to grow. Moreover, mental health professionals have not been content to label only obviously and blatantly dysfunctional patterns of behaving, thinking, and feeling as "mental disorders." Instead, we have defined the scope of psychopathology to include many common problems in living.

Consider some of the "mental disorders" found in the *DSM-IV*: Cigarette smokers have Nicotine Dependence. If you drink large quantities of coffee, you may develop Caffeine Intoxication or Caffeine-Induced Sleep Disorder. If you have "a preoccupation with a defect in appearance" that causes "significant distress or impairment in…functioning" (p. 466), you have Body Dysmorphic Disorder. A child whose academic achievement is "substantially below that expected for age, schooling, and level of intelligence" (p. 46) has a Learning Disorder. Toddlers who throw tantrums have Oppositional Defiant Disorder. Not wanting sex often enough is Hypoactive Sexual Desire Disorder. Not wanting sex at all is Sexual Aversion Disorder. Having sex but not having orgasms or having them too late or too soon is an Orgasmic Disorder. Failure (for men) to maintain "an adequate erection…that causes marked distress or interpersonal difficulty" (p. 504) is Male Erectile Disorder. Failure (for women) to attain or maintain "an adequate lubrication or swelling response of sexual excitement" (p. 502) accompanied by distress is Female Sexual Arousal Disorder.

The past few years have witnessed media reports of epidemics of Internet addiction, road rage, and "shopaholism." Discussions of these new disorders have turned up at scientific meetings and in courtrooms. They are likely to find a home in the next revision of the *DSM* if the media, mental health professions, and society at large continue to collaborate in their construction and if "treating" them and writing books about them become lucrative.

The social constructionist perspective does not deny that human beings experience behavioral and emotional difficulties—sometimes very serious ones. It insists, however, that such experiences are not evidence for the existence of entities called "mental disorders" that can then be invoked as causes of those behavioral and emotional difficulties. The belief in the existence of these entities is the product of the all too human tendency to socially construct categories in an attempt to make sense of a confusing world.

Summary and Conclusions

The debate over the conception or definition of *psychopathology* and related terms has been going on for decades, if not centuries, and will continue, just as we will always have debates over the definitions of truth, beauty, justice, and art. Our position is that *psychopathology* and *mental disorder* are not the kinds of terms whose "true" meanings can be discovered or defined objectively by employing the methods of science. They are *social constructions*—abstract ideas whose meanings are negotiated among the people and institutions of a culture and that reflect the values and power structure of that culture at a given time. Thus, the conception and definition of *psychopathology* always has been and always will be debated and always has been and always will be changing. It is not a static and concrete thing whose true nature can be discovered and described once and for all.

By saying that conceptions of psychopathology are socially constructed rather than scientifically derived, we are not proposing, however, that human psychological distress and suffering are not real or that the patterns of thinking, feeling, and behaving that society decides to label *psychopathology* cannot be studied objectively and scientifically. Instead, we are saying that it is time to acknowledge that science can no more determine the "proper" or "correct" conception of *psychopathology* and *mental disorder* than it can determine the "proper" and "correct" conception of other social constructions such as beauty, justice, race, and social class. We can nonetheless use science to study the phenomena that our culture refers to as psychopathological. We can use the methods of science to understand a culture's conception of mental or psychological health and disorder, how this conception has evolved, and how it affects individuals and society. We also can use the methods of science to understand the origins of the patterns of thinking, feeling, and behaving that a culture considers psychopathological and to develop and test ways of modifying those patterns.

Psychology and psychiatry will not be diminished by acknowledging that their basic concepts are socially and not scientifically constructed—no more than medicine is diminished by acknowledging that the notions of *health* and *illness* are socially constructed (Reznek, 1987), nor economics by acknowledging that the notions of *poverty* and *wealth* are socially constructed. Science cannot provide us with "purely factual, scientific" definitions of these concepts. They are fluid and negotiated matters of value, not fixed matters of fact.

As Lilienfeld and Marino (1995) have said:

Removing the imprimatur of science…would simply make the value judgments underlying these decisions more explicit and open to criticism… heated disputes would almost surely arise concerning which conditions are deserving of attention from mental health professionals. Such disputes, however, would at least be settled on the legitimate basis of social values and exigencies, rather than on the basis of ill-defined criteria of doubtful scientific status. (pp. 418–419)

References

Alarcon, R. D., Foulks, E. F., & Vakkur, M. (1998). *Personality disorders and culture: Clinical and conceptual interactions*. New York: Wiley.

American Psychiatric Association (1994). *Diagnostic and statistical manual of mental disorders* (4th ed.). Washington, D.C.: Author.

American Psychiatric Association (2000). *Diagnostic and statistical manual of mental disorders* (4th ed., rev.). Washington, DC: Author.

Anthony, J. L., Lonigan, C. J., & Hecht, S. A. (1999). Dimensionality of post-traumatic stress disorder symptoms in children exposed to disaster: Results from a confirmatory factor analysis. *Journal of Abnormal Psychology, 108*, 315–325.

Barkley, R. A. (1997). *ADHD and the nature of self-control*. New York: Guilford.

Baumeister, R. F. (1987). How the self became a problem: A psychological review of historical research. *Journal of Personality and Social Psychology, 52*, 163–176.

Baumeister, R. F., & Scher, S. J. (1988). Self-defeating behavior patterns among normal individuals: Review and analysis of common self-destructive tendencies. *Psychological Bulletin, 104*(1), 3–22.

Beall, A. E. (1993). A social constructionist view of gender. In A. E. Beall & R. J. Sternberg (Eds.), *The psychology of gender.* (pp. 127–147). New York: Guilford.

Becker, H. S. (1963). *Outsiders*. New York: Free Press.

Bergner, R. M. (1997). What is psychopathology? And so what? *Clinical Psychology: Science and Practice, 4*, 235–248.

Bohan, J. (1996). *The psychology of sexual orientation: Coming to terms*. New York: Routledge.

Claridge, G. (1995). *Origins of mental illness*. Cambridge, MA: Malor Books/ISHK

Cosmides, L., Tooby, J., & Barkow, J. H. (1992). Introduction: Evolutionary psychology and conceptual integration. In J. H. Barkow, L. Cosmides, & J. Tooby (Eds.), *The adapted mind: Evolutionary psychology and the generation of culture* (pp. 3–17). New York: Oxford University Press.

Costello, C. G. (1993a). *Symptoms of depression*. New York: Wiley.

Costello, C. G. (1993b). *Symptoms of schizophrenia*. New York: Wiley.

Costello, C. G. (1996). *Personality characteristics of the personality disordered*. New York: Wiley.

Cross, S. E., & Markus, H. R. (1999). The cultural constitution of personality. In L. A. Pervin & O. P. John (Eds.), *Handbook of personality: Theory and Research* (2nd ed., pp. 378–396). New York: Guilford.

Cushman, P. (1995). *Constructing the self, constructing America*. New York: Addison-Wesley.

Edens, J. F., Marcus, D. K., Lilienfeld, S. O., & Poythress, N. G. (2006). Psychopathic, not psychopath: Taxometric evidence for the dimensional structure of psychopathy. *Journal of Abnormal Psychology, 115*, 131–144.

Fraley, R. C., & Waller, N. G. (1998). Adult attachment patterns: A test of the typological model. In J. A. Simpson & W. S. Rholes (Eds.), *Attachment theory and close relationships* (pp. 77–114). New York: Guilford.

Gardner, H. (1999). *Intelligence reframed: Multiple intelligences for the 21st century*. Cambridge, MA: Basic.

Gergen, K. J. (1985). The social constructionist movement in modern psychology. *American Psychologist, 40*(3), 266–275.

Gergen, K. J. (1999). *An invitation to social construction*. Thousand Oaks, CA: Sage.

Gilman, S. L. (1988). *Disease and representation: Images of illness from madness to AIDS*. Ithaca, NY: Cornell University Press.

Gorenstein, E. E. (1984). Debating mental illness: Implications for science, medicine, and social policy. *American Psychologist, 39*, 50–56.

Hankin, B. L., Fraley, R. C., Lahey, B. B., & Waldman, I. D. (2005). Is depression best viewed as a continuum or a discrete category? A taxonomic analysis of childhood and adolescent depression in a population-based sample. *Journal of Abnormal Psychology, 114*, 96–110.

Hewitt, J. P. (2002). The social construction of self-esteem. In C. R. Snyder & S. J. Lopez (Eds.), *Handbook of positive psychology* (pp. 135–147). New York: New York University Press.

Holmes, W. C., & Slapp, G. B. (1998). Sexual abuse of boys: Definition, prevalence, correlates, sequelae, and management. *Journal of the American Medical Association, 280*, 1855–1862.

Horwitz, A. V. (2002). *Creating mental illness*. Chicago: University of Chicago Press.

Johns, L. C., & van Os, J. (2001). The continuity of psychotic experiences in the general population. *Clinical Psychology Review, 21*, 1125–1141.

Kelly, L., & Radford, J. (1998). Sexual violence against women and girls: An approach to an international overview. In R. E. Dobash & R. P. Dobash (Eds.), *Rethinking violence against women* (pp. 53–76). Thousand Oaks, CA: Sage.

Keyes, C. L., & Lopez, S. J. (2002). Toward a science of mental health: Positive directions in diagnosis and interventions. In C. R. Snyder & S. J. Lopez (Eds.), *Handbook of positive psychology* (pp. 45–59). London: Oxford University Press.

Kirk, S. A., & Kutchins, H. (1992). *The selling of DSM: The rhetoric of science in psychiatry*. New York: Aldine de Gruyter

Krueger, R F., Markon, K. E., Patrick, C. J., & Iacono, W. G. (2005). Externalizing psychopathology in adulthood: A dimensional-spectrum conceptualization and its implications for DSM-V. *Journal of Abnormal Psychology, 114*, 537–550.

Kutchins, H., & Kirk, S. A. (1997). *Making us crazy: DSM: The psychiatric bible and the creation of mental disorder*. New York: Free Press.

Larsson, H., Andershed, H., & Lichtenstein, P. (2006). A genetic factor explains most of the variation in the psychopathic personality. *Journal of Abnormal Psychology, 115*, 221–230.

Lilienfeld, S. O., & Marino, L. (1995). Mental disorder as a Roschian concept: A critique of Wakefield's "harmful dysfunction" analysis. *Journal of Abnormal Psychology, 104*(3), 411–420.

Livesley, W. J., Jang, K. L., & Vernon, P. A. (1998). Phenotypic and genotypic structure of traits delineating personality disorder. *Archives of General Psychiatry, 55*, 941–948.

Lubinski, D. (2000). Scientific and social significance of assessing individual differences: "Sinking shafts at a few critical points." *Annual Review of Psychology, 51*, 405–444.

Maddux, J. E., & Mundell, C. E. (1999). Disorders of personality: Diseases or individual differences? In V. J. Derlega, B. A. Winstead, & W. H. Jones (Eds.), *Personality: Contemporary theory and research* (2nd ed., pp. 541–571). Chicago: Nelson-Hall.

McNamee, S., & Gergen, K. J. (1992). *Therapy as social construction*. Thousand Oaks, CA: Sage.

Muehlenhard, C. L., & Kimes, L. A. (1999). The social construction of violence: The case of sexual and domestic violence. *Personality and Social Psychology Review, 3*, 234–245.

Neimeyer, R. A., & Raskin, J. D. (2000). On practicing postmodern therapy in modern times. In R. A. Neimeyer & J. D. Raskin (Eds.), *Constructions of disorder: Meaning-making frameworks for psychotherapy* (pp. 3–14). Washington, D.C.: American Psychological Association.

Oatley, K., & Jenkins, J. M. (1992). Human emotions: Function and dysfunction. *Annual Review of Psychology, 43*, 55–85.

Ossorio, P. G. (1985). Pathology. *Advances in Descriptive Psychology, 4*, 151–201.

Parker, I., Georgaca, E., Harper, D., McLaughlin, T., & Stowell-Smith, M. (1995). *Deconstructing psychopathology*. London: Sage.

Patrick, D. (2005). Defining mental disorder: Tautology in the service of sanity in British mental health legislation. *Journal of Mental Health, 14*, 435–443.

Peele, S. (1995). *Diseasing of America: How we allowed recovery zealots and the treatment industry to convince us we are out of control*. San Francisco: Lexington Books.

Persons, J. (1986). The advantages of studying psychological phenomena rather than psychiatric diagnosis. *American Psychologist, 41*, 1252–1260.

Raskin, J. D., & Lewandowski, A. M. (2000). The construction of disorder as human enterprise. In R. A. Neimeyer & J. D. Raskin (Eds.), *Constructions of disorder: Meaning-making frameworks for psychotherapy* (pp. 15–40). Washington, D.C.: American Psychological Association.

Reznek, L. (1987). *The nature of disease*. London: Routledge & Kegan Paul.

Rind, B., Tromovich, P., & Bauserman, R. (1998). A meta-analytic examination of assumed properties of child sexual abuse using college samples. *Psychological Bulletin, 124*, 22–53.

Rosenblum, K. E., & Travis, T. C. (1996). Constructing categories of difference: Framework essay. In K. E. Rosenblum & T. C. Travis (Eds.), *The meaning of difference: American constructions of race, sex and gender, social class, and sexual orientation* (pp. 1–34). New York: McGraw-Hill.

Sadler, J. Z. (1999). Horsefeathers: A commentary on "Evolutionary versus prototype analyses of the concept of disorder." *Journal of Abnormal Psychology, 108*, 433–437.

Sedgwick, P. (1982). *Psycho politics: Laing, Foucault, Goffman, Szasz, and the future of mass psychiatry*. New York: Harper & Row.

Shaywitz, S. E., Escobar, M. D., Shaywitz, B. A., Fletcher, J. M., & Makuch, R. (1992). Evidence that dyslexia may represent the lower tail of a normal distribution of reading ability. *New England Journal of Medicine, 326*(3), 145–150.

Shorter, E. (1997). *A history of psychiatry: From the era of the asylum to the age of Prozac*. New York: Wiley.

Spanos, N. P. (1996). *Multiple identities and false memories: A sociocognitive perspective*. Washington, D.C.: American Psychological Association.

Szasz, T. S. (1974). *The myth of mental illness*. New York: Harper & Row

Wakefield, J. C. (1992a). The concept of mental disorder: On the boundary between biological facts and social values. *American Psychologist, 47*(3), 373–388.

Wakefield, J. C. (1992b). Disorder as harmful dysfunction: A conceptual critique of DSM-III-R's definition of mental disorder. *Psychological Review, 99*, 232–247.

Wakefield, J. C. (1993). Limits of operationalization: A critique of Spitzer and Endicott's (1978) proposed operational criteria for mental disorder. *Journal of Abnormal Psychology, 102*, 160–172.

Wakefield, J. C. (1997). Normal inability versus pathological inability: Why Ossorio's definition of mental disorder is not sufficient. *Clinical Psychology: Science and Practice, 4*, 249–258.

Wakefield, J. C. (1999). Evolutionary versus prototype analyses of the concept of disorder. *Journal of Abnormal Psychology, 108*, 374–399.

Wakefield, J. C. (2006). Personality disorder as harmful dysfunction: *DSM*'s cultural deviance criterion reconsidered. *Journal of Personality Disorders, 20*(2), 157–169.

Wakefield, J. C., Horwitz, A. V., & Schmitz, M. F. (2006). Are we overpathologizing the socially anxious? Social phobia from a harmful dysfunction perspective. *Canadian Journal of Psychiatry, 50*(6), 317–427.

Widiger, T. A. (1997). The construct of mental disorder. *Clinical Psychology: Science and Practice, 4*, 262–266.

Widiger, T. A., & Trull, T. J. (1991). Diagnosis and clinical assessment. *Annual Review of Psychology, 42*, 109–134.

Wilson, M. (1993). *DSM-III* and the transformation of American psychiatry: A history. *American Journal of Psychiatry, 150*, 399–410.

2

Cultural Dimensions of Psychopathology
The Social World's Impact on Mental Disorders[1]

Steven Regeser López and Peter J. Guarnaccia

Over the past several decades, researchers have increasingly examined cultural influences in psychopathology. However, for much of this period the study of culture and mental disorders was a marginal field of inquiry. As we demonstrate in this review, cultural issues have moved to the fore in the study of psychopathology. A landmark event marking this transition came in 1977 when Kleinman heralded the beginning of a "new cross-cultural psychiatry," an interdisciplinary research approach integrating anthropological methods and conceptualizations with traditional psychiatric and psychological approaches. Mental health researchers were encouraged to respect indigenous illness categories and to recognize the limitations of biomedical illness categories, such as depression and schizophrenia. Also, the new cross-cultural psychiatry distinguished between disease, a "malfunctioning or maladaptation of biological or psychological processes", and illness, "the personal, interpersonal, and cultural reaction to disease" (p. 9). The perspective that Kleinman and others (Fabrega, 1975; Kleinman, Eisenberg, & Good, 1978) articulated in the seventies reflected an important direction for the study of culture and psychopathology—to understand the social world within mental illness (see also Draguns, 1980; Marsella, 1980).

Many advances were made during the first decade of the new cross-cultural psychiatry. One was the establishment of the interdisciplinary journal, *Culture, Medicine, and Psychiatry*. This newly founded journal, in conjunction with *Transcultural Psychiatry* in Canada (formerly *Transcultural Psychiatric Research Review*), provided and continues to provide an important forum for cultural research in psychology and psychiatry. Also, during the eighties, large-scale epidemiologic studies were carried out. The second multinational World Health Organization (WHO) study of schizophrenia was launched and preliminary findings were reported (Sartorius et al., 1986). The Epidemiological Catchment Area (ECA) studies were conducted as well (Regier et al., 1984). Some may question how culturally informed these classic studies were (Edgerton & Cohen, 1994; Fabrega, 1990; Guarnaccia, Kleinman, & Good, 1990). However, most reviews of culture, ethnicity, and mental disorders today refer to the findings from the WHO and ECA studies to address how social, ethnic, and cultural factors are related to the distribution of psychopathology. Also during this time, the National Institute of Mental Health funded research centers with the sole purpose of conducting research on and for specific ethnic minority groups (African Americans, American Indians, Latino Americans, and Asian Americans). Some of the research from these centers contributed to the growing cultural psychopathology database (e.g., Cervantes, Padilla, & Salgado de Zinder, 1991; King, 1978; Manson, Shore, & Bloom, 1985; Neighbors, Jackson, Campbell, & Williams, 1989; Rogler, Malgady, & Rodriguez, 1989; Sue, Fujino, Hu, Takeuchi, & Zane, 1991).

Dialogues across disciplines were also initiated during this time. For example, Kleinman and Good's (1985) influential volume, *Culture and Depression*, brought together the research of not only anthropologists, but also of psychologists and psychiatrists as well as historians and philosophers. Another significant indicator of the field's development was and continues to be its success in attracting new investigators. In sum, these first 10 years can be characterized as an exciting and fertile time for the study of cultural psychopathology.

Despite the many advances, the field's main messages were not reaching larger audiences. Investigators were communicating primarily among themselves in their specialty journals and books. On a rare occasion, one would find a special issue on cultural research in a mainstream journal (e.g., Butcher, 1987). Those findings that did manage to be published in widely distributed journals were scattered among a broad array of journals. Thus, from the perspective of mainstream investigators, the developments of the new cross-cultural psychiatry went largely unnoticed. A telling example of this occurred at a joint meeting of the *DSM-IV* Task Force and the Culture and Diagnosis Work Group in 1991. After two days of intensive discussion of the potential contributions of cultural psychopathology research to *DSM-IV*, the chair of the *DSM-IV* Task Force commented that this was really interesting work and that the members of the Culture and Diagnosis Work Group should publish this research—this three years after Kleinman's (1988) *Rethinking Psychiatry* had appeared! In this book, Kleinman provided a comprehensive review of culture, psychopathology, and related research. Drawing on empirical data and theory, he argued that culture matters for the study and treatment of mental disorders. This volume serves as a significant marker in the development of the new cross-cultural psychiatry, which we refer to here as the study of cultural psychopathology.

Key Developments

Conceptual Contributions

Definition of culture Central to the study of cultural psychopathology is the definition of culture. Much of the past and even current research relies on a definition of culture that is outdated. In fact, Betancourt and López (1993) wrote a critical review of cultural and psychological research in which culture was defined as the values, beliefs, and practices that pertain to a given ethnocultural group. The strength of this definition is that it begins to unpack culture. Instead of arguing that a given expression of distress resides within a given ethnocultural group, for example, researchers argue that the expression of distress is related to a specific value or orientation. We see this as a significant advancement. It helps researchers begin to operationalize what about culture matters in the specific context. Further, it recognizes the heterogeneity within specific ethnocultural groups. Knowing that someone belongs to a specific ethnic group provides guidelines to potential cultural issues in psychopathology, but it does not imply that that person adheres to all the cultural values and practices of that group.

At the same time, this definition of culture as values, beliefs, and practices has significant limitations (Lewis-Fernandez & Kleinman 1995). One is that it depicts culture as residing largely within individuals. The emphasis on values and beliefs points out the psychological nature of culture. We argue that culture is manifested in the interaction between people and is highly social in nature. Situating practices (customs and rituals) with values and beliefs gives the impression that the practices in the social world are a function of values and beliefs. For example, people are thought to rely on their family in times of crisis because they are high in *familism* or family orientation. Investigators rarely examine what about the social world facilitates or fosters reliance on family members. Perhaps harsh environmental conditions contribute to families coming together to overcome adversity. When applying the values and beliefs definition of culture, the social world is subjugated to the psychological world of the individual. Contrary to this perspective, we argue that it is action in the social and physical world that produces culture as much as people's ideas about the world. In our view, the social world interacts on an equal footing with the psychological world in producing human behavior.

A second important limitation of this frequently used definition of culture is that it depicts culture as a static and bounded phenomenon. We assert that culture involves process and change and that culture is constantly in flux both in its regions of origin and as people bring their cultures with them as they move around the globe (Garro, 2001; Greenfield, 1997; Guarnaccia & Rodriguez, 1996). Attempts to freeze culture into a set of generalized value orientations or behaviors will continually misrepresent what culture is. Culture is a dynamic and creative process, some aspects of which are shared by large groups of individuals resulting from particular life circumstances and histories. Given the changing nature of our social world and given the efforts of individuals to adapt to such changes, culture can best be viewed as an ongoing process, a system or set of systems in flux.

A related limitation of the values-based definition of culture is that it depicts people as recipients of culture from a generalized "society" with little recognition of the individual's role in negotiating their cultural worlds (Garro, 2000). More recent approaches to culture in anthropology, while not discarding the importance of a person's cultural inheritance of ideas, values, and ways of relating, have focused equally on the emergence of culture from the life experiences and interactions of individuals and small groups. People can change, add to, or reject cultural elements through social processes such as migration and acculturation. A viable definition of culture acknowledges the agency of individuals in establishing their social worlds.

In sum, current views of culture attend much more to people's social world than past views of culture that emphasized the individual. Of particular interest are people's daily routines and how such activities are tied to families, neighborhoods, villages, and social networks. By examining people's daily routines one can identify what matters most to people (Gallimore, Goldenberg, & Weisner, 1993) or what is most at stake for people (Kleinman, 2006; Ware & Kleinman, 1992). Furthermore, this perspective captures the intersubjective and interactional dimensions of culture as it is both a product of group values, norms, and experiences, as well as individual innovations and life histories. The use of this broader definition of culture should help guide investigators away from flat, unidimensional notions of culture, to discover the richness of a cultural analysis for the study of psychopathology. An important component of this perspective is the examination of intracultural diversity. In particular, social class, poverty, and gender continue to affect different levels of mental health both within and across cultural groups.

Goals of cultural research Culture is important in a number of domains within psychopathology research. It is important in the expression of disorder and distress; a cultural analysis can point out the variability in the manner in which mental illness is manifested. Social and cultural factors can also affect the etiology and prevalence of disorder by differentially placing some at more risk than others for developing psychopathology. In addition, the course of disorder, as reflected in the degree of disability, or in the number of clinical relapses, is also related to important cultural factors. We want to encourage all of these lines of inquiry.

Regardless of the specific domain of research, there are two meta-goals of cultural research. Some writers imply that cultural research should test the generality of given theoretical notions. For example, in a thoughtful analysis of cultural research Clark (1987) noted: "Conceptual progress in psychology requires a unified base for investigating psychological phenomena, with culture-relevant variables included as part of the matrix" (p. 465). From Clark's point of view, cross-cultural work can serve to enhance the generality of given conceptual models by adding cultural variables to an existing theoretical model when necessary to explain between group and within group variance. Although Clark acknowledges the possibility that a construct developed in one country may not have a counterpart in another country, at no time does she discuss the value of deriving models of distinct clinical entities found in only one country or ethnocultural group. This suggests that for Clark the main purpose of studying culture is to reinforce the universality of existing psychological models by subsuming cross-cultural variations into the mainstream of research.

In contrast, both Fabrega (1990) and Rogler (1989) criticize researchers for attending insufficiently to the cultural specificity of mental illness and mental health. Fabrega examines researchers' use of mainstream instruments and conceptualizations in studying mental disorders among Latinos and challenges such researchers to be bold in their critiques of "establishment psychiatry." Rogler recommends a framework for mainstream psychiatric researchers that attends more fully to culture. For both Fabrega and Rogler, the risk of overlooking cultural variations is much greater in current psychopathology research than the risk of overlooking cultural similarities. Focusing on culture-specific phenomena at this time is of central importance to the further development of the field.

An important conceptual advancement is the recognition of both positions, that is, studying culture to identify general processes and studying culture to identify culture-specific processes. By focusing only on generalities, we overlook the importance of culture-specific phenomena. On the other hand, by emphasizing culture-specific phenomena we overlook the possibility of generalities. The overall purpose of cultural research, therefore, is to advance our understanding of general processes, culture-specific processes, and the manner in which they interact in specific contexts (see also Beals, Manson, Mitchell, Spicer, & AI-SUPERPFP Team, 2003; Draguns, 1990). Our aim is to identify culture's mark amidst the ubiquity of human suffering.

Major Advances: DSM-IV, the World Mental Health Report, and the Surgeon General's Report on Mental Health: Culture, Race, and Ethnicity

We now turn to selected developments since the mid-1980s in the study of culture and psychopathology. We begin with a discussion of three of the most important projects that were carried out since 1988: the incorporation of cultural factors in the *Diagnostic and Statistical Manual-IV* (*DSM-IV*; American Psychiatric Association, 1994), the publication of the *World Mental Health Report* (Desjarlais, Eisenberg, Good, & Kleinman, 1996), and the release of the *U.S. Surgeon General's Report on Mental Health: Culture, Race and Ethnicity* (U.S. Department of Health and Human Services [USDHHS], 2001).

The National Institute of Mental Health (NIMH) funded the establishment of a Culture and Diagnosis Work Group to inform the development of the *DSM-IV*. The work group's efforts resulted in three main contributions to *DSM-IV*: (1) inclusion of some discussion of how cultural factors can influence the expression, assessment, and prevalence of disorders in each of the disorder chapters; (2) an outline of a cultural formulation of clinical diagnosis to complement the multiaxial assessment; and (3) a glossary of relevant cultural-bound syndromes from around the world. A more complete documentation of the Work Group's findings and contributions is available in a special volume growing out of the group's deliberations (Mezzich, Kleinman, Fabrega, & Parron, 1997), in volume 3 of the *DSM-IV Sourcebook* (Widiger et al., 1997), and in other publications (e.g., Alarcon, 1995; Kirmayer 1998; Mezzich et al., 1996). Another major impact of the Culture and Diagnosis Work Group was the bringing together of a large number of senior and junior investigators that brought new energy to the field of cultural psychopathology. Without a doubt the attention given to culture in *DSM-IV* is a major achievement in the history of the classification of mental disorders. Never before had classification schemas or related diagnostic interviews addressed the role of culture in psychopathology to this degree (López & Núñez 1987; Rogler 1996). See Kirmayer (1998) and Lewis-Fernandez & Kleinman (1995) for a discussion of the limitations of how *DSM-IV* considered culture.

A second major development since the mid-1990s was the publication of the *World Mental Health Report* (Desjarlais, Eisenberg, Good, & Kleinman, 1996). Desjarlais and colleagues compiled research from across the world to identify the range of mental health and behavioral problems (e.g., mental disorders, violence, suicide) particularly among low-income countries in Africa, Latin America, Asia, and the Pacific. The authors derived several conclusions, perhaps the most significant of which was that mental illness and related problems exact a significant toll on the health and well-being of people worldwide, and produce a greater burden based on a "disability-adjusted life years" index than that from tuberculosis, cancer, or heart disease (Murray & Lopez, 1996). Among all physical and mental disorders, depressive disorders alone were found to produce the fifth greatest burden for women and seventh greatest burden for men.

Another important observation was that mental disorders and behavioral problems are intricately tied to the social world and occur in clusters of intimately linked social and psychological problems. For example, the authors identified the social roots of the poor mental health of women. Among the many factors were hunger (undernourishment afflicts more than 60% of women in developing countries), work (women are poorly paid for dangerous, labor intensive jobs), and domestic violence (surveys in some low-income communities worldwide report that up to 50 and 60% of women have been beaten). The research on women's mental health illustrates that psychopathology is as much pathology of the social world as pathology of the mind or body.

Based on their findings, Desjarlais and colleagues make specific recommendations to advance both mental health policy and research to help reduce the significant burden of mental illness across the world. Their consideration of the social world leads easily to recommending specific interventions to address not only mental health problems but also the social conditions which surround and greatly influence such problems. In addressing the poor mental health of women, for example, they call for coordinated efforts to empower women economically and through education, as well as reduce violence against women in all its forms. In addition, women's mental health is identified as one of the top five research priorities worldwide. They call for research to examine the social factors that influence women's health in specific cultural contexts and to identify effective community based interventions in improving their health status (see also Winstead & Sanchez, this volume.)

The most recent development was the *Surgeon General's Supplemental Report on Mental Health* concerning culture, race and ethnicity (USDHHS, 2001). The Surgeon General had previously published a landmark report on the status of the nation's mental health (USDHHS, 1999). Some observers were concerned that insufficient attention was given to the mental health of the country's ethnic and racial minority groups (López, 2003). In response to this concern and under the leadership of the Substance Abuse and Mental Health Services Administration, the Surgeon General published a report on the mental health of the nation's four main minority groups: American Indians/Alaska Natives, African Americans, Asian Americans/Pacific Islanders, and Latino/a Americans. Although the report's focus was mental health care, considerable attention was given to our current understanding of the types of psychopathology common among these groups, based largely on epidemiological and clinical research. One of the major contributions of this report was the synthesis of literature on the mental health of these diverse groups.

The main message of the Surgeon General's report was that "culture counts." "The cultures from which people hail affect all aspects of mental health and illness, including the types of stresses they confront, whether they seek help, what types of help they seek, what symptoms and concerns they bring to clinical attention, and what types of coping styles and social supports they possess." (p. ii) The Surgeon General's report compiled the best available research that culture matters in these domains. For example, evidence was reviewed regarding the relationship between racism and mental health (e.g., Kessler, Mickelson, & Williams, 1999), and ethnicity and psychopharmacology (e.g., Lin, Poland, & Anderson, 1995). In addition, the report outlined future directions to address the mental health needs of these underserved communities, including expanding the science base and training mental health scientists and practitioners. In all, this report served two important functions. It brought together the best available mental health research regarding the main U.S. minority groups. Also, because of the status and visibility of the Office of the Surgeon General, the report alerted the nation to the mental health needs of the four main ethnic and racial minority groups.

Together, the *DSM-IV*, the *World Mental Health Report*, and the *Surgeon General's Supplemental Report on Mental Health* make major contributions to the study of culture and psychopathology and give important visibility and credibility to this important domain of research. At the same time, they illustrate the range of conceptualizations of culture and the importance of the social domain. In *DSM-IV*, culture tends to be depicted as exotic, through its influence on symptom expression, the noted culture-bound syndromes, and that culture largely resides in persons from "culturally different" groups. There is little attention paid to the influence of culture in every clinical encounter—influencing the client, provider, and the broader community context, regardless of the patient's ethnic or racial background.

The *World Mental Health Report*, on the other hand, recognizes the dynamic, social processes linked to culture. Hunger, work, and education, for example, are integrally related to how people adapt or fail to adapt. Clinical phenomena are recognized but so are behavioral problems not traditionally considered in psychiatric classification systems, such as domestic violence and sexual violence. Throughout, the authors recognize cultural variability as a key dimension of culture and mental health and they highlight the moral and health implications of controversial practices, such as female circumcision.

The Surgeon General's report falls between both perspectives. It recognizes the importance of culture in specific clinical entities (both culture bound syndromes and mainstream mental disorder categories). It also acknowledges the importance of the broader social world though the emphasis tends to be more disorder based and less contextually based than the *World Mental Health Report*. Despite the differences in the treatment of culture, these three publications indicate that culture as a subject matter is no longer the exclusive purview of cultural psychologists, psychiatrists, and anthropologists. It is now the subject matter of all users of *DSM-IV*, worldwide policy makers, national health policy makers, mental health researchers, and those who care for people with mental disorders

Disorder-Related Research

We now turn to the examination of selected psychopathology research. We chose the study of anxiety, schizophrenia, and childhood psychopathology because within each of these areas there are systematic studies that examine the cultural basis of the expression of these disorders as well as the social and cultural processes that underlie the development and course of illness.

Anxiety In this area, we chose to focus our attention on one line of research, the study of *ataques de nervios*, though there are important overviews of this broad area of anxiety research (Guarnaccia 1997; Guarnaccia & Kirmayer 1997). The study of *ataques de nervios* is an important line of research because it focuses on a culture-specific phenomenon for which the triangulation of ethnography, epidemiology, and clinical research has made important contributions. Thus, we will be able to examine some ways ethnography informs mainstream research and highlight the important ways culture influences psychopathology.

Ataque de nervios is an idiom of distress particularly prominent among Latinos/Latinas from the Caribbean, but also recognized among other Latino/a groups. Symptoms commonly associated with *ataques de nervios* include: trembling, attacks of crying, screaming uncontrollably, and verbal or physical aggression. Other symptoms that are prominent in some *ataques* but not others are seizurelike or fainting episodes, dissociative experiences, and suicidal gestures. A general feature experienced by most sufferers of *ataques de nervios* is feeling out of control. Most episodes occur as a direct result of a stressful life event related to family or significant others (e.g., death or divorce). After the *ataque*, people oftentimes experience amnesia of what occurred, but then quickly return to their usual level of functioning (American Psychiatric Association, 1994, p. 845).

Guarnaccia and colleagues initiated a program of research by first carrying out open-ended, descriptive interviews in clinical settings with people who had experienced *ataques de nervios* (De La Cancela, Guarnaccia, & Carrillo, 1986; Guarnaccia, Rubio-Stipec, & Canino, 1989). Drawing from the rich description of clinical cases and an understanding of the social history of Puerto Ricans living in the United States, these investigators pointed out an association between social disruptions (family and immediate social networks) and the experience of *ataques*. To build on the ethnographic base, Guarnaccia and colleagues turned to epidemiological research to examine its prevalence in Puerto Rico. They examined data from a large epidemiological study in Puerto Rico (Canino et al., 1987) in which respondents were directly queried as to whether they had suffered an *ataque de nervios* and what the experience was like (Guarnaccia, Canino, Rubio-Stipec, & Bravo, 1993). The prevalence rate was found to be high, 16% of the large community sample (N = 912), and *ataques de nervios* were found to be associated with a wide range of mental disorders, particularly anxiety and mood disorders. The social context continued to be important in understanding *ataques de nervios*. *Ataques* were found to be more prevalent among women, persons older than 45, people from a lower socioeconomic background, and those with disrupted marital relations. More recently, Guarnaccia and colleagues (Guarnaccia, Rivera, Franco, & Neighbors, 1996) returned to the ethnographic mode to explicate the experience of *ataques* among those persons who had reported suffering an *ataque de nervios* in the epidemiological study. Through in-depth interviewing, the full range of symptoms and the specific social contexts were identified. This "experience-near" research approach enabled Guarnaccia and associates to examine carefully how the social world can become part of the physical self as reflected in *ataques de nervios*.

Clinical research has further examined the relationship between *ataques de nervios* and psychiatric diagnoses. Liebowitz and colleagues (1994) carried out clinical diagnostic interviews of 156 Latino/a patients from an urban psychiatric clinic that specializes in the treatment of anxiety. They explicated the relationship between patients having an *ataque de nervios* and meeting criteria for panic disorder, other anxiety disorders, or an affective disorder. Their fine-grained analysis suggests that the different expressions of *ataque de nervios* interact with different coexisting psychiatric disorders. Persons with an *ataque de nervios* who also suffer from panic disorder present largely anxiety symptoms. However, in those with an affective disorder, *ataque de nervios* are characterized by emotional lability, especially anger (Salmán et al., 1998). Thus, in addition to the social factors previously noted, these findings suggest that the clinical context may also play a role in understanding *ataque de nervios*. A more recent clinical study from the same site, but with different data, more clearly delineates the borderlines between *ataque de nervios* and panic disorder (Lewis-Fernandez et al., 2002). The investigators note that key distinguishing features of *ataques* as compared to panic attacks are that *ataques* are most often triggered by some stressful event, that people feel relieved after their *ataques*, and that *ataques* do not follow the same rapid crescendo as panic attacks.

Recently, work on *ataques de nervios* has been extended to children (Guarnaccia, Martinez, Ramirez, & Canino, 2005). In a study of the mental health of children in Puerto Rico, the authors included a question on *ataques de nervios*. They found that *ataques* continue to be reported by Puerto Rican children, particularly adolescent girls. As in adults, *ataques* are more common in children who meet criteria for a range of psychiatric disorders in the anxiety and depression spectrum.

The study of *ataque de nervios* is exemplary for many reasons. What is most striking is the systematic ongoing dialogue between ethnographic, epidemiological, and clinical research methods to advance our understanding of *ataques de nervios* and how the social world interacts with psychological and physical processes in the individual. With the multiple approaches, one observes the shifting of the researchers' lenses (Kleinman & Kleinman, 1991). In the early ethnographic work, Guarnaccia and colleagues drew from a small number of clinical cases and interpreted their findings with broad strokes focusing on the broader social contexts of the individuals, particularly their migration experience and experiences of marginal social status. In the epidemiological research, the investigators used large, representative samples to identify people with *ataques* and the social correlates of that experience. In this research, the social context is reduced to single questions concerning gender, age, educational level, and marital status, which provides some basis for interpretation but certainly lacks the richness of ethnographic material. The clinical studies provide an in-depth profile of patients' symptomatology, and the symptom patterns of those with and without an *ataque*, but they provide less information about the social world of the sufferer. Each approach has its strengths and limitations. What matters though is not a given strength or limitation of a specific study but the weaving of multiple studies with multiple approaches to understand the given phenomenon in some depth.

In addition to the ongoing dialogue between research approaches, the research is also exemplary by placing *ataque de nervios* and related mental disorders in their social context. In almost all studies, *ataque de nervios* is presented not as a popular illness (that is, an illness defined by the community) or clinical entity (that is, a psychologically defined disorder) that resides within individuals, but as a popular illness that reflects the lived experience of women with little power and disrupted social relations. In adopting multiple approaches, the emphasis given to the social domain is likely to shift. Nevertheless, over the several studies, Guarnaccia and his colleagues have maintained considerable attention to the social context. In so doing, they have demonstrated how to include the social world in epidemiological (e.g., Guarnaccia, Canino, et al., 1993) and clinical (Salmán et al., 1998), as well as ethnographic studies. This integration resulted in a proposal for a parallel categorization of psychopathology for Puerto Ricans using popular categories that bring together both the psychiatric and social dimensions of distress (Guarnaccia, Lewis-Fernandez, & Rivera Marano, 2003). Overall, the study of *ataque de nervios* provides a model for the investigation of culture and psychopathology, particularly for research that begins with a culture-specific form of distress (Guarnaccia & Rogler, 1999).

Schizophrenia The cultural conception of the self can influence the manner in which disorders are expressed and understood by others. This is articulated in Fabrega's (1989) thoughtful overview of how past anthropologically informed research contributed to the study of psychosis and how future studies can advance our understanding of the interrelations of culture and schizophrenia. According to Fabrega, the effect of schizophrenia on individuals and communities depends on whether they conceive of the self as autonomous and separate from others or as connected and bound to others (Markus & Kitayama, 1991; Shweder & Bourne, 1984). The research that most directly addresses this notion is that which examines the role of social factors in the course of schizophrenia. Two prominent lines of inquiry include the World Health Organization (WHO) cross-national study of schizophrenia and a series of studies examining the relationship of families' emotional climate to the course of illness. (For an examination of culture and symptom expression in schizophrenia see Brekke and Barrio, 1997; Weisman et al., 2000)

The WHO's *International Pilot Study on Schizophrenia* (IPSS) and the follow-up study *Determinants of Outcomes of Severe Mental Disorder* (DOSMD) represent the largest multinational study of schizophrenia to date (IPSS: 9 countries and 1,202 patients; DOSMD: 10 countries and 1379 patients; Jablensky et al., 1992; World Health Organization, 1979). Many contributions have been made by these investigations, including finding evidence of the comparability of schizophrenia's core symptoms across several countries (for a critique see Kleinman, 1988). The finding that has received the most attention by cultural researchers is that schizophrenia in developing countries has a more favorable course than in developed countries (Weisman, 1997). Some investigators have referred to this basic finding as "arguably the single most important finding of cultural differences in cross-cultural research on mental illness" (Lin & Kleinman, 1988, p. 563). Others have been most critical of methods and interpretations (Cohen, 1992; Edgerton & Cohen, 1994; Hopper, 1991). For example, Edgerton and Cohen (1994) point out that the distinction between "developed" and "developing" countries is unclear. Moreover, they argue that the cultural explanation for the differences in course is poorly substantiated. They also suggest that such research could be more culturally informed through the direct measure of specific cultural factors in conjunction with observations of people's daily lives (see also Hopper, 1991). What is clear is that the WHO findings have provided the basis for an important discussion of method and theory regarding how the course of schizophrenia can be shaped by the social world.

Another line of research addressing culture's role in the course of schizophrenia focuses on families' emotional climate. Based on the early work of George Brown and associates (e.g., Brown, Burley, & Wing, 1972), research has found that hospitalized patients who return to households marked by high *expressed emotion* (EE; criticism, hostility, and emotional involvement) are more likely to relapse than those who return to households that are not so characterized (Bebbington & Kuipers, 1994; Butzlaff & Hooley, 1998; Leff & Vaughn, 1985). This line of investigation is important to the study of culture because it points out the importance of the social world. More specifically, cross-national and cross-ethnic studies have uncovered interesting differences in the level and nature of expressed emotion (Jenkins & Karno, 1992). These studies show that cultural factors in the definitions and experiences of schizophrenia affect the emotional climate of families where ill individuals live. Furthermore, these cultural differences have important effects on mental health outcomes.

The most systematic cultural analysis of families' role in schizophrenia has been carried out by Jenkins and her colleagues. In using both clinical research methods based on the prototypic contemporary study of expressed emotion (Vaughn & Leff, 1976) and ethnographic methods based on in-depth interviews, Jenkins and associates extended this line of study to Mexican-American families in Los Angeles. In the first major report, Karno et al. (1987) replicated the general finding that patients who return to high EE families are more likely to relapse than patients who return to low EE families. Jenkins (1988a) then carried out an in-depth examination of Mexican-American families' conceptualization of schizophrenia, specifically *nervios*, and how this differed from a comparable sample of Anglo-American families who viewed schizophrenia largely as a mental illness (see also Guarnaccia, Parra, Deschamps, Milstein, & Argiles, 1992). Based on both quantitative (coded responses to open-ended questions) and qualitative data, Jenkins (1988b) suggested that Mexican Americans' preference for labeling the family member's schizophrenia as *nervios* is tied to the family members' efforts to decrease the stigma associated with the illness and also to promote family support for the ill individual. In subsequent papers, Jenkins (1991, 1993) critiqued the cultural basis of the expressed emotion construct in general, as well as its components of criticism and emotional overinvolvement in particular. An important theoretical contribution to the study of the course of schizophrenia is that Jenkins situates families' expressed emotion not only in the family members' attitudes, beliefs, or even feelings (which is usually the case among most researchers), but also in the patient–family social interaction. Overall, Jenkins's work has brought much needed attention to how serious mental illness is embedded in specific social and cultural contexts.

Building on Jenkins's work, López and colleagues have further critiqued the notion of expressed emotion with its focus on negative family functioning (López, Nelson, Snyder, & Mintz, 1999). They point out that at an early juncture in the study of families and relapse, investigators (Brown et al., 1972) opted to focus on aspects of family conflict that predict relapse rather than the prosocial aspects of family functioning that buffer relapse. In a reanalysis and extension of the Mexican-American sample (Karno et al., 1987) and a comparable Anglo-American sample (Vaughn, Snyder, Jones, Freeman, & Falloon, 1984), López and associates (2004) found that family warmth predicted relapse for Mexican Americans whereas criticism predicted relapse for Anglo Americans. In other words, Mexican-American patients who returned to families marked by high warmth were less likely to relapse than were those who returned to families characterized by low warmth. For Anglo Americans, high criticism was positively related to relapse, but warmth was unrelated to relapse. Subsequent analyses of the Mexican-American sample (Breitborde, Lopez, Wickens, Jenkins, & Karno, 2007) provided direct evidence that the presence of high warmth and a moderate degree of emotional overinvolvement were associated with less relapse than the usual relapse rate in the study of expressed emotion (Butzlaff & Hooley, 1998). Moreover, a high level of emotional overinvolvement was associated with a greater than usual rate of relapse. Together these findings point out that for this largely immigrant Mexican-American sample, there is an ongoing tension between maintaining close family ties (high warmth and moderate degrees of involvement) without becoming too involved (Jenkins, 1993). Although close family connections may be valued (and beneficial), too much closeness can be problematic (see Kopelowicz et al., 2006, for a behavioral observation study of Mexican-American families' interactions with their ill relatives that found a similar dynamic). This emphasis on family process differs from the emphasis given to family caregivers' negativity in prior expressed emotion research (e.g., Falloon et al., 1982).

López and colleagues (2004) did not attribute the observed ethnic differences in family processes related to relapse to a set of presumed cultural beliefs associated with the "Mexican culture" or a collectivist culture. Instead, they noted that most of the families and patients of Mexican origin were immigrants and that maintaining family ties was crucial to the survival of low-income immigrants living in a foreign and at times hostile environment. Their maintenance of the value of family support was extended to relatives who developed serious mental illness. The latter interpretation is consistent with a view of culture as embedded in the social world, rather than as a set of individual values or beliefs. Research is underway to assess directly what aspects of culture are associated with family caregivers' reactions to their ill relatives.

In conjunction with two other international studies (Italy: Bertrando et al., 1992; Yugoslavia: Ivanović, Vuletic, & Bebbington, 1994), these findings are consistent with the hypothesis that culture plays a role in the manner in which families respond to relatives with schizophrenia, which in turn influences the course of illness. A limitation of these findings is that there was no direct measure of cultural processes. Nevertheless, the importance of this research is that the exploration of possible cultural variability led to the beginning of a line of inquiry that examines what families do to prevent relapse. Such research has the potential to add a much needed balance to family research by focusing on both positive and negative aspects of families' behaviors (see also Weisman, Gomes and López, 2003). The study of caregiving (e.g., Guarnaccia, 1998; Lefley, 1998) and families' day-to-day interactions with ill family members will likely shed further light on the importance of families' prosocial functioning.

Childhood disorders The study of child psychopathology is a rich field of inquiry for those interested in culture. As noted by Weisz and associates (1997), child psychopathology requires attention to the behavior of children as well as the views of adults—parents, teachers, and mental health practitioners—for it is the adults who usually decide whether or not a problem exists. The fact that others determine whether children's behavior is problematic underscores the importance of the social world in defining mental illness and disorders of children and adolescents.

John Weisz and his colleagues have carried out the most systematic research on culture and childhood psychopathology (for a review see Weisz et al., 1997). In their first study, conducted in Thailand and the United States, Weisz, Suwanlert, Chaiyasit, Weiss, and Walter (1987) found that Thai children and adolescents who were referred to mental health clinics reported more internalizing problems than U.S. children and adolescents. In contrast, U.S. children and adolescents reported more externalizing problems than Thai children and adolescents. In follow-up community studies, where the mental health referral process was not a factor in the identification of problem behaviors, the cross-national differences were confirmed for internalizing problems but not for externalizing problems (Weisz, Suwanlert, et al., 1993; Weisz, Weisz, et al., 1987). The prevalence of externalizing problems among U.S. and Thai youth identified in their respective communities did not differ. Weisz and colleagues argue that the findings with regard to internalizing problems are consistent with the idea that culture shapes the manner in which children and adolescents express psychological distress. Because they come from a largely Buddhist religious and cultural background that values self-control and emotional restraint, Thai youth may be more likely than U.S. youth to express psychological distress in a manner that does not violate cultural norms. (For an analysis of the syndromes across the U.S. and Thai samples, see Weisz, Weiss, Suwanlert, & Chaiyasit, 2003).

In addition to these intriguing findings, two other factors stand out in Weisz and colleagues' research: the systematic nature of the research, and the care with which the research has been conducted. Weisz and colleagues began this line of investigation in mental health clinics, and then used a community survey to rule out the possibility of the influence of referral factors (Weisz, Suwanlert, Chaiyasit, Weiss, Achenberg, et al., 1987). Based on these findings, Weisz and Weiss (1991) derived a referability index for specific problem behaviors (e.g., vandalism and poor schoolwork) that specifies the likelihood that a given problem will be referred for treatment, taking into account the problem's prevalence in a given community. In this study, they demonstrated how gender and nationality influence whether or not a problem is brought to the attention of mental health professionals. Subsequently, Weisz and colleagues examined teachers' reports of actual children (Weisz et al., 1989) and both parents' and teachers' ratings of hypothetical cases (Weisz, Suwanlert, Chaiyast, Weiss, & Jackson, 1991). Weisz and colleagues (Weiss, Chaiyasit, Weiss, Eastman, & Jackson, 1995) later found that Thai teachers report more internalizing and externalizing problem behaviors among Thai children than U.S. teachers report among U.S. children. Each of Weisz and colleagues' studies systematically builds on their previous work in advancing an understanding of how adults with differing social roles define children's problem behaviors. Multiple cross-cultural studies using different methods with different research participants provide a rich network of findings to advance our understanding of how the social context shapes the identification of youths' mental health problems.

The care with which Weisz and colleagues carry out their research is best illustrated in the study of teachers' ratings of problem behaviors (Weisz et al., 1995). They found that Thai teachers rate more internalizing and externalizing problem behaviors for Thai students than U.S. teachers rate for their own students. Given that this finding runs counter to the previous clinical and community studies which only found differences for internalizing problems, they devised an innovative observational methodology to assess whether it was something about the children or the teachers that contributed to this contradictory finding. Weisz and associates (1995) employed independent observers of children's school behavior and obtained teacher ratings of the same children who were observed in Thailand and in the United States. One of the independent raters was a bilingual Thai psychologist who had received graduate training in the United States. His participation in both teams of independent observers was critical to assessing the reliability of the Thai and U.S. observers. The relationship between his ratings and those of the other U.S. and Thai raters were equally high, suggesting that the ratings were reliable across both national sites. Interestingly, the observers rated Thai children as having less than half as many problem and off-task behaviors than U.S. children, yet Thai teachers rated the observed students as having many more of these problem behaviors than U.S. teachers rated their students. These data suggest that Thai teachers have a much lower threshold than their U.S. colleagues for identifying problem behaviors in their students. Findings in cross-cultural research are often open to multiple interpretations. By using careful methodology across multiple studies, Weisz and collaborators have discerned the specific meaning of their complex set of findings. In doing so, they have highlighted the importance of contextual factors in the assessment of child psychopathology and demonstrate that it is untenable to view the assessment of child psychopathology as culture-free.

Developmental researchers are examining more closely the influence of culture on the type and degree of problem behaviors of children and adolescents. Weisz and associates extended their research to Jamaica and Kenya (Lambert, Weisz, & Knight, 1989; Weisz, Sigman, Wiess, & Mosk, 1993a). Other investigators have compared rates of internalizing and externalizing problems in other parts of the world (e.g., Denmark: Arnett & Balle-Jensen, 1993; Puerto Rico: Achenbach et al., 1990).

Other researchers have examined specifically internalizing type problem behaviors (Greenberger & Chen, 1996) or externalizing type problem behaviors (e.g., Weine, Phillips, & Achenbach, 1995) in cross-national or cross-ethnic samples. An important trend in this research is that epidemiological research that compares groups cross-nationally and suggests possible cultural explanations is now being complemented by research that examines the psychosocial processes associated with children and adolescents' adjustment or psychopathology. For example, Chen and associates (1998) examined risk factors (parent–adolescent conflict and perceived peer approval of misconduct) and protective factors (parental warmth and parental monitoring) associated with acting-out problems across four groups of adolescents: European Americans, Chinese Americans, Taipei Chinese, and Beijing Chinese. They found both cross-cultural similarities and differences in the way both family and peer factors contributed to misconduct. Generally the predicted risk and protective factors accounted for a significant amount of variance for misconduct in each of the four groups; however, peer influences were less relevant for the Taipei and Beijing Chinese youth.

The strength of the more recent studies is that they examine processes that may explain potential cross-national differences and similarities, including social (family and peers) and psychological (values) processes. Thus, an important step has been taken to understand why differences and similarities may occur in behavior problems cross-nationally. Although the conceptual models used to frame such research are rich, include social processes, and have a strong empirical tradition in psychological research, they are not well informed by cultural-specific processes of the non-U.S. groups under study. Investigators typically apply models developed largely in the United States. Ethnographic research that attempts to identify what about the social and cultural world might play a role in the expression of distress and disorder among children would be especially welcome. This research could then lead to the direct examination of those culture-specific factors that are believed to affect psychopathology within a given conceptual framework as evidenced in the work of some developmental researchers (e.g., Fuligni, 1998), and as advocated by others (e.g., Schneider, 1998). The growing interest of researchers in studying internalizing and externalizing problem behaviors cross-nationally and cross-ethnically attests to the utility of this approach for enhancing our understanding of culture and childhood psychopathology.

Emerging Trends

Among the most significant emerging trends are findings regarding immigration and U.S. ethnic minority groups.

Immigration A number of findings highlight the importance of immigration in understanding mental health and mental disorders. The Los Angeles Epidemiologic Catchment Area study reported that Mexican-born Mexican Americans had significantly lower prevalence rates across a wide range of disorders than U.S.-born Mexican Americans (Burnam, Hough, Karno, Escobar, & Telles, 1987). This finding was replicated in a more recent epidemiologic study comparing the prevalence rates of rural and urban Mexican-origin adults in Fresno and nearby communities (Vega et al., 1998). An important contribution of the Fresno study is that evidence was provided from a Mexico City sample indicating that Mexico City residents had rates of psychological disorders comparable to those of the Mexican immigrant sample, thus countering the "hardy" immigrant hypothesis (see Medina-Mora et al., 2003 for a more complete report of the prevalence rates of mental disorders in Mexico). These and other studies (Ortega, Rosenheck, Alegria, & Desai, 2000) have been interpreted as suggesting that acculturation to the "American" culture may be harmful to Latinos'/Latinas' mental health. More recently, in a large national epidemiology study of over 43,000 adult residents, Grant and colleagues (2004) reported that the acculturation effect applied not only to Mexican-origin residents but also to non-Latino white immigrants when compared to non-Latino whites born in the United States.

Using the same database, Alegria and colleagues (2006) found that the acculturation effect was not as pronounced for Puerto Ricans and Cuban Americans; it was primarily noted in specific substance use disorders but not observed in most mood and anxiety disorders. Marshall and Orlando (2002) provide a counterpoint that acculturation can serve as a protective factor rather than a risk factor, particularly in the domain of dissociation associated with trauma among young Latinos. The social and psychological mechanisms that are responsible for the differing prevalence rates for the immigrant groups at this time are unknown. Nevertheless, available studies indicate that research on immigration and acculturation can contribute much to our understanding of how the social world and psychopathology interrelate (see also Rogler, 1994). A particularly wide-open area of study is the examination of immigration and mental health and disorders among children and adolescents (Gil & Vega, 1996; Guarnaccia & López, 1998; Polo, 2002). Not only will immigration/acculturation research be able to address important conceptual and methodological issues in the study of culture but it will also have important policy implications for the delivery of mental health services to underserved communities (e.g., Salgado de Snyder, Diaz-Perez, & Bautista, 1998).

U.S. ethnic minority groups We are encouraged by the growing interest in the study of psychopathology among U.S. ethnic minority groups. With regard to African Americans, there has been an increase in the study of anxiety disorders since Neal and Turner's (1991) call for research. The more recent studies include clinical studies (Friedman, Paradis, & Hatch, 1994), epidemiologic studies (Horwath, Johnson, & Hornig, 1993), a combined ethnographic and epidemiological study (Heurtin-Roberts, Snowden, & Miller, 1997), and a study of childhood fears (Neal, Lilly, & Zakis, 1993). Although these studies are largely descriptive in nature, there is some attention to the differential social world of African-American and white patients. For example, Friedman and associates (1994) found that, relative to white patients with panic disorder and agoraphobia, African-American patients reported a greater likelihood of having been separated as children from their parents and of having experienced their parents' divorce.

A systematic series of studies has examined the mental health problems of American-Indian children (e.g., Beiser, Sack, Manson, Redshirt, & Dion, 1998; Dion, Gotowiec, & Beiser, 1998) and adults (Maser & Dinges, 1992/1993). Although many of these studies use mainstream models of disorder and distress (O'Nell, 1989), there are growing efforts to contextualize the mental health problems within these communities. In one study, Duclos and colleagues (1998) found that nearly half of the Indian adolescents detained in the juvenile justice system met criteria for mental disorders ranging from substance abuse/dependence (38%) to major depression (10%). These rates were much higher than community surveys of Indian youth and non-Indian youth. These researchers argue that the juvenile justice system has the potential to serve as an important site for treating these high-risk youth, many of whom would go untreated. In another study, O'Nell and Mitchell (1996) found that the line between normal and pathological drinking among adolescent Indians is contextually based. Their ethnographic findings suggest that a rigid model of alcohol abuse defined by biology (frequency and amount of alcohol) or psychology (distress) without significant attention to the sociocultural context (e.g., when and with whom one drinks) is limited in distinguishing between normative and pathological drinking (see also Fals-Stewart & Klostermann, this volume.)

The largest study to date of the mental health of Americans Indians is the American Indian Services Utilization, Psychiatric Epidemiology, Risk and Protective Factors Project (Beals, Manson, Mitchell, Spicer, & AI-SUPERPFP Team, 2003). This project is based on representative samples of adult residents within two reservations (Southwest tribe $N = 1,446$, and Northern Plains tribe $N = 1,638$). Among the early findings reported from this research is that when controlling for various demographic correlates, the American Indian samples reported greater lifetime prevalence rates of alcohol abuse and posttraumatic stress disorder and lower lifetime rates of major depression than a national sample of the United States across ethnicities (Beals, Novins, et al., 2005). Given that ethnographic interviews were also carried out in this large scale project, we expect in the future more nuanced research reports that examine the social world as it relates to trauma and alcohol disorders, for example.

With regard to Asian-American research, Sue and his associates (1991) have had a longstanding interest in treatment issues. Sue and colleagues have broadened their interests to include psychopathology (Sue et al., 1995). Two epidemiologic surveys are of particular importance: the Filipino-American Community Epidemiological Study, a cross-sectional investigation of 2,241 Filipino Americans living in San Francisco and Honolulu (e.g., Gee et al., 2006), and the Chinese American Psychiatric Epidemiologic Study of 1,747 Chinese immigrants and native-born adult residents residing in Los Angeles County (Takeuchi et al., 1998). With regard to the latter study, researchers documented the prevalence rates of traditional depressive and related disorders, as well as neurasthenia (Zheng et al., 1997), a concept that was retired in the classification of mental disorders in the United States, but is still in use in China and other parts of Asia. Neurasthenia usually refers to weakness or fatigue often accompanied by a variety of psychological (e.g., poor concentration) and physical symptoms (e.g., diffuse aches and pains). Of particular interest is the finding that neurasthenia had the highest one-year prevalence rate (6.4%) of any disorder in the Chinese American epidemiologic survey. This was the case even after removing those persons with both neurasthenia and another disorder such as anxiety or depression (pure neurasthenia rate = 3.6%). The study of neurasthenia is another example of how culture can contribute to shaping the expression of disorder.

Most of the research with Latinos/Latinas has involved adults. Vega and colleagues (1995), however, conducted an important study regarding Latino adolescents in Miami, Florida. A significant contribution of this research is that it points out that the relationship between specific acculturative stressors (e.g., language conflicts, perceived discrimination) and problem behaviors varies by immigration status. Specifically, for immigrant youth only language conflicts were associated with increased behavior problems as reported by both parent and teacher. In contrast, for U.S.-born youth, language conflicts, perceived discrimination, and the perception of a closed society were all associated with increased behavior problems. Interestingly these associations were only observed in teachers' reports, not in parents' reports. These findings suggest that the acculturation strains are most relevant to the U.S.-born youth's behavior problems observed in school. In another epidemiologic study of adolescents, this one carried out in the Houston metropolitan area, Roberts and colleagues (Roberts, Roberts, & Chen, 1997) found that of nine ethnic groups, Mexican Americans reported the highest rates of major depression. Both studies are characterized by rigor in sampling schools, multiethnic samples, and large sample sizes. Most recently, Canino and colleagues (2004) examined prevalence rates of psychological disorders among Puerto Rican Island youth, and Bird and colleagues (2006) compared the rates of disruptive behavior disorders among Puerto Rican youth on the Island and in the South Bronx. These studies advance past epidemiologic studies of Latino youth by examining a wider and younger age range (Canino study: 4 to 17 years old; Bird study: 5 to 13 years old) and by applying household sampling methods rather than the previously used school based sampling methods. Some of the key findings of these studies include the low use of services by children with a diagnosable disorder and significant impairment (Canino et al., 2004) and the important role of parent–child relations and peer-relations in predicting disruptive behavior disorders (Bird et al., 2006). Together the child and adolescent epidemiologic studies are addressing the mental health needs of Latino youth.

Much of the past epidemiologic research of ethnic minority groups has focused on specific communities or locales. Several important studies have been completed recently on the mental health of ethnic groups throughout the United States. To expand the scope of epidemiological and services research on the U.S. population from the National Co-Morbidity Study, investigations were funded by the National Institute of Mental Health to examine the mental health of African Americans (Jackson et al., 2004) and Latinos/Latinas and Asian Americans (Alegria, Takeuchi, et al., 2004). These studies promise to provide a rich profile and deeper understanding of how the mental health of our diverse population is influenced by the social worlds that shape the living conditions of people in the United States.

Conclusion

Cultural psychopathology, the study of culture and the definition, experience, distribution, and course of psychological disorders, is now "on the map." Articles are being published in culture focused journals as well as mainstream journals (e.g., *American Journal of Psychiatry, Journal of Abnormal Psychology, Journal of Nervous and Mental Disease, Journal of the American Academy of Child and Adolescent Psychiatry, Child Development*). Substantive areas of psychopathology research are being shaped by cultural research. Efforts to integrate idioms of distress with mainstream constructs are well underway. Examples include studies of *ataques de nervios* and anxiety and affective disorders, and *nervios* and families' conceptualization of serious mental illness. Guarnaccia and Rogler (1999) provide a program for moving some of this research forward. Kleinman's important 1988 book got the message out that culture matters. As evidenced in the Surgeon General's Report, the message has been received; cultural research is providing an innovative and fresh perspective to our understanding of several important aspects of psychopathology.

For cultural researchers to build on the empirical and conceptual foundation that has been established, they need to continue to be critical of how culture is conceptualized and how such conceptualizations guide their research. It is clear from this review that culture can no longer be treated solely as an independent variable or as a factor to be controlled for. Rather, culture infuses the full social context of mental health research. Culture is important in all aspects of psychopathology research—the design and translation of instruments, the conceptual models that guide the research, the interpersonal interaction between researcher and research participants, the definition and interpretation of symptom and syndromes, and the structure of the social world that surrounds a person's mental health problems. Cultural psychopathology research requires a framework that incorporates culture in multifaceted ways. For this reason, it is crucial that cultural research not obscure the importance of other social forces such as gender, class, poverty, and marginality that work in conjunction with culture to shape people's everyday lives. The examination of both social and cultural processes is one way to help guard against superficial cultural analyses that ignore or minimize the powerful political economic inequalities that coexist with culture.

A corollary of the need for a broad framework for research is the need for approaches that integrate qualitative and quantitative methods. Cultural psychopathology research can serve as an important site for integrating ethnographic, observational, clinical, and epidemiological research approaches. Mental health problems cannot be fully understood through one lens. Ethnographic research provides insights into the meaning of mental health problems and how they are experienced in their sociocultural context. Observational research captures people's functioning in their daily lives. Clinical research can provide detailed descriptions of psychopathological processes and can contribute to developing treatments to alleviate suffering at the individual as well as social levels. Epidemiological research can identify who is most at risk for psychopathology and broaden perspectives to more generalized processes and populations. It is the integration of these perspectives, through new mixes of methodologies and in the composition of research teams that will make the cultural psychopathology research agenda succeed.

The ultimate goal of cultural psychopathology research is to alleviate suffering and improve people's lives. This requires attention to the multiple levels of individual, family, community, and the broader social system. Our enhanced notion of culture leads to analysis of the expression and sources of psychopathology at all of these levels. Our commitment to making a difference in peoples' everyday lives argues for the development of treatment and prevention interventions at these multiple levels as well. The increasing cultural diversity of the United States and the massive movements of people around the globe provide both an opportunity and imperative for cultural psychopathology research.

Note

1. This chapter is adapted from Lopez, S. R., & Guarnaccia, P. J. (2000). Cultural psychopathology: Uncovering the social world of mental illness. *Annual Review of Psychology, 51*, 571–598.

References

Achenbach, T. M., Bird, H. R., Canino, G., Phares, V., Gould, M. S., & Rubio-Stipec, M. (1990). Epidemiological comparisons of Puerto Rican and U.S. mainland children: Parent, teacher and self-reports. *Journal of the American Academy of Child & Adolescent Psychiatry, 29*(1), 84–93.

Alarcon, R. D. (1995). Culture and psychiatric diagnosis: Impact on DSM-IV and ICD-10. *Psychiatric Clinics of North America, 18*, 449–465.

Alegria, M., Canino, G., Stinson, F. S., & Grant, B. F. (2006). Nativity and DSM-IV psychiatric disorders among Puerto Ricans, Cuban Americans, and non-Latino Whites in the United Status: Results from the National Epidemiologic Survey on Alcohol and related conditions. *Journal of Clinical Psychiatry, 67*, 56–65.

Alegria, M., Takeuchi, D., Canino, G., Duan, N., Shrout, P., Meng, X. L., et al. (2004). Considering context, place and culture: The National Latino and Asian American Study. *International Journal of Methods in Psychiatric Research, 13*, 208–220

American Psychiatric Association. (1994). *Diagnostic and statistical manual of mental disorders* (4th ed.). Washington, D.C.: Author.

Arnett, J., & Balle-Jensen, L. (1993). Cultural bases of risk behavior: Danish adolescents. *Child Development, 64*, 1842–1855.

Beals, J., Manson, S. M., Mitchell, C. M., Spicer P., AI-SUPERPFP Team. (2003). Cultural specificity and comparison in psychiatric epidemiology: Walking the tightrope in American Indian research. *Culture, Medicine & Psychiatry, 27*, 259–289.

Beals, J., Novins, D. K., Whitesell, N. R., Spicer, P., Mitchell, C. M., & Manson, S. M., T AI-SUPERPFP Team (2005). Prevalence of mental disorders and utilization of mental health services in two American Indian reservation populations: Mental health disparities in a national context. *American Journal of Psychiatry, 162*, 1723–1732.

Bebbington, P., & Kuipers, L. (1994). The predictive utility of expressed emotion in schizophrenia: An aggregate analysis. *Psychological Medicine, 24*, 707–718.

Beiser, M., Sack, W., Manson, S., Redshirt, R., & Dion, R. (1998). Mental health and the academic performance of First Nations and majority-culture children. *American Journal of Orthopsychiatry, 68*, 455–467.

Bertrando, P., Beltz, J., Bressi, C., Clerici, M., Farma, T., Invernizzi, G., et al. (1992). Expressed emotion and schizophrenia in Italy: A study of an urban population. *British Journal of Psychiatry, 161*, 223–229.

Betancourt, H., & López, S. R. (1993). The study of culture, race and ethnicity in American psychology. *American Psychologist, 48*, 629–637.

Bird, H. R., Davies, M., Duarte, C. S., Shen, S., Loeber, R., & Canino, G. J. (2006). A study of disruptive behavior disorders in Puerto Rican youth: II. Baseline prevalence, comorbidity, and correlates in two sites. *Journal of the American Academy of Child & Adolescent Psychiatry, 45*, 1042–1053.

Breitborde, N. J. K., Lopez, S. R., Wickens, T. D., Jenkins, J. H., & Karno, M. (2007). Toward specifying the nature of the relationship between expressed emotion and schizophrenic relapse: The utility of curvilinear models. *International Journal of Methods in Psychiatric Research, 16*, 1–10.

Brekke, J. S., & Barrio, C. (1997). Cross-ethnic symptom differences in schizophrenia: The influence of culture and minority status. *Schizophrenia Bulletin, 23*, 305–316.

Brown, G. W., Birley, J. L. T., & Wing, J. K. (1972). Influence of family life on the course of schizophrenic disorders: A replication. *British Journal of Psychiatry, 21*, 241–258.

Burnam, A., Hough, R. L., Karno, M., Escobar, J. I., & Telles, C. (1987). Acculturation and lifetime prevalence of psychiatric disorders among Mexican Americans in Los Angeles. *Journal of Health and Social Behavior, 28*, 89–102.

Butcher, J. N. (Ed.). (1987). Cultural factors in understanding and accessing psychopathology [Special section]. Journal of Consulting & Clinical Psychology, 55, 459–512.

Butzlaff, R. L., & Hooley, J. M. (1998). Expressed emotion and psychiatric relapse: A meta-analysis. *Archives of General Psychiatry, 55*, 547–552.

Canino, G. J., Bird, H. R., Shrout, P. E., Rubio-Stipec, M., Bravo, M., Martinez, R., et al. (1987). The prevalence of specific psychiatric disorders in Puerto Rico. *Archives of General Psychiatry, 44*, 727–735.

Canino, G. J., Shrout, P.E., Rubio-Stipec, M., Bird, H. R., Bravo, M., Ramirez, R., et al. (2004), The DSM-IV rates of child and adolescent disorders in Puerto Rico: Prevalence, correlates, service use, and the effects of impairment. *Archives of General Psychiatry, 61*, 85–93

Cervantes, R. C., Padilla, A. M., & Salgado de Zinder, V. N. (1991). The Hispanic Stress Inventory: A culturally relevant approach to psychological assessment. *Psychological Assessment, 3*, 438–447.

Chen, C., Greenberger, E., Lester, J., Dong, Q., & Guo, M. (1998). A cross-cultural study of family and peer correlates of adolescent misconduct. *Developmental Psychology, 34*, 770–781.

Clark, L. A. (1987). Mutual relevance of mainstream and cross-cultural psychology. *Journal of Consulting and Clinical Psychology, 55*, 41–70.

Cohen, A. (1992). Prognosis for schizophrenia in the Third World: A reevaluation of cross-cultural research. *Culture, Medicine, and Psychiatry, 16*, 53–75.

De La Cancela, V., Guarnaccia, P., & Carrillo, E. (1986). Psychosocial distress among Latinos. *Humanity Society, 10*, 431–447.

Desjarlais, R., Eisenberg, L., Good, B., & Kleinman, A. (1996). *World mental health: Problems priorities in low-income countries.* Oxford: Oxford University Press.

Dion, R., Gotowiec, A., & Beiser, M. (1998). Depression and conduct disorder in Native and non-Native children. *Journal of the American Academy of Child & Adolescent Psychiatry, 37*, 736–742.

Draguns, J. G. (1980). Disorders of clinical severity. In H. C. Triandis, & J. G. Draguns (Eds.), *Handbook of cross-cultural psychology: Vol. 6. Psychopathology* (pp. 99–174). Boston: Allyn & Bacon.

Draguns, J. G. (1990). Culture and psychopathology: Toward specifying the nature of the relationship. In J. Berman (Ed.), *Nebraska Symposium on Motivation: 1989: Cross-Cultural Perspectives* (pp. 235–277). Lincoln: University of Nebraska Press.

Duclos, C. W., Beals, J., Novins, D. K., Martin, C., Jewett, C. S., & Manson, S. M. (1998). Prevalence of common psychiatric disorders among American Indian adolescent detainees. *Journal of the American Academy of Child & Adolescent Psychiatry, 37*, 866–873.

Edgerton, R., & Cohen, A. (1994). Culture and schizophrenia: The DOSMD challenge. *British Journal of Psychiatry, 164*, 222–2231.

Fabrega, H. (1975). The need for an ethnomedical science. *Science, 189*, 969–975.

Fabrega, H. (1989). On the significance of an anthropological approach to schizophrenia. *Psychiatry, 52*, 45–65.

Fabrega H. (1990). Hispanic mental health research: A case for cultural psychiatry. *Hispanic Journal of Behavioral Science, 12*, 339–365.

Falloon I. R. H., Boyd, J. L., McGill, C. W., Razani, J., Moos, H. B., & Gilderman, A.M. (1982). Family management in the prevention of exacerbations of schizophrenia. *New England Journal of Medicine, 396*, 1437–1440.

Friedman, S., Paradis, C. M., & Hatch, M. (1994). Characteristics of African-American and white patients with panic disorder and agoraphobia. *Hospital and Community Psychiatry, 45*, 798–803.

Fuligni, A. (1998). Authority, autonomy, and parent–adolescent conflict and cohesion: A study of adolescents from Mexican, Chinese, Filipino, and European backgrounds. *Developmental Psychology, 34*, 782–792.

Gallimore, R., Goldenberg, C. N., & Weisner, T. S. (1993). The social construction and subjective reality of activity settings: Implications for community psychology. *American Journal of Community Psychology, 21*, 537–559.

Garro, L. C. (2000). Cultural knowledge as resource in illness narratives: Remembering through accounts of illness. In C. Mattingly & L. C. Garro (Eds.), *Narrative and the cultural construction of illness and healing* (pp. 70–87). Berkeley: University of California Press.

Garro, L. C. (2001). The remembered past in a culturally meaningful life: Remembering as cultural, social and cognitive process. In C. Moore, H. Mathews (Eds.), *The Psychology of Cultural Experience* (pp. 105–147). Cambridge: Cambridge University Press.

Gee, G. C., Chen, J., Spencer, M. S., See, S., Kuester, O., Tran, D., et al. (2006). Social support as a buffer for perceived unfair treatment among Filipino Americans: Differences between San Francisco and Honolulu. *American Journal of Public Health, 96*, 677–684

Gil, A., & Vega, W. A. (1996). Two different worlds: Acculturation stress and adaptation among Cuban and Nicaraguan familias in Miami. *Journal of Social and Personal Relations, 13*, 437–458.

Grant, B. F., Stinson, F. S., Hasin, D. S., Dawson, D. A., Chou, S. P., & Anderson, K. (2004). Immigration and lifetime prevalence of DSM-IV psychiatric disorders among Mexican Americans and non-Hispanic whites in the United States. *Archives of General Psychiatry, 61*, 1226–1233.

Greenberger, E., & Chen, C. (1996). Perceived family relationships and depressed mood in early and late adolescence: A comparison of European and Asian Americans. *Developmental Psychology, 32*, 707–716.

Greenfield, P. M. (1997). Culture as process: Empirical methods for cultural psychology. In J. W. Berry, Y. H. Poortinga, & J. Pandey (Eds.), *Handbook of cross-cultural psychology: Theory and method* (Vol. 1, pp. 301–346). Needham Heights, MA: Allyn & Bacon.

Guarnaccia, P. J. (1997). A cross-cultural perspective on the anxiety disorders. In S. Friedman (Ed.), *Treating anxiety disorders across cultures* (pp. 3–20). New York: Guilford.

Guarnaccia, P. J. (1998). Multicultural experiences of family caregiving: A study of African American, European American and Hispanic American families. In H. Lefley (Ed.), *Families coping with illness: The cultural context* (pp. 45–61). San Francisco: Jossey-Bass.

Guarnaccia, P. J., Canino, G., Rubio-Stipec, M., & Bravo, M. (1993). The prevalence of *ataques de nervios* in the Puerto Rico study: The role of culture in psychiatric epidemiology. *Journal of Nervous and Mental Disease, 181*, 157–165.

Guarnaccia, P. J., De La Cancela, V., & Carrillo, E. (1989). The multiple meanings of *ataques de nervios* in the Latino community. *Medical Anthropology, 11*, 47–62.

Guarnaccia, P. J., & Kirmayer, L. (1997). Culture and the DSM-IV anxiety disorders. In T. Widiger, A. Frances, H. A. Pincus, M. B. First, R. Ross, & W. Davis, (Eds.), *DSM-IV source book* (Vol. 3, pp. 925–932). Washington, D.C.: American Psychiatric Press.

Guarnaccia, P. J, Kleinman, A., & Good, B. J. (1990). A critical review of epidemiological studies of Puerto Rican mental health. *American Journal of Psychiatry, 147*, 449–456.

Guarnaccia, P.J., Lewis-Fernandez, R., & Rivera Marano, M. (2003). Toward a Puerto Rican popular nosology: *Nervios* and *ataques de nervios. Culture, Medicine and Psychiatry, 27*, 339–366.

Guarnaccia, P. J., & López S. (1998). The mental health and adjustment of immigrant and refugee children. *Child & Adolescent Psychiatric Clinics of North America, 7*, 537–553.

Guarnaccia, P. J., Martinez, I., Ramirez, R., & Canino, G. (2005). Are *ataques de nervios* in Puerto Rican children associated with psychiatric disorder? *Journal of the American Academy of Child and Adolescent Psychiatry, 44*, 1184–1192.

Guarnaccia, P. J., Parra, P., Deschamps, A., Milstein, G., & Argiles, N. (1992). Si Dios quiere: Hispanic families' experiences of caring for a seriously mentally ill family member. *Culture, Medicine, and Psychiatry, 16*, 187–215.

Guarnaccia, P. J., Rivera, M., Franco, F., & Neighbors, C. (1996). The experiences of ataques de nervios: Towards an anthropology of emotions in Puerto Rico. *Culture, Medicine, and Psychiatry, 20*, 343–367.

Guarnaccia, P. J., & Rodriguez, O. (1996). Concepts of culture and their roles in the development of culturally competent mental health services. *Hispanic Journal of Behavioral Sciences, 18*, 419–443.

Guarnaccia, P. J., & Rogler, L. H. (1999). Research on culture-bound syndromes: New directions. *American Journal of Psychiatry, 156*, 1322–1327.

Guarnaccia, P. J., Rubio-Stipec, M., & Canino, G. (1989). *Ataques de nervios* in the Puerto Rican Diagnostic Interview Schedule: The impact of cultural categories on psychiatric epidemiology. *Culture, Medicine, and Psychiatry, 13*, 275–295.

Heurtin-Roberts, S., Snowden, L., & Miller, L. (1997). Expressions of anxiety in African Americans: Ethnography and the Epidemiological Catchment Area studies. *Culture, Medicine, and Psychiatry, 21*, 337–363.

Hopper, K. (1991). Some old questions for the new cross-cultural psychiatry. *Medical Anthropology Quarterly, 5*, 299–330.

Horwath, E., Johnson, J., & Hornig, C. D. (1993). Epidemiology of panic disorder in African-Americans. *American Journal of Psychiatry, 150*, 465–469.

Ivanović, M., Vuletić, Z., & Bebbington, P. (1994). Expressed emotion in the families of patients with schizophrenia and its influence on the course of illness. *Social psychiatry and psychiatric epidemiology, 29*, 61–65.

Jablensky, A., Sartorius, N., Ernberg, G., Ankar, M., Korten, A., Cooper, J. E., et al. (1992). Schizophrenia: Manifestations, incidence and course in different cultures. *Psychological Medicine, 20*(Suppl.), 1–97.

Jackson, J. S., Torres, M., Caldwell, C. H., Neighbors, H. W., Nesse, R. M., Taylor, R. J., et al. (2004). The National Survey of American Life: A study of racial, ethnic and cultural influences on mental disorders and mental health. *International Journal of Methods in Psychiatric Research, 13*, 196–207

Jenkins, J. H. (1988a). Conceptions of schizophrenia as a problem of nerves: A cross-cultural comparison of Mexican-Americans and Anglo-Americans. *Social Science & Medicine, 26*, 1233–1243.

Jenkins, J. H. (1988b). Ethnopsychiatric interpretations of schizophrenic illness: The problem of *nervios* within Mexican-American families. *Culture, Medicine, and Psychiatry, 12*, 303–331.

Jenkins, J. H. (1991). Anthropology, expressed emotion, and schizophrenia. *Ethos, 19*, 387–431.

Jenkins, J. H. (1993). Too close for comfort: Schizophrenia and emotional overinvolvement among *Mexicano* families. In A. D. Gaines (Ed.), *Ethnopsychiatry* (pp. 203–221). Albany, NY: State University of New York Press.

Jenkins, J., & Karno, M. (1992). The meaning of expressed emotion: Theoretical issues raised by cross-cultural research. *American Journal of Psychiatry, 149*, 9–21.

Karno, M., Jenkins, J. H., de la Selva, A., Santana, F., Telles, C., Lopez, S., et al. (1987). Expressed emotion and schizophrenic outcome among Mexican-American families. *Journal of Nervous and Mental Disease, 175*, 143–151.

Kessler, R. C., Mickelson, K. D., & Williams, D. R. (1999). The prevalence, distribution, and mental health correlates of perceived discrimination in the United States. *Journal of Health and Social Behavior, 40*, 208–230.

King, L. M. (1978). Social and cultural influences on psychopathology. *Annual Review of Psychology, 29*, 405–433.

Kirmayer, L. J. (1998). Editorial: The fate of culture in DSM-IV. *Transcultural Psychiatry, 35*, 339–342.

Kleinman, A. (1977). Depression, somatization and the "New Cross-Cultural Psychiatry." *Social Science and Medicine, 11*, 3–10.

Kleinman, A. (1988). *Rethinking psychiatry: From cultural category to personal experience*. New York: Free Press.

Kleinman, A. (2006). *What really matters*. New York: Oxford University Press.

Kleinman, A, Eisenberg, L., & Good, B. (1978). Culture, illness, and care: Clinical lessons from anthropologic and cross-cultural research. *Annals of Internal Medicine, 88*, 251–258.

Kleinman, A., & Good, B. J. (Eds.). (1985). *Culture and depression*. Berkeley: University of California Press.

Kleinman, A., & Kleinman, J. (1991). Suffering and its professional transformations: Toward an ethnography of experience. *Culture, Medicine, and Psychiatry, 15*, 275–301.

Kopelowicz, A., Lopez, S. R., Zarate, R., O'Brien, M., Gordon, J., Chang, C., et al. (2006). Expressed emotion and family interactions in Mexican Americans with schizophrenia. *Journal of Nervous and Mental Disease, 19*, 330–334

Lambert, M. C., Weisz, J. R., & Knight, F. (1989). Over- and undercontrolled clinic referral problems of Jamaican and American children and adolescents: The culture-general and the culture-specific. *Journal of Consulting and Clinical Psychology, 57*, 467–472.

Leff, J. P., Vaughn, C. E. (1985). *Expressed emotion in families*. New York: Guilford.

Lefley, H. (Ed.). (1998). *Families coping with illness: The cultural context*. San Francisco: Jossey-Bass.

Lewis-Fernandez, R., Guarnaccia, P. J., Martinez, I. E., Salmán, E., Schmidt, A., & Liebowitz, M. (2002). Comparative phenomenology of *ataques de nervios*, panic attacks, and panic disorder. *Culture, Medicine and Psychiatry, 26*, 199–223.

Lewis-Fernandez, R., & Kleinman, A. (1995). Cultural psychiatry: Theoretical, clinical and research issues. *Psychiatric Clinics of North America, 18*, 433–448.

Liebowitz, M. R., Salmán, E., Jusino, C. M., Garfinkel, R., Street, L., Cardenas, D. L, et al. (1994). Ataque de nervios and panic disorder. *American Journal of Psychiatry, 151*, 871–875.

Lin, K. M., & Kleinman, A. M. (1988). Psychopathology and clinical course of schizophrenia: A cross-cultural perspective. *Schizophrenia Bulletin, 14*, 555–567.

Lin, K. M., Poland, R. E., & Anderson, D. (1995). Psychopharmacology, ethnicity and culture. *Transcultural Psychiatric Research Review, 32*, 3–40.

López, S. R. (2003). Reflections on the Surgeon General's Report on Mental Health: Culture, race and ethnicity. *Culture, Medicine and Psychiatry, 27*, 419–434.

López, S. R, Nelson, K., Polo, A., Jenkins, J. H., Karno, M., Vaughn, C., et al. (2004). Ethnicity, expressed emotion, attributions and course of schizophrenia: Family warmth matters. *Journal of Abnormal Psychology, 113*, 428–439.

López, S. R., Nelson, K., Snyder, K., & Mintz, J. (1999). Attributions and affective reactions of family members and course of schizophrenia. *Journal of Abnormal Psychology, 108*, 307–314.

López, S. R., & Núñez, J. A. (1987). The consideration of cultural factors in selected diagnostic criteria and interview schedules. *Journal Abnormal Psychology, 96*, 270–272.

Manson, S. M., Shore, J. H., & Bloom, J. D. (1985). The depressive experience in American Indian communities: A challenge for psychiatric theory and diagnosis. In A. Kleinman & B. J. Good (Eds.), *Culture and Depression* (pp. 331–368). Berkeley: University of California Press.

Markus, H. R., & Kitayama, S. (1991). Culture and the self: Implications for cognition, emotion, and motivation. *Psychological Review, 98*, 224–253.

Marsella, A. J. (1980). Depressive experience and disorder across cultures. In H. Triandis & J. Draguns (Eds.), *Handbook of cross-cultural psychology: Vol. 6. Psychopathology* (pp. 237–289). Boston: Allyn & Bacon.

Marshall, G. N., & Orlando, M. (2002). Acculturation and peritraumatic dissociation in young adult Latino survivors of community violence. *Journal of Abnormal Psychology, 111*, 166–174.

Maser, J. D., & Dinges, N. (1992–1993). The co-morbidity of depression, anxiety and substance abuse among American Indians and Alaska Natives. *Culture, Medicine, and Psychiatry, 16*, 409–577.

Medina-Mora, M. E., Borges, G., Lara Muñoz, C., Benjet, C., Blanco Jaimes, J., Fleiz Bautista, C., et al. (2003). Prevalence of mental disorders and use of services: Results from the Mexican National Survey of Psychiatric Epidemiology. *Salud Mental, 26*, 1–16.

Mezzich, J. E, Kleinman, A., Fabrega, H., & Parron, D. L. (Eds.). (1996). *Culture and psychiatric diagnosis: A DSM-IV perspective.* Washington, D.C.: American Psychiatric Association.

Mezzich, J. E., Kleinman, A., Fabrega, H., Parron, D. L., Good, B. J., Lin, K., et al. (1997). Cultural issues for DSM-IV. In T. A. Widiger, A. J. Frances, H. A. Pincus, R. Ross, M. B. First, & W. Davis (Eds.), *DSM-IV Sourcebook,* (Vol. 3, pp. 861–1016). Washington, D.C.: American Psychiatric Association.

Murray, C. J. L., & Lopez, A. D. (1996). *The global burden of disease: A comprehensive assessment of mortality and disability from diseases, injuries, and risk factors in 1990 and projected to 2020.* Cambridge, MA: Harvard University Press.

Neal, A. M., Lilly, R. S., & Zakis, S. (1993). What are African American children afraid of? *Journal of Anxiety Disorders, 7*, 129–139.

Neal, A. M., & Turner, S. M. (1991). Anxiety disorders research with African Americans: Current status. *Psychological Bulletin, 109*, 400–410.

Neighbors, H. W., Jackson, J. S., Campbell, L., & Williams, D. (1989). The influence of racial factors on psychiatric diagnosis: A review and suggestions for research. *Community Mental Health Journal, 25*, 301–310.

O'Nell, T. (1989). Psychiatric investigations among American Indians and Alaska Natives: A critical review. *Culture, Medicine, and Psychiatry, 13*, 51–87.

O'Nell, T., & Mitchell, C. M. (1996). Alcohol use among American Indian adolescents: The role of culture in pathological drinking. *Social Science and Medicine, 42*, 565–578.

Ortega, A., N., Rosenheck, R., Alegria, M., & Desai, R. A. (2000). Acculturation and the lifetime risk of psychiatric and substance use disorders among Hispanics. *Journal of Nervous and Mental Disease, 188*, 728–735.

Polo, A. J. (2002). *Mental health problems among Mexican American youth: Socio-cultural and family correlates.* Unpublished doctoral dissertation, University of California, Los Angeles.

Regier, D. A., Myers, J. K., Kramer, M., Robins, L. N., Blazer, D. G., Hough, R. L., et al. (1984). The NIMH Epidemiologic Catchment Area program. *Archives of General Psychiatry, 41*, 934–941.

Roberts, R. E., Roberts, C. R., & Chen, Y. R. (1997). Ethnocultural differences in prevalence of adolescent depression. *American Journal of Community Psychology, 25*, 95–110.

Rogler, L. H. (1989). The meaning of culturally sensitive research in mental health. *American Journal of Psychiatry, 146*, 296–303.

Rogler, L. H. (1994). International migrations: A framework for directing research. *American Psychologist, 49*, 701–708.

Rogler, L. H. (1996). Framing research on culture in psychiatric diagnosis: The case of the DSM-IV. *Psychiatry: Interpersonal & Biological Processes, 59*, 145–155.

Rogler, L. H., Malgady, R. G., & Rodríguez, O. (1989). *Hispanics and Mental Health: A Framework for Research.* Malabar, FL: Krieger.

Salgado de Snyder, V. N., Diaz-Perez, M., & Bautista, E. (1998). Pathways to mental health services among inhabitants of a Mexican village with high migratory tradition to the United States. *Health and Social Work, 23*, 249–261.

Salmán E., Liebowitz, M., Guarnaccia, P. J., Jusino, C. M., Garfinkel, R., Street, L., et al. (1998). Subtypes of ataques de nervios: The influence of coexisting psychiatric diagnosis. *Culture, Medicine, and Psychiatry, 22*, 231–244.

Sartorius, N., Jablensky, A., Korten, A., Ernberg, G., Anker, M., Cooper, J. E., et al. (1986). Early manifestations and first-contact incidence of schizophrenia in different cultures. *Psychological Medicine, 16*, 909–928.

Schneider, B. H. (1998). Cross-cultural comparison as doorkeeper in research on social and emotional adjustment of children and adolescents. *Developmental Psychology, 34*, 793–797.

Shweder, R. A., & Bourne, E. J. (1984). Does the concept of the person vary cross-culturally? In R. A. Shweder, & R. A. LeVine (Eds.), *Culture theory: Essays on mind, self and emotion* (pp. 158–199). Cambridge: Cambridge University Press.

Sue S., Fujino D. C., Hu, L., Takeuchi, D., & Zane, N. (1991). Community mental health services for ethnic minority groups: A test of the cultural responsiveness hypothesis. *Journal of Consulting and Clinical Psychology, 59*, 533–540.

Sue, S., Sue, D., Sue, L., & Takeuchi D. (1995.) Asian American psychopathology. *Cultural Diversity and Mental Health, 1*, 39–51.

Takeuchi, D. T., Chung, R. C. Y., Lin, K. M., Shen, H., Kurasaki K., Chung, C. A., et al. (1998). Lifetime and twelve-month prevalence rates of major depressive episodes and dysthymia among Chinese Americans in Los Angeles. *American Journal of Psychiatry, 155*, 1407–1414.

U.S. Department of Health and Human Services [USDHHS] (1999). *Mental health: A report of the surgeon general*. Rockville, MD: Author.

U.S. Department of Health and Human Services [USDHHS] (2001). *Mental health: Culture, race, and ethnicity—A supplement to Mental health: A report of the surgeon general*. Rockville, MD: Author.

Vaughn, C. E., Snyder, K. S., Jones, S., Freeman, W. B., & Falloon, I. R. H. (1984). Family factors in California of British research on expressed emotion. *Archives of General Psychiatry, 41*, 1169–1177.

Vaughn, C. E., & Leff, J. P. (1976). The influence of family and social factors on the course of psychiatric illness. *British Journal of Psychiatry, 129*, 125–137.

Vega, W., Khoury, E. L., Zimmerman, R. S., Gil, A. G., & Warheit, G. J. (1995). Cultural conflicts and problem behaviors of Latino adolescents in home and school environments. *Journal of Community Psychology, 23*, 167–179.

Vega, W. A., Kolody, B., Aguilar-Gaxiola, S., Aldrete, E., Catalana, R., & Caraveo-Anduaga, J. (1998). Lifetime prevalence of DSM-III-R psychiatric disorders among urban and rural Mexican Americans in California. *Archives of General Psychiatry, 55*, 771–778.

Ware, N., & Kleinman A. (1992). Culture and somatic experience: The social course of illness in neurasthenia and chronic fatigue syndrome. *Psychosomatic Medicine, 54*, 546–560.

Weine, A. M., Phillips, J. S., & Achenbach, T. M. (1995). Behavioral and emotional problems among Chinese and American children: Parent and teacher reports for ages 6 to 13. *Journal of Abnormal Child Psychology, 23*, 619–639.

Weisman, A. (1997). Understanding cross-cultural prognostic variability for schizophrenia. *Cultural Diversity and Mental Health, 3*, 3–35.

Weisman, A. G., Gomes, L., & López, S. R. (2003). Shifting blame away from ill relatives: Latino families' reactions to schizophrenia. *Journal of Nervous and Mental Disease, 175*, 143–151.

Weisman, A. G., Lopez, S. R., Ventura, J., Nuechterlein, K. H., Goldstein, M. J., & Hwang, S. (2000). A comparison of psychiatric symptoms between Anglo-Americans and Mexican-Americans with schizophrenia. *Schizophrenia Bulletin, 26*, 817–824.

Weisz, J. R., Chaiyasit, W., Weiss, B., Eastman, K. L., & Jackson, E. W. (1995). A multimethod study of problem behavior among Thai and American children in school: Teacher reports versus direct observation. *Child Development, 66*, 402–415.

Weisz, J. R., McCarty, C. A., Eastman, K. L., Chaiyasit, W., & Suwanlert, S. (1997). Developmental psychopathology and culture: Ten lessons from Thailand. In S. S. Luthar, J. A. Burack, D. Cicchetti, & J. R. Weisz (Eds.), *Developmental psychopathology: Perspectives on adjustment, risk, and disorder* (pp. 568–592). Cambridge: Cambridge University Press.

Weisz, J. R., Sigman, M., Weiss, B., & Mosk J. (1993a). Parent reports of behavioral and emotional problems among children in Kenya, Thailand, and the United States. *Child Development, 64*, 98–109.

Weisz, J. R., Suwanlert, S., Chaiyasit, W., Weiss, B., Achenbach, T. M., & Eastman, K. L. (1993b). Behavioral and emotional problems among Thai and American adolescents: Parent reports for ages 12–16. *Journal of Abnormal Psychology, 102*, 395–403.

Weisz, J. R., Suwanlert, S., Chaiyasit, W., Weiss, B., Achenbach, T. M., & Trevathan D. (1989). Epidemiology behavioral and emotional problems among Thai and American children: Teacher reports for ages 6–11. *Journal of Child Psychology and Psychiatry & Allied Disciplines, 30*, 471–484.

Weisz, J. R., Suwanlert, S., Chaiyasit, W., Weiss, B., & Jackson, E. W. (1991). Adult attitudes toward over- and undercontrolled child problems: Urban and rural parents and teachers from Thailand and the United States. *Journal of Child Psychology and Psychiatry & Allied Disciplines, 32*, 645–654.

Weisz, J. R., Suwanlert, S., Chaiyasit, W., Weiss, B., & Walter, B. (1987a). Over- and undercontrolled referral problems among children and adolescents from Thailand and the United States: The *wat* and *wai* of cultural differences. *Journal of Consulting & Clinical Psychology, 55*, 719–726.

Weisz, J. R., Suwanlert, S., Chaiyasit, W., Weiss, B., Achenbach, T. M., & Walter, B. R. (1987b). Epidemiology of behavioral and emotional problems among Thai and American children: Parent reports for ages 6 to 11 *Journal of the American Academy of Child & Adolescent Psychiatry, 26*, 890–897.

Weisz, J. R., & Weiss, B. (1991). Studying the "referability" of child clinical problems. *Journal of Consulting & Clinical Psychology, 59*, 266–273.

Widiger, T., Frances, A., Pincus, H.A., First, M.B., Ross, R. & Davis, W. (Eds.). (1997). *DSM-IV Source Book* (Vol. 3). Washington, D.C.: American Psychiatric Press.

Weisz, J. R., Weiss, B., Suwanlert, S., & Chaiyasit, W. (2003). Syndromal structure of psychopathology in children of Thailand and the United States. *Journal of Consulting and Clinical Psychology, 71*, 375–385.

World Health Organization. (1979). *Schizophrenia: An International Follow-up Study*. New York: Wiley.

Zheng, Y. P., Lin, K. M, Takeuchi, D., Kurasaki, K. S., Wang, Y., & Cheung, F. (1997). An epidemiological study of neurasthenia in Chinese-Americans in Los Angeles. *Comprehensive Psychiatry, 38*, 249–259.

3

The Role of Gender, Race, and Class in Psychopathology

Barbara A. Winstead and Janis Sanchez-Hucles

We are considering the occurrence of psychopathology, its etiology, and the effectiveness of its treatment, yet, we generally treat clients and clinicians involved as if they all belong to the same group. We are not unaware of group differences. Most chapters in this textbook intentionally address issues of gender or race as they are related to the psychological disorder being described. And chapter 2 presents a full description of the importance of culture in understanding psychopathology. But the majority of descriptions of disorders, treatments, and research speak of clients and clinicians without reference to their social identities and with the assumption that diagnoses, treatments, and research outcomes can be generally applied to one and all.

This chapter focuses on the differences rather than the universalities. It addresses these questions: (1) Do gender, race, and class affect which psychological disorders individuals experience or how they experience them? (2) Are individuals from different groups treated differently by the mental health system? (3) Do recommended treatments work equally well for individuals from these different groups? (4) Should treatments take the demographic characteristics of the client into account? (5) Do the gender or race of the therapist matter? (6) What difference do gender, race, and class make? (7) And, if they make a difference, why? This chapter tackles these questions. In the end we will discover that these questions raise more questions. Clear-cut answers are scarce, but the questions themselves shed light on the process of psychological diagnosis and the treatment of psychological disorders.

First, a word about terminology: *Race* may be considered an outdated term; scientists are in agreement that biological variation among humans does not fall neatly into "racial" groups. The assumption is often made, however, that group differences in physical or mental health have biological foundations, and persists despite the argument that these categories are socially constructed and represent social relationships, often between those with more power and privilege and those with less (Mullings & Schulz, 2006). The use of the term *race,* then, as opposed to *ethnicity* or *culture,* is meant to remind us of these historical and current assumptions and of the advantages (increasing understanding across groups) and hazards (distancing and pathologizing of the "other") of using race as an identifier. *Gender* is also a problematic term (Pryzgoda & Chrisler, 2000). A distinction has often been made between "sex," meaning biological differences between women and men, and "gender," referring to psychological and sociological differences. But how does one sort these out?

Gender reminds us again that a simple biological explanation will rarely if ever suffice in understanding human mental health or disorder.

Recent Initiatives Focused on Gender, Race, and Class

Concern about the impact of gender, race, and class on mental health and mental health care is expressed in at least three recent and ongoing national efforts. One is the attention currently being paid to racial and ethnic disparities in health and mental health. The second is interest in "cross-cultural issues" as part of the planning process for the fifth edition of *The Diagnostic and Statistical Manual (DSM-V)*. The third is the focus in the training of mental health professionals on cultural competence. Inequities in health and health care based on ethnicity is hardly news; but the attention paid to these inequities at the national level is a relatively recent phenomenon. Chang (2003) writes about the politics of making disparities salient in the mental health community. The publication in 1999 by the U.S. Department of Health and Human Services of *Mental Health: A Report of the Surgeon General* was a first and was intended as "an up-to-date review of scientific advances in the study of mental health and of mental illnesses that affect at least one in five Americans" (USDHHS, 1999, p. 3). In the preface to this report, Surgeon General Dr. David Satcher acknowledged that "Even more than other areas of health and medicine, the mental health field is plagued by disparities in the availability of and access to its services. These disparities are viewed readily through the lenses of racial and cultural diversity, age, and gender" (USDHHS, 1999, p. vi).

While issues of diversity were considered in the report, its main thrust was universalistic, treating diagnosis and treatment of psychological disorders as if current tests and treatments could and should be equally applied to all individuals. Nelba Chavez, the Administrator of Substance Abuse and Mental Health Services Administration (SAMHSA), refused to sign the report on the grounds that insufficient attention was paid to cultural diversity and disparities in mental health care (Chavez, 2003). This led to the development of a supplement to the report, *Mental Health: Culture, Race, and Ethnicity* (USDHHS, 2001), an over 200-page report summarizing available research on the impact of ethnicity on mental health. The report is organized around presentation of information about the four "most recognized" U.S. minority groups: African Americans, American Indians/Alaska Natives, Asian Americans/Pacific Islanders, and Hispanic Americans. Both the initial report and the culture, race, and ethnicity supplement are available online: http://www.surgeongeneral.gov/library/mentalhealth/cre/.

One of two goals of the U.S. health agenda, *Healthy People 2010*, is the elimination of health disparities. The Office of Minority Health (part of Health and Human Services), the National Center on Minority Health and Health Disparities, the Center for Disease Control, the National Institutes of Health, and other federal agencies all support research to understand health and mental health disparities and programs to eliminate them. In 2003, The President's New Freedom Commission on Mental Health issued a report, *Achieving the Promise: Transforming Mental Health Care in America* that speaks explicitly to problems for ethnic minorities in accessing quality mental health care and outlines a plan for research and practice that can close the gap: http://www.nicic.org/Library/020228.

The *Diagnostic and Statistical Manual* published by the American Psychiatric Association is the standard used by all mental health professionals for diagnosis of psychological disorders. Concerns with gender and ethnic bias in the criteria for various disorders have been longstanding (Caplan & Cosgrove, 2004). As the American Psychiatric Association plans for the fifth edition of *DSM*, it has established six workgroups that have published preplanning white papers in *A Research Agenda for DSM-V* (2002): http://appi.org/book.cfm?id=2292. One of these papers by Alarcón, Alegria, Bell, Boyce, Kirmayer, Lin et al. (2002) deals with the influence of culture on psychiatric diagnosis, including the influences of ethnicity, language, education, gender, and sexual orientation.

In the disciplines of counseling and clinical psychology there has been a persistent, but increasing, focus on the cultural competence of practitioners. In fact, psychologists have been concerned about cultural diversity for decades. Training in cultural diversity was recommended at the Vail Conference that established the scientist–practitioner model adhered to by most clinical psychology graduate programs (Korman, 1974); questions regarding training in cultural diversity became a part of the American Psychological Association Accreditation Domains and Standards in 1986 and continue to be a focus of consideration in accreditation of clinical, counseling, and school psychology programs; the American Psychological Association published *Guidelines for Providers of Psychological Services to Ethnic, Linguistic, and Culturally Diverse Populations* (1990) and incorporated awareness of "cultural, individual, and role differences, including those related to age, gender, race, ethnicity, national origin" in its Ethics code in 1992 (p. 1598). In 2002 the American Psychological Association approved *Guidelines on Multicultural Education, Training, Research, Practice, and Organizational Change for Psychologists:* http://www.apa.org/pi/multiculturalguidelines/references.html. The Council of National Psychological Associations for the Advancement of Ethnic Minority Interests published *Psychological Treatment of Ethnic Minority Populations* in 2003: http://www.apa.org/pi/oema/programs/empa_ptemp.pdf with recommendations for treatment of Asian American/Pacific Islanders, African descent populations, Hispanic/Latinos, and American Indians. A joint task force of American Psychological Association Divisions 17 (Society of Counseling Psychology) and 35 (Society for the Psychology of Women) published a draft of *Guidelines for Psychological Practice with Girls and Women* in July 2006: http://www.apa.org/about/division/7%2024%2006%20final%20revised%20tx%20guidelines%20_2_.pdf.

These efforts by the federal government, the American Psychiatric Association, and the American Psychological Association to identify and address the impact of gender, race, and social class on psychological disorders, their diagnosis and treatment, illustrate the importance of the issue and the recognition that mental health practitioners have a clear responsibility to be familiar with the knowledge base concerning gender, race, and class and to develop skills that allow them to be competent in their interactions with and treatment of individuals who may be different from themselves.

Although we and many others stress the importance of taking gender, race, and social class into account in our interactions with and responses to others, the research base for understanding *if* these variables make a difference in prevalence of a disorder or in the effectiveness of an intervention or *how* they make a difference generally deal with one or two variables at a time. Thus, this chapter will present research on gender differences, but the interaction of gender with ethnicity or class may be missing due to limitations in the literature. There may be information on race, but its interaction with gender may not be taken into account. Of great significance when considering race will be whether or not social class, as represented by income and education, is included. In the United States, class and ethnicity are highly interrelated. While 9.1% of whites live below the poverty level, 24.9% of African Americans, 25.7% of American Indian and Alaska Natives, and 22.6% of Hispanics live below the poverty line (U.S. Census, 2003). Analyses of ethnicity that do not include social class are in danger of confounding a difference among ethnic groups with a difference attributable to income. Likewise, although even more often overlooked, there is a connection between gender and poverty. The poverty rate for married-couple families is 4.9%, for single male head-of-household (6% of all families), 13.6%, and for single female head-of-household (17% of all families), 26.5% (Bishaw & Iceland, 2003).

Even in this brief introduction it should be apparent that, although we continually refer to the intersection among gender, race, and social class, other documents refer to some of these, all of these, or these plus various other demographic characteristics. The critical issue is placing the individual within the sociocultural context that best helps us to understand and effectively intervene. So, although this chapter focuses on gender, race, and social class, it is understood that these interact with age, sexual orientation, ability, and other variables to form unique experiences for individuals and that the intersection of these variables with others represents combinations that are perceived differently by society and by mental health professionals.

The Role of Gender, Race, and Class in Diagnosis

To understand and treat a psychological disorder requires accurate diagnosis. The process of diagnosis and treatment is less than perfect, but the goal can be clearly stated: We wish to identify the problem, treat it, and thereby permit the client to lead a more productive and rewarding life. But how do we identify the problem? With physical symptoms physicians are aided by diagnostic tests that identify abnormalities in biochemistry, histology, or anatomy that signal specific disease processes. With psychological problems there are rarely physical signs such as an abnormal cell count. We may use diagnostic tests, but these are likely to be based on the self-reports of clients, not blood chemistry or cell cultures. Often psychological diagnosis is accomplished through interviews, in which clinicians learn about symptoms directly from the client, through psychological tests or through observations of symptoms. What the *Diagnostic and Statistical Manual* (*DSM-IV-TR*; American Psychiatric Association, 2000) provides is a set of agreed upon criteria that help clinicians make diagnoses based on sets of symptoms. Psychological diagnosis, following the medical model, leads to present/absent decisions, although many have argued that a continuous rather than a categorical model is better for understanding psychological disorders (Maddux, 2002). With either model, we want to be able to make an accurate assessment of the individual and to this end we assess the reliability and validity of clinical tests, clinical interviews, and systems for identifying mental disorders (see Widiger, chapter 5, and Garb et al., chapter 6). With a perfectly reliable and valid system we could easily discover if gender, ethnicity, or social class are related to different psychological disorders, if the etiologies or disease courses of these illnesses were similar or different, and ultimately if individuals with different characteristics benefit from similar or different treatments. But with less than perfect diagnostic systems our questions about gender, race, and class become more difficult to answer.

An official nomenclature for identifying mental illnesses was first established in part to create a common language for mental health professionals and researchers (see Widiger, chapter 5). Beginning with *DSM-III* (American Psychiatric Association, 1980), this goal was largely accomplished in the United States, and research on psychological disorders and treatments adopted this system of diagnosis. Efforts to improve the reliability and validity of the *DSM* have led to revised and updated editions, *DSM-III-R* (1987) and the current *DSM-IV-TR* (2000). The purpose of a carefully articulated diagnostic system is to provide clinicians and researchers with an objective-as-possible basis for making decisions about the presence or absence of specific psychopathology. But the question of gender bias in the diagnostic categories themselves (Kaplan, 1983) and of failure to appreciate ethnic and racial variations in perspectives on normality and abnormality (Adebimpe, 1981; Gaines, 1992) were raised almost immediately. Furthermore, to the extent that information relies on the interviewing and interpersonal skills of a diagnostician (as opposed to a standardized survey or interview), the gathering of pertinent information to make this determination may also be influenced by the gender, race, and class of the client and the interviewer. Even items on standardized scales may introduce bias. Finally, although *DSM* guidelines are in black and white, putting all the symptoms together to arrive at a diagnosis may be influenced by clinician expectations and beliefs about the client based on these demographic characteristics.

DSM-IV-TR Information on Gender, Race, and Class

A fundamental issue, for example, is whether or not the prevalence rates of disorders vary by gender or race. *DSM-IV-TR* includes for many disorders a section that presents information regarding the relation of such elements as gender, ethnicity, age, and class to that disorder. Social class is referenced as a link to etiological factors for mental retardation, such as lead poisoning and premature birth, and as a context for understanding undesirable behaviors, such as carrying a weapon or joining a gang, that might be considered indicators of conduct or antisocial disorder but could, in an impoverished or high crime neighborhood, be self-protective. *DSM-IV-TR* also states that undifferentiated somatization disorder is more common in women of lower SES and that conversion disorders are more common among lower SES and rural individuals. Most of the presentation of cultural features simply exhorts the clinician to be sensitive to cultural variations in symptoms and symptom presentation for various disorders. For example, depression might be experienced as "nerves" or headache among Hispanic or Mediterranean clients, "imbalance" in Asian clients, and problems of the "heart" in Middle Eastern clients (p. 353). Specific ethnic differences are presented for alcohol-related disorders: lower in Japanese, Chinese, and Korean populations, equal in whites and African Americans, higher in male Hispanics but lower among female Hispanics. Alcohol abuse is also related to lower education, unemployment, and lower SES, although abuse of alcohol may well have contributed to these variables rather than being an outcome of them. Inhalant abuse (e.g., glue sniffing) is noted as a particular problem for Alaskan natives, especially children and adolescents. Although somatization disorder is relatively rare in men, it occurs at a higher rate in Greek and Puerto Rican men. Finally *DSM-IV-TR* takes note of the research (see below) revealing that African Americans are more often diagnosed with schizophrenia, also noting that whether this is a true difference or the result of bias is unclear. Ethnic differences in bipolar disorder have not been found. Bulimia nervosa is described as "primarily white" (p. 592).

While there is interesting but not extensive information in *DSM-IV* on race or social class differences, Hartung and Widiger (1998) conclude that "[m]ost of the mental disorders diagnosed with the *DSM-IV* do appear to have significant differential sex prevalence rates" (p. 280). According to their analysis, the *DSM-IV-TR* provides information on differential sex prevalence for 101 of its 125 described psychological disorders. Excluding disorders that are, by definition, specific to one sex or the other (e.g., female orgasmic disorder, male erectile disorder), 84% of the *DSM-IV* disorders, for which information on prevalence by sex is available, are reported to occur at different rates in females and males. A general summary of these differences indicates that boys and men are more likely to be diagnosed with the infancy, childhood, and adolescent disorders and with substance-related, sexual, gender identity, and impulsive disorders. Girls and women are more likely to be diagnosed with depression, anxiety, somatization, dissociative, and eating disorders. Diagnoses of personality disorders tend to parallel expected sex differences in personality traits or even gender stereotypes: Females are reported to have higher rates of borderline, histrionic, and dependent personality disorders; males are reported to have higher rates of paranoid, schizoid, schizotypal, antisocial, and compulsive personality disorders.

Gender, Race, and Class Bias

As with the ethnic difference in diagnosis of schizophrenia, much has been written about whether sex differences in prevalence rates represent true differences or bias. In 1997 Garb summarized the research literature on gender, race, and social class bias in clinical judgment. In terms of diagnosis, he concluded that there was race bias for diagnosis of schizophrenia and psychotic affective disorders such that black and Hispanic patients were more likely than white patients to be misdiagnosed with schizophrenia when symptoms suggest psychotic affective disorders and gender bias such that a diagnosis of antisocial personality disorder (APD) is more likely to occur for males and histrionic personality disorder (HPD) for females. Social class was not found to affect diagnoses.

In the following year Widiger (1998) delineated six ways in which diagnoses may reflect bias: (a) biased diagnostic constructs, (b) biased diagnostic thresholds, (c) biased application of the diagnostic criteria, (d) biased sampling of persons with the disorder, (e) biased instruments of assessment, or (f) biased diagnostic criteria" (p. 96). Using these categories as a basis for understanding bias in diagnosis, we will discuss biases in diagnostic standards (e.g., constructs, criteria, and thresholds), biased applications of these diagnostic standards, including assessment instruments, and biased sampling.

Biased Diagnostic Standards Critics of *DSM* have argued that any classification system of psychological disorder represents an ethnocentric construction of what an idealized, or nonpathological, self is. Gaines (1992) suggested that the essential feature of *DSM* diagnoses is absence of self-control, a Western/European ideal. Others argued that the diagnostic constructs were sexist and that women are pathologized by *DSM* diagnostic criteria (Brown, 1992; Caplan, 1991, 1995; Kaplan, 1983; Walker, 1994). HPD and dependent personality disorder (DPD) have been cited as the most egregious examples of gendered, in this case feminine, traits being used to establish the presence of psychopathology (Kaplan, 1983). Kaplan (1983) proposed "independent personality disorder" and "restricted personality disorder" and Pantony and Caplan (1991) suggested "delusional dominating personality disorder" as comparable, but masculine stereotyped, disorders. Others, however, argued that *DSM-III* already included personality disorders that captured maladaptive masculine traits, specifically, APD and compulsive personality disorder (Williams & Spitzer, 1983).

Ross, Frances, and Widiger (1995) suggest: "The *DSM-III/DSM-III-R* personality disorder criteria were constructed, for the most part, by males with little input from systematic empirical research. It would not be surprising to find that male clinicians would have a lower threshold for the attribution of maladaptive feminine traits than for the attribution of maladaptive masculine traits" (p. 212). They go on to describe how the *DSM-IV* Personality Disorders Work Group addressed this problem both by extensive reviews of existing empirical research and by creating more gender-neutral criteria. For example, the HPD item "Inappropriately sexually seductive in appearance or behavior" (*DSM-III-R*, 1987) was changed to "interaction with others is often characterized by inappropriate sexually seductive or provocative behavior." Removing the reference to "appearance" was intended to reduce the possibility that the normal female response to social pressure to appear physically attractive might be viewed as "inappropriately sexually seductive."

Other diagnostic categories also represent a challenge for gender neutrality. Somatization disorder is reported to range from "0.2% to 2% among women and less than 0.2% in men" (*DSM-IV*, 1994, p. 447). Although substantial revisions were made to make criteria less sex biased, *DSM-IV* retains criteria that make a diagnosis in men unlikely. Clients must meet all of the four criteria and the symptoms reported must be found to be not fully explained by a medical condition. Criterion 3 is "one sexual or reproductive symptom other than pain." The examples given include four symptoms that apply exclusively to women ("irregular menses, excessive menstrual bleeding, vomiting throughout pregnancy"), one that applies to men ("erectile or ejaculatory dysfunction") and one that may apply more often to women ("sexual indifference") (*DSM-IV*, 1994, p. 449). Hartung and Widiger (1998) conclude: "Research on the epidemiology of the disorder therefore continues to use a criteria set that is biased against making the diagnosis in males, complicating any identification of the disorder in males" (p. 269). They further point out that the World Health Organization criteria for this disorder, while still including menstrual symptoms, also list gastrointestinal symptoms, abnormal skin sensations, and blotchiness as common symptoms, making it easier for males to be diagnosed with somatization.

The question of criterion bias is further complicated by the issue of the diagnostic validity of specific symptoms for different groups. The purpose of gathering information about a client's feelings, thoughts, and behaviors is to identify a psychological disorder. It may be the case that certain symptoms are predictive of a diagnostic category, future symptoms, or responsiveness to treatment for some groups, but not for others. An example from the arena of physical illness illustrates this problem. Although heart disease is the number 1 killer of both women and men in the United States and more women than men have died from heart disease every year since 1984 (Giardina, 2000), heart disease is still generally regarded as a greater problem for men than for women. It is estimated that 35% of heart attacks in women are unreported. Women having heart attacks are as likely as men to experience chest pain, but they are somewhat more likely to experience other symptoms, such as breathlessness, perspiration, nausea, and a sensation of fluttering in the heart (Giardina, 2000). An unfamiliar constellation of symptoms may prevent women or health professionals from suspecting the presence of heart disease. In the case of heart attacks, although the underlying condition is the same, the presenting symptoms for women and men are somewhat different. It is likely that for some psychological disorders a similar process occurs.

Being able to identify a criterion that is differentially valid for females or males or for a particular ethnic group requires a diagnostic system that is independent of this criterion. In the case of heart disease, whatever the presenting symptoms, the presence or absence of a myocardial infarction can be assessed independently. For psychological disorders there is no similar confirmation. In reference to establishing criteria for personality disorders, Robins and Guze (1970) advocated for validation studies that would "assess the extent to which the criteria select persons who have a history, present, and/or future consistent with the construct of a (particular) personality disorder" (p. 17). One might also suggest a validity test that considers the effectiveness of standard interventions for persons with and without a particular diagnostic criterion.

According to *DSM-IV* (1994), "[t]he definition of *mental disorder*...requires that there be clinically significant impairment or distress" (p. 7). Thresholds for diagnoses should represent the point at which the accumulation of symptoms reaches this level of impairment or distress. But where is it? The issue of thresholds is one of the arguments for a dimensional rather than categorical view of psychopathology (Maddux, 2002), but it remains the case that clinicians and clinical researchers are regularly faced with the task of a present/absent decision in regard to the diagnosis of pathology. Prevalence of a disorder for any particular group will be affected by the setting of this threshold. It is important to note that, for the most part, the number of criteria needed to reach threshold for a DSM-IV diagnosis is established by committee rather than by empirical research that would justify that particular number.

Biased Application of the Diagnostic Criteria Diagnosis may also involve objective tests or structured or semistructured interviews. Although bias often suggests subjectivity in judgment, standardized tests can also contain bias. A 2005 special issue of *Psychological Assessment* includes articles on evidence-based assessment (EBA) of major psychological disorders. In their introduction, Hunsley and Mash (2005) specify, "EBAs need to be sensitive to gender, ethnicity, and cultural factors. Scientific evidence for the applicability of assessment tools needs to be demonstrated, not simply assumed on the basis of generalizations from nonrepresentative samples" (2005, p. 252). Anthony and Rowa (2005) admit that for many of the instruments used to assess anxiety disorders, utility across different populations remains an unanswered question. Similarly, in their article on assessment of couple distress, Snyder, Heyman, and Haynes (2005) conclude: "Given that nearly all measures of couple distress were developed and tested on White middle-class married couples, their relevance to, and utility for, assessing ethnic couples, gay and lesbian couples, and low-income couples is unknown" (p. 302).

Joiner, Walker, Pettit, Perez, and Cukrowicz (2005) cite several studies that have demonstrated no evidence for gender or ethnic bias in the commonly used assessment measures for depression. On the other hand, Sprock and Yoder (1997) reviewed studies that suggest that circumstances and age may affect the validity of these instruments. When scales were described as measures of depression, items were endorsed less often by men than by women; but there was no sex difference when the instruments were described as hassles scales (Page & Bennesch, 1993). In a sample of geriatric patients hospitalized for major unipolar depression, Allen-Burge, Storandt, Kinscherf, and Rubin (1994) found that the BDI and the Geriatric Depression Scale were more likely to detect depression in elderly women than in elderly men. In addition, depressed women report more symptoms of depression than do depressed men, even when clinicians' judgments of severity of depression do not differ, leading Sprock and Yoder (1997) to suggest that the number of criteria for diagnosis of depression should perhaps be greater for women than for men.

Not surprisingly, on the assessment of personality disorders, Widiger and Samuel (2005) present a more complex picture. Self-report inventories can provide gender-biased assessments. Problems occur when self-report instruments use responses that do not reflect dysfunction but do apply to one sex or gender more than the other (Lindsay & Widiger, 1995; Widiger, 1998; Widiger & Samuel, 2005). A biased item occurs when men or women (sex bias) or masculine or feminine persons (gender bias) are more likely to endorse the item. The item itself is not a "symptom," nor is it related to general psychopathology, but it does contribute to a scale that measures a personality disorder. Using college students, Lindsay and Widiger (1995) determined that 13 to 31% of the items from three standardized measures of personality disorder showed some evidence of sex or gender bias according to these criteria.

In a follow-up study Lindsay, Sankis, and Widiger (2000) used outpatients from mental health clinics and updated versions of the instruments: Millon Clinical Multiaxial Inventory-III (MMCI-III), Minnesota Multiphasic Personality Inventory-II (MMPI-II), and Personality Diagnostic Questionnaire-Revised (PDQ-R). Four personality disorder scales (histrionic, dependent, antisocial, and narcissistic) from these instruments were analyzed for sex or gender bias. None of the scale scores from any of the inventories was related to biological sex. Only three scale items showed sex bias (women or men were more likely to endorse them but the item was unrelated to a measure of psychopathology, the Personality Assessment Inventory). However, 36 items suggested gender bias; that is, the item correlated with a measure of femininity or masculinity but not with the measure of psychopathology. An example of an item that demonstrated sex bias and gender bias was "It's very easy for me to make many friends" from the MCMI-III Histrionic scale. This item is not indicative of a psychological problem, but it does contribute to a higher score for histrionic personality disorder. It is also more frequently endorsed by women than men and it correlates positively with measures of femininity. This item would tend to give women and feminine individuals higher scores for HPD when they endorse an item that does not represent a maladaptive trait or behavior. Although the few items (three) demonstrating sex bias were all from the Histrionic scales, more examples of gender bias were from the Narcissistic scale, suggesting that masculine individuals may receive a higher score by endorsing items that reflect adaptive, rather than pathological, characteristics.

Widiger and Samuel (2005) also argue that diagnostic criterion sets themselves are in need of examination for gender bias. Assessment tools based on these criteria as well as interview outcomes will inevitably yield biased outcomes if they are established to diagnose according to definitions of disorder that are inherently biased.

Less attention has been paid to the role of ethnicity in assessment of personality disorder, although Widiger and Samuel note the finding of higher scores for African Americans compared to whites on the paranoid personality disorder scales of the MCMI-III. As they suggest, it is possible but not empirically established, that experiences of discrimination and prejudice lead to greater endorsement of items, such as "I am sure I get a raw deal in life," which contributes to the paranoid personality score but may be a reasonable reflection on a life lived facing barriers imposed by racism.

Regardless of the care taken to establish reliable and valid diagnostic tools, the clinicians using the tools or other sources of clinical information may be biased in making diagnoses. Lopez (1989) reviewed the effect of patient variables on clinical judgment. He found evidence of overpathologizing for cases with low social class and diagnostic category biases for race and, to some extent, gender. But he also argued that clinicians can both overpathologize and underpathologize in their judgments of patients and that errors in judgment affect both oppressed and nonoppressed groups and result from information processing biases, not just prejudice or discrimination. He cites Luebnitz, Randolph, and Gutsch (1982) who found that a lower-class African-American patient was more likely to receive a diagnosis of chronic alcohol abuse than white lower-class or African-American or white higher-class patients. But given the symptoms presented, the error was more in underdiagnosing based on race and class. Similarly, he cites a study by Leinhardt, Seewald, and Zigmond (1982) suggesting that white boys are disproportionately identified as learning disabled. Diagnoses of depression may also be affected by clinician bias. Potts, Burnam, and Wells (1991) compared clinicians' judgments to diagnoses made with a standardized interview assessment and found that there were discrepancies between standardized assessment and clinician judgments in that medical practitioners were less likely to diagnose depression in men and mental health practitioners were more likely to diagnose depression in women. Clearly in the real world of persons interacting with health and mental health practitioners, diagnosis of depression, as with other disorders, is not free of sex bias. Overpathologizing can lead to unnecessary interventions and stigma; underpathologizing can lead to lack of treatment and failure to intervene where needed.

Lopez (1989) noted the power of experimental (or analogue) studies in uncovering bias. In his review, 45% of experimental cases examining severity judgments and 55% examining diagnostic judgments revealed bias. In analogue studies clinicians are presented with case histories that are identical except for the sex or ethnicity of the patient. Many studies have focused on gender bias. In these studies half of the clinicians in the research diagnose the "female patient," half diagnose the "male patient." Given the same information will clinicians come to the same or different conclusions about the presence of psychological disorders? Warner (1978) gave clinicians ambiguous patient profiles, with a mixture of hysterical and antisocial symptoms (e.g., suicide attempts, no close relationships, self-centered, shoplifting with no remorse for crime, flirtatious). Female profiles were more likely than male profiles to be labeled hysterical (76 vs. 49%) and male profiles were more likely than female to be labeled antisocial (41 vs. 22%). It can be argued that with ambiguous information, clinicians rely on base rates (women *are* more likely to be hysterical; men *are* more likely to be antisocial). The base rates themselves, however, may also represent a biased accumulation of data on women and men. If clinicians use stereotyped perceptions of women and men in their diagnoses (as these studies indicate), then the data based on their clinical judgments will be biased.

To circumvent the issue of base rates, subsequent studies presented clinicians with cases that meet the *DSM* criteria for one or more disorders. Ford and Widiger (1989) created cases that met *DSM-III* criteria for HPD or APD or failed to reach diagnostic criteria for either. HPD was more frequently diagnosed in women, even when the case contained more antisocial than histrionic criteria; and APD was less often diagnosed in women. Adler, Drake, and Teague (1990) developed one case history that met the explicit criteria of four diagnoses: histrionic, narcissistic, borderline, and dependent. Men were more likely to receive a diagnosis of narcissistic personality disorder; women, histrionic personality disorder. There were no differences for borderline or dependent (which was rarely used) personality disorder. In research using a case that met the criteria for borderline personality disorder (BPD) and posttraumatic stress disorder, however, women did receive higher ratings for BPD (Becker & Lamb, 1994). Fernbach, Winstead, and Derlega (1989) created separate cases for antisocial and somatization disorders and found that there were no sex-of-vignette differences for somatization disorder; but for APD, although most cases were accurately diagnosed, men (73%) were significantly more likely than women (53%) to receive the diagnosis. Nineteen percent of clinicians made an inaccurate diagnosis of BPD, of these 68% were for the female case and 32% for the male case.

If the diagnostic criteria for a disorder are built into the case description, then the presence of clinician bias represents a failure to adhere to the *DSM* diagnostic criteria. Clinicians are coming up with the "wrong" answer when they indicate a diagnostic category other than the one intended. Ford and Widiger (1989) demonstrated that at the level of individual criteria there is no sex bias. Specific behaviors were rated as indicative of HPD and APD with equal frequency for men and women. But they did find sex bias when assigning clients to one of these diagnostic categories. They concluded that histrionic personality disorder was overdiagnosed in women and underdiagnosed in men (Ford & Widiger, 1989). Morey and Ochoa (1989) and Blashfield and Herkov (1996) looked at clinicians' ratings of *DSM* criteria for their own patients and compared ratings on individual criteria with actual diagnoses of these patients. They found weak associations between clinicians' ratings of criteria and the clinicians' diagnoses, suggesting that giving a diagnosis does not necessarily involve an objective formula based on the presence or absence or the total number of certain criteria. Morey and Ochoa (1989) found that clinicians overdiagnose antisocial personality disorder in men and borderline personality disorder in women; and Blashfield and Herkov (1996) replicated these findings for overdiagnosis. The absence of sex bias for specific criteria in contrast to the presence of sex bias in assigning *DSM*-based labels suggests that dimensional approaches to diagnosis may be less prone to bias than categorical labels, as judgments in the dimensional approach remain at the level of behavioral indicators rather than a summary diagnostic decision.

Crosby and Sprock (2004) further explored the influence of patient sex on under- and overdiagnosing antisocial personality disorder. They provided clinical psychologists with two cases, one meeting minimum criteria for APD, the other used as a distracter. Participants received female cases, male cases, or sex-unspecified cases. Clinicians rated symptoms and diagnoses. Most cases were accurately diagnosed as APD. Female cases were significantly more likely than male cases to receive a diagnosis of borderline personality disorder. When ratings for representativeness of the personality disorders were made, female cases received much higher ratings than male cases for both BPD and HPD. When symptoms, rather than diagnoses, were rated, however, there was a sex-of-patient difference only for histrionic symptoms, and contrary to the results for diagnosis, these symptoms were rated higher for men. When diagnoses for male and female cases were compared with the sex-unspecified case, there were no significant differences for the male case. Female cases, however, were underdiagnosed for APD, and overdiagnosed for BPD.

Another effort to understand the influence of gender on diagnoses of personality disorders had clinicians read one sentence at a time in cases with antisocial, histrionic or mixed criteria (Flanagan & Blashfield, 2005). In general, the findings confirmed previous research showing that clinicians are more likely to apply HPD to women and APD to men, although gender did not affect diagnoses (inaccurate in these cases) of narcissistic or borderline personality disorder. The staged presentation of diagnostic information also demonstrated that clinicians use gender as a context for understanding symptoms. Clinicians tended not to make "gendered" diagnoses in response to background information but only when diagnostic criteria were presented.

A great deal has been written about the overdiagnosis of schizophrenia in African Americans and the underdiagnosis of affective disorders (Adembimpe, 1981; Baker & Bell, 1999; Simon, Fleiss, Gurland, Stiller, & Sharpe, 1973). Neighbors, Trierweiler, Ford, and Muroff (2003) cite numerous studies that have found higher rates of schizophrenia in African Americans and mood disorders in whites. In a study of race disparities in emergency rooms, Kunen, Neiderhauser, Smith, Morris, and Marx (2005) found that, although the observed rate of psychiatric diagnoses (5.27%) was substantially lower than the national prevalence rate (20–28%), African-American patients were particularly likely to be undiagnosed. Anxiety and depression were more likely to be diagnosed for white than for African-American patients and, even though whites were more likely to be diagnosed as psychotic, African Americans were more likely than whites to be diagnosed for schizophrenia. Although differences in prevalence do not necessarily indicate bias, Garb (1997) concluded that bias exists. In a major epidemiological study, no racial differences in prevalence rates for psychotic disorders were reported (Robins & Regier, 1991); researchers used structured interviews in community samples to establish, as objectively as possible, actual rates of psychological disorders.

Unlike research on gender bias, which has relied on analogue studies, most studies supporting racial bias have compared diagnoses by hospital or clinic staff with diagnoses from research investigators using chart reviews or structured interviews (e.g., Mukherjee, Shukla, Woodle, Rosen, & Olarte, 1983; Pavkov, Lewis, & Lyons, 1989; Simon et al., 1973). In an early study, Simon et al. (1973) compared diagnoses made by hospital staff with diagnoses made by researchers using structured interviews. For clinical diagnoses, race (African American vs. white) was a significant factor. African-American patients received more schizophrenia diagnoses and fewer affective disorder diagnoses; but with research diagnoses there were no racial differences. Neighbors et al. (1999) found the agreement between hospital and research diagnoses to be low for both African-American and white patients, but the higher rates of schizophrenia diagnoses for African Americans and of mood disorders for whites remained even with research diagnoses. Nevertheless, racial discrepancies were smaller in the more structured assessment (using a DSM-III checklist) than in the less structured assessment. In a subsequent study using research interviewers, Neighbors et al. (2003) found the same race differences in schizophrenia (African American higher) and bipolar disorder (whites higher), but no differences in major depression or schizoaffective disorder. There were no SES differences between patient groups. In this study they also measured ratings of symptoms and relations between symptoms and diagnoses. Similar profiles were used for diagnosing bipolar disorder, although white patients received higher ratings for hypertalkativeness which may have led to their higher rate of bipolar diagnosis. But for schizophrenia, more symptoms led to the diagnosis for African Americans than for whites, and of particular interest, inappropriate affect, although equally observed in the two groups, was considered an indicator of schizophrenia for African Americans but not whites (Neighbors et al., 2003).

Examining diagnoses of psychotic patients discharged from a state psychiatric hospital, Strakowski, Shelton, and Kolbrener (1993) found more diagnoses of schizophrenia, especially the paranoid subtype, and fewer diagnoses of affective disorders for African-American patients than for white patients. Similarly, in a psychiatric emergency clinic, Strakowski et al. (1995) found more diagnoses for schizophrenia, particularly for African-American men. Focusing on patients with research diagnoses of bipolar disorder or schizoaffective disorder, bipolar-type, with current psychotic mania, Strakowski, McElroy, Keck, and West (1996) found that, adjusting for other sociodemographic variables, African-American patients were significantly more likely than white patients to have received a *clinical* diagnosis of a nonaffective psychosis. They also found that African-American patients were more likely to receive high ratings for first-rank symptoms, such as auditory hallucinations. In another study, using patients recruited for the *DSM-IV* Field Trials for Schizophrenia and Other Psychotic Disorders, they found that African-American patients demonstrated more severe psychotic symptoms, especially first-rank symptoms (i.e., hallucinations, delusions, disordered thinking). There were no differences in rates or severity of affective symptoms (Strakowksi, Flaum, et al., 1996).

In a more recent study, differences in the occurrence of first-rank symptoms were confirmed by Arnold et al. (2004) who used transcripts of audiotapes from structured diagnostic interviews with all cues to ethnicity removed to evaluate the presence of first-rank symptoms and the diagnosis of schizophrenia. In this study, however, they found that the African-American men were more likely than other groups (African-American women and white men and women) to be rated as having first-rank symptoms and greater psychopathology by both raters with and without information about race. There were not, however, differences based on race in diagnoses of schizophrenia; but men were significantly more likely to be diagnosed with schizophrenia and less likely to be diagnosed with depression. The fact that no race differences occurred for diagnoses of schizophrenia, mania, or depression is perhaps due to the use of structured interviews by clinicians with extensive training. The presence of an interaction between race and gender, similar to the one found by Strakowski et al. (1995), reminds us of the importance of intersectionality in understanding psychological disorder.

In summary these studies indicate that less structured assessments (in many cases, clinical assessment) of patients tend to result in higher rates of schizophrenia diagnoses in African Americans compared to whites, whereas more structured (or research) diagnoses show fewer differences. These studies suggest that clinicians may have a bias toward labeling African Americans as schizophrenic. On the other hand, structured assessments and transcripts with race removed (Arnold et al., 2004) suggest that African Americans, especially men, may present with different, perhaps more severe symptoms. The possibility of sociocultural differences in presentation of mental disorder must always be considered.

An exception to the absence of analogue studies to explore racial bias in diagnosis and the exclusive focus on gender in most analogue studies is the work of Kales et al. (2005) and Loring and Powell (1988). Kales et al. (2005) used video vignettes of elderly African-American and white women and men describing symptoms that met criteria for major depression but also included cognitive problems, alcohol use, and paranoid thoughts. The vignettes were viewed by primary care physicians. In this well-controlled study neither gender nor race nor the interaction affected diagnosis or treatment recommendations. These physicians were generally accurate in their diagnoses: 70 to 80% of cases were diagnosed with major depression. They were even more likely to recommend antidepressants as the first-line treatment, 82 to 90%, although interestingly they were unlikely to refer the patient to a psychiatrist or other mental health professional, 9 to 19.5%. The only variables that affected diagnosis were the physician characteristics of being trained at a non-U.S. medical school or being nonwhite. These two variables were highly related to one another and predicted being significantly less likely to make a diagnosis of depression. It is possible that the cultural distance (being foreign or foreign-born) led to less accuracy in diagnosis.

Using written vignettes that included both personality disordered (dependent) and psychotic (undifferentiated schizophrenia) symptoms in the cases to be diagnosed, Loring and Powell (1988) manipulated race (African American vs. white) and gender as demographic characteristics of the case. Cases with no information about ethnicity or sex were also included. Finally, they examined gender and race of the diagnosing psychiatrists as influences on the diagnostic process. They found that modal diagnoses were most accurate in cases *without* information on gender and ethnicity. When this information was introduced, complex patterns of interaction between characteristics of the case and characteristics of the diagnosing psychiatrist occurred. Generally, similarity in race and gender between clinician and client produced the most accurate diagnoses. However, male clinicians overdiagnosed depression in women and histrionic personality disorder in white women; and both male and female clinicians overdiagnosed paranoid schizophrenia and paranoid personality disorder in African-American men. This study reinforces the conclusion that the intersection of race and gender has a powerful influence on diagnosis.

Loring and Powell (1988) suggest that clinicians are more accurate in their diagnosis when the gender and race of the case are the same as those of the clinician. An exception was diagnosis of white female client by white female clinicians that suggested favoring of a less severe diagnosis. Although a full exploration of the interaction of clinician characteristics with patient characteristics is beyond the scope of this chapter, Garb (1997) presents further evidence that clinicians may see less pathology in similar others and more pathology in dissimilar others. For example, Li-Repac (1980) found that white clinicians compared to Chinese-American clinicians gave more negative ratings on depression and interpersonal variables to Chinese-American clients and Chinese-American clinicians rated white clients as having more severe psychopathology. Tseng, McDermott, Ogino, and Ebata (1982) found that American psychiatrists' ratings of Japanese fathers were more negative than Japanese psychiatrists' ratings. A possible source of bias in diagnosis is the actor–observer effect (Jones & Nisbett, 1987) by which we are more likely to explain our own behavior, or the behavior of those with whom we can identify, in terms of situational factors, but the behavior of others in terms of inner causes, such as a psychological disorder (Poland & Caplan, 2005). This may lead clinicians to overpathologize others, perhaps especially those whose sociocultural context is difficult for the clinician to understand; but it can also lead to underdiagnosing similar others.

These studies indicate that clinicians do use sex and race of client as information that affects their judgment about the diagnosis of a case. Some diagnoses are more prone to this bias than others. Although analogue studies allow the researcher to present clinicians with identical information while varying characteristics of the client, the responses of clinicians to paper-and-pencil or even audio or video versions of a patient, cannot completely capture the more interactive process that actually occurs during diagnosis, a process which may be even more susceptible to bias. On the other hand, evidence also suggests that the use of structured interviews can diminish the effects of bias.

Bias in the application of criteria is a reality in the practice of mental health care. Furthermore, to the degree that accurate diagnosis leads to more effective treatment of disorders, biases that lead to inaccurate diagnoses are particularly troublesome.

BIASED SAMPLING The most convenient data for analysis of prevalence rates are data obtained in clinical settings. When individuals come into a clinical setting either of their own volition or as a result of the actions of others (e.g., parent, courts), they generally receive a diagnosis. Assuming diagnoses are accurately obtained, these data would appear to be a good source of information. But do all individuals with a particular disorder show up in a clinical setting? Factors bringing adults into a clinical setting include willingness to acknowledge the symptoms, willingness to seek treatment, or the persuasive or coercive influence of others. Factors bringing children into a clinical setting include parents' and teachers' perceptions of the severity of the problem and of the possibilities for treatment. These factors are likely to be influenced by the gender, race, and class of the affected individual. Women may be more likely to recognize and less resistant to acknowledging that symptoms are indicative of an emotional problem that needs treatment (Yoder, Shute, & Tryban, 1990). Nonwhites are less likely to have access to mental health care, in part due to lack of health insurance, and less likely to use specialized care, often seeking help, when it is sought, from primary care services (USDHHS, 2001). Arnold et al. (2004) suggest that one reason first rank symptoms of schizophrenia may be more pronounced in African-American men is that they have delayed seeking mental health treatment. To the extent that rates of psychological disorder seen in clinical populations are the result of differences in help seeking, problem recognition, tolerance/intolerance for symptoms by self or others or attitude toward mental health care, then differences in prevalence rates in clinical settings will reflect these differences and not just "true" differences in the occurrence of the psychological disorder.

The solution to this dilemma is epidemiological studies with community samples. In these studies, interviewers contact individuals in representative samples and acquire information about symptoms. Diagnosis is accomplished independently of the participants' acknowledgment or concern about the disorder. Whereas differences in clinical populations reflect differences in the psychological disorders plus differences in various nondisordered behaviors such as help seeking, differences in community samples will not have this problem. For numerous disorders, *DSM-IV-TR* (2000) cites discrepancies in community vs. clinical samples or suggests that clinical data may over- or underrepresent different groups due to disorder-specific factors that encourage or discourage treatment seeking. For example, trichotillomania (compulsive hair pulling) is seen more often in women in clinical settings, but women may be more inclined to seek treatment for such an appearance-altering problem. More men than women seek help for gambling, but female gamblers may feel stigmatized and unwilling to seek treatment (Hartung & Widiger, 1998). Ideally, every disorder would have an adequate and current base of epidemiological data from community samples. This is not the case, and often statements about differences in prevalence rates are based on potentially biased clinical samples.

The Role of Gender, Race, and Class in Treatment

While concerns about gender bias have focused on *DSM* criteria as well as bias in application of criteria and sampling, concerns about racial bias have largely focused on questions of how criteria are applied; how racial stereotypes affect diagnosis; how sampling affects outcomes (i.e., are ethnic minorities more disturbed by the time they reach the clinic or hospital); and how culture or subculture affects the presentation of symptoms in clinical settings. It is unlikely that bias has been completely removed from the diagnostic process and it is critical to remember that diagnosis does influence treatment. But independent of diagnosis, is there evidence that gender, race, and class influence the treatment process and treatment outcomes? As with research on diagnosis, most studies of psychotherapeutic process and outcome have treated gender, race, and class as discrete, rather than intersecting, variables. Furthermore in order to thoroughly examine the impact of gender, race, and class on treatment outcomes, we should consider the characteristics of the therapist, the type of therapy, the therapy setting, the type of problem, and even the question of access to any therapy at all.

The question of access, whether individuals from different groups have equal opportunities to seek and receive psychotherapeutic treatment, has been the focus of much research on ethnic minorities or persons with low incomes. In general, the majority of individuals identified through epidemiological studies as having psychological disorders do not receive care for these disorders (USDHHS, 1999). Low income and minority status, however, are additional barriers to receiving mental health care (Cooper-Patrick et al. 1999; USDHHS, 2001). Furthermore, among the poor, lack of access to transportation or inflexible work schedules, can also work against using mental health resources even when they are available through public mental health services—for example, Armistead et al. (2004) increased retention in a community intervention program by providing childcare and transportation. Because publicly funded programs, such as Medicaid, are intended to provide mental health care for the uninsured, the connection between medical insurance and access to care is complicated. For example, racial disparities in use of publicly supported services are generally small but data from the National Medical Expenditure Survey (NMES) revealed that African Americans with private insurance are less likely than whites to use mental health care (Snowden & Thomas, 2000).

Large epidemiological data sets have made it possible to track mental health need (based on diagnostic interviews of study participants) and patterns of care received. Wang, Berglund et al. (2005) found that within a one-year period only 41% of those identified with a psychological diagnosis received any care, most from a general medical provider, but those with treatment from mental health specialties received more visits and more adequate care. Unmet need was greatest for those with low incomes and without insurance and for minorities, the elderly, and rural residents. Controlling for mental health need, they found that several sociodemographic characteristics predicted the use of different mental health care modalities. Women were more likely than men to use general medical services only but less likely to use a psychiatrist only as their source of care; Hispanics were less likely than whites to use psychiatry only; and Hispanics and African Americans were more likely than whites to use human services only. Level of education was positively related to use of psychiatry, other mental health specialties, and human services, but negatively related to general medical only. In these data, family income was not a significant predictor of source of care. For individuals with depressive symptoms as their main reason for a medical visit, Pingitore, Snowden, Sansone, and Klinkman (2001) reported that men, African Americans, other persons of color, and those over 65 were more likely to seek care from a primary care physician, whereas women, whites, and individuals between 45 and 64 years were more likely to visit a psychiatrist. The level of care provided by primary care physicians was significantly less that the care provided by a psychiatrist. Alegría et al. (2002) found that Hispanics, compared to whites, with low SES and African Americans, compared to whites, with higher SES were less likely to use specialty care for mental health problems. Other studies confirm that Hispanics (Cabassa, Zayas,

& Hansen, 2006) and African Americans (Cooper-Patrick et al., 1999; Snowden & Pingitore, 2003) are more likely to receive mental health care from a general medical setting than from a mental health specialist. Richardson, Anderson, Flaherty, and Bell (2003) examined treatment for African Americans and whites who received a primary diagnosis of major depression in outpatient clinics (both medical and mental health). They found that African Americans were more likely than whites to receive psychotherapy from substance abuse clinics, but whites were more likely than African Americans to receive psychotherapy from primary care and specialty mental health clinics. In addition, Kung (2003) found that about 15% of Chinese Americans (in Los Angeles) received mental health specialty care, a figure even lower than that reported for other minority groups. Similarly, Wells, Klap, Koike, and Sherbourne (2001) found that among those with perceived need for treatment of alcoholism, drug abuse, or mental health disorders, African Americans and Hispanics were more likely to report unmet needs and were less likely to be in active treatment. Additionally, Hispanics, compared to whites, reported significantly more delays in treatment and less satisfaction in all components of health care. Using the National Comorbidity Survey Replication, Wang, Berglund et al. (2005) concluded that sociodemographic characteristics that predicted delays in treatment included being male, poorly educated, a member of a racial minority, or married.

Wang, Berglund, and Kessler (2000) found no ethnic or racial differences in access to treatment but they did find that being African American and not having insurance predicted not receiving evidence-based care. Young, Klap, Sherbourne, and Wells (2001) also found that African Americans and Hispanics suffering from anxiety or depression were less likely than whites to receive care congruent with established guidelines. Cabassa et al. (2006) reviewed 16 articles based on seven epidemiological studies and concluded that Hispanic adults compared to non-Hispanic whites both underutilize mental health services and are less likely to receive guideline congruent care.

Examining clinical characteristics and mental health service use patterns of whites, African Americans, Hispanic, and Asians in low and high poverty communities, Chow, Jaffee, and Snowden (2003) found that socioeconomic status does moderate the relationship between ethnicity and service access and use. In high poverty areas, Hispanics and Asians were more likely than whites to use emergency services and whites were more likely to receive a diagnosis of schizophrenia, perhaps reflecting the downward social mobility of poorly functioning whites. In low poverty areas, African Americans and Hispanics were more likely than whites to be referred into mental health services by law enforcement, perhaps reflecting the fact that deviant behavior by minorities in low poverty neighborhoods is more likely to be attended to and constrained. Results were complex but clearly indicate that paths to mental health care differ by both ethnicity and the economic status of one's community.

Kuno and Rothbard (2005) examined not quality of care for the individual, but quality of care provided by community mental health centers (CMHCs) in neighborhoods with different income and racial profiles. Using quality indicators, such as use of atypical antipsychotic prescriptions and intensive case management, they found that CMHCs in high income, white areas had higher quality of care than CMHCs in low income, African-American neighborhoods. This suggests that even when mental health care is available it may not be of similar quality.

It is worth noting that several of these studies, which have explored in some detail the interplay of ethnicity, income, insurance, and need on access to care, nevertheless do not include gender in their studies. When gender is analyzed the results tend to support the general finding that women are more likely to seek mental health care than men. Cabassa et al. (2006), in their review of epidemiological studies of Hispanic adults, found that several studies, but not all, reported that women, after controlling for other factors, were more likely than men to use mental health services, either from mental health professionals or general medical practices. Kung (2003) reported that in their Chinese-American sample, women were significantly more likely than men to seek mental health care. In a large sample of mixed ethnicity, Wang, Berglund et al. (2005) found that women were more likely than men to receive mental health care from general medical services but less likely than men to use psychiatry only. Men are more likely than women to show delays in making treatment contact for disorders (Wang, Lane et al., 2005). These studies support the general consensus that women are more likely than men to seek psychological treatment (Petry, Tennen, & Affleck, 2000).

Beyond issues of access and general quality of care, we also want to know if gender, race, and class affect the type of care delivered and perhaps most importantly the outcomes of treatment. The complexity of the question is revealed if we list some of the other treatment-relevant variables that we might also want to consider: Sociodemographic characteristics of the therapist, type of therapy, length of therapy, type of problem being treated. Many studies do not have the methodological controls that allow for random assignment of clients to therapists and therapists to clients, making therapist or client characteristics nonexperimental variables. In these cases the possibility that unmeasured variables account for the outcomes must always be kept in mind.

Influence of the Client on Therapy Outcomes

In reviewing the impact of client variables on psychotherapy outcomes, Clarkin and Levy (2004) cite studies showing that higher SES is related to staying longer in psychotherapy and that higher levels of education are related to longer treatment for substance abuse programs, although they also found studies in which SES was not related to remaining in treatment. Wierzbicki and Pekarik (1993), in a meta-analysis of psychotherapy drop out, found that race (minority status), low level of education, and low SES all significantly predicted dropping out of therapy. Reis and Brown (1999), in their review of three decades of research on the unilateral terminator (i.e., a "client who terminates treatment before the clinician believes the client is ready," p. 123), conclude that SES is a reliable predictor of unilateral termination and that despite some nonsignificant results, nonwhite clients are also more likely to terminate unilaterally. In a study of individual therapy in a substance abuse clinic, researchers found that being female and African American were independent predictors of early treatment drop out (King & Canada, 2004).

Although the focus of research on race and class has mostly been on access to therapy, quality of therapy, and use of therapy (e.g., staying in or dropping out), some research has also examined the effect of client characteristics on therapeutic outcomes. Clarkin and Levy (2004) conclude that neither race nor gender appear to have much impact on therapy outcome. On the other hand, a review by Lam and Sue (2001), while finding that "improvement in therapy is independent of client gender" (p. 480), reports equal numbers of studies that find no difference in outcomes for African Americans compared to whites and studies that find that African Americans do worse in therapy. They also reference a study that found that American-Indian youth did not benefit as much from substance abuse treatment as whites (Query, 1985). But they conclude that outcomes for Asian Americans and Hispanics may be similar to those of whites. Rosenheck, Fontana, and Cottrol (1995) found that African-American veterans in treatment for posttraumatic stress disorder (PTSD) were more likely to drop out but also less likely to benefit from therapy than white veterans. Despite general conclusions of no sex-of-client effects on therapeutic outcomes, some studies suggest otherwise. Recent studies of substance abuse (Galen, Brower, Gillespie, & Zuker, 2000; Kosten, Gawin, Kosten, & Rounsaville, 1993) and substance abuse plus PTSD (Triffleman, 2001) have found greater severity of disorder for women, compared to men, at the beginning of treatment, but equal levels of functioning at the end of treatment, suggesting that women made greater gains during therapy than did men. Ogrodniczuk, Piper, and Joyce (2004) looked at outcomes of short-term group therapy for depression and complicated grief. Women were found to benefit more from this therapy, but they were also found to be more committed to the therapy groups and to be perceived by other group members as more compatible.

Issues about women's special needs in substance abuse treatment have been discussed (Wilke, 1994). Treatments included in the studies reviewed above were all outpatient programs. Many interventions for substance abuse or addiction rely, however, on inpatient treatment. Some women may be unable to participate in inpatient treatment or need to terminate treatment prematurely because of childcare issues; although the extent of this problem is not known, some women in need of inpatient treatment may be the sole caregiver for their children (Wilke, 1994). Questions have also been raised about differences in the effectiveness of single-sex and mixed-sex treatment groups. Dahlgren and Willander (1989) found that women in a single-sex group reported better social adjustment and lower alcohol consumption at a two-year follow-up than did women in a mixed-sex group.

Client–Therapist Matching

Many studies have examined client–therapist matching in terms of race or gender on the assumption that greater understanding or credibility will occur when therapist and client share these critical social statuses. The review of client variables by Petry, Tennen, and Affleck (2000) reports mixed results from studies of matching for race. Some find that clients stay in treatment longer, others that there is no effect on retention or outcomes. In their review, Lam and Sue (2001) find evidence that matching for African Americans is related to number of sessions (Rosenheck et al., 1995) but not to outcomes; and that matching for Asian Americans and Hispanics is related to less drop out and more therapy (e.g., Gamst, Dana, Der-Karabetian, & Kramer, 2001; Sue, Fujino, Hu, Takeuchi, & Zane, 1991). In subsequent studies, Gamst et al. (Gamst, Aguilar-Kitibutr, et al., 2003; Gamst, Dana, Der-Karabetian, & Kramer, 2004) again found no advantage for ethnic matching for African-American children and adolescents, but greater client satisfaction and better child outcomes for ethnically matched Asian Americans. Sterling, Gottheil, Weinstein, and Serota (2001) found no effects for either race or sex matching in terms of retention or outcome in a study of substance abuse treatment for African-American cocaine-dependent clients. In a general review of the relationship between ethnic match and termination, Maramba and Hall (2002) concluded that while ethnic similarity reduces rates of treatment drop out and increases the length of time in treatment, the effects are small and do not improve clinical outcome.

In a study that examined the outcomes from an empirically based treatment, multisystemic therapy (MST), for youth with antisocial behavior, caregiver–ethnic similarity did matter (Halliday-Boykins, Schoenwald, & Letourneau, 2005). The very large sample was diverse and assignment to therapist was to next available. The analyses revealed that "when caregivers are ethnically matched with therapists, youths demonstrate greater decreases in symptoms, stay in treatment longer, and are more likely to be discharged for meeting treatment goals" (p. 814). This effect was partly mediated by therapists' greater adherence to the MST protocol in ethnically matched cases.

A diverse sample of children and adolescents seen in outpatient services in mental health facilities also found that race and language matching matter (Hall, Guterman, Lee, & Little, 2002). Ethnic match, but not gender match, was related to lower dropout rates for Asian-American, Mexican-American, and African-American children. Language match predicted only for Mexican Americans. Ethnic match predicted more treatment sessions for Mexican Americans and Asian Americans; and language and gender match were additional predictors for Mexican Americans.

Gender matching has also been a focus of research. Jones and Zoppel (1982) obtained self-reports from clients and therapists regarding the results of therapy. They found that female clients paired with female therapists were perceived by both clients and therapists as having experienced the most positive outcomes, suggesting that sex matching made the difference. But other research fails to support benefits from gender matching. Zlotnick, Elkin, and Shea (1998) took advantage of an exceptional opportunity to investigate sex-of-therapist effects in a well-controlled study, the National Institute of Mental Health Treatment of Depression Collaborative Research Program (TDCRP). In this research all clients were experiencing major depression and were assigned randomly to different treatment conditions, but also to either a female or male therapist. Attrition, treatment outcome (based on the

Hamilton Rating Scale for Depression), and client-reported therapist empathy were assessed. Analyses revealed that "among depressed patients, a male or female therapist, or same- versus opposite-gender pairing, was not significantly related to level of depression at termination, to attrition rates, or to the patient's perceptions of the therapist's degree of empathy early in treatment and at termination" (Zlotnick et al., 1998, p. 657). Clients' beliefs about whether a female or male therapist would be more helpful were also assessed prior to therapy, but these beliefs had no impact on outcomes, whether they were assigned to the person they believed would be more helpful or not. Similarly, in a study of clients randomly assigned to one of three cognitive–behavioral treatment conditions for panic disorder, neither gender of the therapist nor gender match had an effect on therapy outcomes (Huppert et al., 2001).

Sue, Zane, and their colleagues, who have written extensively on ethnicity and psychotherapy, have argued that the advantages of ethnic matching, when they occur, probably accrue from similarities in problem perception, coping orientation, and goals for treatment (Zane et al., 2005). In a sample of Asian-American and white outpatients they assessed client and therapist for these factors independently and prospectively and found that "treatment-goals match was predictive of session effect and comfort. Coping-orientation match was predictive of less dysphoria after four sessions of treatment.... [S]imilarities...in perceived distress associated with the problem appeared to result in higher psychosocial functioning at the end of the fourth session" (p. 582). This important study suggests mechanisms by which matching may affect outcomes.

Currently, the emphasis in psychological treatment is on empirically supported treatments (see Stewart & Chambless, chapter 7). An assumption may be that once a treatment has been found to be effective in the research sample we can assume it will be effective universally, but data suggest that this is an assumption that is not being empirically tested. Weisz, Doss, and Hawley (2005) identified 236 studies of randomized trials testing 386 treatments for children and adolescents. They report that "60% of all the articles failed to include any report on the race or ethnicity of their samples, and more than 70% failed to provide any information on family income or socioeconomic status" (p. 348). Numbers that were reported indicated that while African-American youth are generally represented in these samples, other minorities are not. Finally, samples of minority youth are generally too small to adequately test the effectiveness for these groups in comparison to whites. A major review of treatments for depression failed to address the question of effects for gender, race, or class at all, except to acknowledge that since women are prone to depression in the childbearing years, the relative success of psychotherapy without medication is encouraging (Hollon, Thase, & Markowitz, 2002). The research of Halliday-Boykins et al. (2005), however, showing that ethnic matching in MST therapy improves outcomes, is an important antidote to the assumption that gender, race, and class will not matter once we have established ESTs.

Gender, Race, and Class and Pharmacotherapy

In previous decades, the exclusion of women and minorities from clinical trials led to a lack of information about the differential responses of women and minorities to psychopharmacological treatment. In 1994 the federal government issued "NIH Guidelines on the Inclusion of Women and Minorities as Subjects in Clinical Research," including both biomedical and behavioral research.

Evidence suggests that African Americans are both more likely and less likely than whites to receive drug therapy. In a study of visits to primary care providers, Lasser, Himmelstein, Woolhandler, McCormick, and Bor (2002) found that African Americans were less likely to receive antidepressant, antianxiety, or any drug therapy and similar results were found for visits to psychiatrists, except there African-American clients were also less likely to receive antipsychotic prescriptions. Similarly, Snowden and Pingitore (2003) found that visits to a primary care physician with a mental health concern led to less pharmacotherapy for African Americans than whites. On the other hand, in a sample of clients with a primary diagnosis of major depression for whom drug treatments were provided only by specialty mental health clinics, African Americans were more likely than whites to receive pharmacotherapy.

Results have also indicated that African Americans may be less likely to receive the current standard of care. Kuno and Rothbard (2002) found that African Americans treated for schizophrenia were significantly less likely than whites, even when controlling for funding and service types, to be prescribed nontraditional, second-generation antipsychotics. Similarly, Herbeck et al. (2004) found that African-American men, adjusting for clinical, SES, and health-system characteristics, were significantly less likely to receive these drugs and more likely to receive medications that have a greater risk of producing tardive dyskinesia and extrapyramidal side effects. Garb (2005), reviewing research regarding clinical treatment decision making, found that adherence with recommended treatment for schizophrenia was poor and that African-American clients often received "excessively high dosages of antipsychotic medicine, and [were] less likely to be on atypical psychotics" (p. 82).

There are also documented racial differences in attitudes toward psychiatric medication. Schnittker (2003) found that African Americans report less willingness to use psychiatric medications or to give them to children in their care. These attitudes about pharmacotherapy are predicted by beliefs about efficacy and side effects and are not related to SES, knowledge, religiosity, or medical mistrust.

Women are more likely than men to be prescribed psychotropic drugs, even after controlling for other demographics, health status, SES, and diagnosis (Simoni-Wastila, 2000). But this may reflect women's mental health care-seeking behaviors, because Garb's review (1997) of numerous studies using case vignettes did not find gender effects on recommendations for use of psychotropic medications.

Sex and ethnicity may also affect responses to drug treatment. Differences may include absorption, distribution, metabolism, and elimination, all of which affect the bioavailability of the therapeutic substance. Women, for example, tend to have more fat tissue than men, which affects the metabolism and storage of drugs. Women's endogenous (e.g., menstrual cycle, pregnancy, postpartum, menopause) and exogenous hormone levels (e.g., birth control pills, hormone replacement therapy) also affect drug response (Yonkers & Hamilton, 1995). Estrogens, for example, tend to increase the effectiveness of some antipsychotic drugs (Seeman, 1995), meaning that women may be treated with lower doses; but they may also experience more side effects or toxicity from doses that are safe in men (Yonkers & Hamilton, 1995). Estrogen affects metabolic processes and drug response and estrogen has been tried with mixed to positive results, alone and combined with antidepressants, in treatment for women with refractory depression and for postmenopausal women (Casper, 1998; Kornstein, 1997). Research on the effectiveness of antidepressant medication, however, suggests that women respond more poorly than men to tricyclics and better than men to selective serotonin reuptake inhibitors (SSRIs) and monoamine oxidase inhibitors (Kornstein, 1997). On the other hand, female schizophrenics respond better and more rapidly to pharmacological treatment and require lower doses than men in both acute episodes (Szymanski, Lieberman, Alvir, & Mayerhoff, 1995) and ongoing treatment (Tamminga, 1997). Women are also more likely than men to be exposed to more than one psychoactive drug due to a greater incidence of comorbidity and so drug interaction effects must be considered (Casper, 1998).

There is growing interest in ethnopsychopharmacology (Baker & Bell, 1999; Lin & Smith, 2000; Snowden, 2001). Baker and Bell (1999) cite studies that suggest that African Americans, compared to whites, may have reduced responsiveness to beta blockers and are more likely to be nonresponders to fluoxetine, but may respond better and more rapidly to tricyclic antidepressants and to certain benzodiazepines and to need less lithium to control manic symptoms. The presence of sickle cell anemia in some African Americans may also complicate pharmacotherapy. Ethnic differences in therapeutic levels of lithium, clozapine, and antidepressants have been reported as well as differences between Asian Americans and whites to haloperidol (Lin & Smith, 2000).

Finally, psychological disorders, especially depression, frequently occur in women between the ages of 20 and 45, years when women are likely to bear children. The effects of psychopharmacological agents on maternal health, the health of the developing fetus, and lactation must be understood. To date research suggests that benzodiazepines (antianxiety drugs) lead to craniofacial abnormalities and, when taken in late pregnancy, "floppy infant" syndrome; lithium (used in treating bipolar disorder) has been associated with cardiovascular, central nervous system, and mental and physical abnormalities; antidepressant medications have shown no adverse effects in some investigations, but small increased risks of miscarriage or deformities in others; antipsychotics have yielded mixed outcomes (Casper, 1998). Clearly research clarifying the effects of medication during various stages of pregnancy and during lactation is critical.

Possible Exceptions to No Effects for Sex of Client or Therapist

Although most studies have found that sex of client and sex of therapist have relatively little impact on the outcome of psychotherapy, there are particular circumstances in which differences may occur. Liddle (1996) examined therapist sex and sexual orientation as predictors of gay and lesbian clients' reports of therapist practices. She found that gay or bisexual male therapists and gay, bisexual, or heterosexual female therapists were rated as equally helpful but as more helpful than heterosexual male therapists. The fact that men generally have less positive attitudes toward homosexuality than women may help explain why heterosexual male therapists were perceived as least helpful (Liddle, 1996). The therapist's attitude toward client sexual orientation may be a better predictor of outcome than sex or sexual orientation per se.

Certain deleterious effects of psychotherapy are also more likely to occur in some sex-of-thera-pist-sex-of-client combinations. For example, data suggest that sexual relationships occur between therapist and client in 5 to 6% of therapy relationships with 85% of these involving a male therapist with a female client (Lamb & Catanzaro, 1998). This particular negative therapeutic experience is clearly more likely to affect women.

Understanding Gender, Race, and Class

Chang (2003) presents two basic research perspectives for understanding racial (and we would add, gender) differences in mental health and mental health care. The first approach seeks to discover and describe the common factors that predict sociodemographic differences, such as discrimination, poverty, low social status. The second approach assumes that each group is embedded in a complex and unique set of historical, social, and cultural factors and that even when common factors are identified, each group may respond differently to them. This approach requires a group-specific approach.

Common factors that affect women and minorities are discrimination and poverty. A series of studies by Landrine, Klonoff, and colleagues have found that sexist discrimination accounted for more variance in depressive and somatic symptoms than life event or daily hassles (Landrine, Klonoff, Gibbs, Manning & Lund, 1995) and that recent and lifetime sex discrimination accounted for the difference between women and men in depressive, anxious, and somatic symptoms (Klonoff, Landrine, & Campbell, 2000). For African Americans, experiences of racial discrimination are related to low self-esteem, depression, anxiety, and stress-related somatic symptoms (Landrine & Klonoff, 1996, Klonoff, Landrine, & Ullman, 1999). Perceived racial discrimination predicted psychological distress in Hispanic women (Salgado de Snyder, 1987). In a study of urban adolescents in mental health treatment, Surko, Ciro, Blackwood, Nembhard, and Peake (2005) found that perceived racism was associated with exposure to risks, such as violence, sexual abuse and assault, drug use, and to worry about self and others. Racial minorities and women are also more likely than nonminorities and men to live in poverty or have fewer economic resources. Poverty and low income are well established correlates of depression (Belle & Doucet, 2003).

Other research, however, suggests that such elements as belief systems, values, and coping strategies will vary by gender, race, and culture (Brown, Abe-Kim, & Barrio, 2003). Sue and Chu (2003) suggest that "rather than developing broad theories to explain the mental health of ethnic minority groups, it may be wiser to begin an inductive process in which separate ethnic groups are studied and examined before construction of a more general theory" (p. 461).

In this era of evidence-based practice, an equally important debate concerns the universality vs. specificity of treatment effectiveness. Miranda, Nakamura, and Bernal (2003) argue that although evidence-based treatments have generally been developed and tested on white, middle-class samples, they are likely to be effective for minorities as well. They acknowledge that these therapies should continue to be studied to determine what cultural, social, or environmental conditions affect the quality or acceptability of these treatments. Sue and Zane (2006) disagree with this argument. They criticize the lack of attention paid to ethnic and cultural minorities in the research on evidence-based interventions and call for not only more research that is inclusive but also research aimed at explaining the effects of cultural variables. Assuming that interventions can and should be adapted for diverse populations, Muñoz and Mendelson (2005) describe the development and evaluation of prevention and treatment manuals created for low-income minority populations. They used five principles in developing these manuals: (1) including members of the target group in developing the manual; (2) incorporating relevant cultural values; (3) using religion and spirituality when appropriate; (4) dealing with the stress of acculturation (for those adapting to a new culture); and (5) acknowledging the reality of racism, prejudice, and discrimination. Empirical evaluations of the effectiveness of these manuals were positive (Muñoz & Mendelson, 2005).

Cultural Competence

No review of the research literature can completely capture the complexities of gender, race, and class. Indeed to improve diagnosis and treatment of individual clients we might focus less on the client and more on the therapist. Strategies for developing individual and cultural competence in therapists are critical. The American Psychological Association's *Guidelines on Multicultural Education, Training, Research, Practice, and Organizational Change for Psychologists* presents six guidelines for enhancing cultural competence: (1) being aware of one's own attitudes and beliefs that can be detrimental in interacting with others who are different; (2) recognizing the importance of multicultural sensitivity, knowledge, and understanding; (3) employing the constructs of multiculturalism and diversity in educating others; (4) recognizing the importance of conducting culture-centered and ethical research with diverse participants; (5) applying culturally appropriate skill in clinical and applied settings; (6) supporting culturally informed policy development and practices. Sanchez-Hucles and Jones (2007) have reviewed each of these guidelines through the lens of gender. Daniel, Roysircar, Abeles, and Boyd (2004) review research on four elements of cultural competence: self-awareness of attitudes, biases, and assumptions; knowledge about diversity; understanding of gender's interaction with other statuses; and the reality of multiple identities for all individuals. They discuss how these can be incorporated into graduate education and training of clinical psychologists.

Conclusions

This chapter has reviewed the research literature on gender, race, and class as they affect diagnosis and treatment of psychological disorders. Evidence shows that certain diagnoses (schizophrenia in the case of African Americans, histrionic and, perhaps, borderline personality disorders in the case of women, antisocial personality disorder in the case of men) are more likely to be given to some clients. Research on access to mental health care has produced complex findings on the effects of gender, race, and class on use of different services for mental health treatment. Whereas a match between gender of therapist and client may matter in certain situations, there is substantial evidence that matching for race/ethnicity can matter. Research on quality and type of treatment and on pharmacotherapy suggests inequities in treatment and a need for better information about the connections between individual characteristics (including gender and race) and effectiveness of and reactions to psychotropic medications. In an era of establishing and promoting empirically supported treatments, we need to be mindful of the population being treated and we need to ask: Do therapies work equally well with different groups and can psychological interventions be improved by culturally based adaptations? Finally, we need to consider how best to seek greater understanding of the role of gender, race, and class on psychopathology and psychotherapy and we need to continue to focus on developing cultural competence in clinicians.

Despite the title of this chapter, "The Role of Gender, Race, and Class in Psychopathology," the preceding review of research makes it abundantly clear that there are very few studies that actually meet the challenge of considering gender, race, and class. Even where all of these sociodemographic variables are assessed, they are often analyzed as individual factors or possibly two-way interactions and the possibilities of higher order interactions are not pursued. Our discipline's attachment to quantitative, linear, main effect approaches to data may account for this. Research that takes context into account, such as Chow et al.'s (2003) examination of mental health service use by diverse populations in low and high poverty communities and Kuno and Rothbard's study of quality of care at CMHCs in neighborhoods that vary by income and racial composition, demonstrate the value of doing more than collecting individual reports on sociodemographic variables. Snowden and Yamada (2005) acknowledge that we do not yet understand disparities in mental health care. They call for "more studies of treatment—seeking pathways that favor nonspecialty sources of assistance, improve trust and treatment receptiveness, eliminate stigma, and accommodate culturally distinctive beliefs about mental illness and mental health and styles of expressing mental health-related suffering" (pp. 160–161). Mullings and Schulz (2006) suggest that a better understanding of intersectionality may require a more qualitative approach. This view is supported by Lopez (2003) who argues that reporting of quantitative differences among groups may serve to further marginalize minority groups without helping us to understand them. Without qualitative/ethnographic research we may be unable to contextualize and interpret the data.

Mullings and Schulz (2006) point out that "it is often difficult to pinpoint how the interaction, articulation, and simultaneity of race, class, and gender affect women and men in their daily lives, and the ways in which these forms of inequality interact in specific situations to condition health" (p. 6). She suggests that gender, race, and class should be viewed as social relationships rather than as characteristics of individuals. Building on this theme, Martin (2006) criticizes the supplement to the surgeon general's report and its assumption that

> there is something concrete and real in the world (and increasingly in the brain) that corresponds one to one with the major psychiatric diagnosis. Identifying this real thing…is the proper first step in getting [patients] the proper treatment. Identifying observer bias and removing it will clear the way to more frequently correct diagnosis. But there are…troubling aspects of this view. First, what if the categories into which psychiatry divides disorders themselves already have cultural assumptions embedded in them, not fixed for all time…? Second, what if our only route to the real is always through linguistic categories that are necessarily saturated with culturally constituted sets of meanings? (p. 85)

These closing remarks remind us that gender, race, and class are more than sociodemographic characteristics. They constitute essential aspects of the lived experience of individuals who may come to us as clinicians in need of understanding and assistance.

References

Adebimpe, V. (1981). Overview: White norms and psychiatric diagnosis of Black patients. *American Journal of Psychiatry, 138,* 279–285.

Adler, D., Drake, R., & Teague, G. (1990). Clinicians' practices in personality assessment: Does gender influence the use of DAM-III Axis II? *Comprehensive Psychiatry, 31,* 125–133.

Alarcón, R. D. Alegría, M., Bell, C. C., Boyce, C. Kirmayer, L. J., Lin, K-M., et al. (2002). Beyond the funhouse mirrors: Research agenda on culture and psychiatric diagnosis. In D. J. Kupfer, M. B. First, & D. A. Regier (Eds.), *A research agenda for DSM-V™* (pp. 219–266). Washington, D.C.: American Psychiatric Association.

Alegría, M., Canino, G., Ríos, R. Vera, M., Calderón, J., Rusch, D., et al. (2002). Mental health care for Latinos: Inequalities in use of specialty mental health services among Latinos, African Americans, and non-Latino Whites. *Psychiatric Services, 53,* 1547–1555.

Allen-Burge, R., Storandt, M., Kinscherf, D. A., & Rubin, E. H. (1994). Sex differences in the sensitivity of two self-report depression scales in older depressed inpatients. *Psychology and Aging, 9,* 443–445.

American Psychiatric Association. (1980). *Diagnostic and statistical manual of mental disorders* (3rd ed.). Washington, D.C.: Author.

American Psychiatric Association. (1987). *Diagnostic and statistical manual of mental disorders* (3rd ed., rev.). Washington, D.C.: Author.

American Psychiatric Association. (1994). *Diagnostic and statistical manual of mental disorders* (4th ed.). Washington, D.C.: Author.

American Psychiatric Association. (2000). *Diagnostic and statistical manual of mental disorders* (4th ed., Text Rev.). Washington, D.C.: Author.

American Psychological Association. (1990). *Guidelines for providers of psychological services to ethnic, linguistic, and culturally diverse populations.* Washington, D.C.: Author.

American Psychological Association. (2002). *Guidelines on multicultural education, training, research, practice, and organizational change for psychologists.* Washington, D.C.: Author.

American Psychological Association. (2006). *Guidelines for psychological practice with girls and women.* Washington, DC: Author.

Anthony, M. M., & Rowa, K. (2005). Evidence-based assessment of anxiety disorders. *Psychological Assessment, 17,* 256–266.

Armistead, L. P., Clark, J., Barber, C. N., Dorsey, S., Hughley, J., & Favors, M. (2004). Participant retention in the Parents Matter! program: Strategies and outcome. *Journal of Child and Family Studies, 13,* 67–80.

Arnold, L. M., Keck, P. E., Collins, J., Wilson, R., Fleck, D. E., Corey, K. B., et al. (2004). Ethnicity and first-rank symptoms in patients with psychosis. *Schizophrenia Bulletin, 67,* 207–212.

Baker, F. M., & Bell, C. C. (1999). Issues in the psychiatric treatment of African Americans. *Psychiatric Services, 50,* 362–368.

Becker, D., & Lamb, S. (1994). Sex bias in the diagnosis of borderline personality disorder and posttraumatic stress disorder. *Professional Psychology: Research and Practice, 25,* 55–61.

Belle, D., & Doucet, J. (2003). Poverty, inequality, and discrimination as sources of depression among U.S. women. *Psychology of Women Quarterly, 27,* 101–113.

Bishaw, A., & Iceland, J. (2003). *Poverty: 1999: Census 2000 Brief.* Washington, D.C.: U.S. Department of Commerce.

Blashfield, R. K., & Herkov, M. J. (1996). Investigating clinician adherence to diagnosis by criteria: A replication of Morey and Ochoa (1989). *Journal of Personality Disorders, 10,* 219–228.

Brown, C., Abe-Kim, J. S., & Barrio, C. (2003). Depression in ethnically diverse women: Implications for treatment in primary care settings. *Professional Psychology: Research and Practice, 34,* 10–19.

Brown, L. S. (1992). A feminist critique of personality disorders. In L. S. Brown & M. Ballou (Eds.), *Personality and psychopathology. Feminist reappraisals* (pp. 206–228). New York: Guilford.

Cabassa, L. J., Zayas, L. H., & Hansen, M. C. (2006). Latino adults' access to mental health care: A review of epidemiological studies. *Administration and Policy in Mental Health and Mental Health Services Research, 33,* 316–330.

Caplan, P. J. (1991). How do they decide who is normal? The bizarre, but true, tale of the DSM process. *Canadian Psychology, 32,* 162–170.

Caplan, P. J. (1995). *They say you're crazy: How the world's most powerful psychiatrists decide who's normal.* Reading, MA: Addison-Wesley.

Caplan, P. J., & Cosgrove, L. (Eds.). (2004). *Bias in psychiatric diagnosis.* Lanham, MD: Jason Aronson.

Casper, R. (1998). The psychopharmacology of women. In R. C. Casper (Ed.), *Women's health: Hormones, emotions and behavior* (pp. 192–218). Cambridge: Cambridge University Press.

Chang, D. F. (2003). An introduction to the politics of science: Culture, race, ethnicity, and the supplement to the Surgeon General's Report on Mental Health. *Culture, Medicine and Psychiatry, 27,* 373–383.

Chavez, D. F. (2003). Commentary. *Culture, Medicine and Psychiatry, 27,* 391–393.

Chow, J. C., Jaffee, K., & Snowden, L. (2003). Racial/ethnic disparities in the use of mental health services in poverty areas. *American Journal of Public Health, 93,* 792–797.

Clarkin, J. F., & Levy, K. N. (2004). The influence of client variables on psychotherapy. In M. J. Lambert (Ed.), *Bergin and Garfield's handbook of psychotherapy and behavior change* (5th ed., pp. 194–226). Hoboken, NJ: John Wiley.

Cooper-Patrick, L., Gallo, J. J., Powe, N. R., Steinwachs, D. M., Eaton, W. W., & Ford, D. E. (1999). Mental health service utilization by African Americans and Whites: Baltimore Epidemiologic Catchment Area follow-up. *Medical Care, 37,* 1034–1045.

Council of National Psychological Associations for the Advancement of Ethnic Minority Interests (2003). *Psychological treatment of ethnic minority populations.* Washington, D.C.: Association of Black Psychologists.

Crosby, J. P., & Sprock, J. (2004) Effect of patient sex, clinician sex, and sex role on the diagnosis of antisocial personality disorder: Models of underpathologizing and overpathologizing biases. *Journal of Clinical Psychology, 60*, 583–604.

Dahlgren, L., & Willander, A. (1989). Are special treatment facilities for female alcoholics needed? A controlled 2-year follow-up study from a specialized female unit (EWA) versus a missed male–female treatment facility. *Alcoholism: Clinical and Experimental Research, 13*, 499–504.

Daniel, J. H., Roysircar, G., Abeles, N., & Boyd, C. (2004). Individual and cultural-diversity competency: Focus on the therapist. *Journal of Clinical Psychology, 60*, 755–770.

Fernbach, B. E., Winstead, B. A., & Derlega, V. J. (1989). Sex differences in diagnosis and treatment recommendations for antisocial personality and somatization disorders. *Journal of Social and Clinical Psychology, 8*, 238–255.

Flanagan, E. H., & Blashfield, R. K. (2005). Gender acts as a context for interpreting diagnostic criteria. *Journal of Clinical Psychology, 61*, 1485–1498.

Ford, M., & Widiger, T. A. (1989). Sex bias in the diagnosis of histrionic and antisocial personality disorders. *Journal of Consulting and Clinical Psychology, 57*, 301–305.

Gaines, A. D. (1992). From DSM-I to DSM-III-R: Voices of self, mastery, and the other: A cultural constructivist reading of U.S. psychiatric classification. *Social Science and Medicine, 35*, 3–24.

Galen, L. W., Brower, K. J., Gillespie, B. W., & Zucker, R. A. (2000). Sociopathy, gender, and treatment outcome among outpatient substance abusers. *Drug & Alcohol Dependence, 61*, 23–33.

Gamst, G., Aguilar-Kitibutr, Herdina, A., Hibbs, S., Krishtal, E. Lee, R., et al. (2003). Effects of racial match on Asian American mental health consumer satisfaction, *Mental Health Services Research, 5*, 197–208.

Gamst, G., Dana, R. H., Der-Karabetian, A., & Kramer, T. (2001). Asian American mental health centers: Effects of ethnic match and age on global assessment and visitation. *Journal of Mental Health Counseling, 23*, 57–71.

Gamst, G., Dana, R. H., Der-Karabetian, A., & Kramer, T. (2004). Ethnic match and treatment outcomes for child and adolescent mental health center clients. *Journal of Counseling and Development, 82*, 457–465.

Garb, H. N. (2005). Clinical judgment and decision making. *Annual Review of Clinical Psychology, 1*, 67–89.

Garb, H. N. (1997). Race bias, social class bias, and gender bias in clinical judgment. *Clinical Psychology: Science and Practice, 4*, 99–120.

Giardina, E. G. (2000). Heart disease in women. *International Journal of Fertility and Women's Medicine, 45*, 350–357.

Hall, J., Guterman, D. K., Lee, H. B., & Little, S. G. (2002). Counselor–client matching on ethnicity, gender, and language: Implications for counseling school-aged children. *North American Journal of Psychology, 4*, 367–380.

Halliday-Boykins, C. A., Schoenwald, S. K., & Letourneau, E. J. (2005). Caregiver–therapist ethnic similarity predicts youth outcomes from an empirically based treatment. *Journal of Consulting and Clinical Psychology, 73*, 808–818.

Hartung, C. A., & Widiger, T. A. (1998) Gender differences in the diagnosis of mental disorders: Conclusions and controversies of the DSM-IV. *Psychological Bulletin, 123*, 260–278.

Herbeck, D. M., West, J. C., Ruditis, I., Farifteh, R. D., Fitek, D. J., Bell, C. C., et al. (2004). Variations in use of second-generation antipsychotic medication by race among adult psychiatric patients. *Psychiatric Services, 55*, 677–684.

Hollon, S. D., Thase, M. E., Markowitz, J. C. (2002). Treatment and prevention of depression. *Psychological Science in the Public Interest, 3*, 39–77.

Huppert, J. D., Bufka, L. F., Barlow, D. H., Gorman, J. M., Shear, M. D., Woods, S. W. (2001). Therapists, therapist variables, and cognitive-behavioral therapy outcome in a multicenter trial for panic disorder. *Journal of Consulting and Clinical Psychology, 69*, 747–755.

Hunsley, J., & Mash, E. J. (2005) Introduction to the special section on developing guidelines for the evidence-based assessment (EBA) of adult disorders. *Psychological Assessment, 17*, 251–255.

Joiner, T. E., Jr., Walker, R. L., Pettit, J. W., Perez, M., & Cukrowicz, K. C. (2005). Evidence-based assessment of depression in adults. *Psychological Assessment, 17*, 267–277.

Jones, E. E., Krupnick, J. L., & Kerig, P. K. (1987). Some gender effects in brief psychotherapy. *Psychotherapy, 24*, 336–352.

Jones, E. E., & Nisbett, R. E. (1987). The actor and the observer: Divergent perceptions of the causes of behavior. In E. E. Jones, D. E. Kanouse, H. H. Kelley, R. E. Nisbett, & S. Valins (Eds.), *Attribution: Perceiving the causes of behavior* (pp. 79–94). Hillsdale, NJ: Lawrence Erlbaum.

Jones, E. E., & Zoppel, C. L. (1982). Impact of client and therapist gender on psychotherapy process and outcome. *Journal of Consulting and Clinical Psychology, 50*, 259–272.

Kales, H. C., Neighbors, H. W., Valenstein, M., Blow, F. C., McCarthy, J. F., Ignacio, R. V., Taylor, K. K., Gillon, L., & Mellow, A. M. (2005). *Journal of the American Geriatric Society, 53*, 777–784,

Kaplan, M. (1983). A woman's view of DSM-III. *American Psychologist, 38*, 786–792.

King, A. C., & Canada, S. A. (2004). Client-related predictors of early treatment drop-out in a substance abuse clinic exclusively employing individual therapy. *Journal of Substance Abuse Treatment, 26*, 189–195.

Klonoff, E. A., Landrine, H., & Campbell, R. (2000). Sexist discrimination may account for well-known gender differences in psychiatric symptoms. *Psychology of Women Quarterly, 24*, 93–99.

Klonoff, E. A., Landrine, H., & Ulllman, J. M. (1999). Racial discrimination and psychiatric symptoms among Blacks. *Cultural Diversity & Ethnic Minority Psychology, 5*, 329–339.

Korman, M. (1974). National conference on levels and patterns of professional training in psychology: Major themes. *American Psychologist, 29*, 441–449.

Kornstein, S.G. (1997). Gender differences in depression: Implications for treatment, *Journal of Clinical Psychiatry, 58* (Suppl. 15), 12–18.

Kosten, T. A., Gawin, F. H., Kosten, T. R., & Rounsaville, B. J. (1993). Gender differences in cocaine use and treatment response. *Journal of Substance Abuse Treatment, 10*, 63–66.

Kunen, S., Neiderhauser, R., Smith, P. O., Morris, J. A., & Marx, B. D. (2005). Race disparities in psychiatric rates in emergency departments. *Journal of Consulting and Clinical Psychology, 73*, 116–126.

Kung, W. W. (2003). Chinese Americans' help seeking for emotional distress. *Social Service Review, 77*, 110–158.

Kuno, E., & Rothbard, A. B. (2005). The effect of income and race on quality of psychiatric care in community mental health centers. *Community Mental Health Journal, 41*, 613–622.

Kuno, E., & Rothbard, A. B. (2002). Racial disparities in antipsychotic prescription patterns for patients with schizophrenia. *American Journal of Psychiatry, 159*, 567–572.

Lam, A. G., & Sue, S. (2001). Client diversity. *Psychotherapy, 38*, 479–486.

Lamb, D. H., & Catanzaro, S. J. (1998). Sexual and nonsexual boundary violations involving psychologists, clients, supervisees, and students: Implication for professional practice. *Professional Psychology: Research and Practice, 29*, 498–503.

Landrine, H., & Klonoff, E. A. (1996). The schedule of racist events: A measure of racial discrimination and a study of its negative physical and mental health consequences. *Journal of Black Psychology, 22*, 144–168.

Landrine, H., Klonoff, E. A., Gibbs, J., Manning, V., & Lund, M. (1995). Physical and psychiatric correlates of gender discrimination: An application of the schedule of sexist events. *Psychology of Women Quarterly, 19*, 473–492.

Lasser, K. E., Himmelstein, D. U., Woolhandler, S. J., McCormick, D., & Bor, D. H. (2002). Do minorities in the United States receive fewer mental health services than whites? *International Journal of Health Services, 32*, 567–578.

Leinhardt, G., Seewald, A. M., & Zigmond, N. (1982). Sex and race difference in learning disabilities classrooms. *Journal of Educational Psychology, 74*, 835–843.

Liddle, B. J. (1996).Therapist sexual orientation, gender, and counseling practices as they related to ratings of helpfulness by gay and lesbian clients. *Journal of Counseling Psychology, 43*, 394–402.

Lindsay, K. A., Sankis, L. M., & Widiger, T. A. (2000). Gender bias in self-report personality disorder inventories. *Journal of Personality Disorders, 14*, 218–232.

Lindsay, K. A., & Widiger, T. A. (1995). Sex and gender bias in self-report personality disorder inventories: Items analyses of the MCMI-II, MMPI, and PDQ-R. *Journal of Personality Assessment, 65*, 1–20.

Lin, K.M., & Smith, M.W. (2000). Psychopharmacotherapy in the context of culture and ethnicity. In P. Ruiz (Ed.), *Ethnicity and Psychopharmacology* (pp. 1–27). Washington, D.C.: American Psychiatric Association.

Li-Repac, D. (1980). Cultural influences on clinical perception: A comparison between Caucasian and Chinese-American therapists. *Journal of Cross-Cultural Psychology, 11*, 327–342.

Lopez, S. (1989). Patient variable biases in clinical judgment. *Psychological Bulletin, 106*, 184–203.

Lopez, S. (2003). Reflections on the surgeon general's report on mental health, culture, race, and ethnicity. *Culture, Medicine and Psychiatry, 27*, 419–434.

Loring, M., & Powell, B. (1988). Gender, race and DSM-III: A study of the objectivity of psychiatric diagnostic behavior. *Journal of Health and Social Behavior, 29*, 1–22.

Luebnitz, R. R., Randolph, D. L., & Gutsch, K. W. (1982). Race and socioeconomic status as confounding variables in the accurate diagnosis of alcoholism. *Journal of Clinical Psychology, 38*, 665–669.

Maddux, J. E. (2002). Stopping the "madness": Positive psychology and the deconstruction of the illness ideology and the *DSM*. In C. R. Snyder & S. J. Lopez (Eds.), *Handbook of positive psychology* (pp. 13–25). New York: Oxford,

Maramba, G. G., & Hall, G. C. N. (2002). Meta-analyses of ethnic match as a predictor of dropout, utilization, and level of functioning. *Cultural Diversity & Ethnic Minority Psychology, 8*, 290–297.

Martin, E. (2006). Moods and representations of social inequality. In A. Schulz & L. Mullings (Eds.), *Gender, race, class, and health* (pp. 60–88). San Francisco, CA: Jossey-Bass,.

Miranda, M., Nakamura, R., & Bernal, G. (2003). Including ethnic minorities in mental health intervention research: A Practical Approach to a long-standing problem. *Culture, Medicine and Psychiatry, 27*, 467–486.

Morey, L.C., & Ochoa, E. (1989). An investigation of adherence to diagnostic criteria: Clinical diagnosis of the DSM-III personality disorders. *Journal of Personality Disorders, 3*, 180–192.

Mukherjee, S., Shukla, S., Woodle, J., Rosen, A. M., & Olarte, S. (1983). Misdiagnosis of schizophrenia in bipolar patients: A multiethnic comparison. *American Journal of Psychiatry, 140*, 1571–1574.

Mullings, L., & Schulz, A. (2006). Intersectionality and health: An introduction. In A. Schulz & L. Mullings (Eds.), *Gender, race, class, & health* (pp. 3–17). San Francisco, CA: Jossey-Bass.

Muñoz, R. F., & Mendelson, T. (2005). Toward evidence-based interventions for diverse populations: The San Francisco General Hospital prevention and treatment manuals. *Journal of Consulting and Clinical Psychology, 73*, 790–799.

Neighbors, H. W., Trierweiler, S. J., Ford, B. C., & Muroff, J. R. (2003). Racial differences in DSM diagnosis using a semi-structured instrument: The importance of clinical judgment in the diagnosis of African Americans. *Journal of Health and Social Behavior, 43*, 237–256.

Neighbors, H. W., Trierweiler, S. J., Munday, C., Thompson, E. E., Jackson, J. S., Binion, V. J., et al. (1999). Psychiatric diagnosis of African Americans: Diagnostic divergence in clinican structured and semistructured interviewing conditions. *Journal of the National Medical Association, 91*, 601–612.

Ogrodniczuk, J. S., Piper, W. E., & Joyce, A. S. (2004). Differences in men's and women's responses to short-term group psychotherapy. *Psychotherapy Research, 14*, 231–243.

Page, S., & Bennesch, S. (1993). Gender and reporting differences in measures of depression. *Canadian Journal of Behavioural Science, 25*, 579–589.

Pantony, K. L., & Caplan, P. J. (1991). Delusional dominating personality disorder: A modest proposal for identifying some consequences of rigid masculine socialization. *Canadian Psychology, 32*, 120–133.

Pavkov, T. W., Lewis, D. A., & Lyons, J. S. (1989). Psychiatric diagnosis and ethnic bias: An empirical investigation. *Professional Psychology: Research and Practice, 20*, 364–368.

Petry, N. M., Tennen, H., & Affleck, G. (2000). Stalking the elusive client variable in psychotherapy research. In C. R. Snyder & R. E. Ingram (Eds.), *Handbook of psychological change* (pp. 88–108). Hoboken, NJ: John Wiley.

Pingitore, D., Snowden, L., Sansone, R. A., & Klinkman, M. (2001). Persons with depressive symptoms and the treatments they receive: A comparison of primary care physicians and psychiatrists. *International Journal of Psychiatry in Medicine, 31,* 41–60.

Poland, J., & Caplan, P. J. (2004). The deep structure of bias in psychiatric diagnosis. In P. J. Caplan & L. Cosgrove (Eds.), *Bias in psychiatric diagnosis* (pp. 9–23). Lanham, MD: Jason Aronson.

Potts, M. K., Burnam, M. A., & Wells, K. B. (1991). Gender differences in depression detection: A comparison of clinician diagnosis and standardized assessment. *Psychological Assessment, 3,* 609–615.

Pryzgoda, J., & Chrisler, J. C. (2000). Definitions of gender and sex: The subtleties of meaning. *Sex Roles, 43,* 553–569.

Query, J. N. (1985). Comparative admission and follow-up study of American Indians and Whites in a youth chemical dependency unit on the North Central Plains. *International Journal of the Addictions, 20,* 489–502.

Reis, B. F., & Brown, L. G. (1999). Reducing psychotherapy dropouts: Maximizing perspective convergence in the psychotherapy dyad. *Psychotherapy, 36,* 123–136.

Richardson, J., Anderson, R., Flaherty, J., & Bell, C. (2003). The quality of mental health care for African Americans. *Culture, Medicine and Psychiatry, 27,* 487–498.

Robins, E., & Guze, S. B. (1970). Establishment of diagnostic validity of psychiatric illness: Its application to schizophrenia. *American Journal of Psychiatry, 126,* 983–986.

Robins, L. N., & Regier, D. A. (1991). *Psychiatric disorders in America: The epidemiologic catchment area study.* New York: Free Press.

Rosenheck, R., Fontana, A., & Cottrol, C. (1995). Effect of clinician–veteran racial pairing in the treatment of post-traumatic stress disorder. *American Journal of Psychiatry, 152,* 555–563.

Ross, R., Frances, A. J., & Widiger, T. A. (1995). Gender issues in DSM-IV. In J. M. Oldham & M. B. Riba (Eds.), *Review of psychiatry* (Vol. 14, pp. 205–226). Washington, D.C.: American Psychiatric Press.

Salgado de Snyder, V. (1987). Factors associated with acculturative stress and depressive symptomatology among married Mexican immigrant women. *Psychology of Women Quarterly, 11,* 475–488.

Sanchez-Hucles, J., & Jones, N. (2007). Gender issues in applying the mutilcultural guidelines to populations of color in the United States.

Schnittker, J. (2003). Misgivings of medicine: African Americans' skepticism of psychiatric medication. *Journal of Health and Social Behavior, 44,* 506–524.

Seeman, M. V. (1995). Gender differences in treatment response in schizophrenia. In M. V. Seeman (Ed.), *Gender and psychopathology.* Washington, D.C.: American Psychiatric Press.

Simon, R. J., Fleiss, J. L., Gurland, B. J., Stiller, P. R., & Sharpe, L. (1973). Depression and schizophrenia in hospitalized Black and White mental patients. *Archives of General Psychiatry, 28,* 509–512.

Simoni-Wastila, L. (2000). The use of abusable prescription drugs: The role of gender. *Journal of Women's Health and Gender-Based Medicine, 9,* 289–297.

Snowden, L. R. (1999). African American service use for mental health problems. *Journal of Community Psychology, 27,* 303–313.

Snowden, L. R. (2001). Barriers to effective mental health services for African Americans. *Mental Health Services Research, 3,* 181–187.

Snowden, L. R., & Pingitore, D. (2003). Frequency and scope of mental health service delivery to African Americans in primary care. *Mental Health Services Research, 4,* 123–130.

Snowden, L. R., & Thomas, K. (2000). Medicaid and African American outpatient mental health treatment. *Mental Health Services Research, 2,* 115–120.

Snowden, L. R., & Yamada, A-M. (2005). Cultural differences in access to care. *Annual Review of Clinical Psychology, 1,* 143–166.

Snyder, D. K., Heyman, R. E., Haynes, S. N. (2005). Evidence-based approaches to assessing couple distress. *Psychological Assessment, 17,* 288–307.

Sprock, J., & Yoder, C. Y. (1997). Women and depression: An update on the report of the APA task force. *Sex Roles, 36,* 269–303.

Sterling, R. C., Gottheil, E., Weinstein, S. P., & Serota, R. (2001). The effect of therapist/patient race- and sex-matching in individual treatment. *Addiction, 96,* 1015–1022.

Strakowski, S. M., Flaum, M., Amador, X., Bracha, H. S., Pandurangi, A. K., Robinson, D., et al. (1996). Racial differences in the diagnosis of psychosis. *Schizophrenia Bulletin, 21,* 117–124.

Strakowski, S. M., Lonczak, H. S., Sax, K. W., West, S. A., Crist, A., Mehta, R., et al. (1995). The effects of race on diagnosis and disposition from a psychiatric emergency service. *Journal of Clinical Psychiatry, 56,* 101–107.

Strakowski, S. M., McElroy, W. L., Keck, P. E., & West, S. A. (1996). Racial influence on diagnosis in psychotic mania. *Journal of Affective Disorders, 39,* 157–162.

Strakowski, S. M., Shelton, R. C., & Kolbrener (1993). The effects of race and comorbidity on clinical diagnosis in patients with psychosis. *Journal of Clinical Psychiatry, 54,* 96–102.

Sue, S., & Chu, J. Y. (2003). The mental health of ethnic minority groups: Challenges posed by the supplement to the Surgeon General's Report on Mental Health. *Culture, Medicine and Psychiatry, 27,* 447–465.

Sue, S., Fujino, D. C., & Hu, L. (1991). Community mental health services for ethnic minorities: A test of the cultural responsiveness hypothesis. *Journal of Consulting and Clinical Psychology, 59,* 533–540.

Sue, S., & Zane, N. (2006). How well do both evidence-based practices and treatment as usual satisfactorily address the various dimensions of diversity? In J. C. Norcorss, L. E. Beutler, & R. F. Levant (Eds.), *Evidence-based practices in mental health* (pp. 329–337). Washington, D.C.: American Psychological Association.

Surko, M., Ciro, D., Blackwood, C., Nembhard, M., & Peake, K. (2005). Experience of racism as a correlate of developmental and health outcomes among urban adolescent mental health clients. In K. Peake (Ed.), *Clinical and research uses of an adolescent mental health intake questionnaire: What kids need to talk about* (pp. 235–260). Binghamton, NY: Haworth Social Work Practice Press,.

Szymanski, S., Lieberman, J. A., Alvir, J. M., & Mayerhoff, D. (1995), Gender differences in onset of illness, treatment response, course and biologic indexes in first-episode schizophrenic patients, *American Journal of Psychiatry, 152,* 698–703.

Tamminga, C. A. (1997). Gender and schizophrenia, *Journal of Clinical Psychiatry, 58* (Suppl. 15), 33–37.

Thomas, K. C., & Snowden, L. R. (2001). Minority response to health insurance coverage for mental health services. *The Journal of Mental Health Policy and Economics, 4,* 35–41.

Triffleman, E. (2001) Gender differences in a controlled pilot study of psychosocial treatments in substance dependent patients with post-traumatic stress disorder: Design considerations and outcomes. *Alcoholism Treatment Quarterly, 18,* 113–126.

Tseng, W., McDermott, J. F., Ogino, D., & Ebata, K. (1982). Cross-cultural differences in parent-child assessment: U.S.A. and Japan. *International Journal of Social Psychiatry, 28,* 305–317.

U.S. Department of Health and Human Services (1999). *Mental health: A report of the surgeon general.* Rockville, MD: Public Health Service, Office of the Surgeon General.

U.S. Department of Health and Human Services (2001). *Mental health: Culture, race, and ethnicity—A supplement to mental health: A report of the surgeon general.* Rockville, MD: Public Health Service, Office of the Surgeon General.

U.S. Department of Health and Human Services (2005). *New freedom commission of mental health: Subcommittee on evidence-based practice.* Rockville, MD: U.S. Department of Health and Human Services.

Walker. L. E. A. (1994). Are personality disorders gender biased? In S. A. Kirk & S. D. Einbinder (Eds.), *Controversial issues in mental health* (pp. 22–29). New York: Allyn & Bacon.

Wang, P. S., Berglund, P., Olfson, M., Pincus, H. A., Wells, K. B., & Kessler, R. C. (2005). Failure and delay in initial treatment contact after first onset of mental disorders in the National Comorbidity Survey Replication. *Archives of General Psychiatry, 62,* 603–613.

Wang, P. S., Berglund, P., & Kessler, R. C. (2000). Recent care of common mental disorders in the United States. *Journal of General Internal Medicine, 15,* 284–292.

Wang, P. S., Lane, M., Olfson, M., Pincus, H. A., Wells, K. B., & Kessler, R. C. (2005). Twelve-month use of mental health services in the United States: Results from the National Comorbidity Survey Replication. *Archives of General Psychiatry, 62,* 629–640.

Warner, R. (1978). The diagnosis of antisocial and hysterical personality disorders. *Journal of Nervous and Mental Disease, 166,* 839–845.

Weisz, J. R., Doss, A. J., & Hawley, K. M. (2005). Youth psychotherapy outcome research: A review of critique of the evidence base. *Annual Review of Psychology, 56,* 337–363.

Wells, K., Klap, R., Koike, A., & Sherbourne, C. (2001). Disparities in unmet need for alcoholism, drug abuse, and mental health care. *American Journal of Psychiatry, 158,* 2027–2032.

Widiger, T. A. (1998). Invited essay: Sex biases in the diagnoses of personality disorders. *Journal of Personality Disorders, 12,* 95–118.

Widiger, T. A., & Samuel, D. B. (2005) Evidence-based assessment of personality disorders. *Psychological Assessment, 17,* 278–287.

Wierzbicki, M., & Pekarik, G. (1993). A meta-analysis of psychotherapy dropout. *Professional Psychology: Research and Practice, 24,* 190–195.

Wilke, D. (1994). Women and alcoholism: How a male-as-norm bias affects research, assessment, and treatment. *Health and Social Work, 19,* 29–35.

Williams, J. B. W., & Spitzer, R. L. (1983). The issue of sex bias in DSM-III. Critique of "A woman's view of DSM-III" by Marcie Kaplan. *American Psychologist, 38,* 793–798.

Yoder, C. Y., Shute, G. E., & Tryban, G. M. (1990). Community recognition of objective and subjective characteristics of depression. *American Journal of Community Psychology, 18,* 547–566.

Yonkers, K. A., & Hamilton, J. A. (1995). Psychotropic medications. In J. M. Oldham & M. B. Riba (Eds.), *Review of psychiatry* (Vol. 14). Washington, D.C.: American Psychiatric Press.

Young, A. S., Klap, R., Sherbourne, C. D., & Wells, K. B. (2001) The quality of care for depressive and anxiety disorders in the United States. *Archives of General Psychiatry, 58,* 55–61.

Zane, N., Sue, S., Chang, J., Huang, L., Huang, J., Lowe, S., et al. (2005). Beyond ethnic match: Effects of client–therapist cognitive match in problem perception, coping orientation, and therapy goals on treatment outcomes. *Journal of Community Psychology, 33,* 569–585.

Zlotnick, C., Elkin, I., & Shea, M.T. (1998). Does the gender of a patient or the gender of a therapist affect the treatment of patients with major depression? *Journal of Consulting and Clinical Psychology, 66,* 655–659.

4

Biological Bases of Psychopathology

Robert F. Smith

Behavior, including pathological behavior, has its origins in brain functioning. Many of our current treatments for pathological behavior are biological in nature; for example, we use drugs that alter neurotransmitter systems. Increasingly, noninvasive imaging techniques are used to study and diagnose brain abnormalities associated with some forms of psychopathology. Understanding psychopathology must ultimately include an understanding of its biological bases. This chapter will introduce some issues that are important in understanding the biology of psychopathology.

Introduction to Brain

The human brain is the most complex organ known to science, and this chapter cannot do justice to its complexity. We will attempt to just briefly introduce it to students who have never had a course in biological psychology. The bulk of the chapter, however, will focus on our evolving understanding of the role of the brain and related systems in psychopathology, including chemical underpinnings of disorders and developmental origins of those disorders.

Box 4.1 is a minitutorial on brain, including a drawing of some major regions of brain. It is intended to impart a minimal command of some important concepts and terminology; interested readers are referred to textbooks on biological psychology (Carlson, 2007; Meyer & Quenzer, 2005).

Box 4.2 summarizes just a few of the important neurotransmitters, and the concept of second messenger systems, involved in brain function and aspects of psychopathology. As this chapter will emphasize, this summary only reflects our current understanding of the role of particular neurotransmitters, and that understanding is certain to evolve as research reveals new information.

The brain is actually far more complex than these sketches indicate: as an indicator of its complexity, it probably consists of about 100 *billion* neurons, each with up to 10 *thousand* connections to other neurons; any given function or behavior typically involves thousands to millions of these neurons, usually in several different brain areas. Neurons interact in ways that influence other neurons— a simple perception such as an odor may be initially processed in the olfactory system, but a connection to another area of brain may also trigger a distant memory of an experience associated with that odor, and that area may then trigger emotions associated with the earlier experience.

Box 4.1 A Minitutorial on Brain Terminology

Neuron—A nerve cell. Neurons usually have distinctive projections from the cell body, which process information. Neurons also grow in normal development and in response to chemical stimulation by *neurotransmitters*, and produce large numbers of proteins involved in cell structure and information processing. A human brain has around 100 billion neurons.

Dendrite—A projection from a nerve cell that is specialized for receiving incoming signals from other neurons. Dendrites have large numbers of receptors for *neurotransmitters*.

Axon—A projection from a neuron that is specialized for sending signals, sometimes over very long distances—motor neurons in the spinal cord have axons that reach all the way to the toes. An electrical signal (*action potential*) reaching the end of an axon releases chemicals called *neurotransmitters*, which then chemically interact with receptors on dendrites of the next neurons, which may result in a signal in that neuron.

Action potential—An electrical signal conducted down an axon. Action potentials are biological signals that involve both chemicals (movement of ions, or charged particles of sodium and potassium), and the voltage shifts that accompany ion movement. A full review of it is beyond our scope here, but note that both chemical changes and electrical activity can influence signaling, as signaling involves both.

Synapse—The junction between axon and dendrite, where neurotransmitters transmit information between neurons. Interactions at the synapse are so complex that it is difficult to adequately express that complexity. Each neuron may have hundreds to thousands of synaptic inputs, and whether that neuron fires (has an *action potential*) depends on the sum of *excitatory* and *inhibitory* input from a large number of those inputs.

Neurotransmitters—The chemicals which convey information between neurons. This is not just like electrical action. Neurotransmitters may chemically *excite* the next neuron (making it more likely to conduct an electrical signal) or *inhibit* it (making it less likely), and thousands of excitatory and inhibitory synapses may interact on a given neuron. Neurotransmitters may act by opening or closing ion channels (thus altering the electrical charge of the neuron) and by activating chains of chemical events called second messenger systems, which may alter electrical activity, and also metabolic activity, protein synthesis, and gene expression. We think there are about 200 chemicals which serve as neurotransmitters, with just a few of them listed in Box 4.2.

Learning and memory—To the best of our current knowledge, learning consists of changes in synapses. Changes can include strengthening the connections at a pattern of synapses controlling a particular aspect of behavior, and even growing new synapses—even the adult brain is a very dynamic organism, and formation of new connections, breaking of old and less-used ones, and generation and loss of nerve cells seem to be common events. Most of these changes seem to involve the chemical sequences known as second messenger systems. Later in the chapter we'll discuss changes in the brain during development, which have similar mechanisms of change.

Our experiences rely on, and our behavior is a product of, shifting patterns of electrochemical activity wafting across loosely connected networks of neurons, influenced by current events yet also a product of past experiences, with some experiences having only transient effects, and others processed and repeated to the point where they become very persistent parts of us.

Box 4.2 Neurotransmitters and Behavior

Complex chemical processes are used to synthesize neurotransmitters and their *receptors*, which are also complex molecules. Drugs which alter neurotransmitters can act in a variety of ways. They can increase *synthesis* of a transmitter, increase its *release*, slow down its *chemical breakdown* so that it can act for a longer period of time, imitate it to *stimulate receptors*, or *block receptors* to block the transmitter action. Only a small fraction of the 200 or so chemicals thought to be transmitters have been connected to various forms of psychopathology. While the following list is oversimplified, here are some associations between a few transmitters and the functions and malfunctions they are thought to be involved in:

Dopamine—Part of the brain's reinforcement system. Involved in addictions (it's a critical transmitter for perceptions of pleasure), in schizophrenia (antipsychotic drugs block dopamine receptors), and in control of movement—it's the main transmitter associated with Parkinson's disease, which is accompanied by loss of many dopamine-producing cells.

Serotonin—First associated with sleep, now also thought to be involved in depression.

Glutamate—First associated with neural bases of learning, now also thought to be involved in growth and development processes (the processes of growing the brain and forming new connections during learning are fairly similar). Glutamate is a widespread neurotransmitter, and appears to be involved in many forms of learning, including simple associations and complex learning.

GABA—An acronym for gamma-aminobutyric acid, this transmitter inhibits or slows down firing of nerve cells. Antianxiety drugs act mainly to increase GABA activity.

Second messenger systems— Many neurotransmitters, not just the few listed above, act through second messenger systems. Typically, a neurotransmitter (the "first messenger") binds to a receptor, usually located on a dendrite. That receptor then activates an enzyme (the "second messenger") within the dendrite, and the enzyme then chemically changes the shape of one or several proteins within the dendrite. Those changed proteins may do several things, such as activate gene expression to stimulate changes such as growth or production of more receptors, change existing receptors (to make them more sensitive or less sensitive), open or close channels that permit passage of ions and thus directly affect the likelihood of an action potential, or enable a variety of other chemical events in the postsynaptic dendrite. Second messenger systems enable neurotransmitters to have a remarkable range of effects, not just to activate an action potential.

With such a staggering degree of complexity, it is hardly surprising that we don't yet fully understand the brain. Work is actively continuing on such topics as determining the transmitter bases of cue learning in drug addiction, the signals which lead to progressive loss of brain tissue in early-onset schizophrenia, gene expression abnormalities which produce brain malformations characteristic of autism, the transmitter basis of individual differences in aspects of personality such as temperament and sensation-seeking, and mechanisms underlying effects of prenatal drugs and chemicals on brain growth. Despite the complexity, however, research has already revealed much about aspects of brain which function abnormally in several types of psychopathology, and the neurotransmitter basis of some disorders and their drug therapies.

The brain also has more far-reaching effects than one might guess. The brain not only controls behavior, it also controls most hormones by controlling the pituitary gland, including hormones associated with sexual behavior, thyroid function, and reactions to stress (Carlson, 2007). Control of hormones is often influenced by psychological processes such as perceptions of stress and of the degree of personal control over stress, and, as we will see, by developmental events which influence the development of the stress response system. Through hormones and also through direct nerve connections, the brain also strongly influences the immune system (Wrona, 2006). Both hormones and immune signals can signal changes in brain, which has receptors for most or all hormones and immune signals, and they can influence brain activity, and hence behavior. Literally, the state of our health and hormonal systems can influence behavior, and our mental health can influence our hormones and our physical health, acting through now-established biological mechanisms. So, when a person suffering from a psychiatric disorder *also* has a depressed immune system or abnormal levels of stress hormones, the association of psychopathology with disorders of these other systems might go in either direction: pathology in brain function might cause disorders in other systems, *or* disorders in other systems can trigger psychopathology, as later chapters discuss for depression and schizophrenia. This interaction is an underlying mechanism behind the observation that some psychiatric disorders also result in higher levels of physical illness, and it is also the reason that a thorough physical exam is important for individuals with psychopathology: many a person has been prescribed antidepressant medication, while really suffering from a low thyroid hormone level. In general, treating the cause of a disorder is more effective than treating "something else."

Brain Abnormalities Associated with Psychopathology

In recent years, advances have been made in understanding and treating many psychological disorders, using biological techniques. The early, and often accidental, findings that some drugs alleviated some psychiatric symptoms led to development of modern psychotherapeutic drugs, and to the hypotheses of the 1950s and 1960s that many psychiatric disorders were results of "imbalances" in neurotransmitter systems. Early attempts to verify this through postmortem studies found a number of transmitter differences associated with particular disorders; for example, between individuals with schizophrenia and normal controls. We now regard problems associated with these early drug studies, such as a lapse of many hours between death and tissue preservation, sometimes coupled with sketchy diagnostic information, as very problematic for interpretation of the information obtained. In the 1990s, newly available noninvasive imaging technology largely confirmed, and considerably refined and extended, those early hypotheses, and continuing pharmaceutical development allowed us to refine, revise, and focus our hypotheses of the neurochemical bases of many disorders. What exactly do we know today about the neural bases of psychological disorders?

Inferences from Psychiatric Drug Effects

First, we know that we have fairly effective treatments for many disorders. Commonly used treatments for schizophrenia, depression, and anxiety are listed in Table 4.1. Several other disorders have recently been treated successfully with drugs in some individuals, including obsessive-compulsive disorder and some types of addiction. Generally (but see below), the drug treatments tend to be fairly effective, which is good news for professionals treating these disorders, and for their clients. How much information this gives us about each disorder's *cause*, however, varies between disorders. Why? Well, for some disorders, the mode of action of the drugs is rather well established. For schizophrenia, for example, it is well accepted that antipsychotic drugs are dopamine receptor blockers—their therapeutic effect is closely related to their effectiveness in reducing activity in the dopamine neurotransmitter system (Seeman, 1987). That does not, however, necessarily imply that schizophrenia "is" an overactivity in the dopamine system. Why? Treating a *symptom* effectively does not imply that one is treating a *cause* of the symptom. As examples, if you treat an infection-induced fever with aspirin instead of antibiotics, you can reduce the fever without getting rid of the infection. Early treatments for the motor disorder

Parkinson's disease, which is marked by tremor, postural and motor changes, and loss of brain dopamine neurons, included fairly effective use of drugs which block another transmitter, acetylcholine. More modern treatments increase levels of dopamine, but the early treatments had apparent effects by bringing an acetylcholine/dopamine *balance* closer to normal. Even dopamine-based treatments do not address the *cause*, which is a progressive loss of dopamine neurons due to one of several agents or processes which can kill them. So, finding that a drug alleviates a disorder does not necessarily tell us the actual cause of that disorder.

For other effective drugs, the mode of clinical action remains in dispute. For depression, several classes of drugs are listed in Table 4.1. Each of them has been found to alleviate depression in some people (but note that placebos are also effective in many people). None of them is universally effective, which implies that there may be several mechanisms which each cause some cases of depression. Each drug, however, has a number of direct and indirect effects on the brain, and determining which of those effects actually is the therapeutic mechanism has been difficult. There is some consensus, mostly based on improved effectiveness of the selective serotonin reuptake inhibitors (SSRIs) such as Prozac, that depression is a serotonin-based phenomenon, but that is not yet a universally accepted conclusion. Recent research suggests that antidepressants also stimulate neurogenesis, the formation of new neurons (Malberg, Eisch, Nestler, & Duman, 2000), and increase levels of a transmitter involved in neural and dendritic growth, called BDNF (Levinson, 2006; Molteni et al., 2006). When a drug has several chemical effects and also helps depression, it is difficult to determine which of those chemical effects results in the drug's antidepressant action.

Nor is it the case that any given drug for depression is universally effective. Pharmaceutical treatment of depression is largely a matter of conducting experiments on a client until one finds the best treatment. Family history (was there a depressed family member treated successfully with a drug?), particular symptoms, and research findings can inform that decision, but it is still an individual experiment. This frequent observation may imply that depression can have different underlying mechanisms in different individuals.

With these cautions in mind, we can make some statements about what drug therapies suggest about the causes of various disorders. It is moderately clear that effective therapies for schizophrenia reduce activity in the dopamine system, that drugs for anxiety stimulate GABA receptors, and that we don't know exactly what the basis for treatment for depression is. But a caution for the future remains: *what we now think about the underlying chemical bases of mental disorders may prove in the future to be in error.*

Table 4.1 Examples of drugs used for treating psychological disorders

Disorder	Drug action	Generic name	Trade name
Depression	MAO inhibition	Phenelzine	Nardil
	Tricyclic	Amytriptilene	Elavil
		Imipramine	Tofranil
		Desipramine	Elavil
	SSRI	Fluoxetine	Prozac
		Sertraline	Zoloft
		Paroxetine	Paxil
Anxiety disorders	GABA agonist	Diazepam	Valium
Schizophrenia	DA receptor blocker	Haloperidol	Haldol
		Chlorpromazine	Thorazine
		Thiroridazine	Mellaril
		Trifluoperazine	Stelazine
		Clozapine	Clozaril

Noninvasive Imaging Studies

In recent years, techniques for studying the chemistry and blood flow of a living brain have allowed us to study brain structure and activity in the live individual, and thus to compare brains in normal individuals to brains of individuals with specific disorders. Brain areas have long been linked to specific aspects of normal and pathological behavior, new techniques have emerged to largely confirm earlier research and considerably amplify our knowledge. Noninvasive techniques include magnetic resonance imaging (MRI) and its offspring fMRI (the former is like an enhanced X-ray in that it gives a static picture, the latter reflects dynamic changes over time, and both primarily look at blood flow to various brain areas), positron emission tomography (PET), which uses tiny amounts of radioactively labeled chemicals to identify locations of particular neurotransmitter receptors, and a variety of other techniques to spy on the chemistry, metabolism, and electrical activity of the brain (Otte & Halsband, 2006).

Studies using these techniques have largely confirmed some hypotheses about the neurochemical bases of some disorders. For example, D2 dopamine receptors are more numerous in several brain areas of many but not all schizophrenics evaluated (Huizink & Mulder, 2006; Wong et al., 1986), and dopamine release is elevated in many, but not all individuals with schizophrenia (Laruelle et al., 1996), which fits well with the inference from drug studies that schizophrenia might involve an overactivity of some aspect of the dopamine system. Schizophrenic individuals also have a well-documented underactivity of areas of prefrontal cortex, which seems to be related to attentional deficits (MacDonald & Carter, 2003). But the picture of the biological bases of schizophrenia is complicated by a number of apparent discrepancies between different individuals: some schizophrenics have elevated D2 dopamine receptors, while others do not; some have loss of brain tissue, but some do not; some respond to antipsychotic drugs, but some do not; some have acute onset in early adulthood, while some begin deteriorating in middle childhood. Further complicating the picture is that recent work has shown that severe early onset schizophrenia is accompanied by progressive loss of cortical tissue throughout adolescence—literally, children with schizophrenia progressively lose cortical tissue at a rate that far exceeds normal developmental changes (Thompson et al., 2001). While there is no real current consensus on the cause(s) of schizophrenia, it appears that it is a neurodevelopmental disorder in many cases (Rapoport, Addington, Frangou, & Psych, 2005; Rehn & Rees, 2005); that is, a genetic predisposition exacerbated by unknown developmental influences (prenatal viruses and stress are among the possible causes which have been suggested) leads to progressive maldevelopment of the brain. It is entirely possible that early onset and adult onset schizophrenia may represent different disorders with similar symptoms: they differ in degree of brain tissue loss, developmental timing, and responsiveness to drugs.

In recent years, the use of noninvasive imaging to study brains of individuals with various disorders has exploded, and any summary would be quickly out of date. But it is clear that brains of individuals with many kinds of disorders have various kinds of abnormalities of structure or function.

Dyslexic individuals have poorer activity in several brain regions [especially posterior occipital/temporal and parietal/temporal areas] associated with reading. (Shaywitz, Lyon, & Shaywitz, 2006)

Autistic children have malformed brains in a variety of areas, with overgrowth of anterior areas and undergrowth of posterior areas especially common. (Courchesne, Redcay, Morgan, & Kennedy, 2005)

Children with ADHD have less activity than normal children in frontal areas associated with response inhibition. (Booth et al., 2005; see also Konrad, Neufang, Hanisch, Fink, & Herpertz-Dahlmann, 2006; Turkeltaub, Gareau, Flowers, Zeffiro, & Eden, 2003)

Although the picture for depression is complicated, there is evidence that unipolar depression is associated with increased metabolic activity in amygdala and areas of prefrontal cortex, areas associated with emotional processing. (Drevets, 2001)

Few, if any, disorders have biological bases limited to a defined area of brain. That is, psychopathology typically involves several areas of brain, and certainly may involve more than one neurotransmitter. As we will see in discussing brain development, below, this is consistent with the notion of developmental origins of psychiatric disorders, as development of brain typically involves sequential processing of more and more complex information.

Noninvasive imaging has increased both our awareness that many disorders have associated brain changes, and the specificity of our knowledge of how those brain changes might affect a person's behavior, but there are still some limitations to what noninvasive techniques can reveal. In some cases, they cannot clearly imply a cause and effect relationship; for example, early fMRI studies of posttraumatic stress disorder found some reduction in volume of hippocampus, but a later twin study found that both twins had reduced brain volume, even when only one had PTSD (Gilbertson et al., 2002). Such a finding may imply that reduced brain volume indicates susceptibility to developing PTSD in response to a traumatic event, rather than that the event induces a brain volume change. In addition, imaging studies done after diagnosis cannot fully explain how brain abnormalities might come to exist. For that, we turn to a brief discussion on brain development.

Developmental Antecedents of Neurological Disorders

Like the brain itself, the development of the central nervous system is a topic far too complex to adequately discuss in this chapter. Prenatal growth proceeds from a single fertilized egg to differentiation into definable organ systems to growth of the most complex organ known in a remarkably short time, and we only partially understand the processes involved in that growth. In general, however, development of brain is a complicated interaction of *genes, prenatal environment,* and *postnatal environment.*

Genes

Genes appear to largely determine the pattern of brain development that a given organism may undergo. They influence such factors as segmentation of the developing brain (initial division into regions that will eventually become forebrain, hindbrain, spinal cord), types of nerve cells and types of transmitters, and patterns of interconnections that grow between brain areas (Sanes, Reh, & Harris, 2006). Generally, a human embryo will grow a typically organized human brain, which will then function like a typical human brain, but the process of developing a typical human brain is complex enough that there are many possibilities for errors to occur during development.

A large number of studies indicate that there are genetic risk factors for a variety of disorders, including schizophrenia, depression, and substance abuse disorders. With a very few exceptions, such as Huntington's disease, genes do not directly determine who develops a particular disorder, they only influence the probability of that disorder. For example, if a person diagnosed with schizophrenia happens to have an identical twin, the probability of the twin also having the disease is as high as 50% (estimates differ in different studies) (McGue & Gottesman, 1991). That's a much higher risk than that in the general population, but an overlooked part of the meaning of the statistic is that *50% or more of people who have genes identical to a schizophrenic's genes* (by definition, identical twins have identical genes) *do not develop schizophrenia.* So, the genes do not directly cause schizophrenia, although they can make its development much more likely. Please note the distinction between *being a twin,* which does not increase the risk of schizophrenia, and being the twin *of a schizophrenic,* which does.

Gene Expression Genes are not simply "there," they are expressed, that is, become active and synthesize their respective proteins, in response to signals which can activate or silence them. The degree to which a gene is expressed determines how much of its protein is produced, which in turn determines how much of an effect of that gene is produced. For example, D2 dopamine receptors are involved in several behavioral roles, one of which is reinforcement, including perceptions of pleasure in response to addictive drugs. Literally, all addictive drugs activate D2 receptors, and that activation is an important part of the euphoria that can lead to repeated use and addiction (Volkow et al., 2006). Internal chemical conditions which activate the gene that produces the D2 receptor increase sensitivity to addictive drugs. Chemical conditions, such as neurotransmitter activity, which increase expression of the D2 receptor gene, include activation of the dopamine pathways by addictive drugs. Literally, administration of an addictive drug can change the chemistry of the brain that controls reaction to addictive drugs (Volkow et al., 2006), and this change involves both changes in dopamine release and in the D2 receptor. While direct gene expression studies are relatively new, evidence indicates that addictive drugs such as nicotine can induce expression of a variety of genes, involved not only with the dopamine receptors, but also with growth and development processes (Polesskaya, Smith, & Fryxell, 2006). Thus, the chemical environment can control expression of particular genes, and, in the case of addiction, the genes activated by drug consumption lead to brain changes cuing additional drug consumption. Probably, disorders with a partial genetic basis, such as schizophrenia, are induced by a combination of events: having the gene or gene combination necessary for schizophrenia, which is determined by heredity, in conjunction with developmental events which cause a particular level of expression of those genes (this is environmental).

In most cases, we do not yet know specifically what genes are risk factors for specific disorders, and a historical caution is that many past theories of the biological cause of particular disorders have proven to be incorrect. Recent research suggests some possibilities for the genetic basis for depression and schizophrenia: For depression, recent research suggests that many depressed individuals have a different *allele* (form) of a gene which produces a protein involved in transport of serotonin (Caspi et al., 2003); this can result in less efficient activity in the serotonin system. For schizophrenia, research has recently focused on a particular chromosome region (22q11; Shifman et al., 2006), although many other potentially influential genes are being studied. The precise meaning of the possible involvement of the 22q11 region has yet to be determined, and future research will be required to determine whether and which of these possibilities are actually correct.

Prenatal Development

During the prenatal period, exposure to a variety of drugs and toxins can influence brain development. For example, the fetal alcohol syndrome, seen in children born to many women who drink heavily during pregnancy, includes distinctive facial malformations, bone and joint abnormalities, and reduction in brain growth and organization, which causes moderate to severe mental retardation (Mattson, Schoenfeld, & Riley, 2001). Many studies have documented that prenatal exposure to other drugs as varied as cocaine, anticonvulsants, and nicotine can induce abnormal brain development, suggesting a general rule that any drug which can affect brain function or behavior in the adult has the potential to alter prenatal brain development. The data suggest that even very short binge consumption of drugs (the equivalent of as little as getting intoxicated on two occasions) may have striking effects on prenatal physical development (Sulik, Johnston, & Webb, 1981). As a general rule, very little can be done to alleviate brain growth problems caused by prenatal conditions, so prevention is very important—avoidance of addictive drugs and toxic chemicals altogether, minimized use of medically required drugs which alter brain or behavior. Although data are still sketchy, it appears that many conditions that affect prenatal brain development do so by altering expression of genes which control the overall shape and form of the growing brain, the total number of cells produced, the organization of the basic columnar units of cortex, or signals which guide axons and synaptic connections (Sanes et al., 2006). Disorders most often associated with prenatal drug use include mental retardation, and there is evidence that some types of learning and attentional disorders are more likely in children whose mothers used drugs during pregnancy (Huizink & Mulder, 2006). Other severe disorders, such as autism, seem to have their origins in early pregnancy, but the specific reason for brain malformations in autism is not yet clear (Courchesne et al., 2005).

Postnatal Development

Although in humans most brain cells are formed by birth, a tremendous amount of growth in dendrites and in synaptic connections continues for years. Growth lasts particularly long in frontal areas of the brain, involved in inhibitory control of behavior and other complex functions (Cunningham, Bhattacharyya, & Benes, 2002). Growth is not always progressive: around the time of puberty, for example, there is a large reduction in synapses through a "pruning" process (Teicher, Andersen, & Hostetter, 1995). Presumably these are excess synapses, and the pruning may be associated with better focus as a child matures. It now appears that there is a lifelong process of forming and breaking synaptic connections (see "learning" in the minitutorial) and this process is more robust during childhood and adolescence than it is later in adulthood. In the child and adolescent, most growth in connections seems to be in reaction to neural activity in brain systems, which in turn is induced by sensory input from the environment. Examples include older research with cats that demonstrated that visual system cells are "tuned" to the kinds of angled edges that kittens actually see; restricting the visual environment of kittens restricts the angles to which adult brain cells later respond (Blakemore & Cooper, 1970). Experimental data in animals and anecdotal evidence in humans indicate that lack of experience with a particular type of visual stimulation in early childhood severely restricts the ability to perceive that kind of stimulation later in life. The brain has to "learn" to perceive, and if it lacks opportunities to learn some types of perception, its ability to process those kinds of information is severely limited.

More recently, work by Sapolsky, Meaney and others has found that the quality of maternal care for infant rats can affect development of the pituitary–adrenal stress response system. Rat pups which receive more intensive "mothering" develop stress response systems which produce lower levels of adrenal hormones in response to stress (Caldji et al., 1998). Interestingly, this can affect the offspring in adulthood and old age. In adulthood, they are calmer, more attentive mothers, thus giving their own offspring the same attention that kept them calm. Thus, there is mother–daughter transmission of behavior, acting through a nongenetic mechanism (Meaney, 2001). In old age, poorly mothered animals had high levels of stress hormones, which are toxic to brain cells, and they lose brain cells and spatial memory relatively rapidly. Well mothered animals do not have the premature loss of brain cells seen in poorly mothered animals, and well mothered animals preserve their spatial memory capability farther into old age (Meaney, Aitken, van Berkel, Bhatnagar, & Sapolsky, 1988). Thus, the quality of maternal care has important biological impacts on brain development. Good maternal care biases a mother toward being able to provide good maternal care to her own young, and affects both genders on other aspects of behavior, because good maternal care reduces stress responses and preserves brain capabilities longer into old age.

Does this animal data apply to humans, as well? It's hard to say at this point in time, as parallel studies have not yet been done. In general, the developmental trajectories of all mammal brains are similar enough that finding an effect in animals at least "raises a red flag" that a similar effect may occur in humans. In a very small number of cases, parallel studies have been done in humans and animals—the types of effects of prenatal alcohol are quite similar in animals and humans, for example (Driscoll, Streissguth, & Riley, 1990).

Recent research indicates that sensory aspects of development normally include an element of "recruitment"; that is, activity in basic sensory systems recruits higher order systems to process the information in a more sophisticated manner (Chou et al., 2006; Gogtay et al., 2004) . For example, noninvasive imaging studies have found that presentation of words as stimuli to infants induces activity only in the primary visual cortex. In young children who can recognize the lines as combining to produce letters, they induce activity in secondary visual cortex. In elementary school children who recognize that letters combine into words, activity is induced in areas involved in more complex processing (Schlaggar et al., 2002). Recruitment of additional brain areas eventually extends into areas associated with semantic associations of a word, not just its immediate meaning (Chou et al., 2006). This is a developmental trend in many systems—early on, input gets basic processing from primary systems, and the input that gets a lot of basic processing recruits other systems to pay attention to it, and conduct more sophisticated analysis of the input. That more sophisticated analysis leads a 12-year-old to understand more from the visual stimulus AARDVARK than a 3-year-old can understand.

Early experiences thus appear to mold the focus of the developing brain. They influence the responsiveness of various parts of brain to sensory input, and determine the level of processing that a sensory input induces. This is clearly true for strong maternal care versus poor maternal care, and for a lot of normal information processing in brain. We believe that this can also be a substrate for lasting effects of early learning and early traumatic events, as well.

Some disorders clearly have origins in development, and are brain disorders. Autism is associated with poorly developed posterior areas of brain, and overgrown anterior areas, probably resulting in poor information processing efficiency and overfocus on some types of information. ADHD is first detected in young children, and prenatal drug abuse, including maternal smoking, is one risk factor for developing ADHD (Huizink & Mulder, 2006). Childhood-onset schizophrenia is associated with progressive loss of brain tissue during adolescence (more than normal adolescent pruning) which encompasses many areas of cortex (Thompson et al., 2001). Future research may also reveal that additional psychiatric disorders also have a developmental component.

Understanding the origins of mental disorders has significant implications for treating them. One cannot reverse major brain growth errors, and therapies for disorders which do not involve brain growth errors may be very different if the disorder primarily has inappropriate learned behaviors (overt or covert, including emotions) or chemical aberrations as its basis.

The extent to which some disorders may be influenced by early experiences is difficult to determine, and may very well vary from person to person. While it requires some extrapolation from our current knowledge, patterns of thinking (fearful or negative thoughts, recurring unwanted thoughts, etc.) or particular behavioral experiences (trauma or abuse, or enjoyable experiences) that occur during child or adolescent brain development have the potential to sculpt that development in ways that perpetuate problems or strengths that originate during development. That is, childhood fears and obsessions may become persistent ways of thinking in adulthood for that individual; favorite childhood activities may become lifelong interests; and adolescent drug use may become continuing patterns of addiction. While it is certainly not the case that all behavior pathology originates in development, the tendency of experiences to sculpt the development of brain systems suggests that early interventions are more likely to successfully treat and prevent various disorders than are interventions at later points in time.

Pharmacological Treatment of Psychiatric Disorders

Drugs are used to treat the symptoms of psychosis, depression, anxiety and other psychiatric disorders.

Antipsychotic Drugs

Antipsychotic drugs are most often used to treat symptoms of schizophrenia. As a group, they are dopamine receptor blockers (Wong et al., 1986), although they differ from each other in clinical potency, and in relative specificity for the various dopamine receptor types. Table 4.1 lists a few of the many antipsychotic drugs available. Antipsychotic drugs differ in the likelihood of severe side effects such as tardive dyskinesia (a syndrome of persistent and involuntary motor movements seen after years of antipsychotic drug treatment), immediate motor effects such as tremors, and several other side effects. As with antidepressants, fitting the drug and dosage to the individual is often a process of repeated experimentation.

Antidepressant Drugs

Several pharmacologically different types of drugs are effective in treating depression. The earliest group of drugs inhibit monoamine oxidase (MAO), an enzyme involved in the breakdown of several different transmitters, which is involved in regulating amounts of these transmitters within nerve cells. The effectiveness of MAO inhibitors (MAOIs) was discovered accidentally when patients given an MAO inhibitor for treatment of tuberculosis experienced increased mood beyond that accounted for by improvement in chest X-rays. A couple of MAO inhibitors are still used in this country for treatment of depression in patients responding poorly to other medications, but dietary restrictions/ hazards (ingesting some dairy proteins in conjunction with MAOIs can produce life-threatening blood pressure spikes) have reduced their use.

Tricyclic antidepressants reduce reuptake of several neurotransmitters. Individual tricyclics have slightly different actions, in that they focus on serotonergic neurons versus a different class (noradrenergic) of neurons. By slowing reuptake, they make more transmitter available to the postsynaptic neuron, effectively increasing availability of the transmitter. This process, however, is probably not the basis for their antidepressant action because the reuptake effect is immediate, while clinical antidepressant action typically takes two weeks or more to develop. The actual mechanism of symptom improvement is not known.

SSRIs. Selective serotonin reuptake inhibitors, as the name implies, are more selective for serotonergic neurons, and have largely become the drug class of choice for treating symptoms of depression.

Antianxiety Drugs

Diazepam (Valium) and its relatives have become the drugs of choice for treating anxiety disorders. These drugs largely act to stimulate receptors for the neurotransmitter GABA (gamma-aminobutyric acid). GABA is an inhibitory transmitter (large intravenous doses of Valium can even stop an ongoing epileptic seizure). Unlike earlier tranquilizing drugs such as barbiturates, Valium effectively reduces anxiety in doses too small to sedate the client or to negatively affect cognitive functioning. As noted below, antianxiety drugs can have fatal interactions with other drugs, such as alcohol.

Treatment of Bipolar Disorder

On the surface, it would seem that manic and depressive phases of bipolar disorders should be due to different causes, and thus treated by different drugs. The underlying mechanism of bipolar disorder is largely unknown, although noninvasive imaging studies have found that there are large differences in metabolism in brain between manic and depressive episodes, but lithium has proven a fairly effective modulator of both phases of the disorder. The reason for this has yet to be found.

Other Drug Treatments

In recent years, we have seen an increase in the number of disorders for which some drug therapy has become available. Successful reduction of obsessive-compulsive symptoms with SSRIs, and use of

Table 4.2 Examples of side effects of drug

Drug	Common side effects
Antipsychotics	Tardive dyskinesia, liver impairment, hypotension
MAO inhibitors	In combination with tyramine in diet (dairy products and yeasts), can produce life-threatening blood pressure spikes
Tricyclic Antidepressants	Sedation, cardiovascular effects
SSRIs	Insomnia, gastrointestinal problems, sexual dysfunction Possible association with elevated suicide risk under investigation
Antianxiety drugs	Life-threatening synergism if taken with other depressant drugs, such as alcohol

bupropion for treatment of withdrawal from cigarette addiction have been reported. At this time, a vaccine for nicotine addiction is having mixed success. In general, drug treatments address symptoms of some disorders, but they do not actually "cure" the disorder. In some cases (see below) symptom improvement is associated with normalizing brain function, suggesting that the treatment may be addressing the cause, not just the symptoms.

Side Effects

Most psychoactive drugs can have side effects because the signaling systems they affect can also regulate other behaviors and other body tissues. A list of some common side effects is in Table 4.2. Side effects can be severe in some cases. For example, tardive dyskinesia is a motor control disorder that can develop after years of antipsychotic treatment, and it often does not abate when the drug is stopped or altered. Liver damage is common to many drugs taken long-term. Some precautions to avoid drug interactions are very important. Combining antianxiety drugs such as Valium, with other depressants, especially alcohol, can be fatal in surprisingly small doses. Overdose of many drugs, and even some vitamins, can make side effects much more severe. Finally, there has been some recent suggestion of increased suicide risk from Prozac in adolescents taking this drug for depression, although rigorous data are lacking so far. And these are side effects of drugs appropriately prescribed—a *mis*diagnosis and resulting inappropriate prescription may actually worsen some disorders. In general, drugs for psychiatric disorders are sometimes effective, but they also have some risks. They should be taken only when there is a clear diagnosis and good monitoring to detect side effects, with clear instructions to the client regarding the drug's use. The client's compliance with dose instructions, use of other medications, and sometimes with diet instructions can dramatically affect the risk/benefit ratio of psychiatric drugs, so much so that recently the issue of compliance with medication instructions has been seen as a major risk factor for a large number of drugs. Finally, we should caution that many psychiatric drugs are best used in conjunction with complementary therapies—antidepressant medications with cognitive therapies, for example.

Brain Plasticity and Nonpharmacological Treatments

Much of what we now know about the ever-changing circuitry of the brain simplifies to one statement: "*increasing use of a particular brain area or brain system strengthens and increases synaptic connections*." We can follow this with a lot of appropriate caveats: "…but too much activity can trigger activity-induced cell death,"; "…but there are exceptions." But the general statement seems to hold across a variety of brain systems:

- The use of (addictive) drugs, which activates the mesolimbic dopamine (reinforcement) system strengthens the connections of that system, and increases addiction liability, for a variety of behaviors ranging from drug abuse to gambling to sex addiction (Volkow et al., 2006)
- Environmental cues that have been repeatedly associated with drug use (or internal cues such as thoughts of drug use) have similar effects on brain system as actual drug administration (Volkow et al., 2006)
- A focus on one sensory system (e.g., hearing) after loss of another (e.g.,vision) leads to expansion of areas of cortex that respond to and process auditory stimuli (Ptito & Kupers, 2005)
- Particular types of sensory stimuli, ranging from restricting patterns during development to increasing overall stimulation levels in adulthood, affect the sensitivity of neural systems to those stimuli, and can trigger growth in systems being used more extensively, and regression in systems not being used (Blakemore & Cooper, 1970; Ptito & Kupers, 2005).

In addition, at the behavioral level, we see that repetition of behaviors leads to their strengthening, repetition of unwelcome thoughts induces a pattern of thinking, beliefs about control over the situation tend to be self-perpetuating and self-strengthening. All of these behavioral changes probably have underlying neural changes which sustain them.

What can be developed through behavioral or cognitive processes can often be undone using similar processes. There is reason to believe, for example, that therapies targeting information processing can change beliefs, attitudes, and perceptions, almost certainly by altering the neural substrates that produced those mental phenomena in the first place. While describing those approaches to therapy is beyond the scope of this chapter, recent research suggests that many types of therapies which are effective derive that effectiveness from their ability to resculpt patterns of synapses in the brain. A clear example of this comes from the work of Shaywitz et al, who showed that intensive phonological therapy (reading training) for dyslexia can not only improve reading skills, but improve recruitment of higher level comprehension areas of brain (Shaywitz et al., 2004). Other work has indicated that psychotherapies can improve fMRI indices of brain abnormalities associated with anxiety, for example (Roffman, Marci, Glick, Dougherty, & Rauch, 2005), and that treatment of obsessive-compulsive disorder with either medication or psychotherapy improves fMRI indices of frontal lobe hyperactivation that accompanies this disorder (Nakao et al., 2005). These are just a few examples of the emerging research suggesting that treatments which improve aspects of behavior can also improve brain functioning related to that behavior. LeDoux's speculation that therapies essentially 'rewire' the brain (LeDoux, 2002) is gathering some support from emerging evidence.

As behavior has the brain as its underlying substrate, so does behavior pathology. Pathologies can be developed from many different factors affecting brain function—for example, genes or gene expression, patterns of behavior, developmental or environmental events, or drug use. While some pathologies, particularly those of early developmental origin, may be resistant to therapies simply because they have produced irreversible changes in brain organization and brain functioning, others are reversible with medication or effective psycho- or behavior therapy. Even those of early developmental origin may eventually prove to be partly or wholly preventable, as we understand the origins better and develop diagnostic methods for earlier identification.

Pathology, like normal behavior, often involves a confluence of several different influences. In many cases, the interaction of genetic susceptibility with specific environmental conditions that interact with that susceptibility contribute to the development of a disorder. That interaction probably results in a "wiring" of the brain to produce a particular pattern of behavior we label as abnormal or maladaptive. But our understanding of the processes resulting from the convergence of genes and environment suggests that a potential for better understanding and better treatment in the future already exists. Genetic screening to tell us who is at risk, controlling maternal exposure to toxins during pregnancy, remedial work during early brain development—all of these offer some promise of reducing psychopathology. But our emerging understanding of the plasticity of the brain suggests that even when psychopathology has already developed, altering behavior patterns or patterns of thought, and perhaps even drug therapies in a limited number of cases, may effect change by rewiring some areas of brain not functioning optimally.

Biologically, what causes a psychological disorder? There is no single answer to this question. The old notion that behavior is determined both by heredity and environment is still true, but we can now add some detail to that statement, and the contributions of environment are becoming better understood. Certainly a few specific disorders, such as Huntington's disease, can be directly inherited. In many other cases, chemicals such as alcohol, drugs, or stress hormones may alter the expression of genes, thus altering brain and behavioral development. In still other cases, the sensory stimuli and thoughts which an individual processes during early development sculpt the growth of those brain systems which interpret those kinds of stimuli, and this can lead to more complex development of systems stimulated during brain growth, and less complete development of systems deprived of normal stimulation. While the processes which produce psychopathology may be complex, a better understanding of the biological bases of psychopathology increases our ability to understand, prevent, and treat such disorders.

References

Blakemore, C., & Cooper, G. F. (1970). Development of the brain depends on the visual environment. *Nature, 228*(5270), 477–478.

Booth, J. R., Burman, D. D., Meyer, J. R., Lei, Z., Trommer, B. L., Davenport, N. D., et al. (2005). Larger deficits in brain networks for response inhibition than for visual selective attention in attention deficit hyperactivity disorder (ADHD). *Journal of Child Psychology and Psychiatry, 46*(1), 94–111.

Caldji, C., Tannenbaum, B., Sharma, S., Francis, D., Plotsky, P. M., & Meaney, M. J. (1998). Maternal care during infancy regulates the development of neural systems mediating the expression of fearfulness in the rat. *Proceedings of the National Academy of the Sciences U S A, 95*(9), 5335–5340.

Carlson, N. R. (2007). *Physiology of behavior.* Boston, MA: Allyn & Bacon.

Caspi, A., Sugden, K., Moffitt, T. E., Taylor, A., Craig, I. W., Harrington, H., et al. (2003). Influence of life stress on depression: Moderation by a polymorphism in the 5-HTT gene. *Science, 301*(5631), 386–389.

Chou, T. L., Booth, J. R., Burman, D. D., Bitan, T., Bigio, J. D., Lu, D., et al. (2006). Developmental changes in the neural correlates of semantic processing. *Neuroimage, 29*(4), 1141–1149.

Courchesne, E., Redcay, E., Morgan, J. T., & Kennedy, D. P. (2005). Autism at the beginning: Microstructural and growth abnormalities underlying the cognitive and behavioral phenotype of autism. *Developmental Psychopathology,, 17*(3), 577–597.

Cunningham, M. G., Bhattacharyya, S., & Benes, F. M. (2002). Amygdalo-cortical sprouting continues into early adulthood: Implications for the development of normal and abnormal function during adolescence. *Journal of Comparative Neurology, 453*(2), 116–130.

Drevets, W. C. (2001). Neuroimaging and neuropathological studies of depression: implications for the cognitive-emotional features of mood disorders. *Current Opinion in Neurobiology, 11*(2), 240–249.

Driscoll, C. D., Streissguth, A. P., & Riley, E. P. (1990). Prenatal alcohol exposure: Comparability of effects in humans and animal models. *Neurotoxicology and Teratology, 12*(3), 231–237.

Gilbertson, M. W., Shenton, M. E., Ciszewski, A., Kasai, K., Lasko, N. B., Orr, S. P., et al. (2002). Smaller hippocampal volume predicts pathologic vulnerability to psychological trauma. *Nature Neuroscience, 5*(11), 1242–1247.

Gogtay, N., Giedd, J. N., Lusk, L., Hayashi, K. M., Greenstein, D., Vaituzis, A. C., et al. (2004). Dynamic mapping of human cortical development during childhood through early adulthood. *Proceedings of the National Academy of the Sciences USA, 101*(21), 8174–8179.

Huizink, A. C., & Mulder, E. J. (2006). Maternal smoking, drinking or cannabis use during pregnancy and neurobehavioral and cognitive functioning in human offspring. *Neuroscience and Biobehavioral Review, 30*(1), 24–41.

Konrad, K., Neufang, S., Hanisch, C., Fink, G. R., & Herpertz-Dahlmann, B. (2006). Dysfunctional attentional networks in children with attention deficit/hyperactivity disorder: Evidence from an event-related functional magnetic resonance imaging study. *Biological Psychiatry, 59*(7), 643–651.

Laruelle, M., Abi-Dargham, A., van Dyck, C. H., Gil, R., D'Souza, C. D., Erdos, J., et al. (1996). Single photon emission computerized tomography imaging of amphetamine-induced dopamine release in drug-free schizophrenic subjects. *Proceedings of the National Academy of the Sciences U S A, 93*(17), 9235–9240.

LeDoux, J. E. (2002). *Synaptic self: How our brains become who we are.* New York: Viking Penguin.

Levinson, D. F. (2006). The genetics of depression: A review. *Biological Psychiatry, 60*(2), 84–92.

MacDonald, A. W., 3rd, & Carter, C. S. (2003). Event-related fMRI study of context processing in dorsolateral prefrontal cortex of patients with schizophrenia. *Journal of Abnormal Psychology, 112*(4), 689–697.

Malberg, J. E., Eisch, A. J., Nestler, E. J., & Duman, R. S. (2000). Chronic antidepressant treatment increases neurogenesis in adult rat hippocampus. *Journal of Neuroscience, 20*(24), 9104–9110.

Mattson, S. N., Schoenfeld, A. M., & Riley, E. P. (2001). Teratogenic effects of alcohol on brain and behavior. *Alcohol Research and Health, 25*(3), 185–191.

McGue, M., & Gottesman, I. I. (1991). The genetic epidemiology of schizophrenia and the design of linkage studies. *European Archives of Psychiatry and Clinical Neuroscience, 240*(3), 174–181.

Meaney, M. J. (2001). Maternal care, gene expression, and the transmission of individual differences in stress reactivity across generations. *Annual Review of Neuroscience, 24*, 1161–1192.

Meaney, M. J., Aitken, D. H., van Berkel, C., Bhatnagar, S., & Sapolsky, R. M. (1988). Effect of neonatal handling on age-related impairments associated with the hippocampus. *Science, 239*(4841 Pt 1), 766–768.

Meyer, J. S., & Quenzer, L. F. (2005). *Psychopharmacology: Drugs, the brain, and behavior.* Sunderland, MA: Sinauer.

Molteni, R., Calabrese, F., Bedogni, F., Tongiorgi, E., Fumagalli, F., Racagni, G., et al. (2006). Chronic treatment with fluoxetine up-regulates cellular BDNF mRNA expression in rat dopaminergic regions. *International Journal of Neuropsychopharmacology, 9*(3), 307–317.

Nakao, T., Nakagawa, A., Yoshiura, T., Nakatani, E., Nabeyama, M., Yoshizato, C., et al. (2005). Brain activation of patients with obsessive-compulsive disorder during neuropsychological and symptom provocation tasks before and after symptom improvement: a functional magnetic resonance imaging study. *Biology of Psychiatry, 57*(8), 901–910.

Otte, A., & Halsband, U. (2006). Brain imaging tools in neurosciences. *Journal of Physiology Paris, 99*(4–6), 281–292.

Polesskaya, O. O., Smith, R. F., & Fryxell, K. J. (2006). Chronic nicotine doses down-regulate PDE4 isoforms that are targets of antidepressants in adolescent female rats. *Biology of Psychiatry.*

Ptito, M., & Kupers, R. (2005). Cross-modal plasticity in early blindness. *Journal of Integrative Neuroscience, 4*(4), 479–488.

Rapoport, J. L., Addington, A. M., Frangou, S., & Psych, M. R. (2005). The neurodevelopmental model of schizophrenia: update 2005. *Molecular Psychiatry, 10*(5), 434–449.

Rehn, A. E., & Rees, S. M. (2005). Investigating the neurodevelopmental hypothesis of schizophrenia. *Clinical and Experimental Pharmacology and Physiology, 32*(9), 687–696.

Roffman, J. L., Marci, C. D., Glick, D. M., Dougherty, D. D., & Rauch, S. L. (2005). Neuroimaging and the functional neuroanatomy of psychotherapy. *Psychology and Medicine, 35*(10), 1385–1398.

Sanes, D. H., Reh, T. A., & Harris, W. A. (2006). *Development of the nervous system.* San Diego, CA: Academic Press.

Schlaggar, B. L., Brown, T. T., Lugar, H. M., Visscher, K. M., Miezin, F. M., & Petersen, S. E. (2002). Functional neuroanatomical differences between adults and school-age children in the processing of single words. *Science, 296*(5572), 1476–1479.

Seeman, P. (1987). Dopamine receptors and the dopamine hypothesis of schizophrenia. *Synapse, 1*(2), 133–152.

Shaywitz, B. A., Lyon, G. R., & Shaywitz, S. E. (2006). The role of functional magnetic resonance imaging in understanding reading and dyslexia. *Developmental Neuropsychology, 30*(1), 613–632.

Shaywitz, B. A., Shaywitz, S. E., Blachman, B. A., Pugh, K. R., Fulbright, R. K., Skudlarski, P., et al. (2004). Development of left occipitotemporal systems for skilled reading in children after a phonologically-based intervention. *Biology of Psychiatry, 55*(9), 926–933.

Shifman, S., Levit, A., Chen, M. L., Chen, C. H., Bronstein, M., Weizman, A., et al. (2006). A complete genetic association scan of the 22q11 deletion region and functional evidence reveal an association between DGCR2 and schizophrenia. *Human Genetics, 120*(2), 160–170.

Sulik, K. K., Johnston, M. C., & Webb, M. A. (1981). Fetal alcohol syndrome: Embryogenesis in a mouse model. *Science, 214*(4523), 936–938.

Teicher, M. H., Andersen, S. L., & Hostetter, J. C., Jr. (1995). Evidence for dopamine receptor pruning between adolescence and adulthood in striatum but not nucleus accumbens. *Brain Research Developmental Brain Research, 89*(2), 167–172.

Thompson, P. M., Vidal, C., Giedd, J. N., Gochman, P., Blumenthal, J., Nicolson, R., et al. (2001). Mapping adolescent brain change reveals dynamic wave of accelerated gray matter loss in very early-onset schizophrenia. *Proceedings of the National Academy of the Sciences U S A, 98*(20), 11650–11655.

Turkeltaub, P. E., Gareau, L., Flowers, D. L., Zeffiro, T. A., & Eden, G. F. (2003). Development of neural mechanisms for reading. *Nature Neuroscience, 6*(7), 767–773.

Volkow, N. D., Wang, G. J., Telang, F., Fowler, J. S., Logan, J., Childress, A. R., et al. (2006). Cocaine cues and dopamine in dorsal striatum: Mechanism of craving in cocaine addiction. *Journal of Neuroscience, 26*(24), 6583–6588.

Wong, D. F., Wagner, H. N., Jr., Tune, L. E., Dannals, R. F., Pearlson, G. D., Links, J. M., et al. (1986). Positron emission tomography reveals elevated D2 dopamine receptors in drug-naive schizophrenics. *Science, 234*(4783), 1558–1563.

Wrona, D. (2006). Neural-immune interactions: an integrative view of the bidirectional relationship between the brain and immune systems. *Journal of Neuroimmunology, 172*(1–2), 38–58.

5

Classification and Diagnosis
Historical Development and Contemporary Issues

Thomas A. Widiger

Aberrant, dysfunctional, and maladaptive thinking, feeling, behaving, and relating are of substantial concern to many different professions, the members of which will hold an equally diverse array of beliefs regarding etiology, pathology, and intervention. It is imperative that these persons be able to communicate meaningfully with one another. The primary purpose of an official diagnostic nomenclature is to provide this common language of communication (Kendell, 1975; Sartorius et al., 1993).

Official diagnostic nomenclatures, however, can be exceedingly powerful, impacting significantly many important social, forensic, clinical, and other professional decisions (Schwartz & Wiggins, 2002). The predominant languages of psychopathology are to be found in the fourth edition of the American Psychiatric Association's (1994, 2000) *Diagnostic and Statistical Manual of Mental Disorders* (*DSM-IV*) and the 10th edition of the World Health Organization's (WHO) *International Classification of Diseases* (*ICD-10*; WHO, 1992). As such, these nomenclatures have a substantial impact on how clinicians, social agencies, and the general public conceptualize aberrant, problematic, and maladaptive behavior.

Interpreting *DSM-IV* or *ICD-10* as conclusively validated nomenclatures, however, exaggerates the extent of their scientific support (Frances, Pincus, Widiger, Davis, & First, 1990). On the other hand, *DSM-IV* and *ICD-10* are not lacking in credible or compelling empirical support. Both works contain many flaws but they are also well-reasoned, scientifically researched, and well-documented nomenclatures that describe what is currently understood by most scientists, theorists, researchers, and clinicians to be the predominant forms of psychopathology (Nathan & Langenbucher, 1999; Widiger & Trull, 1993). This chapter will provide an overview of the *DSM-IV* diagnostic nomenclature, beginning with historical background, followed by a discussion of major issues facing future revisions.

Historical Background

The impetus for the development of an official diagnostic nomenclature was the crippling confusion generated by its absence (Widiger, 2001). "For a long time confusion reigned. Every self-respecting alienist [the 19th-century term for a psychiatrist], and certainly every professor, had his own classification" (Kendell, 1975, p. 87). The production of a new system for classifying psychopathology became a right of passage in the 19th century for the young, aspiring professor.

> To produce a well-ordered classification almost seems to have become the unspoken ambition of every psychiatrist of industry and promise, as it is the ambition of a good tenor to strike a high C. This classificatory ambition was so conspicuous that the composer Berlioz was prompted to remark that after their studies have been completed a rhetorician writes a tragedy and a psychiatrist a classification. (Zilboorg, 1941, p. 450)

In 1908 the American Bureau of the Census asked the American Medico-Psychological Association (which changed its name in 1921 to the American Psychiatric Association) to develop a standard nosology to facilitate the obtainment of national statistics. This committee affirmed the need for a uniform system.

> The present condition with respect to the classification of mental diseases is chaotic. Some states use no well-defined classification. In others the classifications used are similar in many respects but differ enough to prevent accurate comparisons. Some states have adopted a uniform system, while others leave the matter entirely to the individual hospitals. This condition of affairs discredits the science. (Salmon, Copp, May, Abbot, & Cotton, 1917, pp. 255–256)

The American Medico-Psychological Association, in collaboration with the National Committee for Mental Hygiene, issued a nosology in 1918, titled *Statistical Manual for the Use of Institutions for the Insane* (Grob, 1991; Menninger, 1963). This nomenclature, however, failed to gain wide acceptance. It included only 22 diagnoses that were confined largely to psychoses with a presumably neurochemical pathology. "In the late twenties, each large teaching center employed a system of its own origination, no one of which met more than the immediate needs of the local institution" (American Psychiatric Association, 1952, p. v). A conference was held at the New York Academy of Medicine in 1928 to develop a more authoritative and uniformly accepted manual. The resulting nomenclature was modeled after the *Statistical Manual* but it was distributed to hospitals within the American Medical Association's *Standard Classified Nomenclature of Disease*. Many hospitals used this system but it eventually proved to be inadequate when the attention of the profession expanded well beyond psychotic disorders during World War II.

ICD-6 and DSM-I

The Navy, Army, and Veterans Administration developed their own, largely independent nomenclatures during World War II due in large part to the inadequacies of the *Standard Classified*. "Military psychiatrists, induction station psychiatrists, and Veterans Administration psychiatrists, found themselves operating within the limits of a nomenclature specifically not designed for 90% of the cases handled" (American Psychiatric Association, 1952, p. vi). The World Health Organization (WHO) accepted the authority in 1948 to produce the sixth edition of the *International Statistical Classification of Diseases, Injuries, and Causes of Death* (ICD). *ICD-6* was the first to include a section devoted to mental disorders (Kendell, 1975; Kramer, Sartorius, Jablensky, & Gulbinat, 1979), perhaps in recognition of the many psychological casualties of World War II, as well as the increasing impact and contribution of mental health professions within the broader society. The U.S. Public Health Service commissioned a committee, chaired by George Raines (with representations from a variety of professions and public health agencies) to develop a variant of the mental disorders section of *ICD-6* for use within the United States. The United States, as a member of the WHO, was obliged to use *ICD-6*, but modifications could be made to maximize its acceptance and utility for use within the United States. The resulting nomenclature resembled closely the Veterans Administration system developed by Brigadier General

William Menninger (brother to Karl Menninger, 1963). Responsibility for publishing and distributing this nosology was given to the American Psychiatric Association (1952) under the title: *Diagnostic and Statistical Manual: Mental Disorders* (*DSM-I*).

DSM-I was generally successful in obtaining acceptance, due in large part to its expanded coverage, including somatoform disorders, stress reactions, and personality disorders. However, the New York State Department of Mental Hygiene, which had been influential in the development of the *Standard Nomenclature*, continued for some time to use its own classification. *DSM-I* also included narrative descriptions of each disorder to facilitate understanding and more consistent applications. Nevertheless, fundamental criticisms regarding the reliability and validity of psychiatric diagnoses were also being raised (e.g., Zigler & Phillips, 1961). For example, a widely cited reliability study by Ward, Beck, Mendelson, Mock, and Erbaugh (1962) concluded that most of the poor agreement among psychiatrists' diagnoses was due largely to inadequacies of *DSM-I*.

ICD-6 was less successful. The "mental disorders section [of *ICD-6*] failed to gain [international] acceptance and eleven years later was found to be in official use only in Finland, New Zealand, Peru, Thailand, and the United Kingdom" (Kendell, 1975, p. 91). The WHO therefore commissioned a review by the English psychiatrist, Erwin Stengel, who reiterated the importance of establishing an official nomenclature (1959).

A…serious obstacle to progress in psychiatry is difficulty of communication. Everybody who has followed the literature and listened to discussions concerning mental illness soon discovers that psychiatrists, even those apparently sharing the same basic orientation, often do not speak the same language. They either use different terms for the same concepts, or the same term for different concepts, usually without being aware of it. It is sometimes argued that this is inevitable in the present state of psychiatric knowledge, but it is doubtful whether this is a valid excuse. (Stengel, 1959, p. 601)

Stengel (1959) attributed the failure of clinicians to accept the mental disorders section of *ICD*-6 to the presence of theoretical biases, cynicism regarding any psychiatric diagnoses (some theoretical perspectives opposed the use of any diagnostic terms), and the presence of abstract, highly inferential diagnostic criterion that hindered consistent, uniform applications by different clinicians.

ICD-8 and DSM-II

Work began on *ICD-8* soon after Stengel's (1959) report (*ICD-6* had been revised to *ICD-7* in 1955, but there were no revisions to the mental disorders). Considerable effort was made to develop a system that would be used by all of the member countries of the WHO. The final edition of *ICD-8* was approved by the WHO in 1966 and became effective in 1968. A companion glossary, in the spirit of Stengel's (1959) recommendations, was to be published conjointly, but work did not begin on the glossary until 1967 and it was not completed until 1972. "This delay greatly reduced [its] usefulness, and also [its] authority" (Kendell, 1975, p. 95). In 1965, the American Psychiatric Association appointed a committee, chaired by Ernest M. Gruenberg, to revise *DSM-I* to be compatible with *ICD-8* and yet also be suitable for use within the United States. The final version was approved in 1967, with publication in 1968.

The diagnosis of mental disorders, however, was receiving substantial criticism during this time (e.g., Rosenhan, 1973; Szasz, 1960). A fundamental problem continued to be the absence of empirical support for the reliability, let alone the validity, of its diagnoses (e.g., Blashfield & Draguns, 1976). Researchers, however, took to heart the recommendations of Stengel (1959) by developing more specific and explicit criterion sets (Blashfield, 1984). The most influential of these efforts was produced by a group of neurobiologically oriented psychiatrists at Washington University in St. Louis. Their criterion sets generated so much interest that they were published separately in what has become one of the most widely cited papers in psychiatry (i.e., Feighner et al., 1972). Research has since indicated that mental disorders can be diagnosed reliably and do provide valid information regarding etiology, pathology, course, and treatment (Nathan & Langenbucher, 1999).

ICD-9 and DSM-III

By the time Feighner et al. (1972) was published, work was nearing completion on the ninth edition of the ICD. The authors of *ICD-9* had decided to include a glossary that would provide more precise descriptions of each disorder, but it was apparent that *ICD-9* would not include the more specific and explicit criterion sets used in research (Kendell, 1975). In 1974, the American Psychiatric Association appointed a Task Force, chaired by Robert Spitzer, to revise *DSM-II* in a manner that would be compatible with *ICD-9* but would also incorporate many of the current innovations in diagnosis. *DSM-III* was published in 1980 and was remarkably innovative, including (1) a multiaxial diagnostic system (most mental disorders were diagnosed on Axis I, personality and specific developmental disorders were diagnosed on Axis II, medical disorders on Axis III, psychosocial stressors on Axis IV, and level of functioning on Axis V); (2) specific and explicit criterion sets for all but one of the disorders (schizoaffective); (3) a substantially expanded text discussion of each disorder to facilitate diagnosis (e.g., age at onset, course, complications, sex ratio, and familial pattern); and (4) removal of terms (e.g., *neurosis*) that appeared to favor a particular theoretical model for the disorder's etiology or pathology (Spitzer, Williams, & Skodol, 1980).

DSM-III-R

An ironic advantage of the specificity and explicitness of the *DSM-III* criterion sets was that a number of mistakes quickly became apparent (e.g., panic disorder in *DSM-III* could not be diagnosed in the presence of a major depression). "Criteria were not entirely clear, were inconsistent across categories, or were even contradictory" (American Psychiatric Association, 1987, p. xvii). Many of these errors and problems were due to the fact that there was insufficient research to guide the authors of the criterion sets and only a small minority of the criterion sets were piloted in clinical trials. The American Psychiatric Association therefore authorized the development of a revision to *DSM-III* to make corrections and refinements. Fundamental revisions were to be tabled until work began on *ICD-10*. However, it might have been unrealistic to expect the authors of *DSM-III*-R to confine their efforts to refinement and clarification, given the impact, success, and importance of *DSM-III*.

> The impact of *DSM-III* has been remarkable. Soon after its publication, it became widely accepted in the United States as the common language of mental health clinicians and researchers for communicating about the disorders for which they have professional responsibility. Recent major textbooks of psychiatry and other textbooks that discuss psychopathology have either made extensive reference to *DSM-III* or largely adopted its terminology and concepts. (American Psychiatric Association, 1987, p. xviii)

It was not difficult to find persons who wanted to be involved in the development of *DSM-III*-R, and most of those who were (or were not) involved wanted to have a significant impact. More persons were involved in making corrections to *DSM-III* than were used in its original construction and, not surprisingly, there were many proposals for major revisions and even new diagnoses. Four of the diagnoses approved for inclusion by the authors of *DSM-III-R* (i.e., sadistic personality disorder, self-defeating personality disorder, late luteal phase dysphoric disorder [the name for which was subsequently changed to premenstrual dysphoric disorder], and paraphiliac rapism) generated so much controversy that a special ad hoc committee was appointed by the Board of Trustees of the American Psychiatric Association to reconsider their inclusion. A concern common to all four was that their inclusion might result in harm to women. For example, paraphiliac rapism might be used to mitigate criminal responsibility for rape and self-defeating personality disorder might be used to blame female victims for having been abused. Another concern was the lack of sufficient empirical support to address or offset these concerns. A compromise was eventually reached in which the two personality disorders and late luteal phase dysphoric disorder were included in an appendix (Endicott, 2000; Widiger, 1995); paraphiliac rapism was deleted entirely.

ICD-10 and DSM-IV

By the time work was completed on *DSM-III-R*, work had already begun on *ICD-10*. The decision of the authors of *DSM-III* to develop an alternative to *ICD-9* was instrumental in developing a highly innovative manual (Kendell, 1991; Spitzer et al., 1980). However, its innovations were also at the cost of decreasing compatibility with the *ICD-9* nomenclature that was used throughout the rest of the world, which is problematic to the stated purpose of providing a common language of communication. In May of 1988 the American Psychiatric Association appointed a *DSM-IV* Task Force, chaired by Allen Frances (Frances, Widiger, & Pincus, 1989). Mandates for *DSM-IV* included better coordination with *ICD-10* and improved documentation of empirical support.

The *DSM-IV* committee aspired to use a more conservative threshold for the inclusion of new diagnoses and to have decisions that were guided more explicitly by the scientific literature (Nathan & Langenbucher, 1999). Frances et al. (1989) suggested that "the major innovation of *DSM-IV* will not be in its having surprising new content but rather will reside in the systematic and explicit method by which *DSM-IV* will be constructed and documented" (p. 375). Proposals for additions, deletions, or revisions were guided by 175 literature reviews that used a specific format that maximized the potential for critical review, containing (for example) a method section that documented explicitly the criteria for including and excluding studies and the process by which the literature had been reviewed. Each of these reviews has since been published in three volumes of a *DSM-IV* Sourcebook (Widiger et al., 1994, 1996, 1997). Testable questions that could be addressed with existing data sets were also explored in 36 studies, which emphasized the aggregation of multiple data sets from independent researchers, and 12 field trials were conducted to provide reliability and validity data on proposed revisions. The results of the 36 studies and 12 field trials were published in the fourth volume of the *DSM-IV* Sourcebook (Widiger et al., 1998). Critical reviews of these 223 projects were obtained by sending initial drafts to advisors or consultants to a respective work group, by presenting drafts at relevant conferences, and by submitting drafts to peer-reviewed journals (Widiger, Frances, Pincus, Davis, & First, 1991).

DSM-IV-TR

One of the innovations of *DSM-III* was the inclusion of a relatively detailed text discussion of each disorder, including information on age of onset, gender, course, and familial pattern (Spitzer et al., 1980). This text was expanded in *DSM-IV* to include cultural and ethnic group variation, variation across age, and laboratory and physical exam findings (Frances, First, & Pincus, 1995). Largely excluded from the text was information concerning etiology, pathology, and treatment as this material was considered to be too theoretically specific and more suitable for academic texts. Nevertheless, it had also become apparent that *DSM-IV* was being used as a textbook, and the material on age, course, prevalence, and family history was quickly becoming outdated as new information was being gathered.

Therefore, in 1997, the American Psychiatric Association appointed a *DSM-IV* Text Revision Work Group, chaired by Michael First (Editor of the Text and Criterion Sets for *DSM-IV*) and Harold Pincus (Vice-Chair for *DSM-IV*) to update the text material. No substantive changes in the criterion sets were considered, nor were any new additions, subtypes, deletions, or other changes in the status of any diagnoses implemented. In addition, each of the proposed revisions to the text had to be supported by a systematic literature review that was critiqued by a considerable number of advisors. The *DSM-IV* Text Revision (*DSM-IV-TR*) was published in 2000 (American Psychiatric Association, 2000).

ICD-11 and DSM-V

In 1999, a conference jointly sponsored by the National Institute of Mental Health (NIMH) and the American Psychiatric Association was held to identify the research that would most likely be informative for the authors of *DSM-V*. This conference was cochaired by Drs. Kupfer, First, and Regier (2002). Substantive issues emphasized by research planning work groups developed from this conference included (but were not limited to) cross-cultural issues, gender differences, developmental differences, the distinction between Axis I and Axis II, the definition of mental disorder, the threshold for diagnosis, the use of laboratory findings in diagnosis, the impact of neuroscience, and dimensional models of psychopathology (e.g., Alarcon et al., 2002; First et al., 2002; Rounsaville et al., 2002).

A series of more specific international conferences subsequently followed, details of which can be obtained at the following website: http://www.dsm5.org. However, in the meantime, work has now begun on *ICD-11*, chaired by Bedirhan Ustun. This start on *ICD-11* led to the formation of the *DSM-V* Task Force, chaired by David Kupfer (Darrel Regier is Vice Chair). The first meeting of the *DSM-V* Task Force was in November of 2006, with an anticipated publication date for *DSM-V* in 2011.

Continuing Issues for *DSM-V*

The issues considered by the *DSM-V* research planning work groups (Kupfer et al., 2002) are not unique to *DSM-V*. In fact, some of them concern fundamental issues that have been raised throughout the history of the diagnosis of mental disorders (Blashfield, 1984; Kendell, 1975; Zilboorg, 1941). Five issues worth highlighting in particular are (1) the definition of mental disorder and threshold for diagnosis; (2) categorical versus dimensional models of classification, (3) culture and values; (4) gender; and (5) the inclusion of laboratory tests within diagnostic criterion sets. Each of these issues will be discussed briefly in turn.

Definition of Mental Disorder and Threshold for Diagnosis

The boundaries of the diagnostic manual have been increasing with each edition and there has been vocal concern that much of this expansion represents an encroachment into normal problems of living (Caplan, 1995; Folette & Houts, 1996). Diagnoses proposed for *DSM-IV* were ultimately included within an appendix primarily because they might be below an appropriate threshold for diagnosis, such as mixed anxiety-depressive disorder, age-related cognitive decline, and minor depressive disorder (Widiger & Coker, 2003). A difficult task facing the authors of *DSM-V* will be to establish a meaningful boundary between abnormal and normal psychological functioning (Rounsaville et al., 2002).

Table 5.1 provides the definition of mental disorder provided in *DSM-IV-TR* (American Psychiatric Association, 2000). This definition was the result of an effort by the authors of *DSM-III* to develop specific and explicit criteria for deciding whether a behavior pattern (homosexuality in particular)

Table 5.1 American Psychiatric Association (2000) definition of mental disorder

In *DSM-IV-TR*, each of the mental disorders is conceptualized as a clinically significant behavioral or psychological syndrome or pattern that occurs in an individual and that is associated with present distress (e.g., a painful symptom) or disability (i.e., impairment in one or more important areas of functioning) or with a significantly increased risk of suffering death, pain, disability, or an important loss of freedom. In addition, this syndrome or pattern must not be merely an expectable and culturally sanctioned response to a particular event, for example, the death of a loved one. Whatever its original cause, it must currently be considered a manifestation of a behavioral, psychological, or biological dysfunction in the individual. Neither deviant behavior (e.g., political, religious, or sexual) nor conflicts that are primarily between the individual and society are mental disorders unless the deviance or conflict is a symptom of a dysfunction in the individual, as described above.

Source: American Psychiatric Association, 2000, p. xxxi.

should be classified as a mental disorder (Spitzer & Williams, 1982). The intense controversy over homosexuality has largely abated, but the issues raised in this historical debate continue to apply.

For example, in order to be diagnosed with pedophilia, *DSM-III-R* (American Psychiatric Association, 1987) required only that an adult have recurrent intense urges and fantasies involving sexual activity with a prepubescent child over a period of at least six months and have acted on them (or be markedly distressed by them). Every adult who engaged in a sexual activity with a child for longer than six months would meet these diagnostic criteria. The authors of *DSM-IV* were therefore concerned that *DSM-III-R* was not providing adequate guidance for determining when deviant sexual behavior is the result of a mental disorder. Presumably, some persons can engage in deviant, aberrant, and even heinous activities without being compelled to do so by the presence of psychopathology. The authors of *DSM-IV*, therefore, added the requirement that "the behavior, sexual urges, or fantasies cause clinically significant distress or impairment in social, occupational, or other important areas of functioning" (American Psychiatric Association, 1994, p. 523).

Require Presence of Pathology? Spitzer and Wakefield (1999), however, have argued that the impairment criteria included in *DSM-IV* are inadequate. They concurred with a concern raised by the National Law Center for Children and Families that *DSM-IV* might contribute to a normalization of pedophilic and other paraphilic behavior by allowing the diagnoses not to be applied if the persons who have engaged in these acts are not themselves distressed by their behavior or do not otherwise experience impairment. In response, Frances et al. (1995) had argued that pedophilic sexual "behaviors are inherently problematic because they involve a nonconsenting person (exhibitionism, voyeurism, frotteurism) or a child (pedophilia) and may lead to arrest and incarceration" (p. 319). Therefore, any person who engaged in an illegal sexual act (for longer than six months) would be exhibiting a clinically significant social impairment and would therefore meet the *DSM-IV* threshold for diagnosis. However, using the illegality of an act as a diagnostic criterion is problematic. It undermines the original rationale for the inclusion of the impairment criterion (i.e., to distinguish immoral or illegal acts from abnormal or disordered acts) and it is inconsistent with the definition of a mental disorder that states that neither deviance nor conflicts with the law are sufficient to warrant a diagnosis (see Table 5.1). Spitzer and Wakefield argued that the distinction between disordered and nondisordered abuse of children requires an assessment for the presence of an underlying, internal pathology (e.g., irrational cognitive schema or neurochemical dysregulation).

Wakefield has provided examples of other criterion sets from *DSM-IV* that are less politically or socially controversial than pedophilia, which he suggests also fail to make a necessary distinction between maladaptive problems in living and true psychopathology due to the reliance within the criterion sets on indicators of distress or impairment rather than references to pathology (Wakefield & First, 2003; Wakefield, Horwitz, & Schmitz, 2005). For example, the *DSM-IV* criterion set for major depressive disorder currently excludes most instances of depressive reactions to the loss of a loved one (i.e., uncomplicated bereavement). Depression after the loss of a loved one can be considered a mental disorder though if "the symptoms persist for longer than two months" (American Psychiatric Association, 1994, p. 327). Allowing two months to grieve before one is diagnosed with a mental disorder might be as arbitrary and meaningless as allowing a person to engage in a sexually deviant act only for six months before the behavior is diagnosed as a paraphilia. Similar concerns have been raised by Regier et al. (1998) regarding the diagnosis of common anxiety and mood disorders. They suggested that the prevalence rates for many of the anxiety, mood, and other mental disorders obtained by the NIMH Epidemiologic Catchment Area program (ECA) and the National Comorbidity Survey (NCS) were excessive (Regier & Narrow, 2002). "Based on the high prevalence rates identified in both the ECA and NCS, it is reasonable to hypothesize that some syndromes in the community represent transient homeostatic responses to internal or external stimuli that do not represent true psychopathologic disorders" (Regier et al., 1998, p. 114).

The inclusion of pathology within diagnostic criterion sets (e.g., irrational cognitive schemas, unconscious defense mechanisms, or neurochemical dysregulations) would be consistent with the definition of mental disorder provided in *DSM-IV*, which states that the syndrome "must currently be considered a manifestation of a behavioral, psychological, or biological dysfunction in the individual" (American Psychiatric Association, 2000, p. xxxi; see Table 5.1). However, a limitation of this proposal is that there is currently little agreement over the specific pathology that underlies any particular disorder. There is insufficient empirical support to give preference to one particular cognitive, interpersonal, neurochemical, psychodynamic, or other theoretical model of pathology. The precise nature of this pathology could be left undefined or characterized simply as an "internal dysfunction" (Wakefield, Pottick, & Kirk, 2002) but an assessment of an unspecified pathology is unlikely to be reliable. Clinicians will have very different opinions concerning the nature of the internal dysfunction and quite different thresholds for its attribution.

The assumption that the expansion of the nomenclature is subsuming normal problems in living is itself questionable. Persons critical of the nomenclature have decried the substantial expansion of the diagnostic manual over the past 50 years (e.g., Caplan, 1995; Follette & Houts, 1996; Kirk, 2005). However, it might have been more surprising to find that scientific research and increased knowledge has failed to lead to the recognition of more instances of psychopathology (Wakefield, 1998, 2001). In fact, the current manual might still be inadequate in its coverage despite the expansion. Quite often, the most common diagnosis in general clinical practice is not-otherwise-specified (NOS; Clark, Watson, & Reynolds, 1995). The NOS diagnosis is provided when a clinician has determined that psychopathology is present but the symptomatology fails to meet criteria for any one of the existing disorders. Clinicians providing the diagnosis of NOS for anxiety, mood, personality, and other disorders testifies to the inadequate coverage currently provided (although perhaps one could argue as well that this testifies to a tendency of clinicians to diagnose normal problems in living as being instances of mental disorder).

The assumption that only a small minority of the population currently has, or will ever have, a mental disorder (Regier & Narrow, 2002), might itself be questionable. Very few persons fail to have at least some physical disorders, and all persons suffer from quite a few physical disorders throughout their lifetime. It is unclear why it should be different for mental disorders, as if most persons have been fortunate to have obtained no problematic genetic dispositions or vulnerabilities and have never sustained any psychological injuries or never have experienced significant economic, environmental, or interpersonal stress, pressure, or conflict that would tax or strain psychological functioning.

Optimal psychological functioning, as in the case of optimal physical functioning, might represent an ideal that is achieved by only a small minority of the population. The rejection of a high prevalence rate of psychopathology may reflect the best of intentions, such as concerns regarding the stigmatization of mental disorder diagnoses (Kirk, 2005) or the potential impact on funding for treatment (Regier & Narrow, 2002) but these social and political concerns could also hinder a more dispassionate and accurate recognition of the true rate of a broad range of psychopathology within the population (Widiger & Sankis, 2000).

Harmful Dysfunction or Dyscontrolled Maladaptivity? Wakefield (1992) has developed an alternative "harmful dysfunction" definition of mental disorder where dysfunction is a failure of an internal mechanism to perform a naturally selected function (e.g., the capacity to experience feelings of guilt in a person with antisocial personality disorder) and harm is a value judgment that the design failure is harmful to the individual (e.g., failure to learn from mistakes results in repeated punishments, arrests, loss of employment, and eventual impoverishment). Wakefield's model has received substantial attention and is being considered for inclusion in *DSM-V* (Rounsaville et al., 2002). However, the model has also received compelling criticism (e.g., Bergner 1997; Kirmayer & Young, 1999; Lilienfeld & Marino, 1999). A fundamental limitation is its girding within evolutionary theory, thereby limiting its relevance and usefulness to alternative models of etiology and pathology (Bergner, 1997). Wakefield's model might even be inconsistent with some sociobiological models of psychopathology. Cultural evolution may at times outstrip the pace of biological evolution, rendering some designed functions that were originally adaptive within earlier time periods maladaptive in many current environments (Lilienfeld & Marino, 1999; Widiger & Sankis, 2000). For example, "the existence in humans of a preparedness mechanism for developing a fear of snakes may be a relic not well designed to deal with urban living, which currently contains hostile forces far more dangerous to human survival (e.g., cars, electrical outlets) but for which humans lack evolved mechanisms of fear preparedness" (Buss, Haselton, Shackelford, Bleske, & Wakefield, 1998, p. 538).

Missing from Wakefield's (1999) definition of mental disorder is any reference to dyscontrol. Harm within Wakefield's conceptualization of mental disorder is concerned with the presence of impairment; dysfunction with the presence of pathology. Mental disorders, however, are perhaps better understood as dyscontrolled impairments in psychological functioning (Kirmayer & Young 1999; Klein, 1999; Widiger & Trull, 1991). "Involuntary impairment remains the key inference" (Klein, 1999, p. 424). Dyscontrol is one of the fundamental features of mental disorder emphasized in Bergner's (1997) "significant restriction" and Widiger and Sankis's (2000) "dyscontrolled maladaptivity" definitions of mental disorder. Including the concept of dyscontrol within a definition of mental disorder would provide a fundamental distinction between mental and physical disorder, as dyscontrol is not a meaningful consideration for or a fundamental component of physical disorder.

Fundamental to the concept of a mental disorder is the presence of impairments to feelings, thoughts, or behaviors over which a normal (healthy) person is believed to have adequate control. To the extent that a person willfully, intentionally, freely, or voluntarily engaged in harmful sexual acts, drug usage, gambling, or child abuse, the person would not be considered to have a mental disorder. Persons seek professional intervention in large part to obtain the insights, techniques, skills, or other tools (e.g., medications) that would increase their ability to better control their mood, thoughts, or behavior. In sum, impairment and dyscontrol might provide the optimal means with which to identify a meaningful boundary between, or an important parameter for quantifying, normal and abnormal psychological functioning, if these constructs are more precisely defined, calibrated, and assessed.

Dyscontrol as a component of mental disorder does not imply that a normal person has free will, a concept that is, at best, difficult to verify in scientific or empirical terms (Bargh & Ferguson, 2000; Howard & Conway, 1986). A person with a mental disorder could be comparable to a computer lacking in the necessary software to combat particular viruses or execute effective programs. Pharmacotherapy alters the neural connections of the central nervous system (the hardware), whereas psychotherapy alters the cognitions (the software) in a manner that increases a person's behavioral repertoire, allowing the person to act and respond more effectively. A computer provided with new software has not been provided with free will, but has been provided with more options to act and respond more effectively.

Categorical and Dimensional Models of Classification

"*DSM-IV* is a categorical classification that divides mental disorders into types based on criterion sets with defining features" (American Psychiatric Association, 2000, p. xxxi). The intention of the diagnostic manual is to help the clinician determine which particular disorder is present, the diagnosis of which would indicate the presence of a specific pathology that would explain the occurrence of the symptoms and suggest a specific treatment that would ameliorate the patient's suffering (Frances et al., 1995; Kendell, 1975).

It is evident, however, that *DSM-IV* routinely fails in the goal of guiding the clinician to the presence of one specific disorder. Despite the best efforts of the authors to revise the criterion sets to increase their specificity, multiple diagnoses are the norm (Widiger & Clark, 2000). It is rare for a patient to meet the *DSM-IV-TR* diagnostic criteria for just one mental disorder. The number of multiple diagnoses is even higher when one includes lifetime as well as current functioning and it might be remarkably high if all of the disorders within *DSM-IV-TR* are in fact considered.

In general medicine, the presence of multiple diagnoses would logically suggest the presence of multiple disorders (i.e., comorbidity). However, the frequency with which psychiatric patients routinely meet diagnostic criteria for multiple disorders has raised questions concerning the validity of the psychiatric diagnostic manual. "The greatest challenge that the extensive comorbidity data pose to the current nosological system concerns the validity of the diagnostic categories themselves—do these disorders constitute distinct clinical entities?" (Mineka, Watson, & Clark, 1998, p. 380). Diagnostic comorbidity has become so prevalent that some argue for an abandonment of the term *comorbidity* in favor of a term (e.g., *co-occurrence*) that does not imply the presence of distinct clinical entities (Lilienfeld, Waldman, & Israel, 1994). There are instances in which the presence of multiple diagnoses does suggest the presence of distinct yet comorbid psychopathologies, but in many instances the presence of co-occurring diagnoses does appear to suggest the presence of an etiology or pathology that is shared by the purportedly distinct disorders (Widiger & Clark, 2000).

There has been a substantial amount of research attention given to identifying a specific gene (or other form of specific etiology) for each mental disorder, modeled after the success obtained with many physical disorders. However, the complex disorders of psychopathology appear unlikely to have specific etiologies, or even specific genetic etiologies, and initial successes in identifying specific genes have typically failed to replicate (Faraone, 2002). Most (if not all) mental disorders appear to be the result of a complex interaction of an array of interacting biological vulnerabilities and dispositions with a number of significant environmental, psychosocial events that exert their effects at different points in time (Rutter, 2003). The symptoms and pathologies of mental disorders appear to be highly responsive to a wide variety of neurobiological, interpersonal, cognitive, and other mediating and moderating variables that help to develop, shape, and form a particular individual's psychopathology profile. This complex etiological history and individual psychopathology profile is unlikely to be well described by single diagnostic categories that attempt to make distinctions at nonexistent discrete joints along the continuous distributions (Widiger & Samuel, 2005).

A model for the future diagnosis of all mental disorders might be provided by one of the oldest and best validated diagnoses, mental retardation. The point of demarcation for its diagnosis is an arbitrary, quantitative distinction along the normally distributed levels of the multivariate domain of intelligence. Mental retardation is diagnosed primarily on the basis of having an intelligence quotient (IQ) of 70 or below (American Psychiatric Association, 2000). There are persons with an IQ less than 70 for whom a qualitatively distinct disorder is evident. However, this disorder is not mental retardation, it is a physical disorder (e.g., Down syndrome) that can be traced to a specific biological event (i.e., trisomy 21). Intelligence is itself distributed as a continuous variable. In addition, "in approximately 30%–40% of individuals seen in clinical settings, no clear etiology for the Mental Retardation can be determined despite extensive evaluation efforts" (*DSM-IV-TR*, p. 45). Intelligence is the result of a complex array of multiple genetic, fetal, and infant developmental events, and environmental influences (Neisser et al., 1996). There are no discrete breaks in the distribution of intelligence that would provide an absolute distinction between normal intelligence and abnormal intelligence.

Many researchers are now turning their attention to the identification of underlying spectra of dysfunction that cut across the existing diagnostic categories (Clark, 2005; Krueger, Markon, Patrick, & Iacono, 2005; Watson, 2005; Widiger & Samuel, 2005). The first of the series of international *DSM-V* research planning conferences was in fact devoted to identifying the research that would lead the field to a dimensional classification of personality disorder (Widiger, Simonsen, Krueger, Livesley, & Verheul, 2005). Krueger et al. (2005) and Watson and Clark (2006) suggest a revision of the classification of mood, anxiety, substance use, and personality disorders into two broad dimensions of internalization and externalization that parallel closely the internalization and externalization distinction emphasized many years ago for disorders of childhood by Achenbach (1966, 2002). Costa and Widiger (2002) have proposed a dimensional classification of the personality disorders that would integrate the psychiatric classification of personality disorders with the five-factor model of general personality structure developed within psychology. A five-factor model understanding of the personality disorders is presented in chapter 5 by Lowe and Widiger (this volume).

Culture and Values

It was the intention of the authors of *ICD-10* to provide a universal diagnostic system, but diagnostic criteria and constructs can have quite different implications and meanings across different cultures. *DSM-IV* addresses cultural issues in three ways. First, the text of *DSM-IV* provides a discussion of how each disorder is known to vary in its presentation across different cultures. Second, an appendix of "culture-bound" syndromes describes disorders that are currently thought to be specific to a particular culture. Third, an additional appendix provides a culturally informed diagnostic formulation that considers the cultural identity of the individual and the culture-specific explanations of the person's presenting complaints (Lim, 2006).

There is both a strong and a weak cross-cultural critique of current scientific understanding of psychopathology. The weak critique does not question the validity of a concept of mental disorder but does argue that social and cultural processes affect and potentially bias the

> science of psychopathology and diagnosis: a) by determining the selection of persons and behaviors as suitable material for analysis; b) by emphasizing what aspects of this material will be handled as relevant from a [clinical] standpoint; c) by shaping the language of diagnosis, including that of descriptive psychopathology; d) by masking the symptoms of any putative 'universal' disorder; e) by biasing the observer and would-be diagnostician; and f) by determining the goals and endpoints of treatment. (Fabrega, 1994, p. 262)

These concerns are not weak in the sense that they are trivial or inconsequential but they do not dispute the fundamental validity of a concept of mental disorder or the science of psychopathology. The strong critique, in contrast, is that the construct of mental disorder is itself a culture-bound belief that reflects the local biases of Western society, and that the science of psychopathology is valid only in the sense that it is an accepted belief system of a particular culture (Lewis-Fernandez & Kleinman, 1995).

The concept of mental disorder does include a value judgment that there should be necessary, adequate, or optimal psychological functioning (Wakefield, 1992). However, this value judgment is also a fundamental component of the construct of physical disorder (Widiger, 2002). In a world in which there were no impairments or threats to physical functioning, the construct of a physical disorder would have no meaning except as an interesting thought experiment. Meaningful and valid scientific research on the etiology, pathology, and treatment of physical disorders occurs because in the world as it currently exists there are impairments and threats to physical functioning. It is provocative and intriguing to conceive of a world in which physical health and survival would or should not be valued or preferred over illness, suffering, and death, but this form of existence is unlikely to emerge anytime in the near future. Placing a value on adequate or optimal physical functioning might be a natural result of evolution within a world in which there are threats to functioning and survival. Likewise, in the world as it currently exists, there are impairments and threats to adequate psychological functioning.

It is also provocative and intriguing to conceive of a society (or world) in which psychological health would or should not be valued or preferred, but this form of existence is also unlikely to emerge anytime in the near future. Placing a value on adequate, necessary, or optimal psychological functioning might be inherent to and a natural result of existing in our world. Any particular definition of what would constitute adequate, necessary, or optimal psychological functioning would likely be biased to some extent by local cultural values, but this is perhaps best understood as only the failing of one particular conceptualization of mental disorder (i.e., a weak rather than a strong critique). Valuing adequate, necessary, or optimal psychological functioning could itself still be a logical and natural result of existing in a world in which there are threats to psychological functioning, just as placing a value on adequate, necessary, or optimal physical functioning would be a logical and natural result of existing in a world in which there are threats to physical functioning (Widiger, 2002).

Different societies, cultures, and even persons within a particular culture will disagree as to what constitutes optimal or pathological biological and psychological functioning (Lopez & Guarnaccia, 2000; Sadler, 2005). An important and difficult issue is how best to understand the differences between cultures with respect to what constitutes dysfunction and pathology (Alarcon et al., 2002). For example, simply because diagnostic criterion sets are applied reliably across different cultures does not necessarily indicate that the constructs themselves are valid or meaningful within these cultures (Lewis-Fernandez & Kleinman, 1995). A reliably diagnosed criterion set can be developed for an entirely illusory diagnostic construct. On the other hand, it is perhaps equally unclear why it would be necessary for the establishment of a disorder's construct validity to obtain cross-cultural (i.e., universal) acceptance. Lewis-Fernandez and Kleinman (1995) argue that it is necessary "to produce a comprehensive nosology that is both internationally and locally valid" (p. 435). A universally accepted diagnostic system will have an international social utility and consensus validity (Kessler, 1999) but it is also apparent that belief systems vary in their veridicality. Recognition of and appreciation for alternative belief systems is important for adequate functioning within an international community but respect for alternative belief systems does not necessarily imply that all belief systems are equally valid (Widiger, 2002).

Kirmayer, Young, and Hayton (1995) illustrate well many of the complexities of cross-cultural research. For example, a woman's housebound behavior might be diagnosed as agoraphobic within Western cultures but it would be considered normative (or even virtuous) within a Muslim culture; submissive behavior that is diagnosed as pathologic dependency within Western societies might be considered normative within Japanese culture. However, simply because a behavior pattern is valued, accepted, encouraged, or even statistically normative within a particular culture does not necessarily mean it is conducive to healthy psychological functioning. "In societies where ritual plays an important role in religious life…such societies may predispose individuals to obsessive-compulsive symptoms and mask the disorder when present" (Kirmayer et al., 1995, p. 507). "The congruence between religious belief and practice and obsessive-compulsive symptoms also probably contributes to relatively low rates of insight into the irrationality of the symptoms" (Kirmayer et al., 1995, p. 508). Behaviors diagnosed as disordered within one culture might be normative within another, but what is accepted, allowed, encouraged, or even statistically normative within a culture might still be pathological. On the other hand, it is equally important not to assume that what is believed to be associated with maladaptive (or adaptive) functioning in one culture should also be considered to be maladaptive (or adaptive) within all other cultures (Alarcon et al., 2002). "This possible tension between cultural styles and health consequences is in urgent need of further research" (Kirmayer et al., 1995, p. 517) and it is important for this research to go beyond simply identifying differences in behaviors, belief systems, and values across different cultures. This research also needs to address the fundamental question of whether differences in beliefs actually question the validity of any universal conceptualization of psychopathology or suggest instead simply different perspectives on a common, universal issue (see also chapter 1, Maddux, Gosselin, & Winstead, this volume).

Gender

Differential sex prevalence rates can be highly controversial because gender differences can reflect wider social, political controversies (Eagly, 1995). The diagnoses that generated the most controversy in the development of the recent editions of the *DSM* were problematic largely because of their questionable application to women (Ross, Frances, & Widiger, 1995). The basic charge is that the *DSM* is fundamentally flawed through its imposition of patriarchal or masculine biases over what does or should constitute psychopathology (Caplan & Cosgrove, 2004). In perhaps one of the more widely cited critiques, Kaplan (1983) argued that "our diagnostic system, like the society it serves, is male centered" (p. 791) and that "masculine-biased assumptions about what behaviors are healthy and what behaviors are crazy are codified in diagnostic criteria" (p. 786). Pantony and Caplan (1991) characterized *DSM-IV* as "sex discrimination in one of its most damaging and dangerous forms" (p. 120).

The premenstrual dysphoric disorder diagnosis (previously identified as late luteal phase dysphoric disorder) has been particularly controversial (Ross et al., 1995). A majority of women may suffer from some form of premenstrual dysphoria. Only 3 to 5% of women would meet the *DSM-IV* diagnostic criteria for premenstrual dysphoric disorder but the reliability of the distinction between normal premenstrual dysphoria and premenstrual dysphoric disorder in general clinical practice is questionable. *DSM-IV* requires daily ratings of mood for at least two months before the diagnosis is made (with at least six episodes over the prior 12 months) and it is unlikely that practicing clinicians or patients would actually adhere to this requirement. The pharmaceutical industry might also market treatments to women who are well below the threshold for the diagnosis and attributions concerning the harm, pathology, and impairments of premenstrual dysphoria will often be exaggerated and can be highly stigmatizing (Caplan, 2004).

Histrionic personality disorder has been criticized for being too closely associated with stereotypic traits of femininity (Kaplan, 1983). Kaplan (1983) went so far as to argue that by virtue of being feminine "a healthy woman automatically earns the diagnosis of Histrionic Personality Disorder" (p. 789). There is no research to support the claim that normal, healthy women meet diagnostic criteria for histrionic personality disorder. Studies have indicated that the diagnostic criteria for this disorder include maladaptive variants of stereotypic feminine traits, but it is unclear whether this association is inappropriate for a personality disorder diagnosis. The inclusion of gender-related traits, however, does appear to contribute to the occurrence of gender-biased applications of the diagnostic criteria and gender-biased assessment instruments (Morey, Alexander, & Boggs, 2005; Widiger, 1998).

There may not be a disorder in *DSM-IV* for which gender differences have not been problematic and even controversial (Kaplan, 1983). Concerns about gender bias have been raised for almost every diagnosis, either with respect to the diagnostic criteria, the applications of these diagnostic criteria by clinicians, the assessment instruments used in research and clinical practice, or the populations that have been sampled (Hartung & Widiger, 1998). An issue for the authors of *DSM-V* is whether to revise diagnostic criteria to improve their gender neutrality or develop different criterion sets for males and females (Widiger, in press). Currently, the same diagnostic criteria are used for males and females for all but a few of the disorders (the exceptions being gender identity disorder and sexual dysfunctions) but the text of *DSM-IV* indicates how each respective disorder appears differently in males and females (Frances et al., 1995). Achieving gender neutral diagnostic criteria for many of these disorders might be difficult (Sprock, Crosby, & Nielsen, 2001). On the other hand, separate diagnostic criteria could result in the creation of different disorders for each sex that might have even more problematic implications of gender bias (Wakefield, 1987; Zahn-Waxler, 1993). For example, Zoccolillo (1993) suggested that the diagnostic criteria for conduct disorder were gender biased because they described a masculine way in which the disorder is expressed. She suggested placing relatively more emphasis for girls on rule violations, substance abuse, prostitution, chronic lying, running away from home, and poor school performance and less emphasis on vandalism, fire setting, burglary, use of a weapon in fights, and rape. However, placing more emphasis on rule violations, rebelliousness, and deceitfulness for girls, and violent and aggressive behavior for boys, could have the effect of diagnosing (and stigmatizing) girls at a level of dysfunction that is much lower than is used to diagnose the disorder in boys (Zahn-Waxler, 1993). Zahn-Waxler suggested alternatively that the criterion set appropriately includes gender-related behaviors (e.g., rape) because the disorder is itself related to gender in its etiology and pathology (see also Winstead & Sanchez-Hucles, chapter 3 this volume).

Laboratory Measures, Diagnostic Criteria, and Clinical Diagnosis

"Diagnoses in the rest of medicine are often heavily influenced by laboratory tests" (Frances et al., 1995, p. 22). Laboratory tests within medical practice go beyond the assessment of symptoms. They provide a more direct and objective assessment of an underlying physical pathology. A hope is that laboratory tests could do the same for psychiatry as they have done for other domains of medicine (Rounsaville et al., 2002; Steffens & Krishnan, 2003). "The increasing use of laboratory tests in psychiatric research raises the question of whether and when these tests should be included within the diagnostic criterion sets" (Frances et al., 1995, p. 22).

Substantial attention is being given to structural and functional brain imaging with the expectation that these instruments could be used eventually to diagnose neurophysiological pathology (Drevets, 2002; Epstein, Isenberg, Stern, & Silbersweig, 2002). However, clearly limiting these and other neurophysiological measures' potential for incorporation within diagnostic criterion sets is the virtual absence of research indicating their ability to provide independent, blind diagnoses. Despite the enthusiasm for their potential diagnostic value, there are currently no studies that have assessed the sensitivity and specificity of neuroimaging techniques for the diagnosis or differential diagnosis of specific mental disorders (Steffens & Krishnan, 2003; see also Smith, this volume).

The inclusion of laboratory data in the diagnosis of a disorder has been particularly controversial for the sleep disorders. Most sleep disorder specialists use the International Classification of Sleep Disorders (ICSD) developed by the American Sleep Disorders Association (1990). The 12 *DSM-IV* sleep disorder diagnoses are coordinated with the ICSD, but differ significantly in failing to include polysomnographic diagnostic criteria (e.g., time of onset of rapid-eye movement sleep). Detailed references are made to polysomnographic findings within the text of *DSM-IV*, and it was acknowledged by its authors that "for sleep disorders other than insomnia, such as narcolepsy and sleep apnea, the utility of sleep laboratory testing is widely accepted" (Buysse, Reynolds, & Kupfer, 1998, pp. 1104–1105). Nevertheless, polysomography findings were not required because of the extensive cost of the technology and their lack of availability within many clinical settings (Buysse et al., 1998; Frances et al., 1995).

There is, however, a precedent in *DSM-IV* for the requirement of laboratory test findings obtained by a specialist. Laboratory tests are fundamental components of the diagnostic criteria for learning disorders and mental retardation. For example,

> the essential feature of Mental Retardation is significantly subaverage general intellectual functioning…[and] general intellectual functioning is defined by the intelligence quotient (IQ or IQ-equivalent) obtained by assessment with one or more of the standardized, individually administered intelligence tests (e.g., Wechsler Intelligence Scales for Children, 3rd Edition; Stanford-Binet, 4th Edition; Kaufman Assessment Battery for Children). (American Psychiatric Association, 2000, p. 41)

Psychological tests administered by a trained specialist using standardized equipment are essentially equivalent to the provision of laboratory testing. There are compelling concerns regarding the precise accuracy of IQ tests (Neisser et al., 1996) but routine diagnoses of mental retardation by practicing clinicians without the input of individually administered IQ-tests would be substantially more problematic and controversial.

The precedent established by mental retardation and learning disorders should perhaps be extended to other disorders (Widiger & Clark, 2000). "Although diagnostic criteria are the framework for any clinical or epidemiological assessment, no assessment of clinical status is independent of the reliability and validity of the methods used to determine the presence of a diagnosis" (Regier et al., 1998, p. 114). The *DSM-III* innovation of providing relatively specific and explicit diagnostic criteria is not realized if clinicians do not in fact adhere to the criterion sets and assess them in a comprehensive, systematic, and consistent fashion (Rogers, 2003). Researchers would be hard pressed to get their findings published if they failed to document that their diagnoses were based upon a systematic, replicable, and objective method, yet no such requirements are provided for clinical diagnoses, with the exception of mental retardation and learning disorders. Clinicians generally prefer to rely on their own experience, expertise, and subjective impressions obtained through unstructured interviews (Westen, 1997), but it is precisely this reliance upon subjective and idiosyncratic clinical interviewing that often undermines the reliability and ultimately the validity of clinical diagnoses (Garb, 2006; Rogers, 2003).

One of the new additions to the text of *DSM-IV* was a section devoted to laboratory and physical exam findings. This material was intended to provide the initial step toward the eventual inclusion of laboratory tests within diagnostic criterion sets (Frances et al., 1995). A noteworthy exclusion from this text are references to psychological tests and instruments (Rounsaville et al., 2002; Widiger & Clark, 2000). It is ironic that psychological tests are included already within the criterion sets for mental retardation and learning disorders, yet virtually no reference is made to any psychological tests within the sections devoted to laboratory test findings.

The discussion of laboratory instruments is confined in *DSM-IV* to measures of neurophysiology (e.g., functional brain imaging and the dexamethasone suppression test). Semistructured interviews and self-report inventories that assess cognitive, behavioral, affective, or other components of psychological functioning that comprise explicitly the diagnostic criterion sets for these disorders and for which substantial research already provides specificity and sensitivity rates not obtained by the neurophysiological instruments, should at least be acknowledged along with the neurophysiological measures. The inclusion of additional psychological tests within diagnostic criterion sets might have professional implications for the necessary qualifications to render a clinical diagnosis. For example, it is unclear whether many psychiatrists and even some psychologists are sufficiently trained in the administration and interpretation of the most informative and valid psychological tests. In any case, the American Psychiatric Association has already developed an authoritative manual for the best "psychiatric" instruments for the assessment of each disorder included within *DSM-IV* (Rush et al., 2000).

Conclusions

Nobody is fully satisfied with, or lacks valid criticisms of, *DSM-IV* and *ICD-10*. Zilboorg's (1941) suggestion that budding 19th century theorists and researchers cut their first teeth by providing a new classification of mental disorders still applies, although perhaps the right of passage today is to provide a critique of the *ICD* and/or *DSM*.

None, however, appear to be suggesting that all official diagnostic nomenclatures be abandoned. The benefits do appear to outweigh the costs (Regier et al., 1998; Salmon et al., 1917; Stengel, 1959). Everybody finds fault with this language, but there is at least the ability to communicate disagreement. Communication among researchers, theorists, and clinicians would be much worse in the absence of a common language.

Clinicians, theorists, and researchers will at times experience the frustration of being required to use the *DSM* or the *ICD*. It can be difficult to obtain a grant, publish a study, or receive insurance reimbursement without reference to a *DSM-IV* diagnosis. However, *DSM-IV* also provides a useful point of comparison that ultimately facilitates the development and understanding of a new way of conceptualizing psychopathology. Viable alternatives to particular sections of *DSM-IV* are being developed, some of which will eventually be incorporated within future revisions of the diagnostic manual. Their effective development will have been due in part to the existence of and empirical support for *DSM-IV*. *DSM-IV* and *ICD-10* are the official diagnostic systems because of their substantial empirical support, theoretical cogency, and clinical utility. They provide a well-validated foil for future contenders to overcome.

References

Achenbach, T. M. (1966). The classification of children's psychiatric symptoms: A factor-analytic study. *Psychological Monographs, 80*, (No. 615).

Achenbach, T. M. (2002). Empirically based assessment and taxonomy across the life span. In J. E. Hulzer & J. J. Hudziak (Eds.), *Defining psychopathology in the 21st century. DSM-V and beyond* (pp. 155–168). Washington, D.C.: American Psychiatric Press.

Alarcon, R. D., Bell, C. C., Kirmayer, L., Lin, K-H., Ustun, B., & Wisner, K. (2002). Beyond the fun-house mirrors: Research agenda on culture and psychiatric diagnosis. In D. J. Kupfer, M. B. First, & D. A. Regier (Eds.), *A research agenda for DSM-V* (pp. 219–281). Washington, D.C.: American Psychiatric Press.

American Psychiatric Association. (1952). *Diagnostic and statistical manual. Mental Disorders.* Washington, D.C.: Author.

American Psychiatric Association. (1968). *Diagnostic and statistical manual of mental disorders* (2nd ed.). Washington, D.C.: Author.

American Psychiatric Association. (1980). *Diagnostic and statistical manual of mental disorders* (3rd ed.). Washington, D.C.: Author.

American Psychiatric Association. (1987). *Diagnostic and statistical manual of mental disorders* (3rd ed., rev.). Washington, D.C.: Author.

American Psychiatric Association. (1994). *Diagnostic and statistical manual of mental disorders* (4th ed.). Washington, D.C.: Author.

American Psychiatric Association. (2000). *Diagnostic and statistical manual of mental disorders* (4th ed., rev.). Washington, D.C.: Author.

American Sleep Disorders Association. (1990). *International classification of sleep disorders: Diagnostic and coding manual.* Rochester, MN: Author.

Bargh, J. A., & Ferguson, M. J. (2000). Beyond behaviorism: On the automaticity of higher mental processes. *Psychological Bulletin, 126*, 925–945.

Bergner, R. M. (1997). What is psychopathology? And so what? *Clinical Psychology: Science and Practice, 4*, 235–248.

Blashfield, R. K. (1984). *The classification of psychopathology: Neo-Kraepelinian and quantitative approaches.* New York: Plenum.

Blashfield, R. K., & Draguns, J. G. (1976). Evaluative criteria for psychiatric classification. *Journal of Abnormal Psychology, 85*, 140–150.

Buss, D. M., Haselton, M. G., Shackelford, T. K., Bleske, A. L., & Wakefield, J. C. (1998). Adaptations, exaptations, and spandrels. *American Psychologist, 53*, 533–548.

Buysse, D. J., Reynolds, C. F., & Kupfer, D. J. (1998). DSM-IV sleep disorders: Final overview. In T. A. Widiger, A. J. Frances, H. A. Pincus, R. Ross, M. B. First, W. Davis et al. (Eds.), *DSM-IV sourcebook* (Vol. 4, pp. 1103–1122). Washington, D.C.: American Psychiatric Press.

Caplan, P. J. (1995). *They say you're crazy. How the world's most powerful psychiatrists decide who's normal.* Reading, MA: Addison-Wesley.

Caplan, P. J. (2004). The debate about PMDD and Sarafem: Suggestions for therapists. In J. C. Chrisler (Ed.), *From menarche to menopause: The female body in feminist therapy* (pp. 55–67). New York: Haworth Press.

Caplan, P. J., & Cosgrove, L. (Eds.). (2004). *Bias in psychiatric diagnosis.* Lanham, MD: Jason Aronson.

Clark, L. A. (2005). Temperament as a unifying basis for personality and psychopathology. *Journal of Abnormal Psychology, 114*, 505–521.

Clark, L. A., Watson, D., & Reynolds, S. (1995). Diagnosis and classification of psychopathology: Challenges to the current system and future directions. *Annual Review of Psychology, 46*, 121–153.

Costa, P. T., & Widiger, T. A. (Eds.). (2002). *Personality disorders and the five factor model of personality* (2nd ed.). Washington, D.C.: American Psychological Association.

Drevets, W. C. (2002). Neuroimaging studies of mood disorders. In J. E. Helzer & J. J. Hudziak (Eds.), *Defining psychopathology in the 21st century* (pp. 71–105). Washington, D.C.: American Psychiatric Press.

Eagly, A. H. (1995). The science and politics of comparing women and men. *American Psychologist, 50*, 145–158.

Endicott, J. (2000). History, evolution, and diagnosis of premenstrual dysphoric disorder. *Journal of Clinical Psychiatry, 62* (Suppl. 24), 5–8.

Epstein, J., Isenberg, N., Stern, E., & Silbersweig, D. (2002). Toward a neuroanatomical understanding of psychiatric illness: The role of functional imaging. In J. E. Helzer & J. J. Hudziak (Eds.), *Defining psychopathology in the 21st century* (pp. 57–69). Washington, D.C.: American Psychiatric Press.

Fabrega, H. (1994). International systems of diagnosis in psychiatry. *Journal of Nervous and Mental Disease, 182*, 256–263.

Faraone, S. v. (2002). Defining genetically meaningful classes of psychology. In J. E. Helzer & J. J. Hudziak (Eds.), *Defining psychopathology in the 21st century* (pp. 231–248). Washington, D.C.: American Psychiatric Press.

Feighner, J. P., Robins, E., Guze, S. B., Woodruff, R. A., Winokur, G., & Munoz, R. (1972). Diagnostic criterion for use in psychiatric research. *Archives of General Psychiatry, 26*, 57–63.

First, M. B., Bell, C. B., Krystal, J. H., Reiss, D., Shea, M. T., Widiger, T. A. et al. (2002). Gaps in the current system: Recommendations. In D. J. Kupfer, M. B. First, & D. A. Regier (Eds.), *A research agenda for DSM-V* (pp. 123–200). Washington, D.C.: American Psychiatric Press.

Folette, W. C., & Houts, A. C. (1996). Models of scientific progress and the role of theory in taxonomy development: A case study of the *DSM. Journal of Consulting and Clinical Psychology, 64*, 1120–1132.

Frances, A. J., First, M. B., & Pincus, H. A. (1995). *DSM-IV guidebook*. Washington, D.C.: American Psychiatric Press.

Frances, A. J., Pincus, H. A., Widiger, T. A., Davis, W. W., & First, M. B. (1990). *DSM-IV*: Work in progress. *American Journal of Psychiatry, 147*, 1439–1448.

Frances, A. J., Widiger, T. A., & Pincus, H. A. (1989). The development of *DSM-IV*. *Archives of General Psychiatry, 46*, 373–375.

Garb, H. (2005). Clinical judgment and decision making. *Annual Review of Clinical Psychology, 1*, 67–89.

Grob, G. N. (1991). Origins of *DSM-I*: A study in appearance and reality. *American Journal of Psychiatry, 148*, 421–431.

Hartung, C. M., & Widiger, T. A. (1998). Gender differences in the diagnosis of mental disorders: Conclusions and controversies of *DSM-IV. Psychological Bulletin, 123*, 260–278.

Howard, G. S., & Conway, C. G. (1986). Can there be an empirical science of volitional action? *American Psychologist, 41*, 1241–1251.

Kaplan, M. (1983). A woman's view of *DSM-III. American Psychologist, 38*, 786–792.

Kendell, R. E. (1975). *The role of diagnosis in psychiatry*. London: Blackwell Scientific.

Kendell, R. E. (1991). Relationship between the *DSM-IV* and the *ICD-10. Journal of Abnormal Psychology, 100*, 297–301.

Kessler, R. C. (1999). The World Health Organization International Consortium in Psychiatric Epidemiology: Initial work and future directions—The NAPE lecture. *Acta Psychiatrica Scandinavica, 99*, 2–9.

Kirk, S. A. (Ed.). (2005). *Mental disorders in the social environment: Critical perspectives*. New York: Columbia University Press.

Klein, D. F. (1999). Harmful dysfunction, disorder, disease, illness, and evolution. *Journal of Abnormal Psychology, 108*, 421–429.

Kirmayer, L. J., & Young, A. (1999). Culture and context in the evolutionary concept of mental disorder. *Journal of Abnormal Psychology, 108*, 446–452.

Kirmayer, L. J., Young, A., & Hayton, B. C. (1995). The cultural context of anxiety disorders. *Psychiatric Clinics of North America, 18*, 503–521.

Kramer, M., Sartorius, N., Jablensky, A., & Gulbinat, W. (1979). The *ICD-9* classification of mental disorders: A review of its development and contents. *Acta Psychiatrica Scandinavika, 59*, 241–262.

Krueger, R. F., Markon, K. E., Patrick, C. J., & Iacono, W. G. (2005). Externalizing psychopathology in adulthood: A dimensional-spectrum conceptualization and its implications for *DSM-V. Journal of Abnormal Psychology, 114*, 537–550.

Kupfer, D. J., First, M. B., & Regier, D. A. (Eds.). (2002). *A research agenda for DSM-V*. Washington, D.C.: American Psychiatric Press.

Lewis-Fernandez, R., & Kleinman, A. (1995). Cultural psychiatry: Theoretical, clinical, and research issues. *Psychiatric Clinics of North America, 18*, 433–446.

Lilienfeld, S.O., & Marino, L. (1999). Essentialism revisited: Evolutionary theory and the concept of mental disorder. *Journal of Abnormal Psychology, 108*, 400–411.

Lilienfeld, S. O., Waldman, I. D., & Israel, A. C. (1994). A critical examination of the use of the term "comorbidity" in psychopathology research. *Clinical Psychology: Science and Practice, 1*, 71–83.

Lim, R. F. (Ed.). (2006). *Clinical manual of cultural psychiatry*. Washington, D.C.: American Psychiatric Press.

Lopez, S. R., & Guarnaccia, J. J. (2000). Cultural psychopathology: Uncovering the social world of mental illness. *Annual Review of Psychology, 51*, 571–598.

Menninger, K. (1963). *The vital balance*. New York: Viking Press.

Mineka, S., Watson, D., & Clark, L. A. (1998). Comorbidity of anxiety and unipolar mood disorders. *Annual Review of Psychology, 49*, 377–412.

Morey, L. C., Alexander, G. M., & Boggs, C. (2005). Gender. In J. M. Oldham, A. E. Skodol, & D. S. Bender (Eds.), *The American Psychiatric Publishing textbook of personality disorders* (pp. 541–559). Washington, D.C.: American Psychiatric Press.

Nathan, P., & Langenbucher, J. W. (1999). Psychopathology: Description and classification. *Annual Review of Psychology, 50*, 79–107.

Neisser, U., Boodoo, G., Bouchard, T. J., Boykin, A. W., Brody, N., Ceci, S. J. et al. (1996). Intelligence: Knowns and unknowns. *American Psychologist, 51*, 77–101.

Pantony, K-L., & Caplan, P. J. (1991). Delusional dominating personality disorder: A modest proposal for identifying some consequences of rigid masculine socialization. *Canadian Psychology, 32*, 120–133.

Prigerson, H. G., Shear, M. K., Jacobs, S. C., Reynolds, C. F., Maciejewski, P. K., Davidson, J. et al. (1999). Consensus criteria for traumatic grief: A preliminary empirical test. *British Journal of Psychiatry, 174*, 67–73.

Regier, D. A., Kaelber, C. T., Rae, D. S., Farmer, M. E., Knauper, B., Kessler, R. C. et al. (1998). Limitations of diagnostic criteria and assessment instruments for mental disorders. Implications for research and policy. *Archives of General Psychiatry, 55,* 109–115.

Regier, D. A., & Narrow, W. E. (2002). Defining clinically significant psychopathology with epidemiologic data. In J. E. Hulzer & J. J. Hudziak (Eds.), *Defining psychopathology in the 21st century: DSM-V and beyond* (pp. 19–30). Washington, D.C.: American Psychiatric Publishing.

Rogers, R. (2003). Standardizing *DSM-IV* diagnoses: The clinical applications of structured interviews. *Journal of Personality Assessment, 81,* 220–225.

Rosenhan, D. L. (1973). On being sane in insane places. *Science, 179,* 250–258.

Ross, R., Frances, A. J., & Widiger, T. A. (1995). Gender issues in *DSM-IV*. In J. M. Oldham & M. B. Riba (Eds.), *Review of psychiatry* (Vol. 14, pp. 205–226). Washington, D.C.: American Psychiatric Press.

Rounsaville, B. J., Alarcon, R. D., Andrews, G., Jackson, J. S., Kendell, R. E., Kendler, K. S. et al. (2002). Toward *DSM-V*: Basic nomenclature issues. In D. J. Kupfer, M. B. First, & D. A. Regier (Eds.), *A research agenda for DSM-V* (pp. 1–30). Washington, D.C.: American Psychiatric Press.

Rush, A. J., Pincus, H. A., First, M. B., Blacker, D., Endicott, J., Keith, S. J. et al. (Eds.). (2000). *Handbook of psychiatric measures*. Washington, D.C.: American Psychiatric Publishing.

Rutter, M. (2003, October). *Pathways of genetic influences on psychopathology*. Zubin Award Address at the 18th Annual Meeting of the Society for Research in Psychopathology, Toronto, Ontario

Sadler, J. Z. (2005). *Values and psychiatric diagnosis*. Oxford: Oxford University Press.

Salmon, T. W., Copp, O., May, J. V., Abbot, E. S., & Cotton, H. A. (1917). Report of the committee on statistics of the American Medico-Psychological Association. *American Journal of Insanity, 74,* 255–260.

Sartorius, N., Kaelber, C. T., Cooper, J. E., Roper, M., Rae, D. S., Gulbinat, W. et al. (1993). Progress toward achieving a common language in psychiatry. *Archives of General Psychiatry, 50,* 115–124.

Schwartz, M. A., & Wiggins, O. P. (2002). The hegemony of the *DSMs*. In J. Sadler (Ed.), *Descriptions and prescriptions: Values, mental disorders, and the DSM* (pp. 199–209). Baltimore, MD: Johns Hopkins University Press.

Spitzer, R. L., & Wakefield, J. C. (1999). *DSM-IV* diagnostic criterion for clinical significance: Does it help solve the false positives problem? *American Journal of Psychiatry, 156,* 1856–1864.

Spitzer, R. L., & Williams, J. B. W. (1982). The definition and diagnosis of mental disorder. In W.R. Gove (Ed.), *Deviance and mental illness* (pp. 15–32). Beverly Hills, CA: Sage.

Spitzer, R. L., Williams, J. B. W., & Skodol, A. E. (1980). *DSM-III*: The major achievements and an overview. *American Journal of Psychiatry, 137,* 151–164.

Sprock, J., Crosby, J. P., & Nielsen, B. A. (2001). Effects of sex and sex roles on the perceived maladaptiveness of *DSM-IV* personality disorder symptoms. *Journal of Personality Disorders, 15,* 41–59.

Steffens, D. C., & Krishnan, K. R. R. (2003). Laboratory testing and neuroimaging: Implications for psychiatric diagnosis and practice. In K. A. Phillips, M. B. First, & H. A. Pincus (Eds.), *Advancing DSM: Dilemmas in psychiatric diagnosis* (pp. 85–103). Washington, D.C.: American Psychiatric Publishing.

Stengel, E. (1959). Classification of mental disorders. *Bulletin of the World Health Organization, 21,* 601–663.

Szasz, T. S. (1961). *The myth of mental illness*. New York: Hoeber-Harper.

Wakefield, J. C. (1987). Sex bias in the diagnosis of primary orgasmic dysfunction. *American Psychologist, 42,* 464–471.

Wakefield, J. C. (1992). The concept of mental disorder: on the boundary between biological facts and social values. *American Psychologist, 47,* 373–388.

Wakefield, J. C. (1998). The *DSM*'s theory-neutral nosology is scientifically progressive: Response to Follette and Houts (1996). *Journal of Consulting and Clinical Psychology, 66,* 846–852.

Wakefield, J. C. (2001). The myth of *DSM*'s invention of new categories of disorder: Hout's diagnostic discontinuity thesis disconfirmed. *Behaviour Research and Therapy, 39,* 575–624.

Wakefield, J. C., & First, M. B. (2003). Clarifying the distinction between disorder and nondisorder: Confronting the overdiagnosis (false-positives) problem in *DSM-V*. In K. A. Phillips, M. B. First, & H. A. Pincus (Eds.), *Advancing DSM: Dilemmas in psychiatric diagnosis* (pp. 23–55). Washington, D.C.: American Psychiatric Publishing.

Wakefield, J. C., Horwitz, A. V., & Schmitz, M. F. (2005). Are we overpathologizing the socially anxious? Social phobia from a harmful dysfunction perspective. *Canadian Journal of Psychiatry, 50,* 317–319.

Wakefield, J. C., Pottick, K. J., & Kirk, S. A. (2002). Should the *DSM-IV* diagnostic criteria for conduct disorder consider social context? *American Journal of Psychiatry, 159,* 380–386.

Ward, C. H., Beck, A. T., Mendelson, M., Mock, J. E., & Erbaugh, J. K. (1962). The psychiatric nomenclature: Reasons for diagnostic disagreement. *Archives of General Psychiatry, 7,* 198–205.

Watson, D. (2005). Rethinking the mood and anxiety disorders: A quantitative hierarchical model for *DSM-V. Journal of Abnormal Psychology, 114,* 522–536.

Watson, D., & Clark, L.A. (2006). Clinical diagnosis at the crossroads. *Clinical Psychology: Science and Practice, 13,* 210–215.

Westen, D. (1997). Divergences between clinical and research methods for assessing personality disorders: Implications for research and the evolution of Axis II. *American Journal of Psychiatry, 154,* 895–903.

Widiger, T. A. (1995). Deletion of the self-defeating and sadistic personality disorder diagnoses. In W. J. Livesley (Ed.), *The DSM-IV personality disorders* (pp. 359–373). New York: Guilford.

Widiger, T. A. (1998). Sex biases in the diagnosis of personality disorders. *Journal of Personality Disorders, 12,* 95–118.

Widiger, T. A. (2001). Official classification systems. In W. J. Livesley (Ed.), *Handbook of personality disorders* (pp. 60–83). New York: Guilford.

Widiger, T. A. (2002). Values, politics, and science in the construction of the *DSM*. In J. Sadler (Ed.), *Descriptions and prescriptions: Values, mental disorders, and the DSM* (pp. 25–41). Baltimore, MD: Johns Hopkins University Press.

Widiger, T. A. (in press). *DSM*'s approach to gender: History and controversies. In K. A. Phillips & M. B. First (Eds.), *A sex research agenda for DSM-V*. Washington, D.C.: American Psychiatric Press.

Widiger, T. A., & Clark, L. A. (2000). Toward *DSM-V* and the classification of psychopathology. *Psychological Bulletin, 126,* 946–963.

Widiger, T. A., & Coker, L. A. (2003). Mental disorders as discrete clinical conditions: Dimensional versus categorical classification. In S. M. Turner & M. Hersen (Eds.), *Adult psychopathology and diagnosis* (4th ed.). New York: John Wiley.

Widiger, T., Frances, A., Pincus, H., Davis, W., & First, M. (1991). Toward an empirical classification for *DSM-IV*. *Journal of Abnormal Psychology, 100,* 280–288.

Widiger, T. A. Frances, A. J., Pincus, H. A., First, M. B., Ross, R. R., & Davis, W. W. (Eds.) (1994). *DSM-IV sourcebook* (Vol. 1). Washington, D.C.: American Psychiatric Publishing.

Widiger, T. A., Frances, A. J., Pincus, H. A., First, M. B., Ross, R. R., & Davis, W. W. (Eds.). (1996). *DSM-IV sourcebook* (Vol. 2). Washington, D.C.: American Psychiatric Publishing.

Widiger, T. A., Frances, A. J., Pincus, H. A., Ross, R. R., First, M. B., & Davis, W. W. (Eds.). (1997). *DSM-IV sourcebook* (Vol. 3). Washington, D.C.: American Psychiatric Publishing.

Widiger, T. A., Frances, A. J., Pincus, H. A., Ross, R., First, M. B., Davis, W. W., & Kline, M. (Eds.). (1998). *DSM-IV Sourcebook* (Vol. 4). Washington, D.C.: American Psychiatric Publishing.

Widiger, T. A., & Samuel, D. B. (2005). Diagnostic categories or dimensions: A question for *DSM-V*. *Journal of Abnormal Psychology, 114.* 494–504.

Widiger, T. A., & Sankis, L. M. (2000). Adult psychopathology: Issues and controversies. *Annual Review of Psychology, 51,* 377–404.

Widiger, T. A., Simonsen, E., Krueger, R., Livesley, J., & Verheul, R. (2005). Personality disorder research agenda for the *DSM-V*. *Journal of Personality Disorders, 19,* 317–340.

Widiger, T. A., & Trull, T. J. (1991). Diagnosis and clinical assessment. *Annual Review of Psychology, 42,* 109–133.

Widiger, T. A., & Trull, T. J. (1993). The scholarly development of *DSM-IV*. In J. A. Costa, E. Silva, & C. C. Nadelson (Eds.), *International review of psychiatry* (Vol. 1, pp. 59–78). Washington, D.C.: American Psychiatric Press.

World Health Organization. (1992). *The ICD-10 classification of mental and behavioural disorders: Clinical descriptions and diagnostic guidelines.* Geneva, Switzerland: Author.

Zahn-Waxler, C. (1993). Warriors and worriers: Gender and psychopathology. *Development and Psychopathology, 5,* 79–89.

Zigler, E., & Phillips, L. (1961). Psychiatric diagnosis: A critique. *Journal of Abnormal and Social Psychology, 63,* 607–618.

Zilboorg, G. (1941). *A history of medical psychology.* New York: W.W. Norton.

Zoccolillo, M. (1993). Gender and the development of conduct disorder. *Development and Psychopathology, 5,* 65–78.

6

Psychological Assessment and Clinical Judgment

Howard N. Garb, Scott O. Lilienfeld, and Katherine A. Fowler

What major advances have occurred in the assessment of psychopathology since the early 1980s? Many psychologists would argue that the most important breakthroughs include the development of explicit diagnostic criteria, the growing popularity of structured interviews, and the proliferation of brief measures tailored for use by mental health professionals conducting empirically supported treatments (e.g., Antony & Barlow, 2002). Others would disagree. Even an advance that most mental health professionals have embraced, the use of explicit criteria for making psychiatric diagnoses, has been challenged (Beutler & Malik, 2002). For example, Weiner (2000) referred to the current *Diagnostic and Statistical Manual of Mental Disorders* (*DSM–IV*; American Psychiatric Association, 1994) as "a psychometrically shaky, inferential nosological scheme involving criteria and definitions that change from one revision to the next" (p. 436; see also Widiger, this volume). Controversies abound in the domain of assessment, and most beginning readers of this literature are left with little guidance regarding how to navigate the murky scientific waters.

In this chapter, we intend to provide such guidance. Specifically, we discuss fundamental conceptual and methodological issues in the assessment of psychopathology, with a particular focus on recent developments and advances. We compare different types of assessment instruments, including structured interviews, brief self-rated and clinician-rated measures, projective techniques, self-report personality inventories, and behavioral assessment and psychophysiological methods. We also review research on the validity of assessment instruments and research on clinical judgment and decision making.

Our principal goal in this chapter is to assist readers with the task of becoming well-informed and discerning consumers of the clinical assessment literature. In particular, we intend to provide readers with the tools necessary to distinguish scientifically supported from unsupported assessment instruments and to make valid judgments on the basis of the former instruments.

Psychometric Principles

Before describing the validity of assessment instruments and research on clinical judgment and decision making, we must first clarify the meaning of three key terms: *reliability, validity,* and *treatment utility* (see also American Educational Research Association, American Psychological Association, & National Council on Measurement in Education [AERA, APA, & NCME], 1999).

Reliability refers to consistency of measurement. It is evaluated in several ways. If all of the items of a test are believed to measure the same trait, we want the test to possess good internal consistency: Test items should be positively intercorrelated. If a test is believed to measure a stable trait, then the test should possess test–retest reliability: on separate administrations of the test, clients should obtain similar scores. Finally, when two or more psychologists make diagnoses or other judgments for the same clients, interrater reliability should be high: Their ratings should tend to agree.

Traditionally, interrater reliability was evaluated by calculating the percentage of cases on which raters agree. For example, two psychologists might agree on diagnoses for 80% of the patients on a unit. However, percentage agreement is unduly affected by base rates. In this context, a *base rate* refers to the prevalence of a disorder. When the base rates of a disorder are high, raters may agree on a large number of cases because of chance. For example, if 80% of the patients on a chronic psychiatric inpatient unit suffer from schizophrenia, then two clinicians who randomly make diagnoses of schizophrenia for 80% of the patients will agree on the diagnosis of schizophrenia for about 64% of the cases (.8 × .8 = .64). Thus, a moderately high level of agreement is obtained even though diagnoses are made arbitrarily. By calculating kappa or an intraclass correlation coefficient (ICC), one can calculate the level of agreement beyond the chance level of agreement. This calculation is accomplished by taking into account the base rates of the disorder being rated.

When interpreting kappa and ICC, one generally uses the following criteria: Interrater reliability is poor for values below .40, fair for values between .40 and .59, good for values between .60 and .74, and excellent for values above .75 (Fleiss, 1981, p. 218). However, these criteria are typically used for making judgments (e.g., diagnoses or predictions of behavior), not for scoring test protocols. For scoring protocols, a reliability coefficient of at least .90 is desirable (Nunnally, 1978, pp. 245–246). Reliability should be higher for scoring tests than for making clinical judgments because if a test cannot be scored reliably, judgments based on those test scores will necessarily have poor reliability.

According to the *Standards for Educational and Psychological Testing* (AERA et al., 1999), *validity* refers to "the degree to which evidence and theory support the interpretations of test scores" (p. 9). Put another way, validity is good if the use of a test allows us to draw accurate inferences about clients (e.g., if the use of test scores helps us to provide correct descriptions of traits, psychopathology, and diagnoses).

Reliability and validity differ in important ways. Reliability refers to the consistency of test scores and judgments; validity refers to the accuracy of interpretations and judgments. When reliability is good, validity can be good or poor. For example, two psychologists can agree on a client's diagnosis, yet both can be wrong. Or a client can obtain the same scores on two administrations of a test, yet inferences made using the test scores may be invalid. In contrast, when reliability is poor, validity is necessarily also poor. For example, if two psychologists cannot agree on a client's diagnosis, at least one of them is not making a valid diagnosis.

Different types of evidence can be obtained to evaluate validity. First, evidence can be based on test content (*content validity*). For example, a measure of a specific anxiety disorder, such as obsessive-compulsive disorder, should include an adequate representation of items to assess the principal features of this disorder, in this case obsessions and compulsions. To ensure content validity, many structured interviews contain questions that inquire comprehensively about the DSM criteria for anxiety disorders and other conditions (e.g., Anxiety Disorders Interview Schedule–IV, ADIS–IV; Brown, Di Nardo, & Barlow, 1994). Second, evidence can be based on the relation between tests. A test should show *moderate or high* correlations with other tests that measure the same attribute or diagnosis (*convergent validity*) and *low* correlations with tests that measure other attributes and diagnoses (*discriminant validity*). When test scores are used to forecast future outcomes, psychologists refer to this as *predictive validity*. When these scores are correlated with indices or events measured at approximately the same time, psychologists refer to this as *concurrent validity*. The validity of an assessment instrument can also be evaluated by examining its internal structure (*structural validity*; see Loevinger, 1957). If a test generates many scores that do not intercorrelate as expected, this result may suggest that inferences based on those test scores are wrong. For example, one problem with the Rorschach Inkblot Test is that scores that are purported to reflect psychopathology are highly correlated with the number of responses produced by clients (Lilienfeld, Wood, & Garb, 2000, p. 34). That is, the more responses a client produces on the Rorschach, the greater the likelihood the client will generate responses that ostensibly indicate the presence of psychopathology. For example, a single Rorschach food response is purportedly indicative of dependent personality traits, but the more overall responses a client produces, the greater the likelihood of the client making a food response.

When we describe the content validity, convergent validity, or structural validity of an assessment instrument, we are also describing its construct validity. A construct is a theoretical variable that cannot be measured perfectly. More specifically, constructs are hypothesized attributes of individuals that cannot be observed directly, such as extraversion or schizophrenia (Cronbach & Meehl, 1955). Construct validity is a broad concept that subsumes content validity, convergent validity, and structural validity.

A number of statistics can be used to evaluate the validity of assessment instruments. Researchers commonly calculate correlations between a test and other measures, including scores on related tests. Other statistics can yield even more useful information. For example, results on sensitivity and specificity are presented routinely in the literature on medical tests, but only infrequently in the literature on psychological assessment (Antony & Barlow, 2002). *Sensitivity* is the likelihood that one will test positive if one has a specified mental disorder. *Specificity* is the likelihood one will test negative if one does not have the specified disorder. Ideally, one attempts to maximize both sensitivity and specificity, although there may be cases in which one elects to emphasize one statistic over the other. For example, if one were attempting to predict suicide in a large group of patients, one would probably be more concerned with sensitivity than specificity. Other important statistics are positive and negative predictive power. *Positive predictive power* describes the likelihood of a disorder given the presence of a particular result on an assessment instrument. *Negative predictive power* describes the likelihood of the absence of a disorder given the absence of the particular result on the assessment instrument.

The concepts of sensitivity, specificity, positive predictive power, and negative predictive power are illustrated in Table 6.1. In this scenario, provisional diagnoses of a mood disorder are made when the *T*-score for Scale 2 (Depression) of the MMPI-2 is ≥65 (the standard cutoff for psychopathology on the MMPI-2).[1] In the sample with a base rate of 50% (50% of the clients are depressed), 500 clients are depressed and 500 clients are not depressed. For the 500 clients who are depressed, 425 have a *T*-score ≥65. Thus, sensitivity is equal to 425/500 = 85.0%. Computations for specificity, positive predictive power, and negative predictive power are also presented in the table.

Depending on the statistic used to evaluate validity, accuracy can vary with the base rate of the behavior being predicted (Meehl & Rosen, 1955; also see Greene, 2000, pp. 365–366). As can be seen from Table 6.1, when percentage correct, positive predictive power, and negative predictive power are used to describe validity, accuracy varies with the base rate. For example, percentage correct is 425 + 350 divided by 1000 = 77.5% when the base rate is 50%, and 17 + 686 divided by 1000 = 70.3% when the base rate is 2%. In contrast, when sensitivity and specificity are used to describe validity, accuracy does not vary with the base rate. Put another way, when percentage correct, positive predictive power, and negative predictive power are used to describe accuracy, the same test will be described as having varying levels of accuracy depending on the base rates in different samples. In general, positive predictive power tends to decrease when base rates decrease, whereas negative predictive power tends to

Table 6.1 Effect of base rate on positive predictive power (PPP), negative predictive power (NPP), sensitivity, and specificity

Base Rate = 50%

Scale 2 (D)	Depressed		Total	PPP	=	425/575	=	73.9%
	Yes	No						
T ≥ 65	425	150	575	NPP	=	350/425	=	82.4%
T < 65	75	350	425	Sensitivity	=	425/500	=	85.0%
Total	500	500	1000	Specificity	=	350/500	=	70.0%

Base Rate=2%

Scale 2 (D)	Depressed		Total	PPP	=	17/311	=	5.0%
	Yes	No						
T ≥ 65	17	294	311	NPP	=	686/689	=	99.6%
T < 65	3	686	689	Sensitivity	=	17/20	=	85.0%
Total	20	980	1000	Specificity	=	686/980	=	70.0%

increase when base rates decrease. Thus, statistically rare events (e.g., suicide) are difficult to predict, whereas common events (e.g., no suicide) are relatively easy to predict.

When reading about positive findings for a test score, psychologists should be aware that the score may not work well in their work setting if the base rate in their work setting differs widely from the base rate in the study. If the base rate for a disorder is .5 in a study but .01 in a clinic, one can expect results for positive predictive power to be much less favorable in the clinic. Nevertheless, a large body of psychological research indicates that psychologists tend to (1) neglect or greatly underuse base rates when making judgments and predictions and (2) focus too heavily on whether a client falls above or below a test's cutoff score (Finn & Kamphuis, 1995). As a consequence, clinicians' judgments can sometimes be grossly inaccurate when the base rates of the phenomenon in question are extreme (e.g., very low).

Signal detection theory (SDT) often provides the most useful information regarding the validity of an assessment instrument. SDT is a statistical approach that is used when the task is to detect a signal, such as the presence of major depression in a client. By using SDT, we can describe the validity of an assessment instrument across all base rates and across all cutoff scores (the signal is said to be present when a client's score exceeds the cutoff score). Different clinicians may set different cutoff scores for the same test; it is important that our estimate of the validity of a test not be influenced by the placement of the cutoff score. As observed by McFall and Treat (1999): "There is no longer any excuse for continuing to conduct business as usual, now that SDT-based indices represent a clear and significant advance over traditional accuracy indices such as sensitivity, specificity, and predictive power" (p. 227). Although such indices as sensitivity, specificity, and predictive power are informative, we agree with McFall and Treat that in many cases the use of SDT is more appropriate and comprehensive.

Other important psychometric concepts are norms, incremental validity, and treatment utility. *Norms* are scores that provide a frame of reference for interpreting a client's results. For the assessment of psychopathology, normative data can be collected by administering a test to a representative sample of individuals in the community. If a client's responses are similar to the normative data, psychologists should be very cautious about inferring the presence of psychopathology. When norms for a test do not accurately reflect the population of interest, clinicians may make inaccurate and potentially harmful judgments even if the test is valid. For example, a test may be a good measure of thought disorder, but a clinician interpreting a client's test results may erroneously conclude that the client has a thought disorder if the norms give a false impression of how people in the community do on the test. Historically, problems with norms have been as serious as, if not more serious than, problems with validity (Wood, Garb, & Nezworski, 2007).

Incremental validity describes the extent to which an instrument contributes information above and beyond already available information (e.g., other measures). For example, the use of a psychological test may allow clinicians to make judgments at a level better than chance, but judgments made using interview and test information may not be more accurate than judgments based on interview information only. One major criticism of the Rorschach Inkblot Test is that it does not provide useful information beyond that which can be obtained using more easily administered instruments, such as questionnaires (Lilienfeld et al., 2000).

Treatment utility describes the extent to which an assessment instrument contributes to decisions about treatment that lead to better outcomes. An assessment instrument could have good validity and good incremental validity, yet not lead to improved treatment outcome. Surprisingly, few researchers have examined the treatment utility of assessment instruments (Harkness & Lilienfeld, 1997).

Assessment Instruments

Interviews

Unstructured interviews are used predominantly in clinical practice, whereas structured and semistructured interviews are used predominantly in research. One exception is that structured and semistructured interviews are used for clinical care in a growing number of university-based clinics. When conducting an *unstructured interview*, a psychologist is responsible for deciding what questions to ask. In contrast, when conducting a *structured interview*, questions are standardized. As one might surmise, *semistructured interviews* represent a balance between structured and unstructured interviews, providing guidance for interviewers but affording them some flexibility.

Reliability The interrater reliability of unstructured interviews is generally good as long as a clinician attends to diagnostic criteria (Garb, 1998, pp. 41–42). For example, acceptable levels of interrater reliability were obtained for many, but not all, diagnostic categories in the *DSM–III* (American Psychiatric Association, 1980, pp. 470–471) field trials and in the field trials for the 10th revision of the *International Classification of Diseases* (World Health Organization, *ICD–10*; Sartorius et al., 1993). However, clinicians who participated in the *DSM–III* and *ICD–10* field trials were familiar with, and presumably adhered to, the diagnostic criteria. Other studies indicate that many mental health professionals do not attend to criteria when making diagnoses, but instead make diagnoses by comparing patients with their concept of the typical person with a given mental disorder (e.g., Blashfield & Herkov, 1996; Garb, 1996; Morey & Ochoa, 1989). When psychologists do not adhere to diagnostic criteria, interrater reliability is often poor.

The use of semistructured and structured interviews tends to lead to both good adherence to diagnostic criteria and good interrater reliability (Antony & Barlow, 2002; Rogers, 1995). For example, the *Anxiety Disorders Interview Schedule for DSM-IV* (ADIS–IV; Brown et al., 1994) requires interviewers to inquire about the *DSM–IV* criteria for anxiety disorders. Favorable reliability results have been found for this instrument: kappa values have ranged from .67 to .86 for diagnoses of the *DSM–IV* anxiety disorders (Brown, Di Nardo, Lehman, & Campbell, 2001).

Validity Some psychologists have argued that diagnoses should not be made using the DSM criteria. For example, as already noted, Weiner (2000) argued that the DSM criteria are questionable, in part because they are inconsistent across editions of the manual. However, virtually all mental disorders are *open concepts* marked by (1) intrinsically fuzzy boundaries; (2) an indicator list that is potentially infinite; and (3) an unclear inner nature (Meehl, 1986). Although diagnostic criteria sometimes change in response to changing social norms and political pressures, they more often change as more is learned about a disorder. For example, we may eventually learn that certain individuals who meet the *DSM–IV* criteria for schizophrenia actually have disorders that have not yet been identified. Still, the construct of schizophrenia can be useful even though we are aware that the meaning of the term is somewhat imprecise and will change as more research is conducted. *DSM* diagnoses can be valid and useful even when we possess an incomplete understanding of the nature, etiology, course, and treatment of the conditions categorized.

As already noted, structured and semistructured interviews are used routinely in research. When important discoveries are made about the nature, etiology, course, or treatment of a disorder, they support the validity of the instruments used in the studies. For example, if a structured interview is used to select participants for a study on treatment outcome and the treatment intervention is found to be effective, one can infer that a client who obtains a specific diagnosis on the structured interview is likely to respond to the treatment. Thus, the bulk of the evidence on validity that supports structured and semistructured interviews derives from studies on psychopathology and treatment outcome. Similarly, evidence that supports the validity of the *DSM* criteria supports the validity of assessment instruments that help to determine if a participant satisfies those criteria. Because there is no "gold standard" for evaluating the validity of structured interviews (Faraone & Tsuang, 1994) or other assessment measures in psychopathology research, validity is established by evaluating "the degree to which evidence and theory support the interpretations of test scores" (AERA et al., 1999, p. 9).

There are several reasons to believe that structured interviews are more valid than unstructured interviews, at least when clinicians conducting unstructured interviews do not adhere to diagnostic criteria. First, interrater reliability tends to be better for structured and semistructured interviews, so, all things being equal, they are more likely to be valid. Second, many structured interviews are designed to inquire comprehensively about the *DSM* criteria. To the extent that the *DSM* criteria have been validated, the validity of these structured and semistructured interviews will be supported. Third, when interviews and self-report instruments are used to diagnose personality disorders, clinicians using unstructured interviews typically show the lowest agreement with other assessment instruments. In his review of the literature, Widiger (2002) noted that "the worst median convergent validity coefficient was obtained in the only study to have used unstructured interviews by practicing clinicians" (p. 463).

Additional evidence raises questions about the validity of diagnoses made by many practicing clinicians. Agreement between structured interview diagnoses and diagnoses made in clinical practice is generally poor (e.g., Brockington, Kendell, & Leff, 1978; Molinari, Ames, & Essa, 1994; Steiner, Tebes, Sledge, & Walker, 1995). For example, in one study (Steiner et al., 1995), clinical diagnoses made for 100 patients were compared with diagnoses made by research investigators using a structured interview. An overall weighted kappa coefficient indicated that agreement between the two interview methods was poor (kappa = .25). Values for kappa are typically higher when one structured interview is compared with another, although to a surprising degree this issue has not been studied for some widely used interviews (Rogers, 1995). Thus, based on the available evidence, one *cannot* argue that it makes little difference whether one conducts an unstructured or structured interview.

Although structured interviews generally appear to be more valid than unstructured interviews, their limitations need to be recognized. Because these limitations are shared with unstructured interviews, they do not indicate that unstructured interviews possess advantages over structured interviews. First, it is relatively easy for respondents to consciously underreport or overreport psychopathology on structured interviews (Alterman et al., 1996). Moreover, few structured interviews contain validity scales designed to detect dishonest or otherwise aberrant responding. Second, because memory is fallible, reports in interviews are often inaccurate or incomplete, even when clients are not intentionally trying to deceive the interviewer (Henry, Moffitt, Caspi, Langley, & Silva, 1994). Third, when clinicians are instructed to make use of medical records and other information in addition to structured interviews, considerable clinical judgment is required to describe and diagnose the client because information from different sources may conflict. This requirement is a potential limitation because clinical judgment is fallible.

Finally, an important methodological advance in evaluating the validity of interviews is the LEAD standard. LEAD is an acronym for *longitudinal, expert*, and *all data*. When using the LEAD standard (Spitzer, 1983), diagnoses made by using interviews are compared with diagnoses made by collecting longitudinal data. Using this approach, clients are followed over time to provide longitudinal data for making diagnoses, and diagnoses are made by expert clinicians using all relevant data. Although the LEAD standard can help us learn about the validity of diagnoses, it has rarely been used. Using this approach, one can more accurately evaluate the validity of diagnoses based on unstructured, structured, or semistructured interviews.

Brief Self-Rated and Clinician-Rated Measures

Brief measures have been developed for (1) monitoring psychotherapy progress and (2) providing information necessary to deliver standardized evidence-based interventions. To an extent seldom found for other assessment instruments, treatment utility has been established for measures used to monitor psychotherapy progress.

A number of systems have been developed for monitoring psychotherapy progress, and in particular for identifying clients who have made little or no progress during psychotherapy and who are at risk for deteriorating. For example, research suggests that it can be helpful to administer the Outcome Questionnaire-45 (OQ-45; Lambert & Finch, 1999) to clients prior to every session. The OQ-45 takes about five to seven minutes to complete, and it measures constructs related to level of functioning including: (1) distress and symptoms; (2) interpersonal problems; and (3) problems related to social role performance. Normative data have been collected, making it possible to identify clients who have made less progress than 95% of the clients who obtained the same initial OQ-45 score (Lambert et al., 2005). Results obtained in Germany and the United States demonstrate that clients tend to have better outcomes when therapists are alerted to poorly progressing clients (e.g., Lambert et al., 2003; Percevic, Lambert, & Kordy, 2004). For example, for clients identified as being at risk, deterioration rates decreased from 21 to 13% when therapists were provided with feedback information (Lambert et al., 2003).

A second major use of brief measures can be described: brief self-rated and clinician-rated measures have been constructed to provide information necessary to deliver standardized, evidence-based interventions. For example, the Beck Depression Inventory–II, the Beck Anxiety Scale, and other scales are frequently used to assess depression and anxiety (Beck & Steer, 1990; Beck, Steer, & Brown, 1996). In addition, psychologists who use cognitive behavioral techniques to treat panic disorder frequently use brief measures to describe (1) the severity and frequency of panic-related symptoms; (2) cognitions or beliefs that are frequently associated with panic disorder; (3) clients' perceptions of their control over threatening internal situations; and (4) panic-related avoidance behaviors (e.g., Baker, Patterson, & Barlow, 2002). Because psychologists who use cognitive behavioral techniques are not usually concerned with measuring broad areas of psychopathology and personality, brief self-rated and clinician-rated measures are typically best suited for their needs.

The reliability and validity of many of these measures appears to be adequate. For example, the Panic Disorder Severity Scale (PDSS; Shear et al., 1997) is a seven-item scale that can be completed by either clients or clinicians to describe key features of panic disorder with agoraphobia. When completed by a clinician, the ratings are based on information that has been gathered in interview and therapy sessions. Ratings are made for frequency of panic, anxiety about future panic attacks, magnitude of distress during panic, interference in social functioning, interference in work functioning, and avoidance behaviors. The PDSS possesses excellent interrater reliability (kappa = .87; Shear et al., 1997). In addition, PDSS ratings are correlated significantly with other measures of features of panic disorder. For example, Shear et al. (1997) obtained a correlation of $r = .55$ for the relation between total scores on the PDSS and severity ratings for panic disorder on the ADIS–IV. Equally important is evidence related to the content of the scale items: The PDSS was designed to assess problems that are important for treatment planning. In fact, a reason that brief self-rated and clinician-rated measures are popular is that they evaluate dimensions believed to be important for treatment planning. That is, they are designed to (1) evaluate problems that need to be addressed in treatment and (2) provide information that is required to implement empirically based treatment interventions. Finally, the PDSS can be used to track a client's progress. This use bears important implications for treatment use. For example, if the measure is administered during the course of treatment and indicates that a client is not improving, the clinician should consider trying a different intervention. In one study (Shear et al., 1997), clients were classified as treatment responders and nonresponders on the basis of ratings made by independent evaluators. A different group of evaluators made PDSS ratings for all clients before and after treatment. In contrast to nonresponders, responders showed statistically significant improvement on the PDSS.

Although reliability and validity appear to be fair for many self-rated and clinician-rated measures, the evaluation of their validity has been limited. Rather than compare the results from one of these measures with the results of a structured interview or with another self-rated or clinician-rated measure, it would be helpful to use behavioral assessment methods to evaluate validity. This approach has rarely been used, but the results from one study are provocative. When behavioral assessment methods were used to evaluate the validity of clients' statements, clients were found to overestimate the frequency and intensity of their panic attacks on a structured interview and on a brief self-rated test (Margraf, Taylor, Ehlers, Roth, & Agras, 1987).

Behavioral Assessment Methods and Psychophysiological Assessment

Behavioral assessment methods and psychophysiological assessment can provide valuable information. For example, by using diary measures, one can ask a client to record and rate the frequency and intensity of panic attacks shortly after symptoms occur. Or one can monitor a client's eating or smoking habits. By making ratings shortly after symptoms or behaviors occur, the results are more likely to be accurate than when based on retrospective reports. The increased accessibility of palm-sized computers may eventually render it easier to collect and analyze self-monitoring data (data describing clients' ongoing behavior recorded by the clients themselves).

Behavioral assessment tests and other behavioral observation techniques can also provide valuable information. Behavioral assessment tests (also known as behavioral approach tests and behavioral avoidance tests) involve asking clients to enter situations that typically make them anxious, that they avoid, or both. For example, a client with a phobia can be instructed to approach a feared object (e.g., a spider) and a client with an obsessive-compulsive disorder can be instructed to switch off an electrical appliance and leave the room without checking it. During and after behavioral assessment tests, clients rate their level of anxiety. Other techniques include observing clients in role-play situations and in natural settings (without their being instructed to confront feared situations). For example, observations can be made of children in classrooms or of patients on psychiatric units.

Psychophysiological techniques can also provide valuable information. For example, a polysomnographic evaluation, which is conducted in a sleep lab, can provide valuable information about how well a client is sleeping (Savard & Morin, 2002). Similarly, measures of psychophysiological arousal can provide important information in the assessment of posttraumatic stress disorder, especially with respect to treatment process and outcome (Litz, Miller, Ruef, & McTeague, 2002). One team of investigators found that by playing a tape of combat sounds and measuring participants' heart rates, systolic blood pressure, and muscle tension with a forehead electromyogram, combat veterans with posttraumatic stress disorder could be discriminated from other veterans with 95.5% accuracy (Blanchard, Kolb, Pallmeyer, & Gerardi, 1982). Nevertheless, it will be important to cross-validate these findings in an independent sample. Because the psychophysiological assessment of other disorders has been confined largely to the laboratory, the extent to which these findings generalize to naturalistic settings remains unclear.

Global Measures of Personality and Psychopathology

Projective techniques and self-report personality inventories are designed to measure broad aspects of personality and psychopathology. Projective techniques include the Rorschach, Thematic Apperception Test (TAT), and human figure drawings. Self-report personality inventories include the Minnesota Multiphasic Personality Inventory–2 (MMPI–2; Butcher, Dahlstrom, Graham, Tellegen, & Kaemmer, 1989), the Personality Assessment Inventory (PAI; Morey, 1991), and the Millon Clinical Multiaxial Inventory–III (MCMI–III; Millon, 1994). Projective techniques are relatively unstructured: Stimuli are frequently ambiguous (e.g., inkblots, as in the case of the Rorschach) and response formats are typically open-ended (e.g., telling a story in response to a drawing of individuals interacting, as in the case of the TAT). In contrast, self-report personality inventories are relatively structured: Stimuli are fairly clear-cut (e.g., statements with which a client agrees or disagrees) and response formats are constrained (e.g., on the MMPI–2, one can make a response of "true" or "false"). In general, validity findings are more encouraging for self-report personality inventories than for projective techniques, although exceptions have been found (see Lilienfeld et al., 2000; Wood, Nezworski, Lilienfeld, & Garb, 2003).

Projective Techniques A common argument for using projective techniques is that they can circumvent a client's purported defenses and therefore can be used to evaluate conscious and unconscious processes. For example, some psychologists believe that when clients look at Rorschach inkblots and report what they see, they cannot invent faked responses because they do not know the true meaning of their Rorschach responses. However, research demonstrates that projective techniques are vulnerable to faking. For example, in one study (Albert, Fox, & Kahn, 1980), normal participants were instructed to fake paranoid schizophrenia. Presumed experts in the use of the Rorschach (Fellows of the Society for Personality Assessment) were unable to detect faking of psychosis. Diagnoses of malingering were made for 4% of the psychotic participants, 9% of the informed fakers (they were informed about the nature of disturbed thought processes and paranoid schizophrenia, but not about the Rorschach), 7% of uninformed fakers, and 2% of normal participants who were not instructed to fake. Diagnoses of psychosis were made for 48% of the psychotic participants, 72% of the informed fakers, 46% of the uninformed fakers, and 24% of the normal participants who were not instructed to fake.

A problem with many projective techniques is that they are difficult to score.[2] For example, the Comprehensive System (CS; Exner, 1993) is the most popular system for scoring the Rorschach. Exner (1993, p. 23), the developer of the CS, claimed that interrater reliability is better than .85 for all CS scores. However, results from other studies indicate that this result is true for only about half of the CS scores (Acklin, McDowell, Verschell, & Chan, 2000; Nakata, 1999; Shaffer, Erdberg, & Haroian, 1999; but see Meyer et al., 2002). Furthermore, in one study (Guarnaccia, Dill, Sabatino, & Southwick, 2001), average scoring accuracy was only about 65%. In comparison, scoring is typically excellent for other types of tests (e.g., intelligence tests and personality inventories). For example, interrater reliability coefficients for the scoring of the Wechsler Adult Intelligence Scale, Third Edition (WAIS–III) have a median value of .95 and a minimum value of .90. Reliability for scoring the MMPI–2 is often better than for the WAIS.

Another problem with projective techniques is that psychologists rarely use normative data when interpreting TAT protocols and human figure drawings, even though the availability of normative data can help to prevent the overperception of psychopathology. Furthermore, serious problems have surfaced regarding the normative data for the Rorschach. Exner (2001b) reported that his 1993 CS adult normative sample contained an error of enormous magnitude: The sample was described as being composed of 700 distinct protocols but it actually contained 479 distinct protocols with 221 protocols counted twice. Subsequently, the CS adult normative sample has been revised (Exner, 2001b), but even this sample has been reported to contain errors (Meyer & Richardson, 2001). Moreover, Exner (personal communication, December 8, 2000) refused to make the current CS adult normative sample available for examination, even though J. M. Wood, a prominent critic of the CS, offered to pay for any expenses that this would incur (J. M. Wood, personal communication, August 5, 2000).[3] Finally, and most important, the use of the CS norms is likely to lead to the overperception of psychopathology (Hamel, Shaffer, & Erdberg, 2000; Shaffer et al., 1999; Wood, Nezworski, Garb, & Lilienfeld, 2001b; also see Aronow, 2001; Exner, 2001a; Hunsley & Di Giulio, 2001; Meyer, 2001; Widiger, 2001; Wood, Nezworski, Garb, & Lilienfeld, 2001a). For example, in one study (Hamel et al., 2000), the Rorschach was administered to a group of 100 relatively normal school children. Children were excluded from the study if they had a history of mental disorder. Even though an independent measure (the Conners Parent Rating Scale–92; Conners, 1989) revealed that the children were healthier than average, the results for the Rorschach indicated that the typical child in the sample suffered from "a distortion of reality and faulty reasoning approaching psychosis" and "an affective disorder that includes many of the markers found in clinical depression" (p. 291).

The evidence for the construct validity of most projective techniques is at best mixed. In several meta-analyses, effect sizes for the Rorschach have ranged from $d=.25$ to .35, indicating that some positive findings have been reported (e.g., Garb, Florio, & Grove, 1998; Hiller, Rosenthal, Bornstein, Berry, & Brunell-Neuleib, 1999; Meyer & Archer, 2001; Parker, Hanson, & Hunsley, 1988). However, positive validity findings for the Rorschach, TAT, and human figure drawings have rarely been independently replicated (Lilienfeld et al., 2000).

The following criteria for evaluating construct validity were proposed by Wood, Nezworski, and Stejskal (1996b): (1) test scores should demonstrate a consistent relation to a particular symptom, trait, or disorder; (2) results must be obtained in methodologically rigorous studies; and (3) results must be replicated by independent investigators. Few scores for the Rorschach, TAT, and human figure drawings satisfy these criteria. For the Rorschach, the criteria have been satisfied for scores intended to detect thought disorder and psychotic conditions marked by thought disorder (e.g., schizophrenia), predict psychotherapy outcome, and assess behaviors related to dependency (e.g., Acklin, 1999; Bornstein, 1999; Jorgensen, Andersen, & Dam, 2000; Meyer & Handler, 1997). For the TAT, the criteria have been satisfied for the assessment of achievement motives, the identification of child sexual abuse history, and the detection of borderline personality disorder (Spangler, 1992; Westen, Lohr, Silk, Gold, & Kerber, 1990; Westen, Ludolph, Block, Wixom, & Wiss, 1990). For human figure drawings, the criteria have been satisfied only for distinguishing global psychopathology from normality (Naglieri & Pfeiffer, 1992). Ironically, over half of the indexes that have been empirically supported are rarely used by psychologists in clinical practice. Some of these indexes are difficult to score, whereas others were not incorporated into Exner's Comprehensive System—the Rorschach scoring system that most clinicians use.

Most projective indexes, including those used widely in clinical practice, have received relatively little empirical support. In commenting on the CS, Meyer and Archer (2001) offered a related observation:

> Yet many variables given fairly substantial interpretive emphasis have received little or no attention (Weiner, 2001). These include the Coping Deficit Index, Obsessive Style Index, Hypervigilance

Index, active-to-passive movement ratio, D-*score, food content, anatomy and X-ray content, Intellectualization Index, and Isolation Index.* (p. 496)

Moreover, in a comprehensive review of research on the relation between Rorschach scores and psychiatric diagnoses (Wood, Lilienfeld, Garb, Nezworski, 2000), Rorschach scores did not show a well-demonstrated relationship to major depressive disorder, posttraumatic stress disorder (PTSD), anxiety disorders other than PTSD, dissociative identity disorder, conduct disorder, psychopathy, or personality disorders. Despite these negative findings, the Rorschach continues to be used by psychologists for the diagnosis of these disorders. Similarly, although the Rorschach and human figure drawings are sometimes used by mental health professionals to help decide whether a child has been sexually abused (Oberlander, 1995), their use for this task has not been consistently supported (e.g., Garb, Wood, & Nezworski, 2000; Trowbridge, 1995).

Personality Inventories Self-report personality inventories require clients to indicate whether a statement describes them. However, contrary to widespread claims, self-report personality inventories do not require clients to be able to accurately describe their symptoms and personality traits. The "dynamics" of self-report personality inventories were described by Meehl (1945):

> *A self-rating constitutes an intrinsically interesting and significant bit of verbal behavior, the non-test correlates of which* must be discovered by empirical means. [The approach is free] from the restriction that the subject must be able to describe his own behavior accurately…. The selection of items is done on a thoroughly empirical basis using carefully *selected criterion groups.* (p. 297)

Thus, whereas the validity of brief self-rated tests rests on the content of items, the validity of self-report personality inventories rests on empirical research that relates test items (and test scales) to client characteristics. This approach has met with some success. For example, results from a meta-analysis indicate that the MMPI can be useful for detecting overreporting and underreporting of psychopathology (Berry, Baer, & Harris, 1991).

Scientific support for personality inventories has been mixed. One positive feature is that psychologists who use self-report personality inventories almost always use norms. Also, the norms of major self-report personality inventories, such as the MMPI-2, are representative of American adults or adolescents in the community. There is no evidence that these norms make relatively normal individuals appear pathological.

In contrast, the validity of the primary scales of some tests (e.g., the MMPI-2, the Personality Assessment Inventory) has generally been supported, whereas the validity evidence for the scales of other widely used tests (e.g., the Millon Clinical Multiaxial Inventory–III; MCMI–III) is weaker and less consistent. For example, Rogers, Salekin, and Sewell (1999) reviewed the research on the MCMI–III and concluded that it should not be used in forensic settings (also see Dyer & McCann, 2000; Rogers, Salekin, & Sewell, 2000). Even for the MMPI-2, half of the supplementary scales have not been consistently supported (e.g., Greene, 2000, pp. 218–269). Despite these negative findings, positive results on validity have been consistently replicated by independent investigators for a large number of MMPI-2 scores. For example, research has demonstrated that Scale 4 (Psychopathic Deviate) is correlated positively with criminal behaviors and recidivism risk (see Greene, 2000, p. 148), whereas Scale 9 (Hypomania) is correlated with such characteristics as impulsiveness, extraversion, and superficiality in social relationships (e.g., Graham, Ben-Porath, & McNulty, 1997). In clinical judgment studies, judgments have been more valid when psychologists have been given results from personality inventories than when given results from projective techniques (e.g., Garb, 1989, 1998, 2003). In fact, in several studies, validity actually decreased, at least slightly, when Rorschach results were made available in addition to brief biographical or questionnaire results (e.g., Whitehead, 1985).

On the negative side, evidence for the utility of personality inventories in treatment planning is scarce, and the *very* little evidence that exists has not been supportive. Specifically, when researchers have used manipulated assessment designs to randomly assign some clinicians to receive specific assessment information (e.g., the MMPI-2), and others to not receive such information, they have not detected significant differences in treatment outcome (Lima et al., 2005). Therapists in this study were 25 doctoral students in clinical psychology who each received about three to five hours per week of supervision with a licensed clinical psychologist.

Clinical Judgment and Decision Making

When confronted with evidence regarding the poor validity of specific assessment instruments, such as projective techniques, some clinicians retort that their extensive clinical experience permits them to extract useful inferences from these instruments. In other words, the argument goes, validation studies fail to capture the rich and subtle information that highly seasoned practitioners can obtain from certain assessment measures. For example, in response to review articles demonstrating that a mere handful of Rorschach variables are empirically supported (e.g., Lilienfeld et al., 2000, 2001), several practitioners on messages to the Rorschach Discussion and Information Group maintained that the negative research evidence was largely irrelevant because their numerous years of clinical experience with the Rorschach endowed them with special judgmental and predictive powers.

Experience, Training, and Clinical Judgment

Nevertheless, the above arguments do not withstand careful scrutiny, because the relation between clinical experience and judgmental accuracy has been weak in most studies of personality and psychopathology assessment (Dawes, 1994). For example, when given MMPI (e.g., Graham, 1967) or Rorschach (e.g., Turner, 1966) protocols, clinicians did not produce more valid ratings of psychopathology or personality than did psychology graduate students (see Garb, 1989, 1998, for reviews). Nor is there evidence that presumed experts on certain personality measures outperform other clinicians. In one striking example, Levenberg (1975) asked clinicians to identify children as either normal or abnormal on the basis of their protocols on the Kinetic Family Drawing test, a commonly used human figure drawing measure. Whereas a group of doctoral-level psychologists was correct for 72% of cases, the author of two books on the Kinetic Family Drawing test was correct for only 47% of cases (see also Turner, 1966, for similar findings on the Rorschach).

One potential exception to the finding that experience and accuracy are negligibly related was reported in a study by Brammer (2002). To help them make diagnoses, psychologists and psychology graduate students were allowed to ask questions and ask for specific items of information. Number of years of clinician experience was significantly associated with the number of correct diagnoses made ($r = .33$), as well as with the number of diagnostically specific questions asked ($r = .51$). Brammer's findings raise the intriguing possibility that experience is related to validity on tasks that require clinicians to structure complex tasks, such as formulating a psychiatric diagnosis by honing in on potential problem areas and then asking progressively more specific questions (see also Clavelle & Turner, 1980).

Some clinicians could contend that although the overall relation between experience and accuracy tends to be weak, many clinicians in real world settings know which of their judgments are likely to be accurate. Nevertheless, for the use of projective techniques and some other assessment instruments, the relation between the validity of clinicians' judgments and their confidence in these judgments is generally weak. For example, Albert et al. (1980) found no significant relation between validity and confidence when practitioners were asked to use Rorschach protocols to detect malingering. For the MMPI, there is some evidence that confidence is positively related to the validity of clinicians' judgments, but only when these judgments are reasonably valid (e.g., Goldberg, 1965). That is, when psychologists use the MMPI to assist in making diagnoses, they tend to be able to state correctly which of their diagnostic judgments are most likely to be correct.

In contrast to the dispiriting findings concerning the value of clinical experience for personality assessment judgments, the research literature supports the value of training on certain assessment instruments. For example, in several studies psychologists using MMPI protocols made more valid personality judgments than did lay judges (e.g., Aronson & Akamatsu, 1981; see Garb, 1989, for a review). Nevertheless, research does not support the value of training in the interpretation of projective protocols. For example, in one study (Gadol, 1969), clinical psychologists and undergraduates were equally accurate when asked to make personality ratings of psychiatric patients on the basis of Rorschach protocols. Similar findings emerged when psychologists were compared with lay judges in their ability to distinguish psychopathology from normality on the basis of human figure drawings or sentence completion tests (see Garb, 1989, for a review).

Why Clinicians Often Do Not Benefit from Experience

Why are practitioners often unable to benefit from clinical experience? Although the reasons are manifold (Arkes, 1981; Dawes, Faust, & Meehl, 1989; Garb, 1989), we focus on six here. The first three concern the nature of the feedback available to clinicians, and the remaining three reasons concern cognitive processes that influence the selection and interpretation of this feedback.

Nature of Feedback   First, in contrast to physicians in most domains of organic medicine, psychologists rarely receive clear-cut feedback concerning their judgments and predictions (Meehl, 1973). Instead, the feedback psychologists receive is often vague, ambiguous, and open to multiple interpretations. For example, if a clinician concludes that an adult client was sexually abused in childhood on the basis of an unstructured interview and Rorschach protocol, this judgment is difficult to falsify. If the client were to deny a past abuse history or express uncertainty about it, the clinician could readily maintain that the interpretation may still be correct because the client may have forgotten or repressed the abuse (although the scientific evidence for repression is controversial; see Holmes, 1990). Moreover, when clinicians receive feedback regarding their predictions (e.g., forecasts of violence), it is often substantially delayed, thereby introducing the potential distorting effects of memory.

Second, clinicians typically have access to only a subset of the data needed for accurate judgments, a quandary referred to by Gilovich (1991) as the "missing data problem." For example, clinicians may perceive certain psychological conditions (e.g., nicotine dependence) to be more chronic and unremitting than they are (Schachter, 1982) because they are selectively exposed to individuals who remain in treatment. Cohen and Cohen (1984) referred to this effect as the "clinician's illusion."

Third, some feedback that clinicians receive from clients is misleading. Meehl (1956) referred to an individual's tendency to accept highly generalized but nonobvious personality descriptions as the *P. T. Barnum effect*, after the circus entrepreneur who quipped that "I like to give a little something to everybody" and "A sucker is born every minute." Numerous studies demonstrate that most individuals presented with Barnum descriptions (e.g., "You have a great deal of unused potential"; "At times you have difficulty making up your mind") find such descriptions to be highly compelling, particularly when they believe that these descriptions were tailored for them (Logue, Sher, & Frensch, 1992; Snyder & Larson, 1972). The P. T. Barnum effect demonstrates that personal validation, the informal method of validating test feedback by relying on respondents' acceptance of this feedback, is a highly fallible barometer of actual validity. In addition, because clients are often impressed by Barnum feedback, such feedback can fool clinicians into believing that their interpretations are more valid than they really are. The same process can also explain why astrologers and palm readers are often confident that their interpretations are accurate (see Wood, Nezworski, Lilienfeld, & Garb, 2003).

Cognitive Processes Fourth, a substantial body of literature documents the issue that individuals are prone to *confirmatory bias*; that is, the tendency to selectively seek out and recall information consistent with one's hypotheses and to neglect information inconsistent with these hypotheses. Several investigators have found that clinicians fall prey to confirmatory bias when asked to recall information regarding clients. For example, Strohmer, Shivy, and Chiodo (1990) asked counselors to read three versions of a case history of a client, one containing an equal number of descriptors indicating good self-control and poor self-control, one containing more descriptors indicating good control than poor self-control, and one containing more descriptors indicating poor than good self-control. One week after reading this case history, psychotherapists were asked to offer as many factors they could remember that "would be helpful in determining whether or not [the client] lacked self-control" (p. 467). Therapists offered more information that would be helpful for confirming than disconfirming the hypothesis that the client lacked self-control, even in the condition in which the client was described as characterized primarily by good self-control descriptors.

There also is evidence that clinicians are sometimes prone to *premature closure* in diagnostic decision making: they may tend to reach conclusions too quickly (Garb, 1998). For example, Gauron and Dickinson (1969) reported that psychiatrists who observed a videotaped interview frequently formed diagnostic impressions within 30 to 60 seconds. Premature closure may both reflect and produce confirmatory bias. It may reflect confirmatory bias because clinicians may reach rapid conclusions by searching only for data that confirm preexisting hypotheses. It may produce confirmatory bias by effectively halting the search for data that could disconfirm such hypotheses.

Fifth, investigators have shown that clinicians, like all individuals, are prone to *illusory correlations*, which has generally been defined as the perception of (1) a statistical association that does not actually exist or (2) a stronger statistical association than is actually present. Illusory correlations are likely to arise when individuals hold powerful a priori expectations regarding the covariation between certain events or stimuli. For example, many individuals are convinced that a strong correlation exists between the full moon and psychiatric hospital admissions, even though studies have demonstrated repeatedly that no such association exists (Rotton & Kelly, 1985).

In a classic study of illusory correlation, Chapman and Chapman (1967) examined why psychologists perceive clinically meaningful associations between signs on the Draw-A-Person (DAP) test (e.g., the drawing of large eyes) and psychiatric symptoms (e.g., suspiciousness) even though research has demonstrated that these associations do not exist (Kahill, 1984). They presented undergraduate participants with DAP protocols that were purportedly produced by psychiatric patients with certain psychiatric symptoms (e.g., suspiciousness). Each drawing was paired randomly with two of these symptoms, which were listed on the bottom of each drawing. Undergraduates were asked to inspect these drawings and estimate the extent to which certain DAP signs co-occurred with these symptoms. Chapman and Chapman found that participants "discovered" that certain DAP signs tended to consistently co-occur with certain psychiatric symptoms, even though the DAP signs and symptoms had been randomly paired. For example, participants mistakenly perceived large eyes in drawings as co-occurring with suspiciousness and broad shoulders in drawings as co-occurring with doubts about manliness. Interestingly, these are the same associations that tend to be perceived by clinicians who use the DAP (Chapman & Chapman, 1967). Illusory correlation has been demonstrated with other projective techniques, including the Rorschach (Chapman & Chapman, 1969) and sentence completion tests (Starr & Katkin, 1969). Scientifically minded practitioners need to be aware of the phenomenon of illusory correlation, which suggests that clinicians can be convinced of the validity of assessment indicators in the absence of validity.

Finally, it can be difficult to learn from clinical experience unless one thinks in probabilistic terms (Einhorn, 1988). Unfortunately, this skill can be very difficult to acquire. For example, individuals tend to overestimate the likelihood that they would have predicted an outcome after they have become aware of the outcome, an effect termed *hindsight bias* (Arkes, Faust, Guilmette, & Hart, 1988; Fischhoff, 1975). Thus, if a client commits suicide and an investigation is conducted, the investigators may conclude that the suicide could have been predicted—in part because of hindsight bias. Similarly, when asked to rate the likelihood of (1) one event occurring and (2) the same event plus another event occurring, individuals will often give a higher rating for the likelihood of both events occurring, an effect termed *conjunction bias* (Garb, 2006; Tversky & Kahneman, 1983). For example, for a particular client, if one diagnosis seems likely (e.g., major depressive disorder) and another diagnosis seems unlikely (e.g., antisocial personality disorder), then some clinicians may believe the likelihood of a client having both diagnoses is greater than the likelihood of the client having only the less likely disorder. However, according to probability theory, the probability of events A and B, $P(A \cap B)$, cannot be greater than the probability of event A, $P(A)$, or the probability of event B, $P(B)$. Because clinicians do not naturally think probabilistically, they sometimes engage in deterministic reasoning. Every clinician can generate explanations for why a client behaves a particular way or has a particular disorder, but these explanations may not be correct. Clinicians do not necessarily have complete information about every client and some of the information they do have is likely to contain error. For this reason, we should not unquestioningly accept a theory or case formulation simply because it seems compelling and seems to explain all of the available information.

Group Biases in Judgment   A large number of studies have examined biases related to the demographic characteristics of clients (e.g., their race, sex, or socioeconomic status; for a review, see Garb, 1997). *Bias* occurs when the validity of a clinical judgment or test differs by demographic characteristics of clients (e.g., when the validity of judgments is better for white clients than black clients). The most frequent type of bias discussed by psychologists is slope bias, which involves differences in validity coefficients across groups. When a test or clinical judgment yields a significantly higher validity coefficient in one group than another (slope bias), the test or judgment exhibits "differential validity" (Anastasi & Urbina, 1997). Note that the mere presence of group differences on a test is not sufficient to infer bias; bias requires that the clinical judgment or test be less valid for one group than another. We will briefly describe results for sex bias, race bias, and social class bias.

Sex Bias   Sex-role stereotypes are a cause for concern in the diagnosis of psychopathology, especially for the diagnosis of personality disorders. When two groups of clinicians are given one of two case vignettes, and the case vignettes are identical except for the designation of gender, then histrionic personality disorder is more likely to be diagnosed in women and antisocial personality disorder is more likely to be diagnosed in men. Both male and female clinicians exhibit this bias (e.g., Adler, Drake, & Teague, 1990; Ford & Widiger, 1989). Ford and Widiger found that clinicians were not biased when they made ratings for the individual criteria making up these diagnoses. This finding suggests that the bias is linked to clinicians' perceptions of the diagnoses themselves, not to the *DSM* criteria for these disorders.

Race Bias   In a number of studies conducted in clinical settings, race bias has been shown to occur in psychiatric diagnosis, the prescription of psychiatric medications, violence prediction, and child abuse reporting (Garb, 1997, 1998). When the effect of social class was controlled, race still emerged as an important predictor. African-American and Hispanic patients were less likely to be diagnosed with a psychotic mood disorder and more likely to be diagnosed with schizophrenia compared with white patients exhibiting similar symptoms (e.g., Mukherjee, Shukla, Woodle, Rosen, & Olarte, 1983;

Simon, Fleiss, Gurland, Stiller, & Sharpe, 1973). This occurred even when a diagnosis of schizophrenia was inappropriate. Additionally, African-American patients received a larger number of antipsychotic medications, injections of antipsychotic medications, and psychiatric medications overall. Moreover, clinicians have exhibited race bias when predicting the occurrence of violence in institutional settings, including psychiatric wards and prisons. In these studies, they have overestimated the risk of violence for black inpatients and inmates. However, for clients residing in the community, race bias was not found for the prediction of violence. Race was a potent predictor of failure to report child abuse: Cases of child abuse were less likely to be reported if the child was White than Black (Hampton & Newberger, 1985).

Social Class Bias Social class bias has been demonstrated only sparsely in psychiatric diagnosis and treatment (Garb, 1997, 1998). One finding that has emerged is the relation of social class to psychotherapy decisions. Clinicians were more likely to recommend middle-class individuals than lower-class individuals for psychotherapy and expected them to do better in therapy when both groups were recommended. Additionally, middle-class clients were more likely to be recommended for insight-focused therapy whereas lower-class clients received more recommendations for supportive therapy (see Garb, 1997, for a review).

Methodological Recommendations

Several methodological steps can be taken to improve the quality of psychological assessment and the judgments derived from psychological tests. First, more sophisticated procedures can be used to evaluate validity. For example, to evaluate the validity of diagnoses, one can use the LEAD standard (Spitzer, 1983; also see Garb, 1998, pp. 45–53). Use of the LEAD standard, which was described earlier, allows researchers to ascertain the validity of structured interviews and other assessment instruments. In addition, the criteria proposed by Wood et al. (1996b) should be used to determine if an assessment instrument is valid for its intended purpose. For example, if positive validity findings have been obtained in two studies but not in two others, one would conclude that the assessment instrument does not meet the Wood et al. (1996b) criteria because the results were not consistent.

A second recommendation is that item response theory (IRT) be used to construct and evaluate tests. IRT is an alternative to traditional (classical) test theory. It can be used as a methodological and statistical tool for a number of purposes including test construction, evaluating a test, and using person-fit indexes to assess how well a trait (or construct) describes an individual. For example, using person-fit indexes, one may conclude that a trait is not relevant to a person if the person responds in an idiosyncratic manner (e.g., endorses severe but not moderate symptoms of depression). IRT also permits test constructors to determine which items are most discriminating at different levels of the trait in question. For example, IRT analyses could reveal that a measure of depression adequately distinguishes nondepressed from moderately depressed individuals, but not moderately from severely depressed individuals. Although well-established in achievement and aptitude testing, IRT has been applied infrequently to personality assessment. This is partly because cognitive constructs are better understood than personality constructs. Put another way, construct validity issues have been more formidable for personality measurement. Just the same, in a relatively few studies, IRT has been applied successfully to personality assessment. For example, historically, linear factor analyses have been used to describe the structure of the MMPI and MMPI–2. Because MMPI and MMPI–2 items are dichotomous (true–false), and because linear factor analysis assumes that ratings are normally distributed and not dichotomous, it is more appropriate to use nonlinear factor analysis or multidimensional IRT methods. Using IRT to uncover the factor structure of the MMPI–2, Waller (1998) found important differences between his results and those of previous factor analyses.

Third, the use of computers for making judgments and decisions is becoming increasingly important in the assessment of psychopathology. Findings from a meta-analysis (Grove, Zald, Lebow, Snitz, & Nelson, 2000) suggest that computer programs can be successfully developed for this purpose. The utility of these programs derives from well-established (although still largely neglected) findings that actuarial (statistical) formulas based on empirically established relations between predictors and criteria are almost always superior or at least equal to clinical judgment (Dawes et al., 1989; Grove & Meehl, 1996). However, relatively few well-validated computer programs are available for clinical tasks (Garb, 2000). As observed by Wood, Garb, Lilienfeld, and Nezworski (2002):

> Substantial progress has been made in developing computerized algorithms to predict violence, child abuse and neglect, and recidivism among juvenile offenders.... However, there are still no well-validated algorithms for making diagnoses [or case formulations]...describing personality traits and psychopathology, or making treatment decisions. (p. 534)

Similarly, Snyder (2000) concluded that popular computer programs that have been used for years to interpret test results (e.g., for the MMPI–2 and the Rorschach) are inadequately validated. Research is needed to develop and validate new computer programs that provide valid descriptions of a client's personality and psychopathology.

Conclusions

Assessing psychopathology is an activity fraught with potential error and bias. However, by attending to research findings, psychologists can avoid using test scores that are invalid, and they can become familiar with the strengths and weaknesses of clinical judgment. In this way, errors that are potentially detrimental to clients can be avoided. For example, the use of the CS norms for interpreting Rorschach protocols can lead to false positives in the assessment of psychopathology. By not using the CS norms, or by using them with extreme caution, one can avoid making harmful judgments such as misdiagnosing normal clients as pathological.[4]

Some psychologists argue that although scientific research is important, we should also rely on clinical experience to determine if an assessment instrument is valuable. Indeed, some even argue that when research and clinical experience conflict, we should place a higher premium on the latter. Psychologists are frequently encouraged to use the Rorschach and other projective techniques because they seem to provide rich clinical data (e.g., Karon, 2000). However, clinical experience can be fallible for a host of reasons including biased feedback, illusory correlation, confirmatory bias, and deterministic reasoning (Dawes et al., 1989; Garb, 1998). The scientific method, not clinical experience, is the best method for minimizing error and resolving controversies. Scientific techniques, such as double-blind designs and control groups, are tools that researchers have developed to protect themselves from being misled (Lilienfeld, 2002). As McFall (1991) noted:

> [There is a] commonly offered rationalization that science doesn't have all the answers yet, and until it does, we must do the best we can to muddle along, relying on our clinical experience, judgment, creativity, and intuition (cf., Matarazzo, 1990). Of course, this argument reflects the mistaken notion that science is a set of answers, rather than a set of processes or methods by which to arrive at answers. Where there are lots of unknowns—and clinical psychology certainly has more than its share—it is all the more imperative to adhere as strictly as possible to the scientific approach. Does anyone seriously believe that a reliance on intuition and other unscientific methods is going to hasten advances in knowledge? (pp. 76–77)

Finally, as noted by McFall (cited in Trull & Phares, 2001, p. 62), one feature that should distinguish clinical and counseling psychologists from most other mental health professionals is their scientific training. To ignore research findings because they make us feel uncomfortable is to neglect our most distinctive and positive attribute: our training in, and our willingness to be guided by, science.

Notes

1. We use the term *provisional diagnoses* because formal diagnoses of psychiatric disorders should not be made on the basis of the MMPI-2 alone.
2. In fact, the TAT is rarely scored in clinical practice (see Lilienfeld et al., 2000).
3. There has also been a heated argument over the accessibility of studies that have been cited to support the CS. Unpublished studies sponsored by Rorschach Workshops are frequently cited as evidence supporting the CS, but attempts to obtain copies of papers describing the studies have frequently been unsuccessful (Nezworski & Wood, 1995; Wood, Nezworski, & Stejskal, 1996a, 1996b; but also see Exner, 1995, 1996). Copies of all correspondence will be provided on request.
4. For a case history describing a client who was apparently harmed by interpretations of the Rorschach, see Garb, Wood, Lilienfeld, and Nezworski (2002).

References

Acklin, M. W. (1999). Behavioral science foundations of the Rorschach test: Research and clinical applications. *Assessment, 6*, 319–326.

Acklin, M. W., McDowell, C. J., Verschell, M. S., & Chan, D. (2000). Interobserver agreement, intraobserver reliability, and the Rorschach Comprehensive System. *Journal of Personality Assessment, 74*, 15–47.

Adler, D. A., Drake, R. E., & Teague, G. B. (1990). Clinicians' practices in personality assessment: Does gender influence the use of DSM-III Axis II? *Comprehensive Psychiatry, 31*, 125–131.

Albert, S., Fox, H. M., & Kahn, M. W. (1980). Faking psychosis on the Rorschach: Can expert judges detect malingering? *Journal of Personality Assessment, 44*, 115–119.

Alterman, A. I., Snider, E. C., Cacciola, J. S., Brown, L. S., Jr., Zaballero, A., & Siddiqui, N. (1996). Evidence of response set effects in structured research interviews. *Journal of Nervous and Mental Disease, 184*, 403–410.

American Educational Research Association, American Psychological Association, & National Council on Measurement in Education. (1999). *Standards for educational and psychological testing.* Washington, D.C.: Author.

American Psychiatric Association. (1980). *Diagnostic and statistical manual of mental disorders* (3rd ed.). Washington, D.C.: Author.

American Psychiatric Association. (1994). *Diagnostic and statistical manual of mental disorders* (4th ed.). Washington, D.C.: Author.

Anastasi, A., & Urbina, S. (1997). *Psychological testing* (7th ed.). New York: Macmillan.

Antony, M. M., & Barlow, D. H. (Eds.) (2002). *Handbook of assessment and treatment planning for psychological disorders.* New York: Guilford.

Arkes, H. R. (1981). Impediments to accurate clinical judgment and possible ways to minimize their impact. *Journal of Consulting and Clinical Psychology, 49*, 323–330.

Arkes, H. R., Faust, D., Guilmette, T. J., & Hart, K. (1988). Eliminating the hindsight bias. *Journal of Applied Psychology, 73*, 305–307.

Aronow, E. (2001). CS norms, psychometrics, and possibilities for the Rorschach technique. *Clinical Psychology: Science and Practice, 8*, 383–385.

Aronson, D. E., & Akamatsu, T. J. (1981). Validation of a Q-sort task to assess MMPI skills. *Journal of Clinical Psychology, 37*, 831–836.

Baker, S. L., Patterson, M. D., & Barlow, D. H. (2002). Panic disorder and agoraphobia. In M. M. Antony & D. H. Barlow (Eds.), *Handbook of assessment and treatment planning for psychological disorders* (pp. 67–112). New York: Guilford.

Beck, A. T., & Steer, R. A. (1990). *Manual for the Beck Anxiety Inventory.* San Antonio, TX: Psychological Corporation.

Beck, A. T., Steer, R. A., & Brown, G. K. (1996). *Beck Depression Inventory Manual* (2nd ed.). San Antonio, TX: Psychological Corporation.

Berry, D. T. R., Baer, R. A., & Harris, M. J. (1991). Detection of malingering on the MMPI: A meta-analysis. *Clinical Psychology Review, 11*, 585–598.

Beutler, L. E., & M. L. Malik (Eds.) (2002). *Rethinking the DSM: A Psychological Perspective.* Washington, D.C.: American Psychological Association.

Blanchard, E. B., Kolb, L. C., Pallmeyer, T. P., & Gerardi, R. J. (1982). A psychophysiological study of posttraumatic stress disorder in Vietnam veterans. *Psychiatric Quarterly, 54*, 220–229.

Blashfield, R. K., & Herkov, M. J. (1996). Investigating clinician adherence to diagnosis by criteria: A replication of Morey and Ochoa (1989). *Journal of Personality Disorders, 10*, 219–228.

Bornstein, R. F. (1999). Criterion validity of objective and projective dependency tests: A meta-analytic assessment of behavioral prediction. *Psychological Assessment, 11*, 48–57.

Brammer, R. (2002). Effects of experience and training on diagnostic accuracy. *Psychological Assessment, 14*, 110–113.

Brockington, I. F., Kendell, R. E., & Leff, J. P. (1978). Definitions of schizophrenia: Concordance and prediction of outcome. *Psychological Medicine, 8,* 387–398.

Brown, T. A., Di Nardo, P., & Barlow, D. H. (1994). *Anxiety Disorders Interview Schedule for DSM-IV.* San Antonio, TX: Psychological Corporation.

Brown, T. A., Di Nardo, P. A., Lehman, C. L., & Campbell, L. A. (2001). Reliability of DSM-IV anxiety and mood disorders: Implications for the classification of emotional disorders. *Journal of Abnormal Psychology, 110,* 49–58.

Butcher, J. N., Dahlstrom, W. G., Graham, J. R., Tellegen, A., & Kaemmer, B. (1989). *Manual for the administration and scoring of the MMPI-2.* Minneapolis: University of Minnesota Press.

Chapman, L. J., & Chapman, J. P. (1967). Genesis of popular but erroneous psychodiagnostic observations. *Journal of Abnormal Psychology, 72,* 193–204.

Chapman, L. J., & Chapman, J. P. (1969). Illusory correlation as an obstacle to the use of valid psychodiagnostic signs. *Journal of Abnormal Psychology, 74,* 271–280.

Clavelle, P. R., & Turner, A. D. (1980). Clinical decision-making among professionals and paraprofessionals. *Journal of Clinical Psychology, 36,* 833–838

Cohen, P., & Cohen, J. (1984). The clinician's illusion. *Archives of General Psychiatry, 41,* 1178–1182.

Conners, K. (1989). *Manual for Conners' rating scales.* North Tonawanda, NY: Multi-Health Systems.

Cronbach, L. J., & Meehl, P. E. (1955). Construct validity in psychological tests. *Psychological Bulletin, 52,* 281–302.

Dawes, R. M., Faust, D., & Meehl, P. E. (1989). Clinical versus actuarial judgment. *Science, 243,* 1668–1674.

Dawes, R. M. (1994). *House of cards: Psychology and psychotherapy built on myth.* New York: Free Press.

Dyer, F. J., & McCann, J. T. (2000). The Millon clinical inventories, research critical of their forensic application, and Daubert criteria. *Law and Human Behavior, 24,* 487–497

Einhorn, H. J. (1988). Diagnosis and causality in clinical and statistical prediction. In D. C. Turk & P. Salovey (Eds.), *Reasoning, inference, and judgment in clinical psychology* (pp. 51–70). New York: Free Press.

Exner, J. E. (1993). *The Rorschach: A comprehensive system: Vol. 1. Basic Foundations* (3rd ed.). New York: Wiley.

Exner, J. E. (1995). Comment on "Narcissism in the Comprehensive System for the Rorschach." *Clinical Psychology: Science and Practice, 2,* 200–206.

Exner, J. E. (1996). Comment on "The Comprehensive System for the Rorschach: A Critical Examination." *Psychological Science, 7,* 11–13.

Exner, J. E. (2001a). A comment on "The Misperception of Psychopathology: Problems with the Norms of the Comprehensive System for the Rorschach." *Clinical Psychology: Science and Practice, 8,* 386–388.

Exner, J. E. (2001b). *A Rorschach workbook for the Comprehensive System* (5th ed.). Asheville, NC: Rorschach Workshops.

Faraone, S. V., & Tsuang, M. T. (1994). Measuring diagnostic accuracy in the absence of a "gold standard." *American Journal of Psychiatry, 151,* 650–657.

Finn, S. E., & Kamphuis, J. H. (1995). What a clinician needs to know about base rates. In J. Butcher (Ed.), *Clinical personality assessment: Practical approaches* (pp. 224–235). New York: Oxford University Press.

Fischhoff, B. (1975). Hindsight ≠ foresight: The effect of outcome knowledge on judgment under uncertainty. *Journal of Experimental Psychology: Human Perception and Performance, 1,* 288–299.

Fleiss, J. (1981). *Statistical methods for rates and proportions* (2nd ed.). New York: Wiley.

Ford, M., & Widiger, T. (1989). Sex bias in the diagnosis of histrionic and antisocial personality disorders. *Journal of Consulting and Clinical Psychology, 57,* 301–305.

Gadol, I. (1969). The incremental and predictive validity of the Rorschach test in personality assessments of normal, neurotic, and psychotic subjects. *Dissertation Abstracts, 29,* 3482B. (UMI No. 69-4469).

Garb, H. N. (1989). Clinical judgment, clinical training, and professional experience. *Psychological Bulletin, 105,* 387–396.

Garb, H. N. (1996). The representativeness and past-behavior heuristics in clinical judgment. *Professional Psychology: Research and Practice, 27,* 272–277.

Garb, H. N. (1997). Race bias, social class bias, and gender bias in clinical judgment. *Clinical Psychology: Science and Practice, 4,* 99–120.

Garb, H. N. (1998). *Studying the clinician: Judgment research and psychological assessment.* Washington, D.C.: American Psychological Association.

Garb, H. N. (2000). Computers will become increasingly important for psychological assessment: Not that there's anything wrong with that! *Psychological Assessment, 12,* 31–39.

Garb, H. N. (2003). Incremental validity and the assessment of psychopathology in adults. *Psychological Assessment, 15,* 508–520.

Garb, H. N. (2006). The conjunction effect and clinical judgment. *Journal of Social and Clinical Psychology, 25,* 1048–1056.

Garb, H. N., Florio, C. M., & Grove, W. M. (1998). The validity of the Rorschach and the Minnesota Multiphasic Personality Inventory: Results from meta-analyses. *Psychological Science, 9,* 402–404.

Garb, H. N., Wood, J. M., Lilienfeld, S. O., & Nezworski, M. T. (2002). Effective use of projective techniques in clinical practice: Let the data help with selection and interpretation. *Professional Psychology: Research and Practice, 33,* 454–463.

Garb, H. N., Wood, J. M., & Nezworski, M. T. (2000). Projective techniques and the detection of child sexual abuse. *Child Maltreatment, 5,* 161–168.

Gauron, E. F., & Dickinson, J. K. (1969). The influence of seeing the patient first on diagnostic decision-making in psychiatry. *American Journal of Psychiatry, 126,* 199–205.

Gilovich, T. (1991). *How we know what isn't so.* New York: Free Press.

Goldberg, L. R. (1965). Diagnosticians versus diagnostic signs: The diagnosis of psychosis versus neurosis from the MMPI. *Psychological Monographs, 79.* (9, Whole No. 602).

Graham, J. R. (1967). A Q-sort study of the accuracy of clinical descriptions based on the MMPI. *Journal of Psychiatric Research, 5,* 297–305.

Graham, J. R., Ben-Porath, Y. S., & McNulty, J. L. (1997). Empirical correlates of low scores on the MMPI-2 scales in an outpatient mental health setting. *Psychological Assessment, 9,* 386–391.

Greene, R. L. (2000). *The MMPI-2: An interpretive manual.* Needham Heights, MA: Allyn & Bacon.

Grove, W. M., & Meehl, P. E. (1996). Comparative efficiency of informal (subjective, impressionistic) and formal (mechanical, algorithmic) prediction procedures: The clinical-statistical controversy. *Psychology: Public Policy and Law, 2,* 293–323.

Grove, W. M., Zald, D. H., Lebow, B. S., Snitz, B. E., & Nelson, C. (2000). Clinical versus mechanical prediction: A meta-analysis. *Psychological Assessment, 12,* 19–30.

Guarnaccia, V., Dill, C. A., Sabatino, S., & Southwick, S. (2001). Scoring accuracy using the Comprehensive System for the Rorschach. *Journal of Personality Assessment, 77,* 464–474.

Hamel, M., Shaffer, T. W., & Erdberg, P. (2000). A study of nonpatient preadolescent Rorschach protocols. *Journal of Personality Assessment, 75,* 280–294.

Hampton, R. L., & Newberger, E. H. (1985). Child abuse incidence and reporting by hospitals: Significance of severity, class and race. *American Journal of Public Health, 75,* 56–60.

Harkness, A. R., & Lilienfeld, S. O. (1997). Individual differences science for treatment planning: Personality traits. *Psychological Assessment, 9,* 349–360.

Henry, B., Moffitt, T. E., Caspi, A., Langley, J., & Silva, P. A. (1994). On the "Remembrance of Things Past": A longitudinal evaluation of the retrospective method. *Psychological Assessment, 6,* 92–101.

Hiller, J. B., Rosenthal, R., Bornstein, R. F., Berry, D. T. R., & Brunell-Neuleib, S. (1999). A comparative meta-analysis of Rorschach and MMPI validity. *Psychological Assessment, 11,* 278–296.

Holmes, D. S. (1990). The evidence for repression: An examination of sixty years of research. In J. L. Singer (Ed.), *Repression and dissociation: Implications for personality theory, psychopathology, and health* (pp. 85–102). Chicago: University of Chicago Press.

Hunsley, J., & Di Giulio, G. (2001). Norms, norming, and clinical assessment. *Clinical Psychology: Science and Practice, 8,* 378–382.

Jorgensen, K., Andersen, T. J., & Dam, H. (2000). The diagnostic efficiency of the Rorschach Depression Index and the Schizophrenia Index: A review. *Assessment, 7,* 259–280.

Kahill, S. (1984). Human figure drawing in adults: An update of the empirical evidence, 1967–1982. *Canadian Psychology, 25,* 269–292.

Karon, B. P. (2000). The clinical interpretation of the Thematic Apperception Test, Rorschach, and other clinical data: A reexamination of statistical versus clinical prediction. *Professional Psychology: Research and Practice, 31,* 230–233.

Lambert, M. J., & Finch, A. E. (1999). The Outcome Questionnaire. In M. E. Maruish (Ed.), *The use of psychological testing for treatment planning and outcomes assessment* (2nd ed., pp. 831–869). Mahwah, NJ: Erlbaum.

Lambert, M. J., Harmon, C., Slade, K., Whipple, J. L., & Hawkins, E. J. (2005). Providing feedback to psychotherapists on their patients' progress: Clinical results and suggestions. *Journal of Clinical Psychology/In Session, 61,* 165–174.

Lambert, M. J., Whipple, J. L., Hawkins, E. J., Vermeersch, D. A., Nielsen, S. L., & Smart, D. W. (2003). Is it time for clinicians to routinely track patient outcome? A meta-analysis. *Clinical Psychology: Science and Practice, 10,* 288–301.

Levenberg, S. B. (1975). Professional training, psychodiagnostic skill, and Kinetic Family Drawings. *Journal of Personality Assessment, 39,* 389–393.

Lilienfeld, S. O. (2002). When worlds collide: Social science, politics, and the Rind et al. (1998) child sexual abuse meta-analysis. *American Psychologist, 57,* 176–188.

Lilienfeld, S. O., Wood, J. M., & Garb, H. N. (2000). The scientific status of projective techniques. *Psychological Science in the Public Interest, 1,* 27–66.

Lilienfeld, S. O., Wood, J. M., & Garb, H. N. (2001, May). What's wrong with this picture? *Scientific American, 284,* 80–87.

Lima, E. N., Stanley, S., Kaboski, B., Reitzel, L. R., Richey, J. A., Castro, Y. et al. (2005). The incremental validity of the MMPI-2: When does therapist access not enhance treatment outcome? *Psychological Assessment, 17,* 462–468.

Litz, B. T., Miller, M. W., Ruef, A. M., & McTeague, L. M. (2002). Exposure to trauma in adults. In M. M. Antony & D. H. Barlow (Eds.), *Handbook of assessment and treatment planning for psychological disorders* (pp. 215–258). New York: Guilford.

Loevinger, J. (1957). Objective tests as instruments of psychological theory. *Psychological Reports, 3,* 635–694.

Logue, M. B., Sher, K. J., & Frensch, P. A. (1992). Purported characteristics of adult children of alcoholics: A possible "Barnum Effect." *Professional Psychology: Research and Practice, 23,* 226–232

Margraf, J., Taylor, C. B., Ehlers, A., Roth, W. T., & Agras, W. S. (1987). Panic attacks in the natural environment. *Journal of Nervous and Mental Disease, 175,* 558–565.

Matarazzo, J. D. (1990). Psychological assessment versus psychological testing: Validation from Binet to the school, clinic, and courtroom. *American Psychologist, 45,* 999–1017

McFall, R. M. (1991). Manifesto for a science of clinical psychology. *Clinical Psychologist, 44,* 75–88.

McFall, R. M., & Treat, T. A. (1999). Quantifying the information value of clinical assessments with signal detection theory. *Annual Review of Psychology, 50,* 215–241.

Meehl, P. E. (1945). The dynamics of "structured" personality tests. *Journal of Clinical Psychology, 1,* 296–303.

Meehl, P. E. (1986). Diagnostic taxa as open concepts: Metatheoretical and statistical questions about reliability and construct validity in the grand strategy of nosological revision. In T. Millon & G. Klerman (Eds.), *Contemporary directions in psychopathology* (pp. 215–231). New York: Guilford.

Meehl, P. E., & Rosen, A. (1955). Antecedent probability and the efficiency of psychometric signs, patterns, or cutting scores. *Psychological Bulletin, 52,* 194–216.

Meehl, P. E. (1956). Wanted–A good cookbook. *American Psychologist, 11,* 263–272.

Meehl, P. E. (1973). Why I do not attend case conferences. In P. E. Meehl, *Psychodiagnosis: Selected papers* (pp. 225–302). Minneapolis: University of Minnesota Press.

Meyer, G. J. (2001). Evidence to correct misperceptions about Rorschach norms. *Clinical Psychology: Science and Practice, 8,* 389–396.

Meyer, G. J., & Archer, R. P. (2001). The hard science of Rorschach research: What do we know and where do we go? *Psychological Assessment, 13,* 486–502.

Meyer, G. J., & Handler, L. (1997). The ability of the Rorschach to predict subsequent outcome: A meta-analysis of the Rorschach Prognostic Rating Scale. *Journal of Personality Assessment, 69,* 1–38.

Meyer, G. J., Hilsenroth, M. J., Baxter, D., Exner, J. E., Fowler, J. C., Piers, C. C., & Resnick, J. (2002). An examination of inter-rater reliability for scoring the Rorschach Comprehensive System in eight data sets. *Journal of Personality Assessment, 78,* 219–274.

Meyer, G. J., & Richardson, C. (2001, March). *An examination of changes in Form Quality codes in the Rorschach Comprehensive System from 1974 to 1995.* Presented at the midwinter meeting of the Society for Personality Assessment, Philadelphia.

Millon, T. (1994). *The Millon Clinical Multiaxial Inventory-III manual.* Minneapolis, MN: National Computer Systems.

Molinari, V., Ames, A., & Essa, M. (1994). Prevalence of personality disorders in two geropsychiatric inpatient units. *Journal of Geriatric Psychiatry and Neurology, 7,* 209–215.

Morey, L. C. (1991). *Personality Assessment Inventory: Professional manual.* Tampa: Psychological Assessment Resources.

Morey, L. C., & Ochoa, E. S. (1989). An investigation of adherence to diagnostic criteria: Clinical diagnosis of the DSM-III personality disorders. *Journal of Personality Disorders, 3,* 180–192.

Mukherjee, S., Shukla, S., Woodle, J., Rosen, A. M., & Olarte, S. (1983). Misdiagnosis of schizophrenia in bipolar patients: A multiethnic comparison. *American Journal of Psychiatry, 140,* 1571–1574.

Naglieri, J. A., & Pfeiffer, S. I. (1992). Performance of disruptive behavior-disordered and normal samples on the Draw-A-Person: Screening Procedure for Emotional Disturbance. *Psychological Assessment, 4,* 156–159.

Nakata, L. M. (1999). Interrater reliability and the Comprehensive System for the Rorschach: Clinical and non-clinical protocols (Doctoral dissertation, Pacific Graduate School of Psychology). *Dissertation Abstracts International, 60,* 4296B.

Nezworski, M. T., & Wood, J. M. (1995). Narcissism in the Comprehensive System for the Rorschach. *Clinical Psychology: Science and Practice, 2,* 179–199.

Nunnally, J. (1978). *Psychometric theory* (2nd ed.). New York: McGraw-Hill.

Oberlander, L. B. (1995). Psycholegal issues in child sexual abuse evaluations: A survey of forensic mental health professionals. *Child Abuse & Neglect, 19,* 475–490.

Parker, K. C. H., Hanson, R., & Hunsley, J. (1988). MMPI, Rorschach, and WAIS: A meta-analytic comparison of reliability, stability, and validity. *Psychological Bulletin, 103,* 367–373.

Percevic, R., Lambert, M. J., & Kordy, H. (2004). Computer-supported monitoring of patient treatment response. *Journal of Clinical Psychology, 60,* 285–299.

Rogers, R. (1995). *Diagnostic and structured interviewing: A handbook for psychologists.* Odessa, FL: Psychological Assessment Resources.

Rogers, R., Salekin, R. T., & Sewell, K. W. (1999). Validation of the Millon Clinical Multiaxial Inventory for Axis II disorders: Does it meet the *Daubert* standard? *Law and Human Behavior, 23,* 425–443.

Rogers, R., Salekin, R. T., & Sewell, K. W. (2000). The MCMI-III and the *Daubert* standard: Separating rhetoric from reality. *Law and Human Behavior, 24,* 501–506.

Rotton, J., & Kelly, I. W. (1985). Much ado about the full moon: A meta-analysis of lunar-lunacy research. *Psychological Bulletin, 97,* 286–306.

Sartorius, N., Kaelber, C. T., Cooper, J. E., Roper, M. T., Rae, D. S., Gulbinat, W. et al. (1993). Progress toward achieving a common language in psychiatry: Results from the field trial of the clinical guidelines accompanying the WHO classification of mental and behavioral disorders in *ICD-10. Archives of General Psychiatry, 50,* 115–124.

Savard, J., & Morin, C. M. (2002). Insomnia. In M. M. Antony & D. H. Barlow (Eds.), *Handbook of assessment and treatment planning for psychological disorders* (pp. 523–555). New York: Guilford.

Schacter, S. (1982). Recidivism and self-cure of smoking and obesity. *American Psychologist, 37,* 436–444.

Shaffer, T. W., Erdberg, P., & Haroian, J. (1999). Current nonpatient data for the Rorschach, WAIS-R, and MMPI-2. *Journal of Personality Assessment, 73,* 305–316.

Shear, M. K., Brown, T. A., Barlow, D. H., Money, R., Sholomskas, D. E., Woods, S. W., Gorman, J. M., & Papp, L. A. (1997). Multicenter collaborative Panic Disorder Severity Scale. *American Journal of Psychiatry, 154,* 1571–1575.

Simon, R. J., Fleiss, J. L., Gurland, B. J., Stiller, P. R., & Sharpe, L. (1973). Depression and schizophrenia in hospitalized black and white mental patients. *Archives of General Psychiatry, 28,* 509–512.

Snyder, C. R., & Larson, G. R. (1972). A further look at student acceptance of general personality interpretations. *Journal of Consulting and Clinical Psychology, 38,* 384–388.

Snyder, D. K. (2000). Computer-assisted judgment: Defining strengths and liabilities. *Psychological Assessment, 12,* 52–60.

Spangler, W. D. (1992). Validity of questionnaire and TAT measures of need for achievement: Two meta-analyses. *Psychological Bulletin, 112,* 140–154.

Spitzer, R. L. (1983). Psychiatric diagnosis: Are clinicians still necessary? *Comprehensive Psychiatry, 24,* 399–411.

Starr, B. J., & Katkin, E. S. (1969). The clinician as an aberrant actuary: Illusory correlation and the Incomplete Sentences Blank. *Journal of Abnormal Psychology, 74,* 670–675.

Steiner, J. L., Tebes, J. K., Sledge, W. H., & Walker, M. L. (1995). A comparison of the Structured Clinical Interview for DSM-III-R and clinical diagnoses. *Journal of Nervous and Mental Disease, 183,* 365–369.

Strohmer, D. C., Shivy, V. A., & Chiodo, A. L. (1990). Information processing strategies in counselor hypothesis testing: The role of selective memory and expectancy. *Journal of Counseling Psychology, 37,* 465–472.

Trowbridge, M. M. (1995). Graphic indicators of sexual abuse in children's drawings: A review of the literature. *The Arts in Psychotherapy, 22,* 485–493.

Trull, T. J., & Phares, E. J. (2001). *Clinical Psychology* (6th ed.). Belmont, CA: Wadsworth.

Turner, D. R. (1966). Predictive efficiency as a function of amount of information and level of professional experience. *Journal of Projective Techniques and Personality Assessment, 30,* 4–11.

Tversky, A., & Kahneman, D. (1983). Extensional vs. intuitive reasoning: The conjunction fallacy in probability judgment. *Psychological Review, 90,* 293–315.

Waller, N. G. (1998). Searching for structure in the MMPI. In S. E. Embretson & S. L. Hershberger (Eds.), *The new rules of measurement* (pp. 185–217). Mahwah, NJ: Lawrence Erlbaum.

Weiner, I. B. (2000). Using the Rorschach properly in practice and research. *Journal of Clinical Psychology, 56,* 435–438.

Weiner, I. B. (2001). Advancing the science of psychological assessment: The Rorschach Inkblot Method as exemplar. *Psychological Assessment, 13,* 423–432.

Westen, D., Lohr, N., Silk, K. R., Gold, L., & Kerber, K. (1990). Object relations and social cognition in borderlines, major depressives, and normals: A Thematic Apperception Test analysis. *Psychological Assessment, 2,* 355–364.

Westen, D., Ludolph, P., Block, M. J., Wixom, J., & Wiss, F. C. (1990). Developmental history and object relations in psychiatrically disturbed adolescent girls. *American Journal of Psychiatry, 147,* 1061–1068.

Whitehead, W. C. (1985). Clinical decision making on the basis of Rorschach, MMPI, and automated MMPI report data (Doctoral dissertation, University of Texas Southwestern Medical Center at Dallas, 1985). *Dissertation Abstracts International, 46,* 2828.

Widiger, T. A. (2001). The best and the worst of us? *Clinical Psychology: Science and Practice, 8,* 374–377.

Widiger, T. A. (2002). Personality disorders. In M. M. Antony & D. H. Barlow (Eds.), *Handbook of assessment and treatment planning for psychological disorders* (pp. 453–480). New York: Guilford.

Wood, J. M., Garb, H. N., Lilienfeld, S. O., & Nezworski, M. T. (2002). Clinical assessment. *Annual Review of Psychology, 53,* 519–543.

Wood, J. M., Garb, H. N., & Nezworski, M. T. (2007). Psychometrics: Better measurement makes better clinicians. In S. O. Lilienfeld & W. T. O'Donohue (Eds.), *The great ideas of clinical science: The 17 concepts that every mental health practitioner should understand* (pp. 77–92). New York: Brunner-Routledge.

Wood, J. M., Lilienfeld, S. O., & Nezworski, M. T. (2000). The Rorschach test in clinical diagnosis: A critical review, with a backward look at Garfield (1947). *Journal of Clinical Psychology, 56,* 395–430.

Wood, J. M., Nezworski, M. T., Garb, H. N., & Lilienfeld, S. O. (2001a). Problems with the norms of the Comprehensive System for the Rorschach: Methodological and conceptual considerations. *Clinical Psychology: Science and Practice, 8,* 397–402.

Wood, J. M., Nezworski, M. T., Garb, H. N., & Lilienfeld, S. O. (2001b). The misperception of psychopathology: Problems with the norms of the Comprehensive System for the Rorschach. *Clinical Psychology: Science and Practice, 8,* 350–373.

Wood, J. M., Nezworski, M. T., Lilienfeld, S. O., & Garb, H. N. (2003). *What's wrong with the Rorschach? Science confronts the controversial inkblot test.* San Francisco, CA: Jossey-Bass.

Wood, J. M., Nezworski, M. T., & Stejskal, W. J. (1996a). The Comprehensive System for theRorschach: A critical examination. *Psychological Science, 7,* 3–10.

Wood, J. M., Nezworski, M. T., & Stejskal, W. J. (1996b). Thinking critically about the Comprehensive System for the Rorschach: A reply to Exner. *Psychological Science, 7,* 14–17.

7
Psychotherapy Research

Rebecca E. Stewart and Dianne L. Chambless

The focus of this book is on the study of psychopathology and its assessment. Understanding psychopathology is an important part of the science of psychology in its own right, but it is more than pure science. Psychopathology research plays an important role in the development of interventions to ameliorate mental disorders and to promote well being. Almost every chapter in part II of this text includes material on treatment for the disorders in question, usually based on the outcome of treatment research. Where does this information come from? In this chapter we will describe the process by which psychotherapy research is conducted, and the controversies surrounding the proper nature and role of such research.

Psychotherapy Research

Psychotherapy research is a broad field encompassing a number of streams of research. *Process research*, designed to identify and delineate the important events in therapy, typically addresses what happens in a therapeutic session, and investigates such variables as therapist behaviors, client behaviors, and interactions between the therapist and the client. For example, a common theme in psychoanalytic therapy research is characteristics of the transference (Connolly, Crits-Christoph, Barber, & Luborsky, 2000). *Outcome research* focuses on the effects of psychotherapy, both immediate and long-term changes in the problems for which a person seeks or is referred for treatment as well as improvement on broader variables such as quality of life or interpersonal functioning. Not surprisingly, process research is often linked to outcome research so as to identify factors that may be important in treatment outcome. For example, meta-analyses indicate that the better the client–therapist alliance, the better the treatment outcome, with the alliance accounting for about 5% of the variance in improvement (Martin, Garske, & Davis, 2000).

Yet other questions in psychotherapy research include prediction of treatment outcome—what are the characteristics of clients who do well in this treatment—or, to answer a more sophisticated question, who will do well in this treatment but not in that treatment? For example, Barber and Muenz (1996) showed that in treatment of major depression, interpersonal therapy was better for clients with obsessive-compulsive personality traits, whereas cognitive-behavior therapy was better for clients with avoidant personality traits. Such findings demonstrate *moderation* of treatment outcome by a patient characteristic, in this case, a specific personality disorder. Finally, *mediation* of treatment outcome is an important area of study. Mediation research asks what are the mechanisms underlying treatment efficacy? For example, in a study comparing several forms of treatment for attention deficit hyperactivity disorder Hinshaw and colleagues (2000) found that the impact of treatment on children's social skills at school was mediated by parents' use of negative/ineffective discipline. In other words, to the degree that treatment reduced parents' use of negative/ineffective discipline, children's social skills at school improved. Although all of these forms of psychotherapy research are important, our focus in this chapter will be mainly on psychotherapy outcome research.

A Protypical Psychotherapy Outcome Study

There is no one method of outcome research accepted by all types of psychotherapy researchers. What we describe here is the reigning paradigm for major studies such as those funded by the National Institute of Mental Health in which the efficacy of one or more treatments is tested, as well as the paradigm accepted for research on empirically supported treatments, which will be defined in a later section. We will address some of the controversies about this paradigm later in this chapter. To establish *efficacy*, a psychological intervention is tested under well-controlled circumstances. If it proves to be beneficial in multiple studies, then researchers may turn their attention to *effectiveness* research, in which the generalization of the treatment's benefits to less well controlled, more real world circumstances is examined. Hence, the first efforts have a strong focus on internal validity, whereas later efforts may concentrate on external validity (Moras, 1998).

Research Designs

Both single case experiments (Hersen & Barlow, 1976) and randomized controlled trials (RCTs) allow close controls on the internal validity of research. These experimental methods, properly conducted, permit the investigator to draw causal inferences about the efficacy of a treatment. Because RCTs are far more common, we will focus on this approach here. In RCTs, patients are randomly assigned to the treatment of interest or to one or more control groups or alternative treatments. Without random assignment, it would be impossible to know whether any differences observed among treatments were due to the treatments or to systematic preexisting differences among patients. Control groups are used to determine whether any improvement with treatment might be due simply to effects such as the passage of time, the assessment procedures (e.g., talking at length about your problems with the clinical assessor), or to making a decision to do something about the problem. The simplest control group is a *waiting list condition* where clients receive the treatment under investigation after a prescribed delay during which they participate in assessment. Usually the delay period is for the length of the treatment, but for severely distressed clients, this may be shortened for ethical reasons. Waiting list conditions are similar to the delay many clients undergo when they seek treatment at clinics, but there are drawbacks, including the ethical concern about postponing treatment and the fact that a number of clients will seek treatment elsewhere or lose their resolve to undergo treatment during the waiting period.

Waiting list control conditions permit the researcher to draw an important conclusion that may be all many consumers want to know: Does the treatment work better than no treatment? However, such control groups are unsatisfactory if the researcher or consumer wants to know whether the treatment adds to the so-called nonspecific effects of psychotherapy. That is, does the treatment work because of placebo effects, the belief and hope of change that occur when people think they are getting treatment? Does the treatment work simply because the clients get to talk with a sympathetic person about their problems? If so, there is nothing that is specifically helpful about this treatment versus any other, and no justification for having highly trained psychotherapists versus counselors with less training deliver the treatment. *Placebo control conditions* (e.g., a pill placebo combined with regular meetings with a supportive psychiatrist) and *alternative therapy conditions* (e.g., supportive counseling) provide for another level of analysis than the waiting list control group. However, these control groups are also not without their problems. For ethical reasons, patients given a placebo receive the real treatment at the end of the treatment period, but many may drop out before that time to seek other treatment if it is available. If patients who received supportive counseling are not satisfied with their improvement in treatment, they may get additional treatment during the follow-up period, which precludes controlled assessment of long-term outcome.

Finally, the researcher may choose to compare the treatment of interest to various medications or to other forms of psychotherapy known or thought to be efficacious for the types of problems being treated. Comparisons of two or more types of psychotherapy are less common at this point than is research designed to develop and test the efficacy of one treatment. For many disorders there are not yet two or more psychological approaches that have each been determined to yield satisfactory treatment benefits relative to waiting list or placebo control groups, making such comparisons premature. However, comparisons of psychotherapy with medication and with the combination of medication and psychotherapy are frequently conducted.

Typically in the development of a particular treatment, the research follows this course: First, an uncontrolled study in which the effects of the treatment are tested by comparing clients' status before and after treatment; second, comparisons with waiting list control groups; third, comparisons with placebo or basic counseling; and fourth, comparisons with medication or other efficacious psychotherapies. At each stage, the comparisons become more stringent, and the number of participants required for the research increases. Statistically significant effects between a treatment and waiting list control group may be obtained with 25 patients per condition, but comparisons between two efficacious treatments or between psychotherapy and a medication will require 50 or more patients per group to be able to detect differences in efficacy that are clinically important. Consider that the typical psychotherapy-medication trial includes the following conditions: psychotherapy plus placebo, medication alone, medication plus psychotherapy, pill placebo plus clinical management (meetings with a supportive, encouraging psychiatrist for medication monitoring), and perhaps psychotherapy without pill placebo (to control for any effects of the patients' thinking they are on medication, which may have a positive or negative impact). For such a trial, then, 250 or more patients are required, often requiring multiple treatment sites to obtain enough participants. As a result, these studies are very expensive to mount and virtually impossible to conduct without major government grants. For this reason, psychotherapy research proceeds more slowly than pharmacotherapy research where most of the studies are funded by the pharmaceutical industry, for which there is no psychotherapy equivalent.

Defining the Intervention

For pharmacotherapy researchers, it is fairly easy to define the treatment intervention: Provide the drug (or pill placebo identical in appearance) in the proper therapeutic dosage and monitor its use and side effects. For psychotherapy researchers, the process is more difficult. The researcher must carefully lay out the treatment approaches being studied such that the study therapists and the ultimate readers of the study know exactly what treatment was tested. This is accomplished by writing a treatment manual that details what the principles of this treatment are, and how it is conducted. How structured such manuals are tends to vary with the sort of therapy tested. For example, cognitive-behavioral treatment manuals are often highly detailed, frequently with session-by-session outlines. In contrast, manuals for psychodynamic psychotherapy may rely on broader brush strokes, describing treatment principles and the sorts of conditions under which the therapist chooses one possible intervention over another; for example, when to interpret the patient's behavior versus when to be supportive. Manuals often become more and more highly developed across research trials and end up being book length. Manuals are critical to treatment research in that they permit dissemination of efficacious treatments (others can read how the treatments were done) and because they provide the operational definition of the treatment. Labels for treatments are often not sufficiently informative. For example, there are many versions of psychodynamic treatment, some of which are radically different from others. Just which dynamic treatment approaches were followed in this study? Using manuals also tightens the internal validity of the study by reducing unwanted experimental variance. When therapists have a treatment manual to follow, there is less variability in the outcomes of the individual therapists employed in the treatment trial (Crits-Christoph et al., 1991).

It is not enough that the study therapists are provided with a treatment manual. They must also be trained in delivering this treatment, and then monitored during the study for their adherence to the treatment manual and their competence in carrying out the treatment. Trained raters watch videotapes of treatment sessions and use rating scales to determine whether therapists are following the key procedures of the treatment and are avoiding mixing in other treatments that are not to be included in this study. Expert raters also watch these tapes to code the therapists' skill. Ensuring that the therapists delivered the treatment in at least a minimally competent way is vital to the reception the study will ultimately encounter. Readers can easily reject findings counter to their own beliefs if they can discount the results because therapist competence and adherence were not demonstrated.

Selecting the Treatment Sample and Assessing Outcome

What is the target population for this treatment and for this particular study? Again, an operational definition is required. Earlier in the history of psychotherapy research, the description of the study sample was often quite broad; for example, neurotic outpatients. The present practice is to define study samples more precisely, usually with a specific *DSM* diagnosis (e.g., American Psychiatric Association, 1994) such as borderline personality disorder. However, samples may also be defined on the basis of characteristics other than formal diagnoses. For example, programs for prevention of marital dissatisfaction and divorce target unselected engaged couples, and programs to prevent alcohol abuse and dependence target college students who drink heavily but do not meet the diagnostic criteria for a substance use disorder. The researcher also determines the study's exclusion criteria. Who is omitted? Thus, for example, acutely suicidal patients who require immediate hospitalization are excluded from most outpatient studies for ethical reasons. Alcohol and substance dependent patients are usually excluded from trials for treatment of other disorders they may have until their chemical dependencies have been addressed, because these problems tend to interfere with progress in other areas. In the intake process, the typical RCT screens out about two thirds of the people who initially contacted the project (Westen & Morrison, 2001). This means that for the 250-patient medication versus psychotherapy RCT described earlier, over 750 potential participants would need to be screened for the study.

To determine who enters the study and who improves in treatment, reliable and valid means of assessing the patients' problems and symptom severity are required. Questionnaire measures are often used to assess change in treatment, but interviews are commonly employed to make initial diagnoses as well as to monitor change over time. Interviewers must be carefully trained to be reliable in their assessments, and their reliability across the course of the study must be monitored by another trained rater who is uninformed as to the initial diagnosis or severity rating.

Empirically Validated Treatments

Several of the chapters in part II of this volume mention the terms *empirically validated treatments* or *empirically supported treatments* (ESTs) for the disorders reviewed in that chapter. In general these terms are used interchangeably to refer to treatments that have met the standards set by one or more groups who have reviewed the psychotherapy literature to identify treatments that work for particular disorders or presenting problems (see Chambless & Ollendick, 2001 for a review). These efforts were initiated in the United States by Division 12 (Society of Clinical Psychology) of the American

Psychological Association. Division 12's Task Force on the Promotion and Dissemination of Psychological Procedures (later the Committee on Science and Practice) defined ESTs as treatments that were *probably efficacious* or *efficacious*. Probably efficacious treatments are those that have been found to be superior to waiting list control groups in two or more studies, that have been found to be superior to another treatment in at least one study, or that have been found to be superior to another treatment in multiple studies but only tested by one research group. Efficacious treatments were defined as those that have proved more beneficial than placebo conditions or alternative treatments by more than one research group. (Note that we abbreviate the criteria here, and a complete description may be found in Chambless, Baker et al., 1998.) In both cases, when multiple studies were available, the preponderance of the most exacting evidence had to favor the treatment's efficacy. Moreover, treatments had to be tested according to the methods described in this section for rigorous psychotherapy research.

At the time of their 2001 review, Chambless and Ollendick noted that the various review groups tackling the psychotherapy literature had identified 108 ESTs for adults and 37 for children. The identification of ESTs may be categorized as a part of the *evidence-based practice* movement. According to the principles of evidence-based practice, clinicians are encouraged to integrate the best research evidence regarding possible treatment of a patient with their clinical expertise and consideration of the patient's characteristics and values (Sackett, Straus, Richardson, Rosenberg, & Haynes, 2000). Thus, evidence-based practice includes not only EST research but also any other sort of evidence the practitioner might bring to bear on treatment decisions; for example, knowledge of the importance of building positive expectations for change and of developing a strong working alliance with the client. Compilations of ESTs are intended to serve as quick guides for clinicians, students, and educators who want to learn more about how to effectively treat a variety of disorders but who do not have time or the expertise to conduct extensive literature reviews themselves. With support from the National Institute of Mental Health, a website has been developed to help consumers and therapists access information about ESTs (http://www.therapyadvisor.org). The Committee on Accreditation, which reviews and accredits doctoral programs and internships in professional psychology, requires that at least some of a student's didactic and practical training be devoted to the study of ESTs (Office of Program Consultation and Accreditation, 1996).

A Costly Endeavor

We have covered but a partial list of the requirements for conducting a sound psychotherapy research trial (see Chambless & Hollon, 1998 for a more complete description). However, this should be sufficient for the reader to see that the psychotherapy researcher's efforts must be exhaustive and are exhausting! In addition, such research requires a great deal of patience. Psychotherapy trials often take five years to complete the evaluation of all patients' progress from the beginning to the end of treatment and another two years to complete assessment of treatment response at follow-up. The amount of time required to treat each participant is great, ranging from about 12 sessions of treatment of at least 50 minutes each to a year or more of treatment, for severe psychopathology such as borderline personality disorder. The amount of effort that goes into treating and assessing each patient and the process of treatment, and the requirements for highly trained personnel to carry out these activities make such research a very expensive endeavor. Moreover, one study is not sufficient to convince us that a treatment is efficacious. Multiple replications, especially by other researchers not intimately involved in the development of the treatment, are essential.

Once a treatment's efficacy has been established, it is time to export or disseminate the treatment to the community to test whether it works outside of the hothouse of the research clinic; that is, to conduct effectiveness research. Such tests include determining whether treatments work with the sorts of patients who may not have participated in university-based research trials (e.g., less educated patients), in primary care practices and community mental health centers, when provided by less highly trained personnel, and so forth. Because the focus of such research is on external validity or generalization beyond the research clinic, the designs are often less tightly controlled and may be simple pretest–posttest studies with no control group. In such cases, *benchmarking* may be used. That is, the results of the effectiveness study may be compared to those in published efficacy research. It typically takes many years to move from the initial uncontrolled pilot studies, through efficacy research, to the effectiveness stage of research. However, demonstrating effectiveness of research proven efficacious in RCTs is now a major thrust of the National Institute of Mental Health, and this has served to move research more quickly to tests of effectiveness. Given that psychotherapy research is difficult to conduct and very costly, why do it? We turn to this question next.

The Case for Psychotherapy Research

The Food and Drug Administration requires rigorous testing of medications before they are made available to the public through their physicians. The rationale is that it is important to determine before dissemination whether the drug has harmful effects, and whether its beneficial effects outweigh any harmful effects observed. There is no formal equivalent for testing new psychological interventions. Rather, psychologists' ethical code (American Psychological Association, 2002) exhorts them to let clients know whether a treatment is experimental and to avoid the use of treatments that might be harmful. That is, psychologists are largely expected to police themselves, although occasionally a state licensing board may take action against a psychologist using bogus treatments for which he or she has made unsubstantiated claims.

First, Do No Harm

Some would argue that it is unnecessary to test psychological procedures before their widespread use because psychotherapy is undoubtedly beneficial or, at worst, innocuous. We take issue with this claim on two grounds. First, psychotherapy can be harmful. For example, Dishion, McCord, and Poulin (1999) found that peer group interventions for delinquent teens increased adolescent problem behavior and negative life outcomes in adulthood, compared with control conditions. This research project, and others like it, was critical in determining that a seemingly logical treatment was actually harmful. Bootzin and Bailey (2005) provide other examples of treatments that may produce more harm than good.

Second, an ineffective treatment is in itself harmful. An example is facilitated communication for autistic children, which ostensibly enabled children with developmental disabilities to communicate using a computer keyboard and to demonstrate that they were far more cognitively capable than was apparent. This intervention generated great excitement until controlled research repeatedly demonstrated that the results either did not occur or were created, in all likelihood unknowingly, by the facilitator (e.g., Herbert, Sharp, & Gaudiano, 2002). Without this research, many parents would have continued to have their hopes cruelly and falsely raised, and resources for the treatment of these severely disabled children would have continued to be diverted from programs that might be genuinely helpful and assigned instead to a bogus intervention.

Some disorders worsen without effective treatment. Under these circumstances, providing a patient with an ineffective treatment when effective ones exist is not innocuous. For example, we have seen patients with severe anxiety disorders who had years, even decades of ineffective treatment while they lost their jobs, their friends, their avocations, and their life savings. When the efficacy of cognitive-behavioral treatments for such disorders has been repeatedly demonstrated (see chapter 8, this volume), withholding such treatment in the face of patient deterioration is not a neutral act. The ethics code of the American Psychological Association (2002) requires that psychologists refer clients who are not improving in their care for other treatment. Without psychotherapy research, how does the clinician know what that other treatment might be?

Psychotherapists as Decision Makers

Others claim that psychotherapy research is unnecessary because practicing clinicians know best how to treat their patients based on their clinical training, expertise, and lore. There is a surprising dearth of research on psychotherapists' decision making. However, in a recent survey of psychologists in private practice, clinicians reported that they were most likely to rely on their clinical experiences when making treatment decisions (Stewart & Chambless, 2002). How accurate is clinical judgment? There is a large body of research on clinicians' decision making regarding psychological assessments, much of which suggests clinical experience does not increase practitioners' ability to reach valid conclusions if they rely on clinical judgment rather than empirical data in the assessment process (see Garb et al., this volume). Making a decision about how to treat a new client or a client who is not responding to the present treatment plan is the result of an assessment process and is likely subject to the same errors in judgment if clinical experience is the only guide.

Kadden, Cooney, Getter, and Litt (1989) asked therapists of inpatients with alcohol dependence to predict which of two aftercare treatment programs would be better for their patients. The patients were randomly assigned to one of two treatments, and the authors found that patient data (e.g., severity of psychopathology) predicted which treatment would work better for which patients. In contrast, the inpatient therapists were no better than chance at predicting which treatments would work for which of their patients, despite their extensive contact with these patients—much more contact than an outpatient therapist usually has before embarking upon a treatment plan. Schulte, Kunzel, Pepping, and Schulte-Bahrenberg (1992) randomly assigned patients with phobias to standardized treatment with exposure or to an individualized program of cognitive-behavior therapy of the therapist's device. The same therapists participated in both conditions. Therapists in this study were significantly more effective in treating patients with phobic disorders when they were constrained to use the EST of choice (exposure) than they were when they were allowed to devise their own treatment plan, which plans typically included less exposure than the mandated treatment. These therapists, then, although experienced in treating phobic disorders, thought they could beat the data in developing a treatment plan for their clients. They were wrong. Much more research is needed to test whether clinicians are more effective when they follow the treatment recommended by the research literature rather than when they follow their clinical intuitions, but so far the evidence indicates they should follow the data. This is a distasteful thought to many practitioners.

Why might clinical experience be a less accurate guide to treatment decisions than psychotherapists tend to believe? A variety of forces converge to make decisions about psychotherapy based on unsystematic observation vulnerable to error (Dawes, Faust, & Meehl, 1989). The amount of information that must be processed in psychotherapy is enormous and taxes the cognitive capacity of humans as information processors. This leaves clinicians open to the many cognitive biases that influence the attention, selection, and interpretation of feedback they may receive. It is easy for even the most well-meaning of us to deceive ourselves under such circumstances.

An historical example is known to many a student of abnormal psychology. In the early 1770s, Franz Mesmer developed a technique based on his theory of animal magnetism, which posited the existence of palliative magnetic fluids in nature. With a combination of light, music, and chanting, Mesmer produced *mesmerism*, which allegedly moved the magnetic fluids, curing the body and mind of diseases (Pattie, 1994). Mesmer enjoyed great success and popularity in Europe. What may be less likely to be covered in undergraduate texts is the debunking of mesmerism. King Louis XVI commissioned the French Academy of Sciences, including Benjamin Franklin, then resident in Paris, to investigate Mesmer and his therapeutics. Using an early and literal example of the single blind (wherein patients do not know which treatment they are receiving), the commissioners blindfolded patients so that they would not know whether they were being mesmerized. They discovered that patients' responses depended not on the treatment procedure, but on whether they believed they had been mesmerized, in short, on the placebo effect. Franklin concluded, "Some think it will put an end to Mesmerism, but there is a wonderful deal of credulity in the world, and deceptions as absurd have supported themselves for ages" (cited by Isaacson, 2003, p. 427). The case of mesmerism illustrates the dangers of reliance upon uncontrolled observations of practitioners and patients.

Thinking that a treatment works when it does not is one kind of mistake a therapist may make, but what about the other kind, when therapists think a treatment may be harmful when it is actually beneficial? Prolonged exposure to images, thoughts, and other stimuli associated with the trauma has by far the greatest evidentiary base for treatment of posttraumatic stress disorder (e.g., Foa, Rothbaum, Riggs, & Murdock, 1991). However, despite its strong endorsement by experts, prolonged exposure is underutilized by clinicians in the field, who cite a variety of reasons for their reluctance, none of which is empirically based (Becker, Zeyfert, & Anderson, 2004). In particular, clinicians indicated that prolonged exposure leads to symptom worsening. In contrast, the available evidence shows that patients who receive exposure therapy experience better outcomes and no reliable worsening of symptoms compared to patients in waiting list conditions and other treatments (Cahill et al., 2006).

Garb et al. (this volume) describe a number of cognitive biases that may affect clinicians' decision making in the assessment process. These also come into play in practitioners' assessments of treatment efficacy. Psychotherapists are in a particularly difficult situation, in that unless they make concerted efforts to systematically collect information on their practice, they rarely receive clear-cut feedback on their outcomes. Patients often leave without explanation: some because they are doing better and some because they are dissatisfied. Others may leave saying they are feeling better because they are uncomfortable with telling their therapist that they are disgruntled. Moreover, many factors contribute to patients' improvement or deterioration, only one of which is the patient's psychotherapy, making causal attributions difficult even when it is clear that a patient is doing well or not. Such an information vacuum is fertile ground for cognitive errors. We will consider a few examples here.

First, many problems for which people seek treatment are subject to so-called *spontaneous remission*. That is to say, clients get better because the disorder has run its course or because other forces in their environment or their own efforts have led to improvement. The waiting list control group is designed to detect such improvement and to prevent researchers from concluding that a treatment is efficacious when change would have occurred without the intervention. Practitioners, however, have no control group and thus are subject to the *illusory correlation*, believing that their interventions led to the change when, in fact, there was no causal connection. In addition, once clinicians, like anyone else, begin to believe that an intervention is beneficial for a certain sort of client, they may tend to look for evidence that supports their hypothesis, and ignore evidence to the contrary. This is called the *myside bias*.

The operation of the *availability heuristic* means that certain types of memory errors are likely. When clinicians search their memory bank for an intervention that was helpful in the past for a particular situation, they may recall a salient example of a time the intervention was associated with dramatic improvement and forget all the times it did not help. The availability heuristic may also account for the *clinician's illusion*. Cohen and Cohen (1984) coined this term to describe psychotherapists' beliefs that clinical disorders are more severe and enduring than epidemiological evidence indicates. Vessey, Howard, Jueger, Kächele, and Mergenthaler (1994) demonstrated that most clients stay in psychotherapy for six months or less, but that those clients who do remain long term take up an increasing part of the therapist's practice as they accrue. Thus, it is easy for practitioners to erroneously conclude that most patients who enter treatment are long-term and that psychopathology is generally unremitting because these are the cases that readily come to mind. Absent systematic records, it appears that practitioners cannot accurately calculate the characteristics of their caseloads (Knesper, Pagnucco, & Wheeler, 1985). Yet how long clients stay in treatment seems relatively simple, discrete information compared to the assessment of clients' response to treatment interventions.

Do psychotherapists really know how well their patients are doing? Perhaps not. Lambert, Hansen, and Finch (2001) found that providing clinicians with feedback about their patients' progress throughout treatment improved outcomes and increased retention rates. If clinicians are able to make these calculations without obtaining data on their clients' treatment response, why would feedback improve patient outcomes and ostensibly improve clinician performance? These data speak to the importance of collecting data in clinical practice rather than relying on unsystematic observation.

The purpose of this discussion is not to insinuate that clinicians are incompetent or unresponsive to facts, but rather to make the point that clinicians are subject to the same illusions, biases, and memory distortions as anyone else, and that they deal with very complex data. Nor is this discussion meant to downplay the importance of clinical lore and intuition. Clinical experience is a rich source of hypotheses about disorders and their treatments that, when submitted to experimental testing, have led to a variety of efficacious treatments. Nonetheless, the reliance of many clinicians on clinical judgment is exceedingly problematic in light of the literature on the superiority of data-based predictions over clinical judgment.

Rejection of Psychotherapy Research

As noted previously, some practitioners reject the importance of psychotherapy research for their practice, believing clinical expertise is all that is required. Others object to specific aspects of EST research, the predominant paradigm at present. We will consider a few of those objections here (see also Chambless & Ollendick, 2001; Norcross, Beutler, & Levant, 2006).

Nonspecific Factors Rule

According to some authors, the only important factors in psychotherapy outcome are so-called nonspecific factors that are common to all treatments. These include hope, expectation of change, and a good relationship with the therapist. A great deal of research bears witness to the importance of such factors in treatment outcome (Orlinksy, Grawe, & Parks, 1994), and it is a rare psychologist who would argue that better treatment results are obtained by having an uncaring attitude toward one's clients and communicating to them that therapy is unlikely to work. The controversy, therefore, is not over the importance of the nonspecific factors but rather concerns whether different treatment interventions have an impact above and beyond these factors. In our view, this will depend on whether particular treatments rely on specific and effective treatment interventions attuned to the psychopathology of a disorder. For example, in a recent meta-analysis, Siev and Chambless (2007) demonstrated that cognitive-behavior therapy is significantly more effective for panic disorder than are relaxation-based therapies, whereas this is not the case for generalized anxiety disorder. This difference may arise because the psychopathology of panic disorder is now well understood, and effective treatment interventions have been carefully designed to address that psychopathology. Treatment of generalized anxiety disorder leads to significant change, but the degree to which patients improve remains unsatisfactory. Accordingly, researchers in that area are reconsidering the best approach based on having taken another look at core features of the psychopathology of that disorder. For example, Dugas and his colleagues (Dugas, Schwartz, & Francis, 2004) have highlighted the importance of focusing on these patients' intolerance of uncertainty and have reported very promising preliminary results of treatment that includes such a focus (Dugas & Koerner, 2005).

Researchers in cognitive-behavior therapy have not always included measures of nonspecific factors like the therapeutic relationship, but when they have, the superiority of cognitive-behavior therapy to applied relaxation training is evident despite their equivalence on expectations of improvement and the quality of the therapeutic relationship (e.g., Clark et al., 2006).

Treatment Manuals Are Rigid and Rob Therapists of Creativity

Psychotherapists differ as to whether they consider psychotherapy to be an art, a science, or a mixture of those things. Those who believe therapy is an art have expressed contempt for the constraint implied in treatment that is guided by a manual, a necessary component of EST research (Silverman, 1996). Such practitioners often indicate that they approach each client as an individual and avoid being guided by nomothetic treatment research as channeled through treatment manuals. There seem to be two misconceptions at play here. One is that the practitioner really can approach each client *de novo*, without any ideas about what might be helpful for him or her. After all, if there is nothing a therapist can be taught about how to treat particular clients, then there is no point to training in psychotherapy. Few are likely to agree this is the case. Rather, therapists likely draw on informal observations they learned from their supervisors or conclude from their own clinical experience to be helpful with a particular kind of case. As soon as a psychotherapist says, "In my experience this sort of client is best approached in this way," she or he is making a probabilistic statement. That these observations are unsystematic does not make them idiographic, simply untested. We would argue that there is great value in clearly articulating these clinical observations and testing their validity. This is precisely what is done when a treatment manual is constructed, and an RCT is conducted.

The second misconception is the idea that psychotherapists who use ESTs must follow treatment manuals in a robotic fashion such that they are robbed of their therapeutic creativity and not allowed to use their skills. Certainly some manuals are structured more than others, but it is impossible for the thousands of decisions that each therapist must make to be codified. Although manuals provide extensive descriptions of specific procedures within a treatment, flexibility is inherently necessary so that the therapist can respond to the patient and maintain a good therapeutic relationship (Kendall, Chu, Gifford, Hayes, & Nauta, 1998). Nonetheless, the goal is to detail as many of the treatment decisions as possible so that therapists who are not highly expert in the treatment of a particular disorder are able to learn from the experience of experts to carry out the treatment competently.

ESTs' Efficacy Does Not Generalize to Clinical Practice

The claim is often made that ESTs will not work in clinical practice settings, usually because the clients in practice settings are purported to be more severe or to have more comorbid conditions than clients treated in research studies.

Characteristics of Research Participants Westen and Morrison (2001) estimated that the average inclusion rate for studies of depression, panic disorder, and generalized anxiety disorder ranged from 32 to 36%. They inferred from these data that the more difficult cases were being excluded from research trials and thus the efficacy of ESTs for these disorders was likely overblown. Stirman and colleagues have conducted several studies challenging this conclusion.

In the first of these studies, Stirman, DeRubeis, Crits-Christoph, and Brody (2003) developed the concept of the virtual clinic. That is, they hypothesized that many patients might be excluded from one RCT because they did not have the disorder in question, whereas they would fit inclusion criteria for another RCT being run down the virtual hallway by another researcher. For example, the patient may have applied for treatment of panic disorder and was excluded because she had a primary diagnosis of social phobia. However, she would be eligible for a different RCT in the virtual clinic, the study for social phobia. To test this idea, these authors mapped information from charts of patients seeking treatment through a managed care program to the inclusion and exclusion criteria of nearly 100 RCTs for individual therapies. Of those patients who had diagnoses represented in the RCT literature, 80% of these patients would have been eligible for at least one study. Patients who failed to match to studies in the existing literature mostly would have been excluded not because their case was too complex but because they failed to meet minimum severity criteria.

Another charge is that patients with comorbid conditions are excluded from RCTs. Because people with comorbid conditions are more likely to receive treatment than those with a single disorder (Kessler et al., 1994), it would be difficult indeed to conduct RCT research if this were the case. Nonetheless, the psychotherapy researcher must make a hierarchy of disorders so that the problem most in need of treatment is addressed. In a second study, using records of patients who had been screened out of RCTs, Stirman, DeRubeis, Crits-Christoph, and Rothman (2005) found that all patients who had a primary diagnosis of a disorder represented in the RCT literature would have been included in at least one RCT, regardless of their Axis I or II comorbidity.

Transportability of EST to Clinical Settings A second claim regarding generalization is that ESTs will not work once taken from their ivory tower settings into the real world of clinical practice. This is the domain of effectiveness research, and there is a burgeoning literature on the effectiveness of ESTs. Examples include research testing whether ESTs work with ethnic minority clients (e.g., Carter, Sbrocco, Gore, Marin, & Lewis, 2003), whether they work when administered by clinic personnel instead of highly trained research therapists (e.g., Foa et al., 2005), whether they work in community mental health and primary care settings (e.g., Bedi et al., 2000; Merrill, Tolbert, & Wade, 2003), and whether they work with patients who have not been asked to agree to random assignment to treatment (e.g., Juster, Heimberg, & Engelberg, 1995) or who have refused to be so randomized (e.g., Bakker, Spinhoven, van Balkom, Vleugel, & van Dyke, 2000). We have not made an exhaustive study of effectiveness research. Rather, we have simply compiled articles as they have come to our attention. In this manner we have accrued 10 EST effectiveness studies on treatment of depression and 16 on treatment of anxiety disorders, all of which demonstrated the EST to be beneficial, even if not always as highly beneficial as in research trials. Thus, we conclude that the arguments that ESTs do not generalize to clinical settings and the clients seen therein do not hold water, although more research on effectiveness is clearly needed.

EST Lists Are Unfair Psychologists of some theoretical orientations believe that the EST approach is unfair to their preferred psychotherapy method and argue that, because not all treatments have been tested, the playing field is not level (Greenberg & Watson, 2006). This represents some confusion about what the designation of a treatment as an EST means. That a treatment is empirically supported does not mean that it is portrayed as superior to other treatments. Rather, it has been shown to be efficacious in comparison with control conditions, which might or might not include another type of psychotherapy. Moreover, an untested treatment has not been shown to be lacking in benefit. Its benefits are simply unknown. To the extent that one prefers a treatment with efficacy evidence (and admittedly we do), then ESTs are superior in that sense to treatments without such evidence, but this is a different sort of superiority.

Cognitive-behavioral researchers have been at the forefront of developing treatment manuals and protocols, and the preponderance of EST research has been in cognitive-behavioral treatments. This is not surprising given the traditional emphasis of cognitive-behavioral treatments on specifying procedures and identifying symptoms and treatment goals. Although researchers of other orientations, for example, psychodynamic psychotherapy, have also produced manuals (e.g., Milrod, Busch, Cooper, & Shapiro, 1997), the research on these interventions is limited compared to research on CBT. In part this might account for Stewart and Chambless's (2007) findings that private practitioners with a psychodynamic orientation had less positive attitudes about the utility of EST-type treatment research for their practice than CBT and eclectic therapists.

In their meta-analysis of short-term psychodynamic psychotherapies, Leichsenring, Rabung, and Leibing (2004) concluded that short-term psychodynamic therapy is effective in the treatment of psychiatric disorders in general. However, they reported that the number of RCTs is not yet large enough to perform meta-analyses of short-term psychodynamic therapy for specific disorders, and certain disorders have no research at all. Research on short-term psychodynamic therapy continues, and more dynamic treatments will undoubtedly appear on lists of ESTs in the future. This may make the EST concept more acceptable to psychologists of this orientation. However, controlled research on long-term psychodynamic psychotherapy, which is of great interest to many practitioners, is lacking. This may be due to the greater difficulty of manualizing such treatment, resistance to standardized psychotherapy research, or perhaps low levels of interest. In addition, rates of dropout in long-term treatment research are very high and threaten the internal validity of the research. Perhaps for this reason, funding agencies are reluctant to support research on long-term therapy. As a result, psychodynamic therapists who focus on long-term treatment may rely upon case reports and conceptualizations based on clinical experience as data to inform the theory and practice of therapy.

Conclusions

We began this chapter with a statement that psychopathology research serves psychotherapy research. We end with the observation that psychotherapy research serves psychopathology research. That is, there is a reciprocal feedback loop between these two forms of research that is mutually beneficial. For example, cognitive theory of panic disorder stressed the importance of frightening misinterpretations of bodily sensations to the development and maintenance of this problem (Clark, 1986). Treatment aimed at changing these cognitions has proved to be highly effective (see Chambless & Peterman, 2004 for a meta-analytic review), and, closing the feedback loop, Clark et al. (1994) determined that changing beliefs about bodily sensations was critical to the efficacy of cognitive therapy for panic disorder. Thus, psychopathology research informed treatment, and treatment research confirmed the understanding of the psychopathology of this disorder.

The reciprocal feedback loop can also identify when something is wrong with either the theory or the treatment. For example, it was originally postulated that the "sine qua non of marriage was the quid pro quo" (see Gottman, 1998, p. 181). In other words, in happy couples there was an equitable exchange of positive behaviors. This theory led to the use of contingency contracting in marital behavioral therapy, wherein spouses were trained to contract for a desired behavior on the part of their partner by agreeing to reciprocate by doing something that their partner wanted. However, systematic research on couples' interactions revealed that this was precisely the wrong thing to do. In fact, insistence on the equitable exchange of behaviors actually characterized unhappy marriages. Thus, the increased knowledge about marital satisfaction led to improvements in marital therapy, namely the removal of contingency contracting as a basic intervention.

On the basis of these and many other such examples, we argue that progress in applied clinical psychology occurs when treatments are based on a solid understanding of the psychopathology of a given disorder and when those treatments are rigorously evaluated not only for their efficacy and effectiveness but also for the causal factors underlying their benefits. In this fashion, treatments may be honed more precisely to concentrate on the critical elements in outcome, making psychotherapeutic interventions more efficient and more effective.

References

American Psychiatric Association. (1994). *Diagnostic and statistical manual of mental disorders* (4th ed.). Washington, D.C.: Author.

American Psychological Association. (2002). Ethical principles of psychologists and code of conduct. *American Psychologist, 57*, 1060–1073.

Bakker, A., Spinhoven, P., van Balkom, A. J. L. M., Vleugel, L., & van Dyke, R. (2000). Cognitive therapy by allocation versus cognitive therapy by preference in the treatment of panic disorder. *Psychotherapy and Psychosomatics, 69*, 240–243.

Barber, J., & Muenz, L. R. (1996). The role of avoidance and obsessiveness in matching patients to cognitive and interpersonal psychotherapy: Empirical findings from the Treatment for Depression Collaborative Research Program. *Journal of Consulting and Clinical Psychology, 64*, 951–958.

Becker, C. B., Zeyfert, C., & Anderson, E. (2004). A survey of psychologists' attitudes towards and utilization of exposure therapy for PTSD. *Behaviour Research and Therapy, 42*, 277–293.

Bedi, N., Chilvers, C., Churchill, R., Dewey, M., Duggan, C., Fielding, K. et al. (2000). Assessing effectiveness of treatment of depression in primary care. *British Journal of Psychiatry, 177*, 312–318.

Bootzin, R. R., & Bailey, E. T. (2005). Understanding placebo, nocebo, and iatrogenic treatment effects. *Journal of Clinical Psychology, 61*, 871–880.

Cahill, S. P., Foa, E. B., Jayawickreme, N. Rauch, S. A. M., Resick, P. A., Riggs, D. S., and Rothbaum, B. O. (2006). *Primum non nocere* (first do no harm): Symptom worsening and improvement after prolonged exposure for PTSD. Manuscript submitted for publication.

Carter, M. M., Sbrocco, T., Gore, K. L., Marin, N. W., & Lewis, E. L. (2003). Cognitive-behavioral therapy versus a wait-list control in the treatment of African American women with panic disorder. *Cognitive Therapy and Research, 27*, 505–518.

Chambless, D. L., Baker, M., Baucom, D. H., Beutler, L. E., Calhoun, K. S., Crits-Christoph, P. et al. (1998). Update on empirically validated therapies, II. *The Clinical Psychologist, 51*(1), 3–16.

Chambless, D. L., & Hollon, S. D. (1998). Defining empirically supported therapies. *Journal of Consulting and Clinical Psychology, 66*, 7–18.

Chambless, D. L., & Ollendick, T. H. (2001). Empirically supported psychological interventions: Controversies and evidence. In S. T. Fiske, D. L. Schacter, & C. Zahn-Waxler (Eds.), *Annual Review of Psychology* (Vol. 52, pp. 685–716). Palo Alto, CA: Annual Reviews.

Chambless, D. L., & Peterman, M. (2004). Evidence on cognitive-behavioral therapy for generalized anxiety disorder and panic disorder: The second decade. In R. L. Leahy (Ed.), *Contemporary cognitive therapy* (pp. 86–115). New York: Guilford.

Clark, D. M. (1986). A cognitive approach to panic. *Behaviour Research and Therapy, 24*, 461–470.

Clark, D. M., Ehlers, A., Hackmann, A., McManus, F., Fennell, M., Grey, N. et al. (2006). Cognitive therapy versus exposure and applied relaxation in social phobia: A randomized controlled trial. *Journal of Consulting and Clinical Psychology, 74*, 568–578.

Clark, D. M., Salkovskis, P. M., Hackman, A., Middleton, H., Anastasiades, P., & Gelder, M. (1994). A comparison of cognitive therapy, applied relaxation and imipramine in the treatment of panic disorder. *British Journal of Psychiatry, 164*, 759–769.

Cohen, P., & Cohen, J. (1984). The clinician's illusion. *Archives of General Psychiatry, 41*, 1178–1182.

Connolly, M. B., Crits-Christoph, P., Barber, J. P., & Luborsky, L. (2000). Transference patterns in the therapeutic relationship in supportive-expressive psychotherapy for depression. *Psychotherapy Research, 10*, 356–372.

Crits-Christoph, P., Baranackie, K., Kurcias, J., Beck, A. T., Carroll, K., Perry, K., et al. (1991). Meta-analysis of therapist effects in psychotherapy outcome studies. *Psychotherapy Research, 1*, 81–91.

Dawes, R. M., Faust, D., & Meehl, P. E. (1989). Clinical versus actuarial judgment. *Science, 243*, 1668–1674.

Dishion, T. J., McCord, J., & Poulin, F. (1999). When interventions harm: Peer groups and problem behavior. *American Psychologist, 54*, 755–764.

Dugas, M. J., & Koerner, N. (2005). Cognitive-behavioral treatment for generalized anxiety disorder: Current status and future directions. *Journal of Cognitive Psychotherapy, 19*, 61–81.

Dugas, M. J., Schwartz, A., & Francis, K. (2004). Intolerance of uncertainty, worry, and depression. *Cognitive Therapy and Research, 28*, 835–842.

Foa, E. B., Hembree, E. A., Cahill, S. P., Rauch, S. A. A., Riggs, D. S., Feeny, N. C., et al. (2005). Randomized trial of prolonged exposure for posttraumatic stress disorder with and without cognitive restructuring: Outcome at academic and community clinics. *Journal of Consulting and Clinical Psychology, 73*, 953–964.

Foa, E. B., Rothbaum, B. O., Riggs, D. S., & Murdock, T. B. (1991). Treatment of posttraumatic stress disorder in rape victims: A comparison between cognitive-behavioral procedures and counseling. *Journal of Consulting and Clinical Psychology, 59*, 715–723

Gottman, J. M. (1998). Psychology and the study of marital processes. *Annual Review of Psychology, 49*, 169–197.

Greenberg, L. S., & Watson, J. C. (2006). What qualifies as research on which to judge effective practice? Dialogue: Convergence and contention. In J. C. Norcross, L. E. Beutler, & R. F. Levant, (Eds.) *Evidence-based practices in mental health:Debate and dialogue on the fundamental questions* (pp. 81–89, 112–114). Washington, D.C.: American Psychological Association.

Herbert, J. D., Sharp, I. R., & Gaudiano, B. A. (2002). Separating fact from fiction in the etiology and treatment of autism: A scientific review of the evidence. *The Scientific Review of Mental Health Practice, 1*, 23–43

Hersen, M., & Barlow, D. H. (1976). *Single case experimental designs*. New York: Pergamon.

Hinshaw, S. P., Owens, E. B., Wells, K. C., Kraemer, H. C., Abikoff, H. B., Arnold, L. E., et al. (2000). Family processes and treatment outcome in the MTA: Negative/ineffective parenting practices in relation to multimodal treatment [Special Issue]. *Journal of Abnormal Child Psychology, 28*, 555–568.

Isaacson, W. (2003). *Benjamin Franklin: An American life*. New York: Simon & Schuster.

Juster, H., Heimberg, R. G., & Engelberg, B. (1995). Self selection and sample selection in a treatment study of social phobia. *Behaviour Research and Therapy, 33*, 321–324.

Kadden, R. M., Cooney, N. L., Getter, H., & Litt, M. D. (1989). Matching alcoholics to coping skills or interactional therapies: Posttreatment results. *Journal of Consulting and Clinical Psychology, 57*, 698–704.

Kendall, P. C., Chu, B., Gifford, A., Hayes, C., & Nauta, M. (1998). Breathing life into a manual: Flexibility and creativity with manual-based treatments. *Cognitive and Behavioral Practice, 5*, 177–198.

Kessler, R. C., McGonagle, K. A., Zhao, S., Nelson, C. B., Hughes, M., Eshleman, S. et al. (1994). Lifetime and 12-month prevalence of DSM-III-R psychiatric disorders in the United States: Results from the National Comorbidity Survey. *Archives of General Psychiatry, 51*, 8–19.

Knesper, D. J., Pagnucco, D. J., & Wheeler, J. R. (1985). Similarities and differences across mental health services providers and practice settings in the United States. *American Psychologist, 40*, 1352–1369.

Lambert, M. J., Hansen, N. B., & Finch, A. E. (2001). Patient-focused research: Using patient outcome data to enhance treatment effects. *Journal of Consulting and Clinical Psychology, 69*, 159–172.

Leichsenring, F., Rabung, S., & Leibing, E. (2004). The efficacy of short-term psychodynamic psychotherapy in specific psychiatric disorders. *Archives of General Psychiatry, 61*, 1208–1216.

Martin, D. J., Garske, J. P., & Davis, M. K. (2000). Relation of the therapeutic alliance with outcome and other variables: A meta-analytic review. *Journal of Consulting and Clinical Psychology, 68*, 438–450.

Merrill, K. A., Tolbert, V. E., & Wade, W. A. (2003). Effectiveness of cognitive therapy for depression in a community mental health center: A benchmarking study. *Journal of Consulting and Clinical Psychology, 71*, 404–409.

Milrod, B., Busch, F., Cooper, A., & Shapiro, T. (1997). *Manual of panic-focused psychodynamic psychotherapy*. Washington, D.C.: American Psychiatric Press.

Moras, K. (1998). Internal and external validity of intervention studies. In A. S. Bellack & M. Hersen (Eds.), *Comprehensive clinical psychology* (Vol. 3, pp. 201–224). Oxford: Elsevier.

Norcross, J. C., Beutler, L. E., & Levant, R. F. (Eds.). (2006). *Evidence-based practices in mental health: Debate and dialogue on the fundamental questions*. Washington, D.C.: American Psychological Association.

Office of Program Consultation and Accreditation (1996). *Guidelines and principles for accreditation of programs in professional psychology*. Washington, D.C.: American Psychological Association.

Orlinsky, D. E., Grawe, K., & Parks, B. K. (1994). Process and outcome in psychotherapy. In A. E. Bergin & S. L. Garfield (Eds.), *Handbook of psychotherapy and behavior change* (pp. 270–376). New York: John Wiley.

Pattie, F. A. (1994). *Mesmer and animal magnetism: A chapter in the history of medicine*. Hamilton, NY: Edmonston.

Sackett, D. L., Straus, S. E., Richardson, W. S., Rosenberg, W., & Haynes, R. B. (2000). *Evidence-based medicine: How to practice and teach EBM* (2nd ed.). London: Churchill Livingstone.

Schulte, D., Kunzel, R., Pepping, G., & Schulte-Bahrenberg, T. (1992). Tailor-made versus standardized therapy of phobic patients. *Advances in Behaviour Research and Therapy, 14*, 67–92.

Siev, J., & Chambless, D. L. (2007). Specificity of treatment effects: Cognitive therapy and relaxation for generalized anxiety and panic disorders. *Journal of Consulting & Clinical Psychology, 75*, 513–322.

Silverman, W. H. (1996). Cookbooks, manuals, and paint-by-numbers: Psychotherapy in the 90's. *Psychotherapy, 33*, 207–215.

Stewart, R. E., & Chambless, D. L. (2007). Does psychotherapy research inform treatment decisions in private practice? *Journal of Clinical Psychology, 63*, 267–281.

Stirman, S. W., DeRubeis, R. J., Crits-Christoph, P., & Brody, P. E. (2003). Are samples in randomized controlled trials of psychotherapy representative of community outpatients? A new methodology and initial findings. *Journal of Consulting and Clinical Psychology, 71*, 963–972.

Stirman, S. W., DeRubeis, R. J., Crits-Christoph, P., & Rothman, A. (2005). Can the randomized controlled trial literature generalize to nonrandomized patients? *Journal of Consulting and Clinical Psychology, 73*, 127–135.

Vessey, J. T., Howard, K. I., Lueger, R. J., Kachele, H., & Mergenthaler, E. (1994). The clinician's illusion and the psychotherapy practice: An application of stochastic modeling. *Journal of Consulting and Clinical Psychology, 62*, 679–685.

Westen, D., & Morrison, K. (2001). A multidimensional meta-analysis of treatments for depression, panic, and generalized anxiety disorder: An empirical examination of the status of empirically supported therapies. *Journal of Consulting and Clinical Psychology, 69*, 875–899.

II
Common Problems of Adulthood, Childhood, and Adolescence

8
Anxiety Disorders

S. Lloyd Williams

Understanding anxiety disorder means understanding both *anxiety* and *disorder* as scientific ideas. People are anxious about many different things to many different degrees, but nearly everyone knows anxiety from firsthand experience. We speak of one another as feeling anxious, tense, nervous, afraid, worried, scared, and the like, terms we use not only to describe feelings but to explain behaviors. We say that someone did (or did not do) something because she was afraid or he was nervous. Scientists too have held that fear and anxiety, terms this paper will use as synonyms, cause many behaviors, normal and abnormal, adaptive and maladaptive. This anxiety theory of behavior is widely believed. But the meaning of anxiety, and its power to strongly influence behavior, are far from clear. Disorder is yet more difficult a concept in light of a dimensional alternative, the psychosocial problem.

Anxiety Disorders or Psychosocial Problems?

Problems in consciousness and behavior can be conceived as *mental disorders* or quite differently as *psychosocial problems*.

Anxiety Disorder Theory

Among its other meanings, the word *anxiety* denotes sets of proposed mental disorders called anxiety disorders. Anxiety disorder theory derives from a medical model that considers some psychological problems mental illnesses, mental disorders, symptoms, psychopathology, syndromes, and related diseaselike states. Variant proposed anxiety disorders are defined in leading psychiatric organizations' manuals of mental disorders (e.g., American Psychiatric Association, 1980, *DSM-III*; 1987, *DSM-III-R*; 1994, *DSM-IV*; 2000, *DSM-IV-TR*; World Health Organization, 1992, *ICD-10*). Discussion is lively about the definitions of anxiety disorders. But few question whether they exist. Indeed, the very chapter titles in abnormal psychology textbooks all but acclaim anxiety disorder theory valid. The present chapter bears the same title but it rejects anxiety disorder theory without reservation.

Psychosocial Problem Theory

In the author's preferred psychosocial problem theory (Williams, 2007) derived from social cognitive theory (Williams, 1985; Williams & Cervone, 1998; see also Bandura, 1969, 1978, 1986),

141

mental disorders, including anxiety disorders, do not exist. Rather, psychosocial problems exist. Psychosocial problems differ from mental disorders in fundamental and far-reaching ways.

Personality Is a Unified Field Psychosocial problem theory holds that personality is a unified field, not divided by nature into healthy and ill, or normal and abnormal. One can distinguish normal and abnormal or problematic and nonproblematic as a matter of convenience for a given purpose. But that is far different from saying that human personality consists of two dissimilar domains, disordered and nondisordered, separated by a fixed boundary imposed by human nature. And that measuring personality requires at least two different yardsticks, mental disorders to measure the disordered domain but something else to measure the nondisordered domain. This is scientifically inelegant and psychologically dubious.

Commensurability of Problems and Nonproblems Psychological continuity between problems and nonproblems means that the same psychobiological dimensions apply to both (Bandura, 1978, 1986; Williams, 2007; Williams & Cervone, 1998; cf. see also Maddux, Gosselin, & Winstead, this volume). A single measurement framework is suggested by several observations that apply particularly well to the problems that define anxiety disorders. First, personal attributes, including problems, come in graduated degrees with wide variations in their extent, both between individuals and often within individuals over time and across settings. Second, problems range in severity from zero, meaning no problem, incrementally to as extreme, intense, severe, frequent, distressing, or just plain bad as a problem can be, with a higher "score" or position along a given potential problem dimension meaning a worse problem. Third, people tend to be idiosyncratic in the constellations or mixtures of personality attributes, including problems, that they display. These principles imply a continuity between problems and nonproblems that leaves no place for mental disorder in the explanation of behavior.

Dimensions Are Categories Important to note in passing is that every personality attribute, and hence every psychosocial problem, is both a category and a dimension. Worry is a category, distinct from categories such as phobia, obsession, and panic. Worry is also a graduated psychosocial dimension because people worry to all different degrees. So framing the question as "categories versus dimensions" (e.g., Widiger & Samuel, 2005) is imprecise. ***Disorders*** versus dimensions frames the issue better. We cannot escape from categories of human problems. But are these categories of mental disorders, of graduated dimensions, or of yet other kinds of personality attributes? That is the question.

Dimensions that Define Anxiety Disorder Because people and their problems appear characterized better by dimensions than disorders (Williams, 2007), this chapter will present not the usual proposed anxiety disorders, but the broad psychosocial dimensions that define them. These psychosocial dimensions, namely (1) *phobic avoidance,* (2) *compulsive rituals,* (3) *bothersome thoughts,* (4) *subjective anxiety,* and (5) *physiological hyperarousal,* are compelling realities, problems in their own right, whereas anxiety disorders are abstractions created by committees. Disorders dominate research on psychosocial problems, influencing heavily the ways researchers design studies, select potential participants, structure experimental conditions and treatment interventions, select/create dependent measures, and analyze the results. These practices have broad negative implications because mental disorders do not correspond closely to psychological reality.

Disorders Distort Reality but Dimensions Do Not

Disorders distort psychological reality and degrade information about people in numerous and varied ways (Williams, 2007).

Disorders Are Distorters

We will consider a few distorting features of anxiety disorders before turning to psychosocial problems directly in subsequent sections. Disorders distort in the first instance because, unlike people, they are insensitive to context.

A Fixed Short List of Problems Is Not Possible What constitutes a problem depends a great deal on context, as does human personality in general (Mischel, 1990). There can never be an all-purpose exhaustive short list of problems valid across widely dissimilar contexts because the judgment that something is a problem depends inescapably on both the judge's purposes and the judged person's circumstances. For example, if an assessor wants to measure/predict psychological disability then diagnosing anxiety disorder will not help (e.g., American Psychiatric Association, 2000, p. xxxiii). This is because the dimensions that define anxiety disorder in *DSM-IV* include many that do not indicate functional disability and do not correlate strongly with disability, including panic, danger beliefs, difficulty sleeping, sweating, distressing dreams, shortness of breath, and so on. That people can suffer from even intense anxiety or panic inwardly without being disabled outwardly is common, and accords with decades of research consistently finding anxious feelings and avoidant behaviors to be only modestly correlated (Mineka, 1979; Rachman, 1976; Seligman & Johnston, 1973).

Another example of the limited utility of mental disorder is the care of psychiatric inpatients, for which nurses need to attend mainly to patients' dimensional responses such as their suicidality, their self-care skills, or their assaultiveness, regardless of what mental disorder diagnoses they might have received, if any. A very suicidal or assaultive person can have any abstract diagnosis or none at all, so his or her concrete suicide-related or assaultive responses are far more relevant (McMinn et al., 1994).

Mental disorder theory is thus of limited utility even for significant psychiatric problems. It is less so for the other serious human psychosocial problems that fall outside its self-delimited scope, such as problems that fail to meet diagnostic thresholds, as well as broad problem areas such as criminal behavior and interpersonal aggression. Graduated psychosocial dimensions characterize nearly all behavioral problems, and indeed nearly all of human personality, without arbitrary a priori self-restrictions on their range of applicability.

All Agree that Problems Can Be Dimensions Everybody agrees that human mental and behavioral problems involve graduated dimensions; for example, the number of panic attacks, the extent of phobic avoidance, the amount of time spent in obsessive thinking, and so on. And that measuring such graduated dimensional responses is part of assessing people's problems. But after that, psychosocial problem theory and mental disorder theory diverge sharply. Psychosocial problem theory sees the dimensional responses as the very problems for which people need help, and dimensional measures as sufficient to evaluate, communicate about, and remedy them. In this approach, when a new client's problems have been measured dimensionally, the initial assessment is done. Mental disorder theory is far more complicated.

Disorders Are Unparsimonious Complications Disorder theory prescribes shifting the focus from concrete problem dimensions to abstract mental disorders. This brings vexing scientific and practical complications. In addition to assessing the dimensions, the disorder diagnostician must further determine whether any identified problems are arrayed in certain complex configural constellations at designated threshold levels, and then whether any such constellations are nevertheless disqualified from full or even partial disorderhood by various other complex rules. The entire process, often guided far less by psychometrically objective measures than by clinical judgment, can require much pondering and debate. And for what?

What Is a Disorder More Than Its Dimensions? Anxiety disorder theory lacks a clear explanation of why an anxiety disorder should add predictive accuracy to the dimensions that define it. But the law of parsimony requires that it must. Otherwise, why take all the extra diagnostic trouble? Why not proceed from the dimensional scores alone? The incremental or independent validity of mental disorders over psychosocial dimensions is fundamental to the very existence of mental disorders as meaningful scientific entities. Psychosocial problem theory maintains that dimensions have inherent statistical advantages that make them reliably superior to disorders in measuring and predicting behavior (Williams, 2007).

Dimensions Fit Human Problems

Dimensions fit human problems but disorders do not.

Human Problems Are Graduated Mental disorder is a false dichotomy because psychological problems such as phobic avoidance, compulsive rituals, disturbing intrusive thinking, and anxiety are plainly graduated. They come, as do nearly all personality attributes, in many different degrees. In contrast, an anxiety disorder is all or none: a person either has it or does not have it. Diagnosing anxiety disorder thus means gathering dimensional information about the number of panicky sensations, the amount of time spent ritualizing, and the like, then giving up that information in exchange for a dichotomous illness judgment: disordered or not disordered. This is a very bad trade. Transforming a graduated dimension into a dichotomy is "willful discarding of information. It has been shown that when you so mutilate a variable, you typically reduce its squared correlation with behavior about 36% (Cohen, 1983). Don't do it" (Cohen, 1990, p. 1307).

People and Dimensions Are Flexible but Disorders Are Fixed A disorder is further degraded as a predictor to the extent it defines itself using multiple dimensions, and the damage goes up as the correlation between defining dimensions goes down. The *DSM* diagnosis "panic disorder with agoraphobia," for example, weds two largely uncorrelated dimensions, agoraphobic behavior and panic attacks (Craske & Barlow, 1988; about both of which we have more to say, below), into a joint predictor with fixed relative weights that apply even when far from optimal for a given prediction. The dimensional approach, in contrast, allows optimal weighing of dimensions, including discarding one altogether (i.e., weight=0) if needed to reliably and accurately measure/predict an outcome of interest. The preceding are just two of many statistical advantages psychosocial problems enjoy over mental disorders (Williams, 2007).

Human Problems Come in Idiosyncratic Combinations In psychosocial problem theory problems go with problems, but idiosyncratically. That is, problems tend to spring from, bring on, maintain, and exacerbate diverse other problems, not randomly but in combinations idiosyncratic and varied enough to defy adequate characterization by a few prototypical mental disorders, however carefully crafted. Indeed, people said to have a given anxiety disorder tend to be highly heterogeneous with respect to their actual individual problems (Barlow, 2002). And having almost any problem markedly increases the likelihood of almost any other problem (Boyd et al., 1987), which calls into question the mental disorder ideal of neat clusterings of particular responses into certain disorders, and of those disorders into a few higher-order disorder categories such as mood disorders and anxiety disorders.

Flaws in Anxiety Disorder

The scientific concept of anxiety disorder has serious problems.

No Anxiety Disorder Grouping Exists The term *anxiety disorders* implies falsely that the diverse problems so labeled actually belong together in a special distinctive way. The burden of proof appears to lie heavily on advocates of anxiety disorder theory, because no such cohesive distinctive grouping of problems has been shown empirically to exist. To the contrary, the phobic behaviors, compulsive rituals, anxious and panicky feelings, scary bothersome thoughts, and physiological hyperarousal dimensions that define anxiety disorders are heterogeneous among themselves yet occur frequently in people diagnosed with any anxiety disorder, with no disorder, and with nonanxiety disorders (e.g., Braga, Petrides, & Figueira, 2004; de Waal, Arnold, Eekhof, & van Hemert, 2004; Grant et al., 2004; Gunstad & Phillips, 2003). The concept of anxiety disorder thus captures remarkably little of the psychological responses with which it concerns itself.

This is another way of saying that anxiety disorder lacks formal construct validity (Campbell & Fiske, 1959) because it lacks both convergent validity (anxiety disorder dimensions tend to correlate little with one another) and discriminant validity (anxiety disorder dimensions correlate strongly with ostensibly nonanxiety problems like depressed mood; L. A. Clark, Watson, & Reynolds, 1995; Persons, Roberts, & Salecki, 2003). Multidimensional constructs that lack basic construct validity suffer from a fatal flaw that we ignore at our scientific peril.

Anxiety Disorder Excludes Serious Problems Many psychosocial problems, including phobic avoidance, rituals, bothersome scary thoughts, and fear, mild and severe, are excluded from the scope of mental disorders either outright or by placement in a nonspecific disorder category (e.g., Bienvenu, Nestadt, & Eaton, 1998; Marshall et al., 2001; Widiger & Samuel, 2005), either way denying people the full putative benefits of the disorder-based system. Some call the problems denied true disorderhood "subthreshold disorders," an almost nonsensical term that seems to mean disorders that are not disorders.

Subthreshold whatever-they-ares result in part from arbitrary quasi-stringent cutoff scores that define anxiety disorder. For example, to count an anxiety attack as a panic attack for diagnosing panic disorder, *DSM-IV* requires that some attacks be accompanied by at least four responses from a longer list, although an attack with only one or two such responses (for example, a smothering sensation and a feeling of imminent death) can be intense and have serious psychological sequelae (Katerndahl & Realini, 1993; Margraf, Taylor, Ehlers, Roth, & Agras, 1987). Other official symptoms get excluded from the disorder measurement system, such as those left unmeasured by diagnostic interviews when people say no to diagnostic stem questions. Countless additional problems fall into disorder limbo because they are not on the list of official disorder symptoms and therefore receive relatively little attention (e.g., Maj, 2005).

Anxiety Disorders Are Disconnected From Their Own Responses At the heart of the distorting effects of mental disorders is their extensive disconnection from the psychological responses they consist of. One reason we have mentioned already is that a disorder often conjoins little-correlated problem dimensions, which conjoining alone introduces discord between disorders and their dimensions. The discord grows greater yet when distinct subsets of elevated dimension scores equally yield a positive diagnosis, for example, obsessions with no compulsions or compulsions with no obsessions are both obsessive-compulsive disorder. In such a case, saying someone has a certain anxiety disorder conveys little definite information about the person's problems.

This point is illustrated vividly by the discrepancies between panic attack (the psychosocial dimension) and panic disorder (the proposed mental illness), and between agoraphobic avoidance (the dimension) and agoraphobic disorder (the proposed illness). Panic attack is a sudden surge of intense fear, and agoraphobic avoidance is behavioral avoidance of certain activities/settings in the community

(Marks, 1987; Mathews, Gelder, & Johnston, 1981; Williams, 1985; we will consider some nuances in defining panic and agoraphobia in more detail in later sections).

Striking is that "A *DSM-IV* diagnosis of panic disorder with agoraphobia conveys no information about frequency and intensity of panic attacks and the severity of agoraphobic avoidance" (Brown & Barlow, 2002, p. 325). A person with this alleged mental disorder can suffer from any level of panic attacks including none, and any level of agoraphobic avoidance including none, and indeed can have none of either. In *DSM-IV*, people who either avoid or fear agoraphobic activities have panic disorder whether they have panic attacks or not, as long as they were at least briefly bothered by panic at any past time, however remote. Agoraphobic disorder (i.e., in *DSM-IV*, *panic disorder with agoraphobia* or *agoraphobia without history of panic disorder*) requires only that the person need companionship or feel anxious in agoraphobic settings, not that he or she avoids them (*ICD-10 agoraphobia* requires avoidance). So a person neither panicking nor avoiding can be validly diagnosed as having *DSM-IV* panic disorder with agoraphobia.

Another source of discordance between concrete panic attacks and abstract panic disorder is that panic attacks in both *DSM* and *ICD* often have nothing to do with panic disorder. If panicky people also have obsessions, delusions, compulsions, stress, or any one of diverse phobias, medical conditions, or substance use histories, they might well not have *DSM-IV* panic disorder. If panickers are depressed, phobic of just about anything including agoraphobic, or highly anxious between panic attacks, they definitely do not have *ICD-10* panic disorder. Yet panicky people often suffer from depressed mood, phobias, general stress and anxiety, obsessions, delusions, compulsions and/or meet the various other exclusionary conditions (Barlow, 1987, 2002). The panic attacks occurring in people without official panic disorder become nonspecific responses or disorder nonentities altogether, simply falling off the panic disorder radar screen. Therefore, the panic disorder diagnosis is of little use in studying panic attacks, just as the diagnosis of schizophrenia is not very useful in studying hallucinations (Persons, 1986).

The various anxiety disorder diagnostic rules, quite different between *DSM* and *ICD*, show plainly the arbitrariness of anxiety disorder. And neither set of proposed rules characterizes people's problems very well. Rather than trying to better define anxiety disorder, psychosocial problem theory recommends discarding anxiety disorder altogether, but taking its defining phenomena, namely (1) phobia, (2) compulsion, (3) intrusive thoughts, (4) subjective anxiety, and (5) physiological hyperarousal as starting points for a new dimension-based model of human problems. We turn now to describing these five broad psychosocial problem dimensions.

Problem Dimensions Described

Psychosocial problem theory and social cognitive theory conceive personality as reflecting the reciprocal interaction between persons, their behaviors, and their environments (Williams & Cervone, 1998). The psychological person consists of the individual's consciousness and physiological states, as well as social roles and identifying attributes. Behavior refers mainly to a person's potentially publicly observable outward actions. The environment is the person's physical, social, and cultural circumstances. The environmental context is part of personality and of psychosocial problems because people are highly sensitive, and idiosyncratically so, to variations in situations (Mischel, 1990), a phenomenon illustrated vividly by the problems under consideration here (Williams, 1985).

Overt behavior is a critically important personality domain because people's paths through life, and their inward fulfillments and sufferings along the way, have much to do with what they do, and fail to do, outwardly (Williams & Cervone, 1998). Outward behavior is fundamental to how others perceive and judge us, as well as to how we meet our responsibilities, manage our social circumstances, and achieve our most valued personal goals. To suffer anxiety in grocery stores or social gatherings is bad indeed, but to be unable to go into them is worse, undermining people's very ability to look after their own needs and foreclosing any chance of a near-normal life. Phobic avoidance and compulsive rituals torture people by robbing them of social and recreational possibilities and even of their livelihoods, by humiliating and depressing them, and by lowering their self-esteem and quality of life (Bandura, 1978; Steketee & Barlow, 2002; Marks, 1987). So this is not to belittle the sometimes extreme suffering that inner emotional distress can entail, but to point to our special responsibility to help people regain outward behavioral functioning, which is a key to relieving their inner suffering too in many cases (Bandura, 1997; Williams, 1995, 1996a).

Phobic Avoidance

Needless avoidance in at least mild and transitory forms is widespread in psychological life, but when avoidance is marked and persistent one speaks of *phobia*. Phobia illustrates the "neurotic paradox" of self-defeating behavior in which a person is unable to do an ordinary activity although she is otherwise capable, wishes to function normally, and is well aware that her limitation is senseless. Phobias can involve gross disability, such as outright inability to cross a street or speak to a stranger or be in a room with a small spider, for example. People with phobias also refrain from doing things they could do but would rather not. In *DSM*, but not *ICD*, unwarranted fear toward an activity or object is a phobia even if the person does not avoid. This chapter loosely refers to either excessive fear or avoidance of something as phobia, but needless avoidance is the classical hallmark of phobia.

Avoidance in phobia usually is accompanied by some degree of anxiety toward the avoided activity, but one of the most important and well-established findings in phobia research is that anxious feeling and avoidant behavior are not highly correlated (Carr, 1979; Lang, 1985; Mineka, 1979; Rachman, 1976). We will discuss this lack of correlation in more detail later. The present section emphasizes phobic behavior, while later sections address the subjective anxiety and scary thoughts that can variably accompany it.

Phobias vary widely in object, severity, and generality. Some phobias are of highly specific objects or activities (e.g., riding elevators or encountering cats or loud people), whereas generalized phobic patterns can encompass a wide range of seemingly dissimilar activities. Any specific phobia can be a generalized problem when it is severe enough or when the feared object/activity is found in diverse places (e.g., spiders or strangers; Bandura, 1978; Marks, 1987). Specific phobias tend to occur with other specific phobias, so the distinction between specific and generalized phobias can be difficult to make in any case (Hoffman, Lehman, & Barlow, 1997; Lipsitz, Barlow, Mannuzza, Hoffman, & Fyer, 2002).

Phobias can occur in constellations such as agoraphobia, in which a person is simultaneously phobic of at least a few and possibly many or all of about 15 or so distinct community activities such as leaving home alone, using public transportation, shopping, tolerating heights, crossing bridges, riding elevators or escalators, driving a car, and being in an audience. The validity of agoraphobia as a psychological entity has received some support from factor analyses (e.g., Arrindell, Pickersgill, Merckelbach, Ardon, & Cornet, 1991). But a person need have only a few phobias to earn the label (two in *ICD*), and people with agoraphobia also have many social fears, specific phobias, and indeed many varied problems (Barlow, 2002; Williams, 1985), so as Doctor (1982) put it succinctly, "heterogeneity abounds" (p. 210).

Phobias of social scrutiny or of being embarassed or of causing embarassment to others are common in agoraphobia and apart from it, and can vary tremendously in form, generality, and severity between individuals and across different cultural contexts (Hoffman & Barlow, 2002). Great variation exists in the number, kinds, and patterning of individuals' phobias and in the diverse other problems that can accompany them, such as sad mood, panic attacks, hypochondriacal concerns, and many others (Brown & Barlow, 2002; Williams, 1985). Even a specific phobia can be heterogeneous: A dental-phobic person might dread the confinement, the needle, the drilling, the scents, allergic reactions, panic attacks, or various scary social possibilities (e.g., Moore, Brodsgaard, & Birn, 1991), so the term *dental phobia* conveys limited information.

Phobic avoidance and/or fearful feelings about particular things are common far beyond the problems that diagnostic manuals deem official phobic disorders. All widely proposed anxiety disorders, including obsessive-compulsive disorder, generalized anxiety disorder, and various stress and separation disorders, are defined in significant part by behavioral avoidance of, or fearful feelings about, specifiable activities or objects, in other words, by phobias. Beyond the anxiety disorders, some sexual phobias are called sexual dysfunctions; some phobias of having a bodily deformity, body dysmorphic disorder; some disease phobias, hypochondriasis, some phobias of gaining weight, anorexia nervosa, and so on. Avoidant behaviors and frightened feelings toward different particular activities/objects certainly can have individual distinctive psychological features and thematic concerns not shared among all phobias. But they are nonetheless phobias. A psychosocial problem can be simultaneously an eating problem and a phobia.

Compulsive Rituals

An important variant of dysfunctional avoidance behavior is compulsive behavioral ritualizing, such as excessive cleaning, repeating, checking, counting, arranging, hoarding, doubting, or other action that the person carries out beyond reason. One cannot easily exaggerate the heartbreaking extent of impairment and strangeness of behavior in people with severe compulsions (Rachman & Hodgson, 1980; Steketee & Barlow, 2002). Less debilitating but still troubling compulsions appear to be quite common (Muris, Merckelbach, & Clavan, 1997). And diverse problem behaviors other than those defined by *DSM* or *ICD* as obsessive-compulsive disorder, such as tics, hair pulling, rituals connected with self-starvation, dysmorphophobia, and other problems can be clearly compulsive in nature (Yaryura-Tobias & McKay, 2002).

Compulsive behaviors tend to be accompanied by certain patterns of thought and feeling; for example, by obsessive thoughts, by a feeling of fear or discomfort that declines with the compulsive behavior, by a sense that the compulsions prevent harm or danger, and by recognition that the behavior is excessive. But none of these correlated features is invariably present or necessary (Rachman & Hodgson, 1980; Steketee & Barlow, 2002). Noteworthy is that neither anxiety nor any other emotion is required either in *DSM-IV* or *ICD-10* for a diagnosis of obsessive-compulsive disorder. For example, compulsions alone are sufficient for the diagnosis, and these are defined only by actions, not by feelings.

Phobia and compulsion are closely related, and can be viewed for some purposes as passive and active variants, respectively, of avoidance, with phobia avoiding by not doing and compulsion avoiding by doing. Phobic and compulsive behaviors often co-occur and overlap (Rachman & Shafran, 1998). For example, a woman who dreaded burglars remained fully dressed in bed every night atop the bedcovers (phobia), and spent much time before bed checking and rechecking her window and door locks (compulsion).

Although most people with phobias do not have marked compulsions, they often engage in self-protective rituals, as first described and shown experimentally by Williams (1985) and Williams and Zane (1989) and later by Salkovskis (1991). Most people with marked compulsions are phobic about compulsion-provoking circumstances, such as compulsive handwashers who avoid contact with potential contaminating objects like door handles (Rachman & Shafran, 1998). Cognitive (or "covert") compulsions also exist, in which people perform rituals in thought, such as checking, counting, reciting, or arranging, perhaps in order to neutralize, undo, or counteract a previous unacceptable thought or action.

Compulsions can occur in response to external circumstances or in response to obsessions, intrusive unwanted thoughts, images, or impulses often experienced as aversive, alien, or frightening. At times external situations and obsessive thoughts operate in concert to provoke rituals. For example, when one man stepped off a curb he had to not think "Damn God!" else he would be eternally damned; usually unsure if he had done it right, he had to step back and repeat it over and over.

As maladaptive repetitive thoughts, cognitive compulsions can be difficult to distinguish from obsessions (Steketee & Barlow, 2002). Obsessive thoughts and compulsive thoughts and behaviors demonstrate complex patterns of interplay (Frost & Steketee, 2002), and factor analyses of obsessive-compulsive inventories often find factors other than obsessions and compulsions. Dimensional obsession scales correlate highly with compulsion scales (e.g., D. A. Clark, Antony, Beck, Swinson, & Steer, 2005). Among people with either obsessions or compulsions, perhaps 80% have a mixture of both, but some have only obsessions and others have only compulsions. Either can predominate, and theories and treatments concerning each differ (Rachman, 1998; Salkovskis, 1996a; Steketee & Barlow, 2002). The severity of someone's compulsions and obsessions would be characterized far better by separate dimensional scores than by the diagnosis, or not, of obsessive-compulsive disorder.

Bothersome Thoughts

The obsessive thinking we have been discussing is but one of many possible distinctive conscious thought patterns that can be observed often in people with marked fears or dysfunctional avoidance. Some characteristic thoughts are also proposed cognitive mechanisms of fear and avoidance (e.g., Bandura, 1997; Beck, 1976), which we consider in the section on causes. This section considers cognitions that are problems in their own right.

Troublesome intrusive thoughts, difficult to control or dismiss, can come not only as obsessive preoccupations but as excessive worries, scary images, mad impulses, catastrophic expectations, or horrifying recollections, among others (e.g., Borkovec, Shadick, & Hopkins, 1991; Frost & Steketee, 2002; Rapee & Barlow, 1991). Some bothersome thoughts are neither fear-provoking nor resisted but simply consume too much time and thereby interfere with the person's life, whereas others can be alien repugnant ideas that the person tries to avoid by phobic maneuvers or to undo by neutralizing rituals or thoughts (Steketee & Barlow, 2002). Problematic thoughts can arise with almost any pattern of notable avoidance or fear. People with phobias, for example, often perceive the phobic object/activity as dangerous, and worry, obsess, intrusively remember, fearfully anticipate, and have nightmares about it too (Bandura, 1978; Marks, 1987).

Indeed, bothersome thoughts such as obsessions, worries, intrusions, and even hallucinations and delusions, are common in psychological life generally (Johns & Van Os, 2001; Norton, Cox, & Malan, 1992). Rachman and Hodgson (1980) proposed that "necessary and sufficient for defining a thought, impulse, or image as obsessional are intrusiveness, internal attribution, unwantedness, and difficulty of control" (p. 251). Obsessions seem to be a normal part of thought, occurring in most people who have no serious problems, virtually indistinguishable in content from seriously problematic obsessions, although the latter are more frequent and intense, and occasion greater anxiety, avoidance, and compulsive rituals (Borkovec et al., 1991; Craske, Rapee, Jackel, & Barlow, 1989; Rachman & de Silva, 1978; Rachman & Shafran, 1998; Salkovskis & Harrison, 1984). Whether worrisome thoughts become problems depends partly on their perceived controllability (Borkovec et al., 1991; Craske et al., 1989) and one's self-perceived efficacy to manage worrisome future possibilities (Aikins & Craske, 2003; Benight & Bandura, 2004; Davey & Levy, 1998). Noteworthy is the pronounced situational specificity of thinking, that it can vary markedly as a function of circumstances, with most individuals finding that particular settings or activities evoke more obsessions, worries, catastrophic thoughts, or the like, than do others.

One can examine countless different dimensions of thought for different purposes, but the boundaries between the worrisome and the obsessive are not hard and fast. Worries and obsessions are similar in being excessive, repetitive, and time-consuming, having recurrent themes, and often being experienced as uncontrollable and bothersome. Worry and obsession are correlated and can be hard to tell apart. Although some average differences are found (Turner, Beidel, & Stanley, 1992), there appears to be a worry–obsession continuum with many patterns of bothersome thinking showing elements of prototypical worries and prototypical obsessions (Freeston et al., 1994; Wells & Papageorgiou, 1998). Maladaptive worry is also not always clearly distinct from constructive preparatory problem solving, as both involve considering possible dangers and how to deal with them (Craske, 1999).

Nor are the boundaries between the excessive, the unreasonable, and the delusional entirely sharp. People with avoidance, panic, or scary thoughts often recognize that these are out of proportion to objective facts, but such "insight" is highly variable between individuals and even within individuals across different circumstances (e.g., Rachman & Shafran, 1998; Williams, Turner, & Peer, 1985; Williams & Watson, 1985). Why *DSM-IV* requires full insight in specific and social phobic disorders and partial insight in obsessive-compulsive disorder, but ignores insight in other anxiety disorders, is unclear. But this inconsistency adds incoherence to the anxiety disorder concept.

People with obsessions and compulsions, as well as thoughts of danger and dysfunctional avoidance, might or might not accept that their thoughts and actions are senseless. Some obsessions are plainly delusional (O'Dwyer & Marks, 2000; Steketee & Barlow, 2002; Yaryura-Tobias & McKay, 2002). People with psychotic problems frequently display obsessions, compulsions, phobias, panic, and traumatic stress reactions (Braga, Petrides, & Figueira, 2004; Cassano, Pini, Saettoni, & Dell'Osso, 1999; Cosoff & Hafner, 1998; Pallanti, Quercioli, & Hollander, 2004). Panic, worry, and anxiety are prominent in psychosis (Freeman & Garety, 2004; Goodwin, Ferguson, & Horwood, 2004; Owens, Miller, Lawrie, & Johnstone, 2005). These findings support the hypothesis that psychosocial problems combine idiosyncratically and with little regard for official diagnostic boundaries.

Anxiety

Anxiety has long been a principal proposed cause in theories of avoidance behavior, but anxiety is potentially a serious problem in its own right. What is anxiety? Current usage of the term is anything but clear or consistent.

Unimodal, Multimodal, and Polymodal Anxiety Scientists have conceived anxiety in diverse ways (Hersen, 1973; Lang, 1985). It can be defined *unimodally* by a single kind of response such as subjective fear intensity (Walk, 1956) or physiological arousal (Mowrer, 1960). More commonly anxiety is defined *multimodally* by subjective fear and physiological responses and sometimes by certain ideas. The most multimodal definition I call *polymodal* anxiety because its expansive contents include not only all the usual anxiety responses, but also behavior and much else (Lang, 1985). Because putative anxiety responses in one mode tend to be markedly disassociated from those in a different mode, psychosocial problem theory holds that for most purposes the dissimilar responses are better kept separate terminologically rather than being lumped into an all-purpose but not very meaningful anxiety category (Williams, 1987).

Subjective Anxiety Intensity Being afraid means above all feeling afraid, consciously, without which anxiety has no meaning. Fear in consciousness is difficult to describe, but people can indicate how intensely afraid they feel by rating a scale, for example, from 0 (not anxious or afraid) to 10 (extremely anxious and afraid) in one-point increments. Simple unidimensional fear intensity scales from 0 to 8, 0 to 10, or 0 to 100, with simple instructions to rate one's current fear, are in wide use. This sort of definition has the large advantage of not imposing meanings on anxiety other that what people themselves mean by simple anchor terms like *afraid* or *tense*. Subjective anxiety has meaning in relation to the psychological context in which people experience it, and their anxiety intensity ratings indicate straightforwardly how much particular activities frighten them (Williams, 1985; 1987).

Panic Anxiety Panic attacks are sudden rushes of intense anxiety (or discomfort in *DSM*) that can be disturbing and can leave a lasting residue of dread and disability (Barlow, 2002; Craske, 1999; Rachman & Maser, 1988). Yet people can have panic attacks but not develop serious problems in connection with them (Norton et al., 1992; Wilson et al., 1992). Panic attacks vary widely in intensity, duration, frequency, number and kind of accompanying sensations/reactions, and other graduated dimensions (Craske, 1999). Controversy exists as to whether panic differs fundamentally from simply rapidly mounting intense anxiety (Barlow, 2002). The similarities seem large (Craske, 1999), but Barlow (2002) points to possible differences, especially in neurobiological substrates, that caution against prematurely dismissing the distinction.

The concept of spontaneous (or uncued or unexpected) panic was proposed by Klein (1980) as being importantly different from ordinary phobic anxiety or from cued panic because it was un-linked to particular stimuli. Panic attacks vary dimensionally in their apparent relation to specific environmental circumstances, with some seeming unprovoked and others being more or less likely in certain settings. Early theories considered uncued panic to be a biological event (Barlow, 2002; Klein, 1980). Apart from people's perception of a cue, cued and uncued panic attacks are indistinguishable (Craske, 1991, 1999).

The social cognitive view is that even unexpected anxiety and panic often occur in relation to discrete events, but these can be cognitive events such as catastrophic interpretations of perceived bodily states (e.g., D. M. Clark, 1986; D. M. Clark, Salkovskis et al., 1997; Craske, 1991) and loss of self-efficacy for maintaining cognitive control (Williams & LaBerge, 1994). Panic can be highly re-sponsive to environmental and psychological manipulations and interventions (D. M. Clark, 1993; Craske, 1999; Rapee, 1993, 1995).

Although panic, like ordinary anxiety, is conventionally defined and conceived in part as bodily arousal, the actual relationship between bodily arousal and panic, like that between bodily arousal and anxiety, is not very strong, with many reported panic attacks having no accompanying autonomic arousal, and with high rapid autonomic arousal often not experienced as scary or panicky by an indi-vidual (Barlow, 2002; Craske, 1999; Ehlers, 1993; C. B. Taylor, Sheikh et al., 1986). As the essence of anxiety is the subjective feeling of anxiety, the essence of panic is the subjective feeling of panic. We will consider some aspects of the anxiety disorder theory approach to panic, below.

Trait Anxiety Theorists have conceived subjective anxiety not only as a transitory feeling state but an enduring personality trait, a disposition to generally see circumstances as threatening and to react with fear (e.g., Cattell & Scheier, 1961; Spielberger, 1983). Trait anxiety is usually measured by asking people to indicate the self-descriptiveness of various brief general statements (Hersen, 1973). Variant trait conceptions and traitlike inventories abound that measure anxiety-in-general, without respect to context.

People certainly differ from one another in how much they are generally distressed (or disabled, or bedeviled by intrusive thoughts, etc.), but in every case they are troubled by certain definite things and not by others (e.g., Chambless, Beck, Gracely, & Grisham, 2000). Small changes in context, like the approach of a cat to a severe cat phobic, or a chance reminder of childhood diseases to a worry-ing mother, can produce marked shifts in behavior, thought, and feeling (Beck, 1976; Mischel, 1990; Williams & Cervone, 1998). This sort of marked variation in an individual's problem responses across similar situations, which pervades the phenomena we are considering, is simply ignored by generalized traits, as is the idiosyncratic configuration of problem responses from one person to another. Neither kind of variation can be explained even in principle by a general tendency to feel negative affect, think catastrophic thoughts, or fear perceived bodily arousal (Williams, 1985).

Trait scores have some predictive ability, but they rarely explain even 15% of the variance in be-havior, and often explain far less (Bandura, 1986; Mischel, 1990; Williams & Cervone, 1998). Because psychological treatments involve the person having direct mental and physical commerce with the specific things he or she fears, avoids, ritualizes over, or intrusively thinks about, and not with most other things (Barlow, 2002; Craske, 1999), knowing someone's tendency to be anxious-in-general gives little useful information for helping people change. Psychosocial problem theory advocates measuring problem responses directly in problem circumstances when feasible, and otherwise in a psychologically circumscribed context (Williams & Cervone, 1998). Context-sensitive cognitions predict and explain problem behaviors well, as we will see later.

Physiological "Anxiety" Anxiety is widely conceived partly as a physiological response, mainly autonomic arousal and its associated neurochemical mechanisms. Because autonomic arousal per se can be measured physically, without reference to people's consciousness, it is a favored index of fear among investigators who judge subjective feelings to be private events inaccessible to science and therapy (e.g., Lang, 1985). Defining anxiety as physiological arousal gets people's unscientific inner feelings out of the way, but at a high price. Although people commonly describe fear in part by describing how their heart raced or they began to sweat, their bodily perceptions often do not match their bodies (Hoehn-Saric, McLeod, Funderburk, & Kowalski, 2004). Strong emotions of all kinds tend to come with bodily arousal, and phobic people respond differently physiologically than do nonphobic people when doing tasks that the phobic people fear (Alpers, Wilhelm, & Roth, 2005). But that arousal does not distinguish between fears and other strong emotions (Hoehn-Saric, 1998; Lacey, 1967; Zajonc & McIntosh, 1992). Frightened and panicky people show many patterns of physiological arousal, including no arousal at all (Barlow, 2002; Carr, 1979; Ehlers, 1993; Margraf et al., 1987; Morrow & Labrum, 1978; C. B. Taylor, Sheikh et al., 1986).

Physiological arousal without subjective fear is common, as when people exercise, feel sexual interest, or merely hear a familiar voice (Lang, 1985). Calling some instances of autonomic arousal "anxiety" creates confusion about how anxious someone is because different autonomic indices can correlate little with one another and can even change in opposite directions in an individual during treatment (Bandura, 1969; Morrow & Labrum, 1978; Rachman & Hodgson, 1974). The large gap between physiology and subjective feeling means that bodily responses per se cannot be anxiety, but must be considered on their own terms (Williams, 1987).

Anxiety as Perception of Physiological Arousal Social cognitive theory holds that physiological arousal per se has less impact on behavior than does the person's perception and interpretation of physiological arousal (Cioffi, 1991; D. M. Clark, 1986; Salkovskis & Warwick, 1986). Bodily perceptions can become a focus of obsessive worrying and can give rise to defensive actions, such as seeking medical help for a racing heart or ritually carrying a bottle of water against a possible dry mouth. Bodily perceptions are implicated in panic attacks and illness phobias (Clark, 1986; Salkovskis & Warwick, 1986). Yet people, including those with avoidance and fear-related problems, are not very accurate at perceiving how much they are sweating or their heart is beating (Barlow, 2002; Ehlers, 1993; Hoehn-Saric et al., 2004; Mandler, 1962; Pennebaker, 1982). The inaccuracy of bodily perceptions is curiously ignored by *DSM-IV* and *ICD-10*, which allow diagnosticians to measure accelerated heart rate either by a biometric apparatus or by the diagnosed person's subjective impressions, two little-related indicants.

Anxiety in Mental Disorder Theory Manuals of mental disorders rely on anxiety as a description, a cause, and an effect of diverse mental illnesses, but are unclear and inconsistent in how they formally define anxiety and in how they use the concept. In disorder theory, anxiety is multimodal, and comes in three different forms: the phenomenon of anxiety, the proposed symptoms of anxiety disorder, and panic attacks. Each of these three forms of anxiety is viewed rather differently by *ICD-10* and *DSM-IV*.

1. *Anxiety as a proposed disorder-related phenomenon.* In *DSM-IV*'s glossary, anxiety is "the apprehensive anticipation of future danger or misfortune accompanied by a feeling of dysphoria or somatic symptoms of tension" (p. 764). *ICD-10*'s definition of anxiety is looser (note the term *usually* in what follows) yet more elaborate: "Primary symptoms of anxiety...usually involve elements of (a) apprehension (worries about future misfortunes, feeling 'on edge', difficulty in concentrating, etc.); (b) motor tension (restless fidgeting, tension headaches, trembling, inability to relax); and (c) autonomic overactivity (lightheadedness, sweating, tachycardia...dizziness, drymouth, etc." (p.140). Note that neither definition incorporates avoidance behavior.

The requirement for danger thoughts in *DSM-IV* anxiety, and their optional inclusion in *ICD-10* anxiety (and in *DSM-IV* panic too, by the way), transform danger thoughts from anxiety's cause into its very definition, thereby transforming Beck's (1976; Beck et al., 1985) perceived danger theory of anxiety into the meaningless claim that anxiety causes itself. Better to keep danger thoughts out of the definition of feeling afraid so one can explore the possible role of danger thoughts in making people feel afraid.

2. *Anxiety as symptom of anxiety disorder.* *DSM-IV* and *ICD-10* each propose that dozens of different cognitive, emotional, behavioral, physiological, and perceptual responses (somewhat different between the two manuals) are anxiety disorder symptoms. So according to each manual's definition of anxiety (see the preceding section above), some proposed anxiety disorder symptoms are anxiety, whereas other anxiety disorder symptoms are not anxiety. Examples of the former are fearful subjective feelings and physiological overarousal, and of the latter, avoidant behavior and obsessive thoughts. Because the terms *anxiety* and *anxiety symptoms* are used widely as synonyms, mental disorder manuals' efforts to set things straight seem to have only further beclouded anxiety's already foggy meaning.

3. *Anxiety as panic attack.* Disorder manuals also emphasize panic attacks, a variant form of anxiety we discussed earlier. *DSM-IV* defines a panic attack as a discrete period of rapidly mounting intense anxiety or discomfort accompanied by certain thoughts, feelings, perceptions, and physiological or other sensations numbering about two dozen, grouped into 13 categories, with responses from at least 4 categories needed to call a fear attack a panic attack. Notably, *DSM-IV* lists 7 classic agoraphobic fears but none of the 7 is required for diagnosing agoraphobia. Rather, the person's fears or avoidance must be of "places or situations," almost any places or situations evidently, in which the person would feel trapped or helpless in the face of a "Panic Attack or panic-like symptoms" (p. 396). This makes Klein's (1980) panic hypothesis of agoraphobia true by circular definition.

Multimodal and Polymodal Anxiety: Three Systems and Beyond The preceding kinds of anxiety consist mainly of nonbehavioral responses. The three-systems analysis (Lang, 1985) went further and threw in maladaptive behavior itself, the very phenomenon anxiety was supposed to explain. Lang (1985) proposed that "the data of anxiety" consist of "verbal reports of distress, fear related behavioral acts," and "patterns of visceral and somatic activation" (Lang, 1985, pp. 133–134). People no doubt think, feel, act, and respond physiologically, all at once, in nearly every facet of their lives. But as a theory of avoidant behavior the three systems are stillborn. The emotion of anxiety was to be the cause of problem behavior. Asserting that the emotion and the behavior are one and the same, namely anxiety, robs both of meaning.

The three-systems' verbal report category is sometimes called the cognitive system, but this is ironic because it consists not of actual cognitions but of "verbal reports of distress, i.e., reports of anxiety, fear, dread, panic, and associated complaints of worry, obsessions, inability to concentrate, insecurity, and the like" (Lang, 1985, p. 133). Lang (1985) states that these verbal distress reports are of little scientific or therapeutic value: "Feeling states are completely private and represent a poor data resource for the clinician preparing to undertake treatment," and "their unavailability to...observers appears to deny any possibility of scientific investigation" (p.131). But fortunately, "peculiarities of behavior" and "a variety of [physiological] symptoms…are more yielding to objective analysis" (Lang, 1985, p. 131).

This behavioristic rejection of private experience is profoundly anticognitive, and jarringly out of tune with psychology's cognitive revolution in which even rigorous scientists started taking inner experience seriously on its own terms (e.g., Bandura, 1969). The three systems analysis expanded anxiety to include avoidance, but it did not explain avoidance. To explain avoidance, bioinformational theory elaborated the alleged three systems into a vast polymodal fear network (Lang, 1985), to be discussed with causal theories, next.

Causes of the Problems

This review focuses on current psychological causes of the various problems, although developmental and biological causes certainly have a role and have been studied extensively (Bandura, 1997; Barlow, 2002; Craske, 1999; Rapee & Spence, 2004).

Causes of Phobic Avoidance

Our discussion will focus on phobia as prototypical of maladaptive avoidance. Sometimes phobias develop straightforwardly; for example, instated by brief social modeling experiences in monkeys (Mineka et al., 1984) or emerging full-blown from a single brief traumatic experience. Scary verbal information alone can engender enduring fear (Field & Lawson, 2003; Muris, Bodden, Merckelbach, Ollendick, & King, 2003; Rachman, 1977, 2004). However, most phobias have unclear developmental histories, and multiple biological, social, psychological, and environmental factors appear to play a role (Rachman, 1991). In the social cognitive approach, biological and past influences operate mainly via cognitive processes that sustain avoidance, and that can be measured in conjunction with avoidance, here and now.

Avoidance and rituals are correlated to some extent with countless specific inner states, including feelings, cognitions, sensations, and perceptions (Barlow, 2002; Steketee & Frost, 2002), any of which in principle could cause avoidant behavior. Isolating inner psychological causes of avoidance behavior requires identifying inner states that correlate strongly with behavior, as only these are likely to emerge as independent causes of behavior. Finding strong inner predictors of avoidance behavior took a long time because for decades anxious feelings, not problematic thoughts, dominated the research agenda.

Anxiety Theory of Avoidance Maladaptive avoidance behavior was a principal psychological phenomenon that the concept of anxiety was originally intended to explain. Anxiety was the hypothetical cause and avoidant behavior the explained effect. The psychoanalytic conception that an anxiety drive arising from unconscious threats found symbolic expression in particular phobic or other neurotic behaviors was reformulated in learning terms by two-factor theory (Mowrer, 1960), which proposed that anxiety comes to control avoidant behavior in a two-part process consisting of classical conditioning plus operant conditioning. First the person learns by classical conditioning to be afraid of a previously neutral stimulus after experiencing it paired with an aversive stimulus. Then the anxiety provoked by the now-conditioned stimulus motivates the person to avoid the stimulus, which avoidance is rewarded (operant conditioning) by the decline in anxiety it brings (Mowrer, 1960; Wolpe, 1958). Important to note is that an actual decline in "hot" fear is required to reinforce the avoidance. This was to become two-factor theory's downfall.

Two-factor theory dominated the study of avoidance for decades and continues to have loyal adherents, although a series of important reviews in the late 1960s and 1970s (Bandura, 1969; Bolles, 1975; Carr, 1979; Mineka, 1979; Rachman, 1976; Rachman & Hodgson, 1974; Schwartz, 1978, 1989; Seligman & Johnston, 1973) pointed to fundamental problems that two-factor theory never solved.

Because it relies on hot anxiety as both the instigator and the motivator of avoidance, two-factor theory inherently cannot explain why maladaptive avoidance often takes place with little or no fear, both in research animals (Mineka, 1979; Schwartz, 1989; Seligman & Johnston, 1973) and in severely disabled phobic and compulsive people.

ICD-10 states the point explicitly: "It must be remembered that some agoraphobics experience little anxiety because they are consistently able to avoid their phobic situations" (p. 136; see also Carr, 1979; Rachman, 1976; Spitzer & Williams, 1985). Many bridge phobic commuters fearlessly leave home hours early each day and calmly drive far around large bridges (Williams, 1985). Indeed, most human avoidance behavior is fearless (Carr, 1979): people usually fill fuel tanks and lock doors in perfect emotional calmness. Easily executed, apparently effective avoidance maneuvers, even highly maladaptive ones, can leave nothing to be afraird of. Sustained phobic avoidance or compulsive behavior without hot fear is bluntly incompatible with two-factor theory, as is the sustained hot fear without phobic avoidance seen, for example, in some panicky frequent fliers. In the social cognitive analysis to be discussed in detail below, phobic avoidance is caused not primarily by fearful feelings, but by dysfunctional thoughts.

Mower (1960) defined anxiety operationally as autonomic arousal to avoid the then-devastating charge of mentalism leveled at measures of subjective experience. But physiology is as little related to phobic or compulsive behaviors as it is to subjective fear (Bandura, 1969; Lang, 1985; Mineka, 1979; Schwartz, 1989; Seligman & Johnston, 1973; Williams, 1987). Subjective anxiety is better correlated with avoidant behavior (e.g., Williams, Dooseman, & Kleifield, 1984; Williams et al., 1985), but it too usually accounts for relatively little variance in avoidance (Lang, 1985).

Anxiety researchers widely cite Lang's (1985) correct observation that indices of subjective anxiety and of physiological anxiety are poorly correlated with avoidance behavior, but they almost never draw the inescapable further conclusion that therefore anxiety could be at most only a weak cause of avoidance behavior. Causes come in various strengths, and axiomatically any cause cannot be stronger than its correlation with a possible effect. Weak correlation means at best weak causation, so anxiety is inherently weak in explaining avoidance behavior.

We will see below in discussing social cognitive theory that cool thoughts about possible future anxiety have considerably stronger relationship with avoidant behavior than do hot feelings of current anxiety. But such cool thoughts are not two-factor theory. Yet more accurate cognitive predictors of phobic behavior are people's judgments of self-efficacy, i.e., their sense of their own ability to enact the avoided behaviors (Williams, 1995, 1996a). But conditioning theories, including two-factor theory, seek to explain anxious feelings and avoidant behaviors with external conditioning stimuli alone, avoiding mentalism as far as possible; subjective anxiety is already mentalistic enough, never mind the "c" word.

Cognition in consciousness functions better scientifically than do the mechanistic unconditioned stimuli (USs) and conditioned responses (CRs) of two-factor theory (Seligman & Johnston, 1973; Bandura, 1997; Williams, 1996b). So attempts to resurrect two-factor theory cannot ignore the expectations, appraisals, and other conscious processes that social cognitive theory developed and advanced. But they can reanalyze cognitions into conditioning elements after all (e.g., Foa & McNally, 1996; Davey, 1992). Rehabilitating outmoded theories by reframing cognitive advances in conditioning terms was aptly labeled "post-hoc parsimony" by Wilson (G. T. 1978, p. 227). I question putting new cognitive wine in old conditioning bottles (Williams, 1996b). Why bother saving the old awkward language of USs and CRs when the more straightforward and hence more parsimonious language of conscious thought is now available?

Panic Theory of Avoidance A variation on the anxiety theory of avoidance, embodied in *DSM-IV* but not in *ICD-10*, holds that agoraphobic avoidance is caused by panic attacks or by nonpanic but paniclike attacks. As panic and paniclike attacks are similar to hot anxiety, so panic theory founders on the same rock that sank two-factor anxiety theory; namely, that panic does not correlate much with agoraphobic behavior (Craske & Barlow, 1988). Panic can be accompanied by extensive phobias, but often it is not, and agoraphobia is common without current panic and without a history of panic attacks (e.g, Magee, Eaton, Wittchen, McGonagne, & Kessler, 1996). Panic is also common with a host of problems other than agoraphobia (Barlow, 1987; Cosoff & Hafner, 1998) and occurs in people who have no particular problems at all (Norton et al., 1992). We will review findings that the anticipation of possible future panic, unlike panic per se, has a strong relationship to avoidance behavior. But again that conscious cognitive process is not the two-factor anxiety theory of avoidance or its panic-oriented counterpart.

Bioinformational Theory of Avoidance The three-anxiety-systems view was mainly a listing of proposed anxiety responses, but bioinformational theory (Lang, 1985) elaborated that the three-system responses reflect a fear structure (also called a fear program or emotion prototype) that underlies avoidance. The fear structure is a largely unconscious associative network of memory nodes containing dozens of interacting language and meaning elements linked to diverse neurophysiological substrates. In this theory "emotions…are fundamentally to be understood as behavioral acts" (Lang, 1985, p. 140) insofar as the deep emotional prototype initially produces a fear reaction unified across the three proposed anxiety systems (i.e., overt behavior, language behavior, and physiology), but inhibitory neural pathways selectively abort some fear responses before they are expressed (Lang, 1985).

Transmuting fearful feelings into avoidant behaviors would be quite a feat of psychic alchemy, given their well-established empirical disassociation. Why the fear prototype would abort its own efferent signals and why evolution would construct special neural pathways to achieve this self-cancelling objective are hard to fathom. Barlow (2002) wrote well that accepting bioinformational theory's deep unity of fear and avoidance "demands a leap of faith" (p. 57). Bioinformational theory incorporates the latest terminology from neuroscience, cognitive science, and cyberscience, but it is a big step backward. Its polyform phenomena governed by countless unconscious and neurobiological mechanisms can tell us little about people's problems. In contrast, social cognitive theories are testable and of proven value.

Social Cognitive Theory of Avoidance Psychosocial problem theory emphasizes social cognitive theory and a family of related theories that explain phobic and compulsive behavior, anxiety, panic, hyperarousal, and bothersome thoughts in terms of people's conscious appraisals of themselves and their circumstances (e.g., Bandura, 1997; Beck, 1976; Beck, Emery, & Greenberg, 1985; D. M. Clark, 2001; Leary & Kowalski, 1995; Rachman, 1998; Salkovskis, 1996a, 1998; Williams, 1995, 1996a; Williams & Cervone, 1998). I call these collectively *social cognitive theories* because they explain psychosocial problems by people's beliefs, expectations, and judgments about particular things, as representable vividly to themselves in awareness, and about which they potentially can communicate openly. Social cognitions are not generalized traitlike cognitive or information-processing styles, but context-specific thoughts, which specificity enables them to predict the idiosyncratic patterning of avoidance and fear across situations and time.

Despite important differences among them, all social cognitive theories view cognitive factors as underlying both anxiety and avoidance (Bandura, 1997). Different social cognitive theories emphasize different kinds of conscious thought, of which outcome expectations and self-efficacy judgments are especially important (Bandura, 1986; Beck, 1976; Beck et al., 1985; Salkovskis, 1996b; Williams & Cervone, 1998). Outcome expectations refer to people's beliefs about the future outcomes of their own possible actions, and these can be of several kinds. People can anticipate possible physical or social danger. Danger ideas are central to theories derived from the work of Beck (1976), which holds them mainly responsible for the avoidance, fear, and other problems seen in phobia, panic, obsession, compulsion, and traumatic stress (e.g., Beck et al., 1985; D. M. Clark, 1986, 1999, 2001; Salkovskis, 1998). *Perceived danger* is expressed as the likelihood of a harmful outcome, for example, being certain that walking past a dog would result in being bitten.

A group of social cognitive theories holds that fear of fear, an aversion to becoming afraid, panicky, or physiologically aroused, can underlie avoidance (Chambless & Gracely, 1989; Kirsch, 1990; Smits, Powers, Cho, & Telch, 2004). For example, people can anticipate that walking by the dog might make them afraid or might provoke panic. In rating their *anticipated anxiety*, people indicate the level of anxiety they think they would reach if they did a certain task; in rating *anticipated panic* people indicate the likelihood, from 0% to 100%, that doing a task would result in a panic attack. Important to note once again is the fundamental difference between a theory that avoidance is prompted by relatively cool appraisals of possible future fear, and a theory that avoidance is driven by current hot fear.

A different type of social cognition, *perceived self-efficacy*, concerns not the outcomes of an action but one's perceived ability to execute the action irrespective of any outcome that might result, for example, seeing oneself as unable to walk past a dog. Self-efficacy theory (Bandura, 1988, 1997; Williams, 1995, 1996a) holds that avoidance, fear, and scary thoughts arise in relation to an activity largely because people have a diminished sense that they can act effectively and exercise behavioral and cognitive control (Leary & Kowalski, 1995; Maddux, 1995a; Maddux, Norton, & Leary, 1988; Schwarzer, 1992; Williams, 1995, 1996a). Perceived control is intimately related to self-efficacy because a person cannot feel in control without feeling able to enact controlling responses. A sense of control markedly lessens anxiety and panic (Barlow, 2002; Borkovec et al., 1991; Craske et al., 1991; Mineka & Kelly, 1989).

The power of social cognitions to predict phobic behavior has been compared in diverse studies (summarized in Williams, 1995, 1996; see also Öst, Ferebee, & Furmark, 1997; Zollner, Echinerri, & Craske, 2000). Before and after treatment, severe phobics completed cognitive measures including perceived self-efficacy, anticipated anxiety, anticipated panic, and perceived danger in relation to behavioral avoidance tests. Self-efficacy was consistently the most accurate predictor of behavioral avoidance, usually accounting for more than half the variance in behavior. Anticipated anxiety and anticipated panic proved also to be strong predictors of avoidance, but both were consistently somewhat less accurate than was self-efficacy (Williams, 1996a).

Thoughts of danger, rated as the percent likelihood of a specified harmful outcome, were weak predictors of behavior. Importantly, self-efficacy consistently remained strongly predictive of phobic behavior when the other cognitive factors, such as anticipated anxiety, anticipated panic, and perceived danger were held constant, whereas the other factors consistently failed to significantly predict behavior when self-efficacy was held constant (Öst et al., 1997; Williams, 1995, 1996a; Williams, Doosefield, & Kleifield, 1984; Williams, Turner, & Peer, 1985; Williams, Kinney, & Falbo, 1989).

Self-efficacy remains an accurate predictor of future behavior even when relevant past behavior is controlled statistically or does not exist, and when noncausal interpretations of the efficacy-behavior link can be ruled out (Bandura, 1997; Williams, 1995, 1996a; Williams et al., 1989). These data make clear that people's self-perceptions of their abilities influence their avoidance.

Causes of Anxiety

Even if anxiety is not the main cause of avoidance behavior, it requires explanation in its own right. In this section we will briefly consider some social cognitive causes of subjective anxiety and panic, and some information-processing causes of anxiety.

Social Cognitive Causes of Anxiety The preceding section compared possible social cognitive causes of behavior. One can also compare the same possible social cognitions as causes of subjective anxiety. In the studies summarized above (see Williams, 1995, 1996a), participants rated their subjective anxiety during the behavioral tests, which enabled testing how well their social cognitions predicted their anxiety. Anticipated anxiety and anticipated panic were strong predictors of anxiety rated during the behavioral test, accounting for over half of the variance in subjective anxiety ratings, whereas self-efficacy accounted for only about one-quarter of the variance. Anticipated anxiety and anticipated panic each continued to strongly predict subjective anxiety when either self-efficacy or perceived danger was held constant, whereas the latter two lost significant predictiveness with anticipated anxiety or anticipated panic held constant.

Important to note is that people can express high self-efficacy for doing a task but high anticipated anxiety for it as well, in which case they are likely to do the task easily but with high anxiety (Williams, 1985, 1986, 1996a). Bandura (1988) proposed that lack of self-efficacy for controlling scary thoughts (cf. Kent & Gibbons, 1984; Salkovskis & Harrison, 1984) also gives rise to anxiety. Such "thought-control self-efficacy" indeed predicts performance anxiety better than does "task-performance self-efficacy" (Zane & Williams, 1993). But anticipated anxiety or anticipated panic remain the overridingly accurate predictors of performance anxiety. This result suggests that seeing oneself as vulnerable to anxiety (or to panic) causes one to actually experience anxiety (Kirsch, 1990; Williams, 1986), although how this connection comes about is not clear (cf. Bandura, 1995; Maddux, 1995b). In any case, self-efficacy perceptions are the overriding strong cognitive predictors of avoidance behavior, and anticipated anxiety and anticipated panic are the overriding strong cognitive predictors of performance anxiety.

Danger perceptions are generally weak predictors of the level of anxiety people experience during phobia-related behavioral tests (Williams, 1995, 1996a). In addition, contrary to Beck's (1976) theory that danger thoughts should preoccupy phobic people confronting what they dread, agoraphobics facing the worst expressed many anxious feelings but very few thoughts of danger (Williams, Kinney, Harap, & Liebmann, 1997). It is a puzzle that danger thoughts seem only dimly related to feeling afraid and to phobic avoidance (see also Roth, Wilhelm, & Pettit, 2005).

Social Cognitive Causes of Panic Much work has been done on social cognitive factors in panic attacks (e.g., Clark, 1986; Rapee, 1993). Most early research on panic focused on physiological causes (Barlow, 2002), and indeed a variety of physical influences, including sodium lactate, carbon dioxide, caffeine, vigorous exercise, rapid breathing, and others can induce panic in vulnerable individuals. The sheer variety of apparent bodily influences on panic suggests the possibility of common psychological mechanisms (Clark, 1986; Margraf et al., 1986). Psychological models of panic generally conceive it as resulting from perception of threat (Beck et al., 1985), in particular, a vicious cycle of perceiving bodily sensations, interpreting them catastrophically, therefore feeling afraid and apprehensive, which provokes more bodily sensations to be interpreted catastrophically, and so on (Clark, 1986; Rapee, 1993). (But for a skeptical view of theories of panic, including some social cognitive theories, see Roth et al., 2005).

A self-efficacy analysis places emphasis not just on cognized bad outcomes, but also on the person's self-reflective sense of control or coping, the belief that he or she can marshall inner resources to prevent or limit panic by controlling the thoughts that give rise to it (Williams & LaBerge, 1994). Evidence supports a role for cognition in panic, including for a sense of control (Barlow, 2002; Casey, Oei, & Newcombe, 2004; Williams & Falbo, 1996). Cognitive processes seem to mediate the effects of psychological and environmental manipulations on biological panic induction (Clark, 1993; Rapee, 1993; Margraf et al., 1986) and many of the beneficial effects of treatment interventions.

Cognitive Bias Causes of Anxiety Information processing approaches attribute anxiety partly to cognitive biases, both conscious and unconscious, in anxious people's attention to, perception of, interpretation of, and memory for fear-related information, compared with nonanxious people and compared with non-fear related information in anxious people (Mathews & McLeod, 1994, 2002;

McNally, 1999). In a typical study people selected for having or not having anxiety, such as a high trait anxiety score or a certain anxiety disorder diagnosis, view briefly presented words related to danger and other themes, and their reaction times on subtasks ostensibly unrelated to the word meanings reveal how they deployed attention as a function of different thematic content. Typically, anxious individuals are more attentive to negative items related to their anxiety than are nonanxious individuals for the same items (Mathews & McLeod, 1994, 2002; McNally, 1999). Not all kinds of cognitive operations are equivalently biased in anxious individuals. For example, anxious individuals tend not to show information-processing biases on explicit memory tasks (Mathews & McLeod, 1994, 2002; McLeod, 1999; McNally, 1999).

Social cognitive theories concur that people process information differently in relation to their problems than do people without those problems. And that such biases can contribute to the development of problems and can operate with restricted conscious awareness. But information processing research has limitations. It examines information processing in multidimensional psychological states, such as elevated trait anxiety or anxiety disorder diagnostic status, whose complexity and indefiniteness can leave unclear how processing biases relate to people's fears, intrusive thoughts, and avoidance behaviors. It often uses pallid problem-relevant stimuli consisting of brief verbal material or static visual material in a safe laboratory context, and it measures experimental responses, such as latency to detect a probe or to name a color appearing on a computer screen, rather than problem responses per se.

Traitlike biases for seeing broad classes of information as threatening, like personality traits of all kinds, have little ability to explain the idiosyncratic patterning of people's problems across situations. Bias effects can be complex and subject to divergent interpretations, and many are less than robust, being eliminated or even reversed in direction by theoretically minor variations in experimental stimuli, participants, or responses (Lim & Kim, 2005; Mathews & McLeod, 1994, 2002; McNally, 1999). And whereas processing of complex meaning information with awareness is powerful, processing such information with no awareness is weak, and can be hard to demonstrate convincingly (e.g., Kouider & Depoux, 2004). No evidence exists that any unconscious processing bias predicts avoidance behavior or fear remotely as accurately as do conscious social cognitions (Williams, 1996a).

Finally, processing biases, like other inner causes, need to be shown to have an independent effect on behavior and feeling. Recent work has established that induced information-processing biases can lead to anxiety directly (Mathews, 2006; Mathews & McLeod, 2002). The social cognitive view is that fear and avoidance reflect cognitive biases in the processing of information not only about possible threat, but about self-efficacy, about vulnerability to anxiety, and about maladaptive social cognitions generally.

Causes of Bothersome Thoughts

Social cognitive theories hold that bothersome thoughts such as obsessions and worries occur in the normal stream of consciousness (Rachman & de Silva, 1978), but become problematic as people interpret and respond to them maladaptively. Recent theorizing has emphasized an excessive sense of responsibility for preventing potential harmful effects and a corresponding impulse to take neutralizing actions. When people try to avoid or suppress a bothersome intrusion, their neutralizing rituals can increase the thought's frequency and undermine the sense of control, increasing anxiety and spurring greater efforts to exert control, continuing in a vicious cycle (Rachman, 1998; Salkovskis, 1996a). General cognitive deficit theories of obsession fail because, like traits, they are unable to account for the pronounced situational specificity of obsessions (Salkovskis, 1996a).

Theories of worry view it as reinforced by anxiety reduction, by a sense of control, or by perceived risk reduction (Borkovec, et al., 1991; Craske, 1999). To the extent that a sense of control over scary thoughts is important, self-efficacy for exercising such control should be important as well (Bandura, 1988; Kent & Gibbons, 1987). Lack of self-efficacy for remembering actions, distinguishing imagined from real past actions, etc., also called "cognitive confidence" or "thought control confidence," has been implicated in obsessions and compulsions (Hermans, Martens, De Kort, Pieters, & Eelen, 2003), and lack of self-efficacy for solving problems, in generalized anxiety and worry (Aikins & Craske, 2003).

Bodily Causes Do Not Make Problems Mental Disorders

The present brief overview omits the ever-burgeoning literature on the biological substrates of the problems under discussion, not because they have no relevance but only because they lie outside the chapter's overburdened scope. Nevertheless, the relationship between bodily causes and mental disorders is a point of such widespread confusion that it deserves comment. When a problem behavior is found to be correlated with a biometric assessment of a bodily state, the claim is heard that the finding validates mental illness theory. It does not. It perhaps tends to validate physiological theory. But mental illnesses, including anxiety disorders, are neither defined by nor validated by bodily processes measured biometrically, with few and isolated exceptions. Bodily processes affect nearly every human state, physiological, mental, and behavioral, whether problematic or not, so bodily influence says nothing about disease. When a bodily process affects a bodily organ, logically that does not mean the bodily organ is diseased. Likewise, when a bodily process affects a mental state or behavior, logically that does not mean the mental state or behavior is diseased.

Mental states in their own right can explain problem behaviors, so must be understood on their own terms (Bandura, 1986, 1997; Salkovskis, 1996b; Williams & Cervone, 1998). We have seen that measures of people's consciousness enable predicting their future anxious feelings and avoidant behaviors remarkably accurately, indeed, far more accurately than do any biometric measures. But even if bodily influences on avoidant behavior were strong, phobia would not thereby become a mental disorder.

Treatment of the Problems

Psychological approaches to helping people overcome avoidance and rituals, subjective fear and panic attacks, and worries, obsessions, and intrusive bothersome thoughts have achieved notable successes in recent decades, although much room for improvement remains (Barlow, 2002; Chambless & Peterman, 2004; Craske, 1999; Frost & Steketee, 2002). Nevertheless, the findings make clear that behavioral, social, and cognitive factors influence these responses strongly.

Treatment of Phobic Avoidance and Compulsive Rituals

Helping people overcome behavioral disabilities is important in its own right, of course, but also because reducing avoidance behaviors robustly reduces the subjective fear, panic, obsessions, intrusive thoughts, and depressed mood that often go with it.

Performance-Based Treatments Treatment focused entirely on guiding the person to engage in a phobic activity, with minimal explicit attention to thinking or feeling, can enduringly eliminate specific phobias and their negative cognitive and emotional accompaniments within a few hours in most cases, and with widely generalized benefits (Bandura, Blanchard, & Ritter, 1969; Craske, 1999; Öst, 1996). Such methods are also central elements in the treatment of more generalized phobias and compulsions (Rachman & Hodgson, 1980; White & Barlow, 2002). But they are also central to the treatment of subjective anxiety, panic and stress reactions, and bothersome intrusive thoughts, because these all appear to be sustained at least partly by subtle or gross avoidance behaviors that insulate people from corrective learning experiences (Williams, 1985; Williams & Zane, 1989; see also Clark, 1999; Keane & Barlow, 2002; Salkovskis, 1991).

Historically pivotal to phobia and compulsion treatment was *systematic desensitization* (Wolpe, 1958) and related methods that have people imagine doing their avoided activities, and vicarious methods (e.g., Bandura, Grusec, & Menlove, 1965) in which people watch others doing the activities. The next major advance was *performance-based treatment* (sometimes called "*in vivo exposure*"), in which people directly perform their avoided activities (e.g., Agras, Leitenberg, & Barlow, 1968; Bandura, Blanchard, & Ritter, 1969). In performance-based treatment of compulsive rituals, the person engages in ritual-provoking activities (e.g., touches the contaminated door handle or thinks "Damn God!") but then refrains from the rituals, a method also called *exposure and response prevention* (Rachman & Hodgson, 1980). Performance-based methods are reliably more effective than methods based on only imagining or viewing the activities (Bandura et al., 1969; Emmelkamp & Wessels, 1975; Steketee & Barlow, 2002; White & Barlow, 2002).

Exposure Concept of Treatment   Treatments based on imagining, watching, or actually doing phobia-related activities are sometimes called collectively exposure treatment. The exposure concept likens treatment to classical extinction, with unreinforced exposure to the conditioned fear stimulus deconditioning the fear and avoidance (e.g., Foa & McNally, 1996; Marks, 1978). Commerce with relevant stimuli is required for learning just about anything, but identical durations of commerce with phobic stimuli routinely produce highly disparate degrees of change in phobic behavior between treatment groups and between individuals within groups (e.g., Bandura, Jeffrey, & Wright, 1974; Williams, Dooseman, & Kleifield, 1984; Williams, Turner, & Peer, 1985; Williams & Zane, 1989). The exposure idea cannot explain this variability because it casts treatment in passive mechanistic terms and points to fixed outer stimuli instead of flexible inner mental processes.

Guided Mastery Treatment   Treatment based on self-efficacy theory or *guided mastery treatment* (Williams, 1990; Williams, Dooseman, & Kleifield, 1984) seeks to build a strong sense of self-efficacy by fostering people's performance accomplishments. Although belief that one can do an activity is a cognition, the best way to acquire such a cognition is from firsthand success at doing the activity (Bandura, 1997). Therefore, the guided mastery therapist assists people to succeed at tasks that otherwise would be too difficult, while guiding them to do the tasks proficiently, free of embedded rituals and restrictions that limit their perception of success (Williams, 1985, 1990). Assisting people usually produces better results than does simply encouraging them to expose themselves to scary stimuli (Abramowitz, 1996; Bandura, Jeffrey, & Wright, 1974; Feske & Chambless, 1995; Öst, Salkovskis, & Hellstrom, 1991; Williams et al., 1984; Williams, Turner, & Peer, 1985; Williams & Zane, 1989).

Cognitive Therapies   Cognitive therapies designed to help people change their overestimates of danger and to adopt alternative ways of construing events are widely used in combination with performance-based exposure methods to treat behavioral avoidance and rituals (Beck et al., 1985), but these do not seem to have much impact beyond that achieved by performance exposure methods alone (Feske & Chambless, 1995; Fischer & Wells, 2005; Hoffman, 2004; Hope, Heimberg, & Bruch, 1995; McLean et al., 2001; Öst, Thulin, & Ramnerö, 2005; Williams & Falbo, 1996; Williams & Rappoport, 1983).

Treatment of Anxiety

People usually feel afraid of something in particular, and often avoid it as well. As mentioned earlier, mastering the avoidance behavior alone often eliminates any accompanying subjective anxiety as a by-product (e.g., Bandura et al., 1969; Ost et al., 1991; Williams et al., 1984).

Treatment of Subjective Anxiety When people's anxiety fails to come to an end despite doing an activity for some time, social cognitive theory suggests counteracting subtle avoidance maneuvers, defensive activities, or self-protective rituals that circumscribe people's sense of mastery and thereby prolong their fear (Williams, 1985; Williams & Zane, 1989; Zane & Williams, 1993).

This phenomenon was originally identified and studied from the perspective of self-efficacy theory (Williams, 1985, pp. 123–124; Williams & Zane, 1989). Williams and Zane (1989) showed experimentally that when agoraphobic people were given guided mastery assistance to stop the defensive activities and to perform in a proficient varied manner, their anxiety went away more than when they simply exposed themselves to scary stimuli for the same duration (Williams & Zane, 1989). More recently this phenomenon has been interpreted in light of danger theory, and the self-protective maneuvers recast in stimulus terms as focusing on safety signals (Clark, 2001; Salkovskis, 1991). Of course subjective anxiety has long been successfully treated by guiding people to imagine themselves encountering stressors and coping effectively with them, and by a variety of relaxation and cognitive reappraisal treatment methods (Barlow, 2002; Craske, 1999).

Treatment of Panic Attacks Most people with panic attacks display some avoidance, gross or subtle, and defensive behaviors as mentioned in the preceding paragraph (Williams, 1985; Williams & Falbo, 1996), so performance-based therapies for avoidance can have a notable impact on any accompanying panic attacks (Barlow, 2002; Williams & Falbo, 1996; Michelson, Mavissakalian, & Marchione, 1988). Several treatment methods focused specifically on panic include cognitive therapies designed to increase rational appraisal and to decatastrophize thinking, somatic interventions to induce autonomic arousal or other bodily responses in panic (sometimes called interoceptive exposure), and breathing and relaxation techniques designed to normalize and calm physiological arousal (Craske, 1999; Rachman & Maser, 1988; White & Barlow, 2002).

A meta-analysis of 13 studies of panic treatment with cognitive-behavioral therapies, with diverse selection criteria, found rates of panic-free participants after treatment ranging from 53 to 85%, with a weighted mean of 71% (Chambless & Peterman, 2004). But cognitive-behavioral panic therapies have been evaluated mostly in panic victims with few phobias and mild depression, because panic researchers routinely exclude depressed, agoraphobic, or socially phobic panickers from treatment studies. Panickers with few phobias are easier to treat (Williams & Falbo, 1996), so the high level of benefit in nondepressed, phobia-free panickers probably overestimates the benefit average panic cases experience.

Treatment of Bothersome Thoughts

Helping people with bothersome thoughts often involves a combination of elements administered together. Worries and obsessions are directed toward specific activities or stimuli, and are often accompanied by mental or behavioral avoidance reactions or neutralizing rituals, reassurance-seeking, and other actions that paradoxically maintain and increase inward intrusions (Craske, 1999; Keane & Barlow, 2002; Rachman, 1998; Salkovskis, 1996a). Thus the most widely used technique, regardless of whether the thoughts are worries, obsessions, flashbacks, or visualized future calamities, is with enactive or imaginal performance of avoided activities, with response prevention as appropriate for rituals (e.g., de Silva, Menzies, Shafran, 2003; Taylor, Thorardson et al., 2003). Thus, a person can deliberately think an intrusive thought then practice not mentally reacting to it. Cognitive treatments (Clark, 1999; Craske, 1999; Rachman & Shafran, 1998) contain a variety of verbal elements including dialogue aimed at conveying that obsessions are normal, challenging excessive responsibility beliefs and catastrophic meanings, increasing tolerance of uncertainty, as well as methods to try to alter problem imagery, but without trying to decrease the number of intrusive thoughts directly (Clark, 1999; Salkovskis, 1996a).

Prevalence of Disorder of Distribution of Dimension Scores?

The extent to which psychological problems occur in the community has been measured as prevalence rates of mental disorders rather than as frequency distributions of dimensional scores. Probably just about everybody has experienced needless avoidance, fears, and unpleasant thoughts now and again, so their prevalence as mental disorders is largely in the eye of the beholder, dependent on which responses and cutoffs one chooses to define disorder and on how assessors actually operationalize them. For example, in one analysis the prevalence of *DSM-III* generalized anxiety disorder dropped from 45% to 9% of the population when the required duration of anxiety increased from one month to six months and the number of defining responses increased from three to six (Breslau & Davis, 1985).

Prevalence of social phobic disorder ranges from about 2% to 19% of the population, depending on cutoff scores and on the way in which interviewers pose their questions (Stein, Walker, & Forde, 1994). Markedly varying prevalence rates are found for posttraumatic stress disorder mainly because of *DSM*'s imprecise nonoperational definitions (e.g., Kessler, Sonnega, Bromet, Hughes, & Nelson, 1995). The prevalence of obsessive-compulsive disorder using *DSM-IV*'s definition is about one half of that using *DSM-III*'s definition (Crino, Slade, & Andrews, 2005). The impact of ambiguous psychodiagnostic decision rules is evident in a reanalysis of epidemiological findings applying the *DSM-IV* clinical significance criterion, which lowered the United States national prevalence of mental illnesses by 19.2 million people at a single stroke (Narrow, Rae, Robins, & Regier, 2002).

Plainly, the extent of problems in the population would be characterized far better by distributions of problem dimension scores than by the percent of the population having arbitrarily severe mental disorders. But however one might interpret epidemiological findings, they show beyond doubt that serious psychological problems of the kinds we have been considering are common (Kendler, 1994).

Conclusion

I have encouraged readers to approach anxiety disorders by questioning both anxiety and disorders. Calling psychological phenomena by their own proper names without a pseudo-unifying anxiety label removes a comforting illusion of understanding, but helps us see problems more clearly on their own terms. Although we say glibly that phobic people avoid because they are anxious, the evidence favors the far different conclusion that phobic people avoid, and are anxious, because they entertain maladaptive thoughts.

Perhaps more important is to question disorder theory. Most critics of mental disorder diagnosis oddly conclude with a wish to use psychological dimensions to develop better measures of mental disorders. I disagree fundamentally. Here and now psychosocial dimensions do everything good that disorders do, only better, and without all the distortions. The study of phobia, compulsion, bothersome thoughts, subjective anxiety, and physiological hyperarousal is only determined by working these dimensions into fixed dichotomous complex mental disorders. Far from subordinating psychological science to the disorder model, which would be like the victorious General Grant surrendering his army to the defeated General Lee in Mark Twain's tall tale, scientists can celebrate the triumph of dimensions over disorders and never look back.

References

Abramowitz, J. S. (1996). Variants of exposure and response prevention in the treatment of obsessive-compulsive disorder: A meta-analysis. *Behavior Therapy, 27,* 583–600.

Agras, W. S., Leitenberg, H., & Barlow, D. H. (1968). Social reinforcement in the modification of agoraphobia. *Archives of General Psychiatry, 19,* 423–427.

Aikins, D. E., & Craske, M. G. (2003). Cognitive theories of generalized anxiety disorder. *Psychiatric Clinics of North America, 24,* 57–74.

Alpers, G. W., Wilhelm, F. H., & Roth, W. T. (2005). Psychophysiological assessment during exposure in driving phobic patients. *Journal of Abnormal Psychology, 14,* 126–139.

American Psychiatric Association. (1980). *Diagnostic and statistical manual of mental disorders* (3rd ed.). Washington, D.C.: Author.

American Psychiatric Association. (1987). *Diagnostic and statistical manual of mental disorders* (3rd ed., rev.). Washington, D.C.: Author.

American Psychiatric Association. (1994). *Diagnostic and statistical manual of mental disorders* (4th ed.). Washington, D.C.: Author.

American Psychiatric Association. (2000). *Diagnostic and statistical manual of mental disorders* (4th ed., rev.). Washington, D.C.: Author.

Arrindell, W. A., Pickersgill, M. J., Merckelbach, H., Ardon, A. M., & Cornet, F. C. (1991). Phobic dimensions III: Factor analytic approaches to the study of common phobic fears: an updated review of findings obtained with adult subjects. *Advances in Behaviour Research and Therapy, 13,* 73–130.

Bandura, A. (1969). *Principles of behavior modification.* New York: Holt, Rinehart, & Winston.

Bandura, A. (1978). On paradigms and recycled ideologies. *Cognitive Therapy and Research, 2,* 79–103.

Bandura, A. (1986). *Social foundations of thought and action: A social cognitive theory.* Englewood Cliffs, NJ: Prentice-Hall.

Bandura, A. (1988). Self-efficacy conception of anxiety. *Anxiety Research, 1,* 77–98.

Bandura, A. (1995). On rectifying conceptual ecumenism. In J. E. Maddux (Ed.), *Self-efficacy, adaptation, and adjustment* (pp. 347–375). New York: Plenum.

Bandura, A. (1997). *Self-efficacy: The exercise of control.* New York: Freeman.

Bandura, A., Blanchard, E. B., & Ritter, B. (1969). Relative efficacy of desensitization and modeling approaches for inducing behavioral, affective, and attitudinal changes. *Journal of Personality and Social Psychology, 13,* 173–199.

Bandura, A., Grusec, J. E., & Menlove, F. L. (1967). Vicarious extinction of avoidance behavior. *Journal of Personality and Social Psychology, 5,* 16–23.

Bandura, A., Jeffrey, R. W., & Wright, C. L. (1974). Efficacy of participant modeling as a function of response induction aids. *Journal of Abnormal Psychology, 83,* 35–64.

Barlow, D. H. (1987). The classification of anxiety disorders. In G. L. Tischler (Ed.), *Diagnosis and classification in psychiatry* (pp. 223–242). Cambridge: Cambridge University Press.

Barlow, D. H. (2002). *Anxiety and its disorders.* New York: Guilford.

Beck, A. T. (1976). Cognitive therapy and the emotional disorders. New York: International Universities Press.

Beck, A. T., Emery, G., & Greenberg, R. L. (1985). *Anxiety disorders and phobias: A cognitive perspective.* New York: Basic Books.

Beck, A. T., Epstein, N., Brown, G., & Steer, R. A. (1988). An inventory for measuring clinical anxiety: Psychometric properties. *Journal of Consulting and Clinical Psychology, 56,* 893–897.

Benight, C. C., & Bandura, A. (2004). Social cognitive theory of posttraumatic recovery: The role of perceived self-efficacy. *Behaviour Research and Therapy, 42,* 1129–1148.

Bienvenu, O. J., Nestadt, M. B., & Eaton, W. W. (1998). Characterizing generalized anxiety: Temporal and symptomatic thresholds. *Journal of Nervous and Mental Disease, 186,* 51–56.

Borkovec, T. D., Shadick, R. N., & Hopkins, M. (1991). The nature of normal and pathological worry. In R. M. Rapee & D. H. Barlow (Eds.), *Chronic anxiety: Generalized anxiety disorder and mixed anxiety-depression* (pp. 29–51). New York: Guilford.

Boyd, J. H., Burke, J. D., Gruenberg, E., Holzer, C. E., Rae, D. S., George, L. K., et al. (1987). The exclusion criteria of *DSM-III.* In G. L. Tischler (Ed.), *Diagnosis and classification in psychiatry* (pp. 403–424). Cambridge: Cambridge University Press.

Braga, R. J., Petrides, G., & Figurira, I. (2004). Anxiety disorders in schizophrenia. *Comprehensive Psychiatry, 45,* 460–468.

Breslau, N., & Davis, G. C. (1985). Further evidence on the doubtful validity of generalized anxiety disorder. *Psychiatry Research, 16,* 177–179.

Brown, T. A., & Barlow, D. H. (2002). Classification of anxiety and mood disorders. In D. Barlow (Ed.), *Anxiety and its disorders* (pp. 292–327). New York: Guilford.

Campbell, D. T., & Fiske, D. (1959). Convergent and discriminant validation by the multitrait-multimethod matrix. *Psychological Bulletin, 56,* 81–105.

Carr, A. T. (1979). The psychopathology of fear. In W. Sluckin (Ed.), *Fear in animals and man* (pp. 199–235). New York: Van Nostrand Reinhold.

Casey, L. M., Oei, T. P. S., & Newcombe, P. A. (2004). An integrated cognitive model of panic disorder: The role of positive and negative cognitions. *Clinical Psychology Review, 24,* 529–555.

Cassano, G. B., Pini, S., Saettoni, M., & Dell Osso, L. (1999). Multiple anxiety disorder comorbidity in patients with mood spectrum disorders with psychotic features. *American Journal of Psychiatry, 156,* 474–476.

Cattell, R. B., & Scheier, I. H. (1961). *The meaning and measurement of neuroticism and anxiety.* New York: Ronald Press.

Chambless, D. L., Beck, A. T., Gracely, E. J., & Grisham, J. R. (2000). Relationships of cognitions to fear of somatic symptoms: A test of the cognitive theory of panic. *Depression and Anxiety, 11,* 1–9.

Chambless, D. L., & Gracely, E. J. (1989). Fear of fear and the anxiety disorders. *Cognitive Therapy and Research, 13,* 9–20.

Chambless, D. L., & Peterman, M. (2004). Cognitive behavior therapy for generalized anxiety disorder and panic disorder: The second decade. In R. L. Leahy (Ed.). *New frontiers of cognitive therapy.* New York: Guilford.

Cioffi, D. (1991). Beyond attentional strategies: A cognitive-perceptual model of somatic interpretation. *Psychological Bulletin, 109,* 25–41.

Clark, D. A., Antony, M. M., Beck, A. T., Swinson, R. P., & Steer, R. A. (2005). Screening for obsessive and compulsive symptoms: Validation of the Clark-Beck Obsessive Compulsive Inventory. *Psychological Assessment, 17,* 132–143.

Clark, D. M. (1986). A cognitive approach to panic. *Behaviour Research and Therapy, 24,* 461–470.

Clark, D. M. (1993). Cognitive mediation of panic attacks induced by biological challenge tests. *Advances in Behaviour Research and Therapy, 15,* 75–84.

Clark, D. M. (1999). Anxiety disorders: Why they persist and how to treat them. *Behaviour Research and Therapy, 37* (Suppl.), S5–S27.

Clark, D. M. (2001). A cognitive perspective on social phobia. In W. R. Crozier & L. E. Alden (Eds.), *International handbook of social anxiety: Concepts, research, and interventions relating to the self and shyness* (pp. 405–430). Chichester: Wiley.

Clark, D. M., Salkovskis, P. M., & Chalkley, A. J. (1985). Respiratory control as a treatment for panic attacks. *Journal of Behavior Therapy and Experimental Psychiatry, 16,* 23–30.

Clark, D. M., Salkovskis, P. M., Ost, L.-G., Breitholtz, E., Koehler, K. A., Westling, B. E., et al. (1997). Misinterpretation of body sensations in panic disorder. *Journal of Consulting and Clinical Psychology, 65,* 203–213.

Clark, L. A., Watson, D., & Reynolds, S. (1995). Diagnosis and classification of psychopathology: Challenges to the current system and future directions. *Annual Review of Psychology, 46,* 121–153.

Cohen, J. (1983). The cost of dichotomization. *Applied Psychological Measurement, 7,* 249–253.

Cohen, J. (1990). Things I have learned (so far). *American Psychologist, 45,* 1304–1312.

Cosoff, S. J., & Hafner, R. J. (1998). The prevalence of comorbid anxiety in schizophrenia, schizoaffective disorder and bipolar disorder. *Australian and New Zealand Journal of Psychiatry, 32,* 67–72.

Craske, M. G. (1991). Phobic fear and panic attacks: The same emotional states triggered by different cues? *Clinical Psychology Review, 11,* 599–620.

Craske, M. G. (1999). *Anxiety disorders: Psychological approaches to theory and treatment.* Boulder, CO: Westview.

Craske, M. G., & Barlow, D. H. (1988). A review of the relationship between panic and avoidance. *Clinical Psychology Review, 8,* 667–685.

Craske, M. G., Rapee, R. M., Jackel, L., & Barlow, D. H. (1989). Qualitative dimensions of worry in *DSM*-III-R generalized anxiety disorder subjects and nonanxious controls. *Behaviour Research and Therapy, 27,* 397–402.

Crino, R. C., Slade, T., & Andrews, G. (2005). The changing prevalence and severity of obsessive-compulsive disorder criteria from *DSM*-III to *DSM*-IV. *American Journal of Psychiatry, 162,* 876–882.

Davey, G. C. L. (1992). Classical conditioning and the acquisition of human fears and phobias: A review and synthesis of the literature. *Advances in Behaviour Research and Therapy, 14,* 29–66.

Davey, G. C. L., & Levey, S. (1998). Catastrophic worrying: Personal inadequacy and a perseverative iterative style as features of the catastrophizing process. *Journal of Abnormal Psychology, 107,* 576–586.

de Silva, P., Menzies, R. G., & Shafran, R. (2003). Spontaneous decay of compulsive urges: The case of covert compulsions. *Behaviour Research and Therapy, 41,* 129–137.

de Waal, M. W. M., Arnold, I. A., Eekhof, J. A. H., & van Hemert, A. M. (2004). Somatoform disorders in general practice. *British Journal of Psychiatry, 184,* 470–476.

Doctor, R. (1982). Major results of a large-scale survey of agoraphobics. In R. L. DuPont (Ed.), *Phobia: A comprehensive summary of modern treatments* (pp. 203–214). New York: Brunner-Mazel.

Ehlers, A. (1993). Interoception and panic disorder. *Advances in Behaviour Research and Therapy, 15,* 3–21.

Emmelkamp, P. M. G., & Wessels, H. (1975). Flooding in imagination vs. flooding in vivo: A comparison with agoraphobics. *Behaviour Research and Therapy, 13,* 7–15.

Feske, U., & Chambless, D. L. (1995). Cognitive behavioral versus exposure only treatment for social phobia: A meta-analysis. *Behavior Therapy, 26,* 695–720.

Field, A. P., & Lawson, J. (2003). Fear information and the development of fears during childhood: Effects on implicit fear responses and behavioural avoidance. *Behaviour Research and Therapy, 41,* 1277–1293.

Foa, E. B., & McNally, R. J. (1996). Mechanisms of change in exposure therapy. In R. Rapee (Ed.), *Current controversies in the anxiety disorders* (pp. 329–343). New York: Guilford.

Freeman, D., & Garety, P. A. (2003). Connecting neurosis and psychosis: the direct influence of emotion on delusions and hallucinations. *Behaviour Research and Therapy, 41,* 923–947.

Freeston, M. H., Ladouceur, R., Rheaume, J., Letarte, H., Gagnon, F., & Thibodeau, N. (1994). Self-report of obsessions and worry. *Behaviour Research and Therapy, 32,* 29–36.

Frost, R. O., & Steketee, G. (2002). *Cognitive approaches to obsessions and compulsions: Theory, assessment, and treatment.* Elsevier: Oxford.

Goodwin, R. D., Ferguson, D. M., & Horwood, L. J. (2004). Panic attacks and psychoticism. *American Journal of Psychiatry, 161,* 88–92.

Grant, B. F., Stinson, F. S., Dawson, D. A., Chou, P. et al. (2004). Prevalence and co-occurrence of substance use disorders and independent mood and anxiety disorders. *Archives of General Psychiatry, 61,* 807–816.

Gunstad, J., & Phillips, K. A. (2003). Axis I comorbidity in body dysmorphic disorder. *Comprehensive Psychiatry, 44,* 270–276.

Hermans, D., Martens, K., De Kort, K., Pieters, G., Eelen, P. (2003). Reality monitoring and metacognitive beliefs related to cognitive confidence in obsessive-compulsive disorder. *Behaviour Research and Therapy, 41,* 383–401.

Hersen, M. (1973). Self-assessment of fear. *Behavior Therapy, 4,* 241–257.

Hoehn-Saric, R. (1998). Psychic and somatic anxiety: Worries, somatic symptoms, and physiological changes. *Acta Psychiatrica Scandinavica, 98* (Suppl. 393), 32–38.

Hoehn-Saric, R., McLeod, D. R., Funderburk, F., & Kowalski, R.W. (2004). Somatic symptoms and physiologic responses in generalized anxiety disorder and panic disorder. *Archives of General Psychiatry, 61,* 913–921.

Hoffman, S. G. (2004). Cognitive mediation of treatment change in social phobia. *Journal of Consulting and Clinical Psychology, 72,* 393–399.

Hoffman, S. G., & Barlow, D. H. (2002). Social phobia (social anxiety disorder). In D. H. Barlow (Ed.), *Anxiety and its disorders* (pp. 454–476). New York: Guilford.

Hoffman, S. G., Lehman, C. L., & Barlow, D. H. (1997). How specific are specific phobias? *Journal of Behavior Therapy and Experimental Psychiatry, 28*, 233–240.

Holden, A. E., & Barlow, D. H. (1986). Heart rate and heart rate variability recorded in vivo in agoraphobics and nonphobics. *Behavior Therapy, 17*, 25–42.

Hope, D. A., Heimberg, R. G., & Bruch, M. A. (1995). Dismantling cognitive-behavioral group therapy for social phobia. *Behaviour Research and Therapy, 33*, 637–650.

Johns, L. C., & Van Os, J. (2001). The continuity of psychotic experiences in the general population. *Clinical Psychology Review, 21*, 1125–1141.

Katerndahl, D. A., & Realini, J. P. (1993). Lifetime prevalence of panic states. *American Journal of Psychiatry, 150*, 246–249.

Keane, T. M., & Barlow, D. H. (2002). Posttraumatic stress disorder. In D. H. Barlow (Ed.), *Anxiety and its disorders* (pp. 418–453). New York: Guilford.

Kendler, K. S. (1994). Lifetime and 12-month prevalence of *DSM-III-R* psychiatric disorders in the United States: Results from the National Comorbidity Survey. *Archives of General Psychiatry, 51*, 8–19.

Kent, G., & Gibbons, R. (1987). Self-efficacy and the control of anxious cognitions. *Journal of Behavior Therapy and Experimental Psychiatry, 18*, 33–40.

Kessler, R. C., Sonnega, A., Bromet, E., Hughes, M., & Nelson, C. B. (1995). Posttraumatic stress disorder in the National Comorbidity Survey. *Archives of General Psychiatry, 52*, 1048–1060.

Kirsch, I. (1990). *Changing expectations.* Belmont, CA: Brooks-Cole.

Klein, D. F. (1980). Anxiety reconceptualized. *Comprehensive Psychiatry, 21*, 411–427.

Kouider, S., & Dupoux, E. (2004). Partial awareness creates the "illusion" of subliminal semantic priming. *Psychological Science, 15*,

Lacey, J. I. (1967). Somatic response patterning and stress: Some revisions of activation theory. In M. H. Appley & R. Trumbull (Eds.), *Psychological stress: Issues in research* (pp. 14–42). New York: Appleton Century Crofts.

Lang, P. J. (1985). The cognitive psychophysiology of emotion: Fear and anxiety. In A. H. Tuma & J. D. Maser (Eds.), *Anxiety and the anxiety disorders* (pp. 131–170). Hillsdale, NJ: Erlbaum.

Lang, P. J., Cuthbert, B. N., & Bradley, M. M. (1998). Measuring emotion in therapy: Imagery, activation, and feeling. *Behavior Therapy, 29*, 655–674.

Leary, M. R., & Kowalski, R. M. (1995). The self-presentational model of social phobia. In R. G. Heimberg, M. R. Liebowitz, D. A. Hope, & F. R. Schneier (Eds.), *Social phobia: Diagnosis, assessment, treatment* (pp. 94–112). New York: Guilford.

Lim, S.-L., & Kim, J.-H. (2005). Cognitive processing of emotional information in depression, panic, and somatoform disorder. *Journal of Abnormal Psychology, 114*, 50–61.

Lipsitz, J. D., Barlow, D. H., Mannuzza, S., Hoffman, S. G., & Fyer, A. J. (2002). Clinical features of four *DSM-IV*-specific phobia subtypes. *Journal of Nervous and Mental Disease, 190*, 471–478.

MacLeod, C. (1999). Anxiety and anxiety disorders. In T. Dalgleish & M. J. Power (Eds.), *Handbook of cognitive emotion* (pp. 447–477). New York: Wiley.

Maddux, J. E. (Ed.) (1995a). *Self-efficacy, adaptation, and adjustment: Theory, research, application.* New York: Plenum.

Maddux, J. E. (1995b). Looking for common ground: A comment on Kirsch and Bandura. In J. Maddux (Ed.), *Self-efficacy, adaptation, and adjustment: Theory, research, application* (pp. 377–385). New York: Plenum.

Maddux, J. E., Norton, L. W., & Leary, M. R. (1988). Cognitive components of social anxiety: An investigation of the integration of self-presentational theory and self-efficacy theory. *Journal of Social and Clinical Psychology, 6*, 180–190.

Magee, W. J., Eaton, W. W., Wittchen, H.-U., McGonagne, K. A., & Kessler, R. C. (1996). Agoraphobia, simple phobia, and social phobia in the National Comorbidity Survey. *Archives of General Psychiatry, 53*, 159–168.

Maj, M. (2005). "Psychiatric comorbidity": An artefact of current diagnostic systems? *British Journal of Psychiatry, 186*, 182–184.

Mandler, G. (1962). Emotion. In R. Brown, E. Galanter, E. Hess, & G. Mandler (Eds.), *New directions in psychology* (Vol. 1, pp. 269–343). New York: Holt, Rinehart, & Winston.

Margraf, J., Taylor, C. B., Ehlers, A., Roth, W. T., & Agras, W. S. (1987). Panic attacks in the natural environment. *Journal of Nervous and Mental Disease, 175*, 558–565.

Marks, I. M. (1978). Behavioral psychotherapy of adult neurosis. In S. L. Garfield & A. E. Bergin (Eds.), *Handbook of psychotherapy and behavior change* (pp. 493–547). New York: Wiley.

Marks, I. M. (1987). *Fears, phobias, and rituals.* New York: Oxford.

Marshall, R. D., Olfson, M., Hellman, F., Blanco, C., Guardino, M., & Struening, E. L. (2001). Comorbidity, impairment, and suicidality in subthreshold PTSD. *American Journal of Psychiatry, 158*, 1467–1473.

Mathews, A. M. (2006). Toward an experimental cognitive science of CBT. *Behavior Therapy, 37*, 314–318.

Mathews, A. M., Gelder, M. G., & Johnston, D. W. (1981). *Agoraphobia: Nature and treatment.* New York: Guilford.

Mathews, A. M., & MacLeod, C. (1994). Cognitive approaches to emotion and emotion disorders. *Annual Review of Psychology, 45*, 25–50.

Mathews, A., & MacLeod, C. (2002). Induced processing biases have causal effects on anxiety. *Cognition and Emotion, 16*, 331–354.

McLean, P. D., Whittal, M. L., Thordarson, D. S., Taylor, S., Sochting, I., Koch, W. J. et al. (2001). Cognitive versus behavioral therapy in the group treatment of obsessive compulsive disorder. *Journal of Consulting and Clinical Psychology, 69*, 205–214.

McMinn, B., Lunza, M. L., Kayne, H. L., Pattison, I., Hicks, C., & Islam, S. (1994) Predicting violence: Nursing diagnosis versus psychiatric diagnosis. *Nursing Diagnosis, 5*, 151–158.

McNally, R. J. (1999). Panic and phobias. In T. Dalgleish and M. J. Power (Eds.), *Handbook of cognition and emotion* (pp. 479–496). New York: Wiley.

Michelson, L., Mavissakalian, M., & Marchione, M. (1988). Cognitive, behavioral, and psychophysiological treatments of agoraphobia: A comparative outcome investigation. *Behavior Therapy, 19*, 97–120.

Mineka, S. (1979). The role of fear in theories of avoidance learning, flooding, and extinction. *Psychological Bulletin, 86*, 985–1010.

Mineka, S., Davidson, M., Cook, M., & Keir, R. (1984). Observational conditioning of snake fear in rhesus monkeys. *Journal of Abnormal Psychology, 93*, 344–372.

Mineka, S., & Kelly, K. A. (1989). The relationship between anxiety, lack of control and loss of control. In A. Steptoe and A. Appels (Eds.), *Stress, personal control and health* (pp. 163–191). New York: Wiley.

Mischel, W. (1990). Personality dispositions revisited and revised: A view after three decades. In L. A. Pervin (Ed.), *Handbook of personality: Theory and research* (pp. 111–164). New York: Guilford.

Moore, R., Brodsgaard, I., & Birn, H. (1991). Manifestations, acquisition and diagnostic categories of dental fear in a self-referred population. *Behaviour Research and Therapy, 29*, 51–60.

Morrow, G. R., & Labrum, A. H. (1978). The relationship between psychological and physiological measures of anxiety. *Psychological Medicine, 8*, 95–101.

Mowrer, O. H. (1960). Learning theory and behavior. New York: Wiley.

Muris, P., Bodden, D., Merckelbach, H., Ollendick, T. H., & King, N. (2003). Fear of the beast: A prospective study on the effects of negative information on childhood fear. *Behaviour Research and Therapy, 2003*, 195–208.

Muris, P., Merckelbach, H., & Clavan, M. (1997). Abnormal and normal compulsions. *Behaviour Research and Therapy, 35*, 249–252.

Narrow, W. E., Rae, D. S., Robins, L. N., Regier, D. A. (2002). Revised prevalence estimates of mental disorders in the United States. *Archives of General Psychiatry, 59*, 115–123.

Norton, G. R., Cox, B. J., & Malan, J. (1992). Nonclinical panickers: A critical review. *Clinical Psychology Review, 12*, 121–139.

O'Dwyer, A., & Marks, I. M. (2000). Obsessive-compulsive disorder and delusions revisited. *British Journal of Psychiatry, 176*, 281–284.

Öst, L.-G. (1996). Long term effects of behavior therapy for specific phobias. In M. R. Mavissakalian & R. F. Prien (Eds.), *Long term treatments of the anxiety disorders*. Washington, D.C.: American Psychiatric Press.

Öst, L.-G., Ferebee, I., & Furmark T. (1997). One-session group therapy of spider phobia: Direct versus indirect treatments. *Behaviour Research and Therapy, 35*, 721–732.

Öst, L.-G, Salkovskis, P., & Hellstrom, K. (1991). One-session therapist-directed exposure vs. self-exposure in the treatment of spider phobia. *Behavior Therapy, 22*, 407–422.

Öst, L.-G., Thulin, U., Ramnerö, J. (2004). Cognitive behavior therapy vs exposure in vivo in the treatment of panic disorder with agoraphobia. *Behaviour Research and Therapy, 42*, 1105–1127.

Owens, D. G. C., Miller, P., Lawrie, S. M., & Johnstone, E. C. (2005). Pathogenesis of schizophrenia: A psychopathological perspective. *British Journal of Psychiatry, 186*, 386–393.

Pallanti, S., Quercioli, L., Hollander, E. (2004). Social anxiety in outpatients with schizophrenia: A relevant cause of disability. *American Journal of Psychiatry, 161*, 53–58.

Pennebaker, J. W. (1982). *The psychology of physical symptoms*. New York: Springer-Verlag.

Persons, J. (1986). The advantages of studying psychological phenomena rather than psychiatric diagnoses. *American Psychologist, 11*, 1252–1260.

Persons, J. B., Roberts, N. A., & Zalecki, C. A. (2003). Anxiety and depression change together during treatment. *Behavior Therapy, 34*, 149–163.

Rachman, S. (1976). The passing of the two-stage theory of fear and avoidance: Fresh possibilities. *Behaviour Research and Therapy, 14*, 125–131.

Rachman, S. (1977). The conditioning theory of fear acquisition: A critical examination. *Behaviour Research and Therapy, 15*, 375–387.

Rachman, S. (1991). Neo-conditioning and the classical theory of fear acquisition. *Clinical Psychology Review, 11*, 155–173.

Rachman, S. (1998). A cognitive theory of obsessions: Elaborations. *Behaviour Research and Therapy, 36*, 385–401.

Rachman, S. (2004). Fear of contamination. *Behaviour Research and Therapy, 42*, 1227–1255.

Rachman, S., & de Silva, P. (1978). Abnormal and normal obsessions. *Behaviour Research and Therapy, 16*, 233–248.

Rachman, S., & Hodgson, R. (1974). I. Synchrony and desynchrony in fear and avoidance. *Behaviour Research and Therapy, 12*, 311–318.

Rachman, S., & Hodgson, R. (1980). *Obsessions and compulsions*. Englewood Cliffs, NJ: Prentice-Hall.

Rachman, S., & Maser, J. D. (Eds.) (1988). *Panic: psychological perspectives*. Hillsdale, NJ: Lawrence Erlbaum.

Rachman, S., & Shafran, R. (1998). Cognitive and behavioral features of obsessive-compulsive disorder. In R. P. Swinson, M. M. Anthony, S. Rachman, & M. A. Richter (Eds.), *Obsessive-compulsive disorder*. New York: Guilford.

Rapee, R. M. (1993). Psychological factors in panic disorder. *Advances in Behavior Research and Therapy, 15*, 85–102.

Rapee, R. M. (1995). Psychological factors influencing the affective response to biological challenge procedures in panic disorder. *Journal of Anxiety Disorders, 9*, 59–74.

Rapee, R. M., & Barlow, D. H. (Eds.) (1991). *Chronic anxiety*. New York: Guilford.

Rapee, R. M., & Spence. S. (2004). The etiology of social phobia. Empirical evidence and an initial model. *Clinical Psychology Review, 24*, 737–767.

Roth, W. T., Wilhelm, F. H., & Pettit, D. (2005). Are current theories of panic falsifiable? *Psychological Bulletin, 131*, 171–192.

Salkovskis, P. M. (1991). The importance of behaviour in the maintenance of anxiety and panic: A cognitive account. *Behavioural Psychotherapy, 19*, 6–19.

Salkovskis, P. M. (1996a). Cognitive-behavioral approaches to the understanding of obsessional problems. In R. M. Rapee (Ed.), *Current controversies in the anxiety disorders* (pp. 103–133). New York: Guilford.

Salkovskis, P. M. (1996b). Understanding of obsessive-compulsive disorder is not improved by redefining it as something else. In R. M. Rapee (Ed.), *Current controversies in the anxiety disorders* (pp.191–200). New York: Guilford.

Salkovskis, P. M. (1998). Psychological approaches to the understanding of obsessional problems. In R. P. Swinson, M. M. Anthony, S. Rachman, & M. A. Richter (Eds.), *Obsessive-compulsive disorder: Theory, research, and treatment* (pp. 33–50). New York: Guilford.

Salkovskis, P. M., & Harrison, J. (1984). Abnormal and normal obsessions: A replication. *Behaviour Research and Therapy, 22,* 549–552.

Salkovskis, P. M., & Warwick, H. M. C. (1986). Morbid preoccupations, health anxiety and reassurance: A cognitive behavioural approach to hypochondriasis. *Behaviour Research and Therapy, 24,* 597–602.

Schwartz, B. (1978). *Psychology of learning and behavior.* New York: Norton.

Schwartz, B. (1989). *Psychology of learning and behavior* (3rd ed.). New York: Norton.

Seligman, M. E. P., & Johnston, J. C. (1973). A cognitive theory of avoidance learning. In F. J. McGuigan & D. B. Lumsden (Eds.), *Contemporary approaches to conditioning and learning* (pp. 69–110). Washington, D.C.: Winston & Sons.

Smits, J. A. J., Powers, M. B., Cho, Y., & Telch, M. J. (2004). Mechanism of change in cognitive-behavioral treatment of panic disorder: Evidence for the fear of fear mediational hypothesis. *Journal of Consulting and Clinical Psychology, 72,* 646–652.

Spielberger, C. D. (1983). *Manual for the State-Trait Anxiety Inventory.* Palo Alto, CA: Consulting Psychologists.

Spitzer, R. L., & Williams, J. B. W. (1985). Proposed revisions in the *DSM-III* classification of anxiety disorders based on research and clinical experience. In A. H. Tuma & J. D. Maser (Eds.), *Anxiety and the anxiety disorders* (pp. 759–773). Hillsdale, NJ: Lawrence Erlbaum.

Stein, M. B., Walker, J. R., & Forde, D. R., (1994). Setting diagnostic thresholds for social phobia: Considerations from a community study of social anxiety. *American Journal of Psychiatry, 152,* 408–412.

Steketee, G., & Barlow, D. H. (2002). Obsessive-compulsive disorder. In D. H. Barlow (Ed.), *Anxiety and its disorders* (pp. 516–550). New York: Guilford.

Taylor, C. B., Sheikh, J., Agras, W. S., Roth, W. T., Margraf, J., Ehlers, A., et al. (1986). Ambulatory heart rate changes in patients with panic attacks. *American Journal of Psychiatry, 143,* 478–482.

Taylor, S., Thordson, D. S., Maxfield, L., Fedeoroff, I. C., Lovell, K., & Ogrodniczuk, J. (2003). Comparative efficacy, speed, and adverse effects of three PTSD treatments. *Journal of Consulting and Clinical Psychology, 71,* 330–338.

Turner, S. M., Beidel, D., & Stanley, M. A. (1992). Are obsessional thoughts and worry different cognitive phenomena? *Clinical Psychology Review, 12,* 257–270.

van den Hout, M., Kindt, M. (2003). Repeated checking causes memory distrust. *Behaviour Research and Therapy, 41,* 301–316.

Walk, R. D. (1956). Self ratings of fear in a fear-invoking situation. *Journal of Abnormal and Social Psychology, 52,* 171–178.

Wells, A., & Papageorgiou, C. (1998). Relationships between worry, obsessive-compulsive symptoms and metacognitive beliefs. *Behaviour Research and Therapy, 36,* 899–913.

White, K. S., & Barlow, D. H. (2002). Panic disorder and agoraphobia. In D. H. Barlow, *Anxiety and its disorders* (pp. 328–379). New York: Guilford.

Widiger, T. A., & Samuel, D. B. (2005). Diagnostic categories or dimensions? A question for the *Diagnostic and Statistical Manual of Mental Disorders*—Fifth Edition. *Journal of Abnormal Psychology, 114,* 494–504.

Williams, S. L. (1985). On the nature and measurement of agoraphobia. *Progress in Behavior Modification, 19,* 109–144.

Williams, S. L. (1986, August). Self-appraisal determinants of defensive behavior and emotional arousal. In R. Ganellen (Chair), *Agoraphobia: Cognitive contributions.* Symposium conducted at the meeting of the American Psychological Association, Washington, D.C.

Williams, S. L. (1987). On anxiety and phobia. *Journal of Anxiety Disorders, 1,* 161–180.

Williams, S. L. (1990). Guided mastery treatment of agoraphobia: Beyond stimulus exposure. *Progress in Behavior Modification, 26,* 89–121.

Williams, S. L. (1995). Self-efficacy, anxiety, and phobic disorders. In J. Maddux (Ed.), *Self-efficacy, adaptation, and adjustment: Theory, research, and application* (pp. 69–107). New York: Plenum.

Williams, S. L. (1996a). Therapeutic changes in phobic behavior are mediated by changes in perceived self-efficacy. In R. Rapee (Ed.), *Current controversies in the anxiety disorders* (pp. 344–368). New York: Guilford.

Williams, S. L. (1996b). Overcoming phobia: Unconscious bioinformational deconditioning or conscious cognitive reappraisal? In R. Rapee (Ed.), *Current controversies in the anxiety disorders* (pp. 373–376). New York: Guilford.

Williams, S. L. (2007). *Psychosocial dimensions surpass mental disorders in measuring people's problems.* Manuscript in preparation, University of Basel, Switzerland.

Williams, S. L., & Cervone, D. (1998). Social cognitive theories of personality. In D. F. Barone, M. Hersen, & V. B. Van Hasselt (Eds.), *Advanced personality* (pp. 173–207). New York: Plenum.

Williams, S. L., Dooseman, G., & Kleifield, E. (1984). Comparative effectiveness of guided mastery and exposure treatments for intractable phobias. *Journal of Consulting and Clinical Psychology, 52,* 505–518.

Williams, S. L., & Falbo, J. (1996). Cognitive and performance-based treatments for panic attacks in people with varying degrees of agoraphobic disability. *Behaviour Research and Therapy, 34,* 253–264.

Williams, S. L., Kinney, P. J., & Falbo, J. (1989). Generalization of therapeutic changes in agoraphobia: The role of perceived self-efficacy. *Journal of Consulting and Clinical Psychology, 57,* 436–442.

Williams, S. L., Kinney, P. J., Harap, S., & Liebmann, M. (1997). Thoughts of agoraphobic people during scary tasks. *Journal of Abnormal Psychology, 106,* 511–520.

Williams, S. L., & LaBerge, B. (1994). Panic disorder with agoraphobia. In C. G. Last & M. Hersen (Eds.), *Adult behavior therapy casebook* (pp. 107–123). New York: Plenum.

Williams, S. L., & Rappoport, A. (1983). Cognitive treatment in the natural environment for agoraphobics. *Behavior Therapy, 14*, 299–313.

Williams, S. L., Turner, S. M., & Peer, D. F. (1985). Guided mastery and performance desensitization treatments for severe acrophobia. *Journal of Consulting and Clinical Psychology, 53*, 237–247.

Williams, S. L., & Watson, N. (1985). Perceived danger and perceived self-efficacy as cognitive determinants of acrophobic behavior. *Behavior Therapy, 16*, 237–247.

Williams, S. L., & Zane, G. (1989). Guided mastery and stimulus exposure treatments for severe performance anxiety in agoraphobics. *Behaviour Research and Therapy, 27*, 237–247.

Wilson, G. T. (1978). The importance of being theoretical: A commentary on Bandura's "Self-efficacy: Toward a unifying theory of behavioral change." *Advances in Behaviour Research and Therapy, 1*, 217–230.

Wilson, K. G., Sandler, L. S., Asmundson, G. J. G., Ediger, J. M., Larsen, D. K., & Walker, J. R. (1992). Panic attacks in the non-clinical population: an empirical approach to case identification. *Journal of Abnormal Psychology, 101*, 460–468.

Wolpe, J. (1958). *Psychotherapy by reciprocal inhibition.* Stanford, CA: Stanford University Press.

World Health Organization (1992). *The ICD-10 classification of mental and behavioural disorders: Clinical description and diagnostic guidelines.* Geneva: Author.

Yarura-Tobias, J. A., & McKay, D. (2002). Obsessive compulsive disorder and schizophrenia: A cognitive perspective of shared pathology. In R. O. Frost & G. Steketee (Eds.), *Cognitive approaches to obsessions and compulsions: Theory, assessment, and treatment* (pp. 251–267). Oxford: Pergamon.

Zajonc, R. B., & McIntosh, D. N. (1992). Emotions research: Some promising questions and some questionable promises. *Psychological Science, 3*, 70–74.

Zane, G., & Williams, S. L. (1993). Performance-related anxiety in agoraphobia: Treatment procedures and cognitive mechanisms of change. *Behavior Therapy, 24*, 625–643.

Zoellner, L. A., Echiverri, A., & Craske, M. G. (2000). Processing of phobic stimuli and its relationship to outcome. *Behaviour Research and Therapy, 38*, 921–931.

9

Mood Disorders

Rick Ingram and Lucy Trenary Smith

Depression is not a recent phenomenon. Although descriptions of conditions resembling depression can be found in the Old Testament of the Bible, it was Hippocrates in the fourth century B.C. who hypothesized that "Melancholia" stemmed from an imbalance of black bile. Even more "modern" conceptions of depression were suggested by Araetus of Cappadocia around 120 A.D., who described melancholia as being characterized by sadness, a tendency toward suicide, feelings of indifference, and psychomotor agitation. It was not until the early 20th century that theorists such as Abraham (1911/1960) and Freud (1917/1961) began to recognize the importance of psychological and emotional factors in the development of depression.

Today depression is not only widely recognized as a significant public health concern, but its prevalence rates may be increasing (Kessler at al., 2003), so much that some researchers have argued that the public faces a depression epidemic (e.g., Seligman, 1990). Variations in diagnostic criteria used to assign diagnoses across different generational cohorts make it difficult to know definitively that this increase is authentic, but the evidence to date is consistent with a genuine increase in prevalence (Goodwin, Jacob, Bittner, & Wittchen, 2006). Depression is also associated with a wide variety of problems including social withdrawal, occupational disability, and interpersonal turmoil, as well as with a significant economic cost to society (Simon, 2003). Furthermore, depression is frequently a chronic condition; relapse and recurrence rates are high (Ingram, Miranda, & Segal, 1998; Kessler, 2002), and individuals who experience recurrent depression are also at considerable risk for developing dysthymia (a less severe but longer lasting form of depression), as well as other psychiatric conditions. Apart from the emotional misery linked to depression, suicide and suicide attempts are not uncommon during depressive episodes. Even over and above suicide rates, data also show that depression is related to earlier mortality (Irwin, 2002; Saz & Dewey, 2001).

In this chapter we examine a number of facets of mood disorders. Although mood disorders include both *unipolar depression* and *bipolar disorder*, given the high prevalence rates for unipolar depression and the relatively low rates for bipolar disorder, the majority of our focus is on unipolar depression. We start by briefly describing the various mood disorders presented in the fourth, revised edition of the *Diagnostic and Statistical Manual of Mental Disorders* (*DSM-IV-TR*; American Psychiatric Association, 2000), noting the approach taken by the *DSM* as well as discussing some limitations. We next move to a discussion of the epidemiology of depression, and then provide some perspectives on gender differences and cultural issues in depression. Following this, we examine theory and research on depression. In particular, we discuss the role of stress in depression with specific reference to diathesis-stress hypotheses, and then examine biologically and psychologically based models of depression. We conclude with an examination of data on the prevention of depression and data on biological and psychological approaches to treatment.

Definitions and Descriptions of Mood Disorders

Psychopathological constructs such as depression can be viewed in a variety of different ways. For instance, psychologists have argued that the term *depression* can be used to refer to a mood state, a *symptom* (e.g., being sad), a *syndrome* (a constellation of signs and symptoms that cluster together), a label applied to a group of individuals with a specific mental disorder, or a disease that is associated with biochemical or genetic abnormalities (Kendall, Hollon, Beck, Hammen, & Ingram, 1987; Nurcombe, 1992). Although each of these terms is a legitimate description of a condition, the variety of uses can be a source of confusion.

Issues in Defining Mood Disorders

Adding to possible confusion, a number of specific subtypes of depression have been proposed. For instance, a relatively early distinction differentiated between *reactive depressions*, which were thought specifically to be associated with stressful events, and *endogenous depression*, which was less related to stress and more associated with internal dysregulation. Other distinctions can be theoretically based; for example, Abramson and Alloy (2006) have proposed a cognitive subtype of depression where dysfunctional thinking patterns play a primary causal role, and differentiate this subtype from those where thinking may not be causally significant. With few exceptions, however, there has been little agreement on the nature of specific subtypes. This is not to suggest, however, that subtypes do not exist, but rather that these subtypes are difficult to conceptually define and empirically identify. Adding to this confusion is that depression itself is a label for a heterogeneous group of conditions that exhibit a similar symptom constellation, but that may have very different causes and courses. Despite this uncertainty over the nature of the various types of depression, the most widely used set of definitions of depression is incorporated in *DSM-IV-TR* (2000).

The *DSM* is a taxonomic system of behavior categorization. Specifically, diagnostic categories in the *DSM* reflect an attempt to develop a taxonomy that differentiates and then classifies dysfunctional behavior. It is important to note, however, that such taxonomic systems are not fixed but rather evolve as concepts and paradigms shift and, correspondingly, become more complex with a deeper appreciation of natural phenomena (Kessler et al., 2005). Indeed, psychiatric taxonomy illustrates just such an evolutionary process; since its introduction in 1952, the *DSM* has undergone several extensive revisions with depression being defined in somewhat different ways in each edition (see also Widiger, this volume.)

DSM Defined Diagnoses

Mood disorders can be conceptualized as falling into two main categories: *unipolar* and *bipolar* disorders. In brief, *DSM-IV-TR* includes diagnoses for *unipolar depression, dysthymic disorder, bipolar disorder,* and *cyclothymic disorder,* as well as more "minor" categories that include depressive disorder not otherwise specified, bipolar disorder not otherwise specified, mood disorder due to a general medical condition, substance-induced mood disorder, and mood disorder not otherwise specified. We focus here on a brief description of the major categories of mood disorders.

Unipolar Depression In unipolar depression, an individual suffers from one or more major depressive episodes. A major depressive episode is defined as persisting for a period of at least two weeks, with the experience of at least one of two cardinal features. These two cardinal features are depressed mood and *anhedonia*, which is defined as a loss of pleasure in activities that are usually enjoyable. In total, individuals must endorse five of the following nine symptoms: depressed mood, anhedonia, appetite or weight changes, insomnia or hypersomnia, psychomotor agitation or retardation, loss of energy, feelings of worthlessness or guilt, diminished ability to concentrate or indecision, or suicide ideation. It is important to note that the "depressed" mood exemplifies a change from the person's normal functioning. In addition, symptoms and altered functioning must be associated with significant distress or impairment.

Dysthymic Disorder Dysthymic disorder can best be thought of as a chronic, low grade depression lasting a minimum of two years. The same symptoms as in a major depressive episode are present, but fewer and less severe symptoms are required for a diagnosis. Because of the chronicity of dysthymic disorder, the depressed mood and associated symptoms often become integrated into a person's normal functioning (American Psychiatric Association, 1996). After the first two years of depressed mood, if a major depressive episode also occurs, the combination is referred to as *double depression*. Data have suggested that between 20 and 40% of individuals receiving a diagnosis of depression will also evidence dysthymia (Goodwin et al., 2006)

Bipolar Disorder Bipolar disorder is divided into bipolar I and bipolar II disorder. The presence of a *manic episode* or *mixed episode* (depression and mania) defines bipolar I, with a manic episode defined as a period of at least one week where mood is abnormally expansive, elevated, or irritable. Three (or four if mood is irritable only) out of seven symptoms must be experienced: inflated self-esteem or grandiosity, decreased need for sleep, more talkative than usual, flight of ideas, distractibility, increase in goal-directed activity, and excessive involvement in pleasurable activities that are likely to have adverse consequences. Individuals with bipolar I disorder often show poor judgment and may engage in a number of risky activities. A mixed episode also qualifies for a bipolar I disorder diagnosis. A mixed episode lasts at least a week, during which the criteria are met for both a major depressive episode and a manic episode on a daily basis with the individual's mood state alternating between these extremes. Delusions and hallucinations might also be present in bipolar I disorder. In these cases, the disorder is characterized as having *psychotic features*, which are further specified as *mood-congruent* (consistent with the theme of the manic, mixed, or depressive episode) or *mood-incongruent* (not consistent with the theme of the mood episode).

Bipolar II disorder is characterized by one or more major depressive episodes accompanied by at least one *hypomanic* episode. Though similar to a manic episode, hypomanic symptoms last for a minimum of four days, rather than the week required for mania. Although Bipolar II individuals experience the same number and types of symptoms as mania, functioning is not as greatly impaired and psychotic features are not present.

Cyclothymic Disorder Like dysthymia, cyclothymia is a chronic disorder (lasting at least two years) during which an individual fluctuates between depressive and hypomanic symptoms. Both classes of symptoms are of insufficient number, severity, and duration to warrant a diagnosis of a major depressive episode or hypomania. No major depressive, manic, or mixed episode can occur during the first two years, though they may co-occur with the cyclothymia once this initial period has passed.

Additional Classifications A number of additional well-recognized classifications exist. For example, *seasonal affective disorder*, a condition in which individuals experience depression concomitantly with the approach of winter, is acknowledged by most researchers as a legitimate subtype of depression (Rosenthal & Rosenthal, 2006). *Psychotic depression* is a severe disorder in which hallucinations or delusions are present, and may reflect a distinct disorder from nonpsychotic depression (Flores & Schatzberg, 2006).

Alternatives to the DSM

The *DSM* has become the gold standard in psychopathology research and practice, but it is important to note that the *DSM* represents only one of many potential ways to conceptualize the construct of depression. To further understand this issue, consider the different ways to conceptualize mood disorders. For example, depression can be seen as representing a distinct category or a mood dimension. The *DSM* employs a categorical perspective, delineating distinct classes of mood disorders with definitive boundaries between them. A category is an "either-or" construct—either an individual is depressed, or is not. Major, or clinical, depression is also seen as qualitatively distinct from the mildly depressed mood states that many people experience. Conversely, the dimensional approach views these disorders as existing on a continuum, ranging from less to more severe, without any clear and definitive boundaries or categories (Flett, Verdenburg, & Krames, 1997; see also Widiger, this volume).

Like any classification system, the categorical method has both advantages and disadvantages. An advantage is the fact that distinct categories facilitate clear communication about a particular disorder. For example, the severity and general clinical picture are fairly clear based on the common language that the *DSM* provides between and among clinicians and researchers. Hence, the categorical perspective simplifies the conceptualization of psychopathology and expedites clinical and research decision making (Kendell, 1975; Trull, Widiger, & Guthrie, 1990). On the other hand, problems inherent in such a system are due to the fact that categories can force a vague and unclear phenomenon into specific and fixed compartments. Mood states are seen as qualitatively different from one another, when in fact they, or at least varying components of them, might exist on a continuum. A related point hinges upon the apparent simplicity of a diagnosis. Although a categorical system makes communication easier, it may also disguise important differences. For instance, two cases of major depressive episode could manifest in very different manners, having completely distinct etiologies, symptom patterns, clinical courses, and treatment outcomes. It is important to keep in mind that although it is a real phenomenon, or set of phenomena, "depression" means what we define it to mean. As illustrated by the different editions of *DSM*, definitions and underlying assumptions of these definitions may change with further research and progress.

Course of Mood Disorders

Major depressive episode symptoms often develop over days to weeks, often beginning with a mild form that later escalates into a full-blown episode. The length of each individual episode can vary greatly from person to person, and can depend on a number of factors (e.g., prior episodes), but untreated depressive disorders can last as long as six months to a year (Dorzab, Baker, Winokur, & Cadoret, 1971; Keller, Shapiro, Lavori, & Wolfe, 1982). In some cases individuals may experience significant symptoms for up to two years (Goodwin & Jamison, 1990). Many individuals will completely recover from their symptoms, entering a period of full remission. Approximately 20 to 30% of individuals experiencing a major depressive disorder will remit only partially from the episode, and will remain in a low-grade depressive state.

Unipolar Depression Unipolar depression has an average age of onset into the early to mid-20s, although some data suggest that the average age of first onset is decreasing (Kessler, 2002). Typically, the number of previous episodes is a good predictor of the probability of future episodes. Similarly, periods of remission tend to shorten with each passing episode. High-end estimates have suggested that more than 80% of individuals who experience a major depressive episode will experience recurrent episodes (Kessler, 2002), although data from other sources suggest recurrence rates in the 40 to

50% range (Goodwin et al., 2006). Even lower-end estimates, however, suggest that depression is a recurrent disorder for a great many people. Additionally, data show that although stress is strongly associated with initial episodes of depression, the link becomes considerably weaker with subsequent episodes. Some researchers have suggested that this disassociation indicates that depression becomes increasingly independent of stress, while others have suggested the possibility that considerably less stress is needed to trigger recurrent episodes (Monroe & Harkness. 2005).

Individuals with only partial remission are more likely to develop additional episodes, and are also more likely to only partially remit in between future episodes. *DSM-IV-TR* notes naturalistic studies showing that one year after being diagnosed with a major depressive episode, 40% of individuals still met criteria for major depression, 20% of individuals were in partial remission, and the remaining 40% evidenced no symptoms of depression (American Psychiatric Association, 1996). Chronic medical conditions are also a risk factor for a more persistent course of the disorder. For example, Parkinson's disease, strokes, and thyroid conditions are all associated with depressive symptoms.

Bipolar Disorder Among the individuals diagnosed with bipolar I disorder, approximately 90% have more than one manic episode. Even though bipolar I does not necessarily include a major depressive episode, up to 70% of manic (or hypomanic in bipolar II) episodes occur immediately before or after a major depressive episode. Typically, individuals with bipolar disorders have more total episodes (including both depressive and manic or hypomanic) in their lives than those with unipolar depression. The time between episodes tends to decrease with increasing age. In addition, the presence of psychotic features indicates a greater likelihood of incomplete recovery between episodes, as well as indicating a greater propensity toward psychotic features in subsequent manic episodes.

Epidemiology, Culture, and Gender

Epidemiology Based on clinical interviews, estimates of the current occurrence of major depression (a point prevalence rate) are found to be 2 to 4% for adults (Kessler, 2002). Lifetime prevalence rates for major depression, on the other hand, have been found to range anywhere from 6% to 25% (Kessler, 2002). Researchers suggest three reasons for this wide variation in lifetime prevalence estimates. The first is a true increase in the incidence of depression in more recent cohorts. Second, these more recent cohorts are also more willing to admit their depressive symptoms, thereby leading to an increase in prevalence findings. Lastly, methodological differences between diagnostic interviews may account for the discrepancy: more recent studies employ more refined diagnostic interviews that are better able to detect mood disorders (Kessler, 2002)—Kessler (2002) notes that the most accurate prevalence rate is probably in the neighborhood of 17%.

Epidemiological studies have also found substantial comorbidity between depression and other disorders. The Epidemiologic Catchment Area Study (ECS) and the National Comorbidity Survey (NCS) are two large epidemiological studies that describe depression. Both use diagnostic interviews in assessing the population, and both showed comorbidity rates of approximately 75% (Kessler, 2002). The most frequent Axis 1 comorbid conditions with depression are anxiety disorders, particularly generalized anxiety disorder, panic disorder, and posttraumatic stress disorder. Axis II personality disorders are also frequently comorbid with depression.

GENDER DIFFERENCES Mood disorders, particularly unipolar depression, are characterized by substantial gender differences (Keyes & Goodman, 2006). About twice as many women as men (1.7–2.7; Kessler et al., 2003) suffer from major depression or dysthymia, and women tend to report more severe depression as well as greater distress than men (Kornstein & Sloan, 2006). Moreover, this gender difference persists across demographic and cultural groups as well as in different countries (Nolen-Hoeksema, 2002). Gender differences generally begin to arise around the age of 12 or 13 years (possibly coinciding with the onset of puberty); before this time depression is uncommon, but boys and girls are usually equally affected. Additionally, data from epidemiological studies show that adult gender differences are due to a greater number of initial onsets of depression in women, as opposed to a difference in length or frequency of depressive episodes (Nolen-Hoeksema, 2002).

Possible explanations of these gender differences include biological, psychological, and social processes (Nolen-Hoeksema, 2002). Biological views include hormonal explanations, genetic factors, biological stress reactivity. For example, hormonal hypotheses note that many women experience the onset of mood disorders at times of peak hormonal change, such as puberty, the premenstrual phase of the menstrual cycle, and the postpartum period. Although data such as these are suggestive, research has yet to confirm the causal validity of these possibilities. Psychological theories hinge upon women's greater interpersonal orientation and a tendency to ruminate. For individuals with an interpersonal orientation, relationships become a central focus and a strong determinate of self-worth (Brems, 1995). Women tend to be socialized to be more likely than men to look excessively to others for reassurance. *Rumination* (persistent and obsessive thought about a certain topic) may propel women into a vicious cycle of negative affect, spiraling downward into a depressive state. Lastly, social explanations focus on the greater likelihood that women have suffered from traumatic events (abuse) or chronic negative events (such as poverty or sexual harassment). Despite the plausibility of the different hypotheses, none has received unambiguous empirical support. Gender differences in depression will thus undoubtedly be best explained by a model that integrates biological, psychological, and social explanations.

In unipolar depression, greater comorbidity between depression and anxiety disorders are found in women, with greater comorbidity with substance disorder found in men. With regard to bipolar disorders, few gender differences in incidence are found. Some differences however, have been found in the type of bipolar disorder experienced. For example, women are typically diagnosed first with a major depressive episode and men with a manic episode. Correspondingly, women typically have more major depressive episodes while men typically have more manic episodes (American Psychiatric Association, 1996; see also Winstead & Sanchez, this volume.)

Cultural Factors Although depression seems ubiquitous, culture can affect both the conceptualization and manifestation of the disorder. There are two main approaches that researchers take to understand these culturally based manifestations: ethnographic and biomedical. The ethnographic approach, typically taken by anthropologists, argues that persons in non-Western cultures may indeed experience the same symptoms that are defined as depressive in Western cultures, but that these symptoms may have different meanings and expression. In contrast to the ethnographic stance, the biomedical approach assumes that if the particular symptoms are present, then the disorder exists. For example, numerous studies of depressive symptomatology in non-Western cultures have documented high rates of depressive disorders as they are defined by the constellation of depressive symptoms articulated in the *DSM*. Although the biomedical approach does not entirely discount the role of culture, cultural meanings of symptoms are deemphasized. Psychologists and psychiatrists tend to be more likely to employ a biomedical approach.

There are significantly varied meanings of depression across cultures. Tsai and Chentsova-Dutton (2002) delineate three ways in which Western culture has influenced the definition of depression. First, Western culture values positive emotions and feeling good about oneself, and definitions hinge upon the absence of such positive feelings for a diagnosis of depression. Second, Western cultures tend to view a healthy individual as independent and autonomous, thereby explaining depression as an internal disturbance. In non-Western cultures, where connectedness among people is apt to be more highly valued than individuation, depressive symptoms are more likely to be seen as the result of interpersonal difficulties. This is not to say that depression in Western societies does not involve interpersonal difficulties, but rather that compared to the non-Western world, autonomy is likely to be valued more than interconnectedness.

Numerous factors may be responsible for variations in prevalence rates and frequency of symptoms across cultures, across ethnic groups, and even across geographic locations (e.g., actual differences in depression rates; varying degrees of poverty; different ways of thinking about depression; identifying certain depressive symptoms as another illness; methodological differences in the assessment of depression, etc.; Tsai & Chentsova-Dutton, 2002). It is thus important to keep in mind that "depression" goes beyond *DSM*'s definition and its manner of operationalizing the construct and may have very different meanings in different cultural groups (see also Lopez & Guarnaccia, this volume).

Theory and Research in Depression

Contemporary theory and research recognize that depression is caused by multiple factors that interact in complex ways. Genes, biochemistry, social skills, negative life events, interpersonal interactions, cognitive, and affective processes are all involved in varying ways and degrees in the development and course of depression, and distinctions among models emphasizing various perspectives have become increasingly blurred. For example, life events are recognized as the cornerstone in many episodes of depression, but various life event models now attempt to explicitly integrate notions of vulnerability, cognitive mediation, interpersonal behavior, and brain function (Ingram et al., 1998). However, although some progress has been made toward an integration of the various aspects of depression, few integrative models of depression exist. Thus, in this chapter we will examine contemporary approaches according to single variable points of origin, but it is important to bear in mind that even though we individually describe these various origins, they in fact interact to varying degrees in different cases of depression.

The Role of Stress in Depression

The link between an adverse social environment and depression has been recognized for centuries. Although there are a number of different aspects of social adversity (e.g., poverty), stressful life events are typically considered to be a core correlate of depression. The majority of research examining this link has focused on stress and the onset of depression, and consistently finds a strong relationship between the experience of stressful life events and the onset of depression (Monroe & Hadjiyannakis, 2002). Even though the link between stress and depression is well-documented, the nature of this link is complex and far from completely understood. Stress is anything but a simple concept, and it defies comprehensive exposition in a single chapter. Yet, we will discuss several important themes and questions that are important to recognize in understanding the relationship between stress and depression. As noted by Monroe and Hadjiyannakis (2002), although most models emphasize the role of stress in the etiology of depression, it is also important to ask whether or what role stress plays in different subtypes of depression, as well as if stress plays a role in the course of depression (e.g., degree and duration of symptoms, remission and recovery, relapse or recurrence). Even this discussion, however, barely touches on the complexities of stress. For example, must the stress that is proposed by some models to trigger depressive reactions be characterized by a major life event, several major life events, or is a series of chronic minor life events sufficient? Stress may consist of events that independently "happen" to people, but data have also shown that depressed individuals may play a role in generating stress that prolongs depression and that may predispose to future depression (Hammen, 1991).

Some data have suggested that approximately 50% of individuals diagnosed with depression have experienced severe stress before onset (Mazure, 1998). Such data convincingly show that stress plays a role in depression, but they just as convincingly also show that other factors are important. For example, not all individuals who experience significant stress develop depression, nor do all individuals who develop depression experience significant stress. To account for these facts, many modern theories of depression rely on *diathesis-stress models*. The idea of a diathesis has a long history and, in fact, probably dates back to the ancient Greeks (Monroe & Simons, 1991). Diathesis refers to a predisposition, or vulnerability, to an illness, and although not all models of depression emphasize a diathesis, most contemporary theories do make use of the idea to some degree. There is also general agreement that events perceived as stressful increase vulnerability to future psychopathology (Ingram et al., 1998). Stress and diathesis processes may be closely intertwined. For instance, perceptions of stress can affect stress responsivity; that is, psychological or biological predispositions to depression may affect how stress is perceived (Foley, Neale, & Kendler, 1996). Thus, individuals who might have a predisposition to depression might also have a predisposition to either perceive or experience stress in an exaggerated way. Furthermore, some models suggest an inverse relationship between stress and diatheses, such that as the degree or severity of the diathesis increases, less stress is necessary to initiate a depressive episode (Ingram et al., 1998). Alternatively, some perspectives argue that both severe stress *and* a strong diathesis are necessary to elicit depression (Monroe & Hadjiyannakis, 2002). Whatever its nature, the diathesis–stress idea is one that we will come back to frequently as we discuss theory and research in depression.

Biomedical Models of Depression

Biomedical models encompass several different areas of assumption and inquiry. Although related in important ways, we individually examine genetic approaches to depression, biological approaches, and neuroscience perspectives and data (see also Smith, this volume.)

Genetic Approaches Genetic models argue that at least some of the variance in the onset of depression is linked to genetic factors (Wallace, Schneider & McGuffin, 2002). Data that inform genetic models come from one of three different sources: family studies, twin studies, and adoption studies. Family study methods are based on the observation that depression runs in families, and that to the extent that depression vulnerability is inherited, mood disorders should cluster within a family. The most direct approach to evaluating this clustering is to interview family members using a standardized diagnostic interview to determine the number and type of mood related disorders that occur among relatives (Faraone, Tsuang, & Tsuang, 1999). The more familial history there is of mood disorders, the more evidence there is that the disorder, or the propensity to the disorder, is inherited. However, because families share not only genes, but also share environments, family studies have difficulty disentangling genetic factors from environmental factors.

Twin studies are in some respects an extension of family studies, but compare concordance rates for *monozygotic* twins, who are genetically *identical*, to *dizygotic* twins whose genes are similar (about 50% on average) but not identical. Concordance rates refer to the likelihood that both twins will be diagnosed with the disorder; to the extent that genetically identical monozygotic twins have higher concordance rates than genetically similar dizygotic twins, genetic factors are thought to play a significant role in the disorder. For example, McGuffin, Katz, and Rutherford (1991) found concordance rates of 58% in monozygotic twins as compared to 28% in dizygotic twins. Likewise, Kendler, Neale, Kessler, Heath, and Eaves (1992) found rates of 44% in monozygotic twins and 19% in dizygotic twins. In both cases the degree of concordance was about twice as high for monozygotic twins, and thus strongly suggests a genetic component to depression.

Although superior to family studies, twin studies are not without limitations. For example, twin studies rely on the assumption that similarity of environment is the same for monozygotic and dizygotic twins. This may not always be the case if, for example, twins who are identical in appearance are treated more similarly than twins who look like same aged siblings. Hence, environment cannot be completely ruled out as a contributing factor in concordance rates, although environmental influences are in most cases probably reasonably similar (Kendler & Gardner, 1998). Other methodological issues (e.g., small Ns in many studies, questions about generalizibility to nontwins) may also limit the validity of twin studies (Wallace et al., 2002).

Adoption studies are a powerful method for examining genetic effects. Adopted children are genetically quite similar to their biological parents, and while having nothing genetically in common with their adoptive parents, they share a psychosocial environment with their adopted family. Evidence for a genetic role in depression is thus found when adopted children with a biological family history of depression are also more likely to experience a mood disorder. This is particularly true if children are adopted at a young age and have had less opportunity to be exposed to the psychosocial environment of the biological family, which may be confounded with purely genetic influences. The disadvantage of these studies is more pragmatic than methodological in that such studies are costly and difficult to conduct. As a result, relatively few adoption studies on genetic factors in depression have been published, and those that have suffer from the types of problems that might be expected to result from logistically difficult to conduct studies (e.g., small sample sizes).

Although each of these methods has limitations, when taken together, these data have provided some estimates of the degree to which depression is influenced by genes. Kendler et al. (1992) have suggested that the heritability of milder forms of depression ranges anywhere from 20 to 45%, and based on a review of several twin studies, Sullivan, Neale, and Kendler (2000) estimated approximately 37% of the variance in depressive disorder is accounted for by heritability. However, estimates for more severe cases of depression (e.g., those requiring hospitalization) range as high as 70% (Malhi, Moore, & McGuffin et al., 2000). Genetic contributions for recurrent or chronic cases of depression may also be higher than those for single episodes. Thus, depending on the type and severity of the disorder, data suggest that the heritability of depression is anywhere from moderate to high. Even this range, however, is mitigated by other factors, such as gender differences; for example, heritability appears to be stronger in women than in men.

Family, twin, and adoption studies are informative about the degree of heritability of depression, but they are not particularly informative about the nature or role of genes in depression, nor are they informative about what gene or genes may contribute to depression. Data on specific gene contributions will likely be derived through molecular genetics, which is a relatively recent development in genetic approaches to depression, at least as compared to methods used to estimate the degree of genetic heritability for depression. Combined with data on the efficacy of drugs that target certain neurotransmitters, molecular genetic research has identified several plausible genes, such as those that appear to be associated with the serotonergic systems, although this is not the only neurotransmitter system where genes may be implicated (Wallace et al., 2002).

Even though genes clearly play a role in depression, given the complexity of depression and its recognized subtypes, it is unlikely that a single gene will ever be found that is linked to depression. Moreover, there is a reasonably broad consensus that depression is not inherited, but that a predisposition or vulnerability to depression is. Other factors such as stress will determine whether this susceptibility ever becomes realized in a diagnosable depressive disorder. Thus, even though heritability does play a potentially large role in at least some forms of depression, and probably plays at least some role in most depressions, environmental features also have a considerable part in the etiology of depression. Genes may set the stage more or less for depression and its various forms, but in line with diathesis-stress concepts, a variety of other factors are likely to determine whether depression occurs.

Biological Bases of Depression

Both biological function and genetics are intricately tied to brain structure and functioning (which we examine in the next section). Rendering these variables even more complicated is the fact that biological processes cannot be separated from neuroanatomical function and structure. For example, some researchers have suggested that people who are at risk for depression may have neurons that are unable to tolerate diminished levels of neurotransmitters whereas healthy individuals have neurons that can tolerate lower levels of neurotransmitters with few ill effects (Delgado & Moreno, 2006). For ease of understanding, we discuss the role of neurotransmitters and neuroanatomy in depression separately, but it is important to keep in mind that these, and other, variables are closely intertwined. Additionally, given their central emphasis in much of the literature, we focus on norepinephrine, serotonin, and cortisol, but it is important to note that other biological variables (e.g., neuropetides) have been suggested to play a role in depression in some studies (see also Smith, this volume).

NOREPINEPHRINE Data from a variety of perspectives have causally implicated both *catecholamine norepinephrine* (NE) and *indoleamine serotonin* (5-HT) (Delgado & Moreno, 2006). Current thinking centers on several possible areas of pathophysiological processes in depression linked to 5-HT and NE (Thase, Jindal, & Howland, 2002). For example, a subgroup of depressed individuals appear to excrete low levels of a metabolite for NE (3-methoxy-4hydroxyphenylglycol, or MHPG), thus suggesting that a reduction in NE may be involved in some depressions (Ressler & Nemeroff, 1999). Such findings, however, appear to be limited to subsets of depressed patients.

Just as low levels of a metabolite for NE have been found for some patients, another set of findings show that low levels of a metabolite for 5-HT are found in some subgroups of depressed individuals (Maes & Meltzer, 1995). Tryptophan depletion studies have served as an important source of data for the role of 5-HT in depression. *Tryptophan* is a precursor to 5-HT and when depleted, serves to diminish the availability of 5-HT. Studies have shown that depressed individuals who have responded well to selective serotonin reuptake inhibitors (SSRIs) are more likely to experience a return of symptoms with tryptophan depletion, and some, but not all, studies have shown that tryptophan depletion causes moderate symptoms in nondepressed individuals with a history of depression (Sobczak et al., 2002). However, depressed patients not taking SSRIs do not appear to experience a worsening in their symptoms with tryptophan depletion. Diminished 5-HT function appears then to be related to some subset of depressed patients, but by no means all who are depressed. Diminished 5-HT function does appear to be related to behaviors that may be characteristic of some cases of depression (e.g., suicidality), although these behaviors may characterize other disorders as well. As such, 5-HT disruption may be a more general deficit in psychopathology rather than one specifically linked to depression.

CORTISOL High levels of cortisol (a hormone) have been found in some groups of depressed individuals. Cortisol is regulated by the adrenal cortex and is known to be excreted in times of stress. However, cortisol also returns to normal levels when the individual is no longer depressed (Seidman, 2006). Interestingly, when a synthetic cortisol known as *dexamethasone* is administered, nondepressed people show a suppression of naturally occurring cortisol, a procedure known as a dexamethasone suppression test (DST). However, this suppression is not observed in a subset of depressed people. For these particular depressed individuals, hypercortisol secretion may reflect an exaggerated stress response that is not seen in individuals who experience stress without becoming depressed. Although the DST was originally thought to have great potential as a diagnostic indicator of depression, the fact that only some, but not all, depressed people fail to suppress cortisol has diminished this enthusiasm. Nevertheless, these data do suggest that sustained or excessive cortisol secretion may reflect an important biological process in some depressions (Seidman, 2006).

SLEEP A growing body of evidence suggests that sleep neurophysiology and circadian rhythms may be disturbed in depression (Buysse, Germain, Nofzinger, & Kupfer, 2006). Research has found some evidence to suggest that decreased slow wave sleep, and the intensification of rapid eye movement (REM) sleep are seen in depression. REM sleep occurs several times throughout the night at approximately 90 minute intervals. Some research suggests that the first REM sleep interval for some depressed people occurs earlier than the normal 90 minutes. Moreover, some depressed people show evidence of all three sleep abnormalities. Such sleep disturbances, along with other factors such as hypercortisol excretion, may reflect a disruption in circadian rhythms, although it is unclear if this disruption plays an etiological role in depression, or if it is the result of a more primary dysregulation in biological functioning.

An intriguing line of data has suggested that sleep disturbance may be a precursor to depression, and for patients who are depressed, sleep disturbances may predict a worse outcome (Buysse et al., 2006). For example, Weissman et al. (1979) found that individuals with insomnia were substantially more likely to experience later depression than those without insomnia, although other data (e.g., Mallon, Broman, & Hetta, 2000) found that such a relationship held for women but not men. It is important to note, however, that insomnia does not predict the onset of depression for all who experience it, and many patients do not show evidence of sleep disturbance prior to depression. Just as with other biologically relevant variables that we have discussed, disturbed sleep appears to be a potent factor for some but not all subsets of depression.

SUMMARY Such data clearly show evidence of biological dysregulation in depression. However, several qualifications are in order. Although data have shown a variety of biological processes that appear to be disturbed in depression, these processes do not characterize all cases of depression, nor are they necessarily specific to depression. Some biological processes appear to be stable in some depressions, such as decreased 5-HT and some sleep disturbances such as decreased slow wave sleep. Other processes, however, appear to be more characteristic of the depressed state (e.g., hypercortisol), and tend to normalize as individuals recover. In many but not all cases, the subgroup of individuals who show evidence of these diffuse biological disturbances tend to be older, more severely depressed, have more vegetative symptoms, and experience recurrent episodes of depression. Moreover, rather than a cause of depression, some investigators have suggested that disrupted neurotransmitter or sleep function serve as risk factors for depression rather than as primary causal agents, and that the onset of biological dysregulation may be the result of stress rather than a variable causally linked to depression (Delgado & Moreno, 2006). Hence, many of these processes may reflect the effect of stress that is severe and/or sustained. A related way to conceptualize disrupted biological function, within a diathesis-stress framework, is that these variables may be necessary for the onset of depression (at least in some individuals), but are not sufficient in and of themselves to bring about the disorder.

All cases of depression have both biological and psychosocial components. Although it is an over-simplification to suggest that some depressions are of a biological origin whereas other depressions are psychosocial in nature, data showing that biological dysregulation characterizes some but not all cases of depression indicate that some forms of depression may have a much stronger biological component, particularly those depressions that are quite severe. These cases also tend to be those where many of these abnormalities run in families and thus appear to have a genetic component. Other types of depression that are disabling but not as severe may have a stronger psychosocial component in their causal chain.

Affective Neuroscience Affective neuroscience focuses on the neural processes that are linked to emotion. Research in affective neuroscience uses a variety of methods such as examining the link between brain damage and impaired functioning. However, the use of imagining techniques such as functional magnetic resonance imaging (fMRI) has become increasingly common in recent years. fMRI creates images of the oxygen in the blood flow to brain areas that are active and can thus be used to assess the role and function of brain structures and regions during various tasks. Mapping this activation provides a window into how the brain functions in depressed (and nondepressed) states and can thus help to chart the brain circuitry that may be involved in depression (Mayberg, 2006). Knowledge of this circuitry may have implications for understanding various patterns of cognitive and behavioral deficits in depression, and ideally might also provide insight into the onset, maintenance, and remission of depression.

Affective neuroscience approaches to depression have tended to focus most attention on the prefrontal cortex, the anterior cingulate cortex, the hippocampus, and the amygdala (Davidson, Pizzagalli, & Nitschke, 2002), although other anatomical variables (e.g., glial cells; Rajowska, 2006) have sometime been indicated. Even though the prefrontal cortex, anterior cingulate cortex, hippocampus, and amygdala serve numerous functions and are interconnected in complex ways (and to other brain structures as well), we will underscore several functions that may be particularly involved in depression. In general, the prefrontal cortex is that part of the cortex that is most evolved in primates and that plays a substantial role in goal directed activities such as planning and formulating strategies. To accomplish these goals, the prefrontal cortex sends signals to other parts of the brain, inhibiting some areas and disinhibiting others. The anterior cingulate cortex is typically involved in selective attention and emotion and thus appears to be involved in the perception of emotionally relevant information. The hippocampus is a part of the limbic system, and is involved in the consolidation of memory and is linked to the representation of emotion-evoking events, which may be particularly important in understanding the neural circuitry underlying an emotional state such as depression. The amygdala is also part of the limbic system. This structure is also involved in the memory for emotionally significant events, and is also connected to other brain regions and serves to signal to these areas when stimuli that are important to the person require additional processing (Davidson et al., 2002; see also Smith, this volume.)

Although knowledge of the brain circuitry of depression is far from complete, several promising findings have emerged. For example, depressed individuals have been found to exhibit decreased activation in the prefrontal cortex (Drevets, 1998). In particular, left-side activation deficits have been found in depression (Davidson, 1993), and these deficits may reflect the disruption of goal directed activities that frequently characterize depression. Interestingly, some studies have found that the young children of depressed mothers exhibit a similar pattern of left side hypoactivation (Hammen, 2001), suggesting the possibility of a genetic link to this brain abnormality. Further suggesting a genetic link in at least some forms of depression, Drevets et al. (1997) reported that the prefrontal cortices of depressed individuals with a family history of depression were significantly smaller than the prefrontal cortexes of nondepressed controls. No such differences were found in comparisons between depressed individuals without a family history and normal controls.

Like the prefrontal cortex, decreases in the activation of the anterior cingulate cortex has also been found in depressed individuals and may be linked to the social withdrawal, poor coping, and anhedonia that is sometimes seen in depression (Davidson et al., 2002). Some data have also shown reduced hippocampal volume in depressed patients. One hypothesis concerning this reduced volume is that the hippocampus may atrophy because it contains high levels of cortisol (a glucocorticoid) receptors; glucocorticoids, which are known to be neurotoxic, lead to cell loss. Indeed, some data suggest that hippocampal atrophy is correlated with depression duration (Sheline, Gado, & Kraemer, 2003). Because the hippocampus is involved in encoding environmental context, one result of this atrophy in depression may be deficits in the ability to process social information, leading to the preservation of depressed mood in situations that should provoke positive or neutral affect (Davidson et al., 2002).

The hippocampus is strongly connected to the amygdala, which is another brain region that has been closely linked to depression (Drevets, 2001). In particular, the amygdala has been shown to be hyperactivated in depressed individuals, and has been hypothesized by some investigators to be responsible for the maintenance of the sad mood that is a hallmark of depression (Doughety & Rauch, 1997). Siegle, Steinhauer, Thase, Stenger, and Carter (2002) have summarized the research suggesting that, not only is the amygdala linked to the perservation of sad mood, amygdala hyperactivation may result from the failure of the prefrontal cortex to inhibit this region. Recall that one function of the prefrontal cortex (PFC), which may become hypoactive in depression, is to regulate other areas of the brain to initiate the attainment of goals. Thus failure of the PFC to inhibit the amygdala may precipitate the maintenance of emotional information processing in depression that not only perpetuates sad mood, but also interferes with adaptive functioning. Moreover, Siegle et al. (2002) have shown evidence of sustained activity of the amygdala in depressed people in a manner that is consistent with observations of the rumination of negative information. Rumination has long been theorized to be an important process in depression (Beck, 1967; Ingram, 1984).

The prefrontal cortex, anterior cingulate cortex, hippocampus, and amygdala form a circuit that is extensively interconnected. Certainly other areas of the brain are involved in depression, but this circuit appears to play a key role in at least some forms of depression, and may have a genetic link. It is important to note, however, that much remains to be learned about the neural circuitry of depression. For example, although some data have suggested that neural deficits continue after depression has remitted, it is still unclear if these deficits are linked to the cause of depression, might co-occur with depression, or might arise as a result of depression. This is true for the entire circuitry that has been mapped so far, but can also be true for each of the more specific regions of the circuit; some parts may reflect causality, whereas others may be concomitants or consequences of depression (recall that hippocampus atrophy has specifically been suggested to be a consequence of the depressed state). Moreover, because these brain regions are densely connected, it is difficult to determine whether one region is primarily linked to depression, while other connected regions are of a more secondary nature. Likewise, it may be that the abnormalities that are linked to depression may reside in the *connections* between structures rather than in the structures themselves. Furthermore, dysfunction in these structures, or their connections, may vary with different types of depression, although data so far have been unable to map these dysfunctions onto any of the recognized categories of depression. Some researchers hold out hope that the patterns of brain abnormality may themselves lead to different subtypes of depression. Despite these questions and the complexity of the issues that are inherent in affective neuroscience, significant strides have been made in gaining some insight into how the brain functions in depression.

Psychosocial Approaches to Depression: Cognitive Models

Cognitive approaches to the conceptualization, assessment, and treatment of depression have expanded rapidly over the past several decades and are probably the predominant psychosocial approach to depression today. Even though there are several specific cognitive models of depression, the primary assumption underlying all cognitive models is that certain cognitive negative processes are related in some fashion to vulnerability, onset, course, or alleviation of the disorder.

Irrational Beliefs The earliest cognitive theories tended to emphasize a relatively simple linear association between thinking errors and the onset of emotionally troublesome states. They can be traced to the development of the pioneering cognitive-behavioral interventions that focused on the treatment of psychological dysfunction through procedures designed to correct errors in thinking. Albert Ellis's rational-emotive therapy is probably the first and most enduring example of this model. In the most recent revision of the theory (Ellis, 1996), Ellis argues that depression-prone people tend to hold overly rigid standards that are applied to one's own performance, the performance of others, and life events. Because these standards are too rigid, they are considered to be irrational. Consequently, the person who (irrationally) expects too much of him- or herself, other people, or life in general, is likely to be disappointed and, ultimately, become depressed.

Learned Helplessness and Hopelessness Theory The helplessness theory of depression represents a theory that has evolved from an earlier emphasis on learned helplessness in depression. This work began with Seligman who observed that animals who were unable to control negative events often developed behaviors that "looked like" depressive symptoms. Based on these observations, Seligman developed a theory of human depression that focused on depressed individuals' expectations that they were helpless to control aversive outcomes (Seligman, 1975). Perhaps because of its intuitive appeal and apparent simplicity, learned helplessness theory generated an enormous amount of research (Abramson, Seligman, & Teasdale, 1978).

Even though much of the research on learned helplessness was supportive of the basic tenets of the theory (e.g., that depressed people tended to display more features of helplessness than nondepressed people), other research highlighted some substantial shortcomings. In response to these shortcomings, the theory was reformulated in 1978 as an *attributional theory* which focused on how attributions about the causes of events were linked to depression (Abramson et al., 1978). In particular, making global, stable, and internal attributions for negative events, and making specific, unstable, external attributions for positive events, was proposed to lead to depression. In 1989, Abramson, Metalsky, and Alloy (1989) refined this theory into the *hopelessness theory* of depression and suggested that hopelessness depression represented a specific subtype of depression that was caused by the expectation that highly desired outcomes will not occur, or that highly aversive outcomes will occur and that no response available to the individual will change the likelihood of these outcomes (Abramson & Alloy, 2006).

Cognitive Schemas The most widely known cognitive model of depression was proposed by Beck (1963, 1967, 1987). The model has been elaborated and refined several times (e.g., Beck, 2002), but the basic elements have remained the same. In particular, the model argues that dysfunctional cognitive self-structures, or *schemas*, are the central elements in the onset and maintenance of depression.

Although definitions vary somewhat, schemas have generally been viewed as a stored body of knowledge that interacts with incoming information to influence selective attention and memory search. Self-schemas organize the personal meaning that individuals assign to information. In the case of depression, these schemas incorporate a significant amount of negative self-relevant information, and guide how information is abstracted from social settings and processed. That is, the information to which attention is drawn becomes increasingly congruent with the schematic knowledge structures directing the search (Segal, 1988; Segal & Ingram, 1994). As a result, these dysfunctional schemas are thought to become self-perpetuating and increasingly biased over time because input that may disconfirm or contradict the information encoded in a schema receives insufficient processing. Schemas are also closely linked with affective structures, and in the case of depression, are hypothesized to form the genesis of the disorder because they cause and perpetuate negative cognitive tendencies (Ingram et al., 1998).

Even though the focus of Beck's theory is on schemas and negative thinking in general, he has also articulated two specific types of concepts represented within cognitive structures that are hypothesized to reflect different subtypes of depression. In particular, *sociotropic* individuals value positive interchange with others, and focus on acceptance, support, and guidance from others. Moreover, these individuals also tend to be highly self-critical, which some authors have suggested to be the reason why sociotropy might be related to depression (Blatt & Homann, 1992). Autonomous individuals, on the other hand, value independence, mobility, and achievement. Blatt and colleagues (Blatt, 1974; Luyten, Corveleyn, & Blatt, 2005) have suggested somewhat similar ideas and have argued that depressed individuals can be either *anaclitic* or *introjective*. Anaclitic depression is characterized by feelings of helplessness, weakness, depletion, and being unloved while introjective depression is characterized by feelings of being unworthy, unlovable, guilty, and having failed to live up to expectations and standards. In all cases, when stressors congruent with these themes are experienced (e.g., the dissolution of a relationship for anaclitic or sociotropic individuals), dysfunctional structures become active and depression results. Research has tended to support a link between these dimensions and depression

(Frewen & Dozois, 2006; Lindsay & Scott, 2005). although there is something of a consensus that the sociotropic/anaclitic dimensions may be more strongly related to depression than the remaining dimensions (Enns & Cox, 1997).

Interacting Cognitive Subsystems Teasdale and colleagues (Barnard & Teasdale, 1991; Teasdale, 1993, 1999; Teasdale & Barnard, 1993) have proposed a comprehensive information processing model of depression called the interacting cognitive subsystems (ICS) framework. This framework attempts to account for virtually all aspects of information processing (Siegle & Ingram, 1996) and suggests that different aspects of experience are represented by patterns of different kinds of information, or mental codes. For example, at a superficial level, experience is coded in visual, auditory, and proprioceptive inputs, but at deeper levels, patterns of sensory codes are represented by intermediate codes (e.g., sensory data that form letters are represented by combinations of letters into words and sentences). At deeper levels of encoding, mental codes are formed that create meaning (e.g., a sentence conveys both information and meaning) that can be linked to emotions. In the ICS framework, emotional reactions are produced when patterns of low level meanings and patterns of sensory-derived input produce emotion-laden representations of the self. Production of a depressed state occurs when these depressogenic schematic models are created, and is maintained because these models are continually reproduced in day-to-day experience. When the production of these models stops, the depression abates.

Cognitive Vulnerability Most cognitive models, either directly or indirectly, make statements about the processes that make individuals vulnerable to depression. These models are important not only because they might specify some of the factors that are linked to the emergence of depression, but because these processes are also relevant to core issues about causality.

Vulnerability processes are typically conceptualized as having developmental antecedents (Ingram & Price, 2001). For example, among the earliest descriptions of his cognitive mode, Beck (1967) identified the geneses of vulnerability to depression in key developmental events.

> In childhood and adolescence, the depression-prone individual becomes sensitized to certain types of life situations. The traumatic situations initially responsible for embedding or reinforcing the negative attitudes that comprise the depressive constellation are the prototypes of the specific stresses that may later activate these constellations. (p. 278)

Although not all reported literature has supported these vulnerability ideas, the bulk of available studies clearly suggest cognitive processes that are operating in the way Beck and other cognitive theorists have suggested. That is, dysfunctional cognitions that are not present in the nondepressed state consistently emerge in depression-vulnerable individuals when key activating events occur (see Scher, Ingram, & Segal, 2005 for a review). Other ways to assess vulnerability are seen in behavioral high-risk paradigms of the sort typified by the Temple-Wisconsin Cognitive Vulnerability to Depression Project (Alloy & Abramson, 1999). This longitudinal study examined the proposals of both the hopelessness model and cognitive schema theory as represented by Beck's (1967) model. Specifically, a group of individuals were assessed who, upon entry into college, were identified as possessing negative inferential styles or negative self-schemas. Among their findings, those identified as being at high cognitive risk were in fact more likely to experience depression at some point in the future (Abramson & Alloy, 2006). Hence, data from this project suggest that cognitive factors do in fact predict the eventual onset of depression.

Evaluation of Cognitive Models An enormous body of research has empirically investigated the various claims of various cognitive models. Support for numerous aspects of these models is quite strong. For example, there is little doubt that when depressed, individuals do in fact experience the types of negative cognition that is hypothesized to result from depressive schemas, or to emanate from dysfunctional attributional styles (Ingram et al., 1998). Moreover, studies have found consistent results regardless of whether these cognitive constructs are assessed using self-report methods or performance based information processing tasks. Related lines of research have also suggested that adverse early experiences may create some of the cognitive conditions that are thought to be related to the experience of depression (Ingram, 2001; Ingram et al., 1998).

Recent research has begun to provide substantial support for the causal elements of cognitive models. For example, vulnerability research as illustrated by the Temple-Wisconsin Cognitive Vulnerability to Depression Project provides support for the role of negative cognitions predicting the eventual onset of depression. A key piece of the causal puzzle is also being filled in by research reported by Segal and colleagues. For example, Segal, Gemar, and Williams (1999) and Segal et al. (2006) have provided evidence that depressotypic cognitions not only can be activated, but that they may in fact be related to the onset of depression. Specifically, these studies asked depressed patients who had recovered after being treated with either cognitive-behavior therapy or pharmacotherapy to complete ratings of dysfunctional attitudes. This was done both before and after a negative mood induction that was intended to model the emotional effects of stress. Several years after this initial testing, a follow-up assessment found that cognitive reactions to the mood induction predicted relapse; those who showed the strongest cognitive reactions to the mood were also the most likely to relapse. This line of research provides substantial support for a key element of schema theories of depression.

Despite the growing support for central tenets of cognitive models of depression, significant questions remain. For instance, much of the research that has examined vulnerability has assessed individuals who have been depressed in the past. It is unclear then if the presumed cognitive diatheses that emerge played a role in the initial onset, or whether they were created in whole or in part by the processes involved in the initial onset. This does not diminish the importance of these factors as causal variables but does raise questions as to whether they were initially causal. We have noted throughout this chapter that depression is a heterogeneous disorder with many possible subtypes. Some authors (e.g., Abramson & Alloy, 2006) have suggested a specific negative cognition subtype that is different from others in that cognitions play a key causal role. Research has not yet substantiated whether the cognitions that have been documented to play an important role characterize all or most kinds of depression, or are specific to a negative cognition subtype (should it exist). These important caveats do not diminish the impressive amount of research that has begun to support crucial elements of cognitive models, but do suggest that the process of empirical verification of cognitive models of depression is not yet complete.

Psychosocial Approaches to Depression: Interpersonal Approaches

While the cognitive approach focuses on the internal processes involved in depression, other approaches suggest that people get depressed because of problematic interactions with others. In particular, interpersonal approaches focus on the behaviors, especially the social behaviors, of the depressed individual and suggest that these behaviors have real significance for why people become, and stay, depressed. Before discussing this approach, however, it is important to clarify that perspectives on the social origins and nature of depression do not necessarily represent a specific model of depression. As Hammen (1999) has aptly noted, this approach is not sufficiently theoretically articulated to be considered a psychosocial model.

There is little doubt that the interpersonal functioning of depressed individuals can be significantly disrupted. A large body of research shows that depressed individuals are prone to marital and relationship difficulties (Whisman, 2001), occupational problems (Tennant, 2001), impaired parenting (Garber & Flynn, 2001), and difficulties in daily interpersonal functioning (Dill & Anderson, 1999).

It is easy to see how the features of the depressed state may be linked to some of these interpersonal problems. For example, not only is social withdrawal considered a pervasive feature of depression, some specific symptoms of depression, such as concentration difficulties, may pave the way for problems in relating to others.

A large and growing body of research has sought to examine the interpersonal context in which depression occurs. The first ideas on the interpersonal nature of depression were proposed by Coyne (1976) who assigned a central role to the manner in which the social environment responds to the interpersonal behavior of the depressed individual. According to Coyne's proposals (1976, 1999), the occurrence of stressful life events leads to a display of depressive symptoms by the depressed individual. These symptoms include withdrawal from interactions, expressions of helplessness and hopelessness, and irritability and agitation. The goal of the depressed person is to gain reassurance regarding his or her self-worth and acceptance by others. Initially, individuals respond with genuine concern and support for the person. The effects of this reassurance, however, are short-lived, and the depressed person continues to seek reassurance of his or her self-worth. The persistence of a depressive display, however, eventually becomes aversive to others, and some people in the depressed person's social network may express anger and irritation at the depressed person while others start to find suitable excuses to avoid further interactions. The depressed person accurately interprets these behaviors as rejection, leading to intensified efforts by the depressed person to seek reassurance. Thus, a cycle based on the perceived or actual rejection by others is generated that is unpleasant to both the depressed person and to others who continue to remain in the depressed person's social environment.

Interpersonal perspectives thus argue that depression is fundamentally interpersonal in nature (Joiner & Coyne, 1999). Interpersonal approaches have also been refined and extended since Coyne's original work. For example, investigators have focused on interpersonal topics in depression ranging from life stress and coping, the role of self-esteem, and the relationships between cognitive models and interpersonal approaches (Gotlib & Hammen, 1992). In this last regard, a promising line of research has resurrected the idea of working models embodied in attachment theory to offer a number of proposals regarding the link between cognitive schemas and interpersonal functioning in depression (Ingram et al., 1998).

Causal Factors in the Interpersonal Approach With regard to the possible causal factors of depression, Joiner (2002) has argued that interpersonal factors may create risk for depression in three ways. First, deficits in social skills may represent a risk factor, specifically that individuals who are prone to depression may have impaired social skills that cause the interactional disruptions which lead to depression. Although there is little doubt that many individuals who are depressed do display limited social skills, and the idea that social skill deficits characterize depression prone people has been around for awhile (e.g., Lewinsohn, 1985; Lewinsohn & Amenson, 1978), thus far there are few data which show that these deficits precede depression. Such temporal antecedence is a necessary condition for demonstrating that a factor is causally related to depression (Garber & Hollon, 1991); a variable must occur before the disorder if it plays some role in causing the disorder.

A related but second possibility is that depression prone individuals evidence general interpersonal inhibition, which creates risk for depression. Such inhibition would suggest that depressed individuals tend to be socially avoidant or shy, and that these inhibitions lead to disrupted social functioning and depression. Although data reliably show that these inhibitions occur in the depressed state (Joiner, 2002), little research has addressed the possibility that these processes lead to depression.

A third possibility, and one that is associated with cognitive models, is that an excessive amount of interpersonal dependency creates risk for depression. A number of studies have shown a link between depressive symptoms and dependency (Blatt & Homann, 1992; Zuroff & Fitzpatrick, 1995), making it a reasonable candidate for creating risk. Some research has supported this proposition. For instance,

Stader and Hokanson (1998) demonstrated that feelings of dependency preceded elevations in depressive symptoms, although these feelings remained even after the depressive symptoms diminished. Although data such as these are suggestive, more extensive longitudinal research will be necessary to determine how much of a role dependency plays in the onset of depressive episodes.

It is important to note that the onset of depression is only one element of the causal cycle in depression (Ingram et al., 1998). Perhaps an equally important perspective on causality is the fact that depression is a condition that can last for months or years, sometimes even with treatment. Interpersonal processes may play a critical role in maintaining the depressed state. The excessive reassurance seeking that is the cornerstone of interpersonal models suggests pathways whereby depression may be maintained. The interference with social bonds that this process may lead to indicates that social support will be diminished, and interpersonal rejection will be increased. Data have repeatedly demonstrated this process in depressed individuals (Joiner, 2002). Moreover, these behaviors may also be related to increases in the experience or the generation of stress (Hammen, 1991), thus making depression more difficult to escape. Regardless of whether these problematic interactions are involved in the onset of depression or in the maintenance of depression, there is little doubt that the interpersonal approach is an important perspective in understanding depression.

Treatment and Prevention

Treatment of depression after it has reached clinical significance will always be a method used by mental health professionals. On the other hand, some researchers have argued that a better approach to treatment is prevention of the disorder before it has occurred (Albee, 2000).

Prevention

There is little argument that preventing depression would provide considerably greater benefits to society and to individuals than does the treatment of one depressed individual at a time. Prevention has traditionally been divided into three types. *Primary prevention* is aimed at relatively large populations that do not necessarily display a risk factor (e.g., televised antismoking commercials aimed at adolescents). *Secondary prevention* programs specifically target high-risk individuals. *Tertiary prevention* programs aim to prevent relapse after the occurrence of a disorder. Though the lines that define the types of prevention are frequently blurred, there is little doubt that investigation of prevention in any form may lead to important strategies for preventing the onset of depression, or perhaps diminishing its severity if it does occur.

For the most part, prevention trials to date have proven somewhat successful in reducing the incidence of depression (Munoz, Le, Clarke, & Jaycox, 2002). Moreover, the data tend to show that those who are most helped by prevention programs are children and adolescents (Ingram, Odom, & Mitchusson, 2004). The majority of prevention research has focused on psychosocial treatment methods, frequently with an emphasis on modifying cognitive factors. Research suggests the promise of these methods, and offers individuals the possibility of new learning and of modifying cognitive and behavioral functioning that may have lasting effects.

Though psychopharmacological approaches have not been the focus of nearly as much prevention research as psychological methods, such approaches may prove useful for depression prevention in some situations. For instance, the appearance of *prodromal* (early) symptoms presents a rationale for using psychopharmacological treatment to interrupt a developing depressive episode, an approach that empirical research has suggested can be effective in adults (e.g., Rapaport & Judd, 1998). Although few data on the use of these methods to prevent depression in children and adolescents have been reported, data do suggest that they can be effectively used for treatment in already depressed children and adolescents. Hence, there is reason to believe that psychopharmacological methods might effectively aid in preventing the full blown development of depression in children and adolescents who might be experiencing early signs of the disorder. Such results are particularly important in light of the fact that the average age of depression onset is in late adolescence.

Biologically Based Treatments Pharmacotherapy to treat depression has become increasingly common. Indeed, because of their demonstrated effectiveness, the prevalence of antidepressants as the front-line treatment against depression has soared. Antidepressant medications fall into the categories of monoamine oxidase (MAO) inhibitors, tricyclic antidepressants, and selective serotonin reuptake inhibitors (SSRIs). All of these drugs work by increasing the levels of norepinephrine and/or serotonin. Researchers, however, are still unsure as to the exact mechanisms by which these medications have their effects (see also Smith, this volume).

Monoamine Oxidase Inhibitors MAOIs were the first antidepressant medications, accidentally discovered in the 1950s when one such drug (iproniazid) failed to cure tuberculosis but inadvertently ameliorated the patient's depressive symptoms (Pinel, 2000). This class of drugs increases the level of monoamines (e.g. serotonin and norepinephrine) by inhibiting the enzymes that would otherwise break down these neurotransmitters. Currently, MAOIs have been relegated to third- or fourth-line antidepressants, mostly due to dietary restrictions that are required with their use (Gitlin, 2002). Such dietary restrictions have been termed the "cheese effect" since certain foods that contain an amine called tyramine cannot be eaten because they can raise blood pressure dangerously high (wine and cheese are two such restricted foods). In addition, MAOIs have potentially perilous drug to drug interactions that can lead to hypertension or death (these other medications include over the counter cold remedies, as well as SSRIs). Other, less serious, side effects include anxiety, nausea, dizziness, insomnia, weight gain, and sexual dysfunction. MAOIs, as with other antidepressant medications such as tricyclic medications, can be lethal when overdosed and have been used by depressed patients to commit suicide. SSRIs are less toxic and are less frequently associated with suicide (Potter, Paich, Rudorfer, & Krishnan, 2006).

Tricyclic Antidepressants So named because of their three-ringed structure, tricyclic antidepressants were also developed in the 1950s. Similar to the MAOIs, these were accidentally discovered when imipramine was unsuccessful as an antischizophrenic medication but appeared to have antidepressant effects in this population (Pinel, 2000). Tricyclics function by blocking the reuptake of serotonin and norepinephrine, thereby causing an increase in these neurotransmitters. These antidepressants consistently show good efficacy and are therefore frequently used as the reference drugs in evaluating new treatments (Gitlin, 2002). Disadvantages of tricyclics include the need to slowly increase the dosage to full effect, as well as several deleterious side effects. Side effects include heart arrhythmias, tachycardia, constipation, urinary problems, sedation, weight gain, blurry vision, and dry mouth (Gitlin, 2002).

Selective Serotonin Reuptake Inhibitors Developed in the 1990s, SSRIs are currently the most commonly prescribed antidepressants, and include brand names such as Prozac, Paxil, and Zoloft. As the name implies, SSRIs inhibit the reuptake of serotonin, thereby increasing the level of serotonin in the brain. Their widespread use is due to the fact that they only require one dose daily as well as to their limited side effects, such as nausea, insomnia, nervousness, sedation, and sexual side effects (Gitlin, 2002). Quite often, the nausea, insomnia, and nervousness diminish after the first few weeks of treatment. Despite a widespread public perception that SSRIs are more effective than earlier antidepressants, SSRIs are in fact roughly equal in effectiveness to tricyclics. Their main advantage lies in fewer side effects than other antidepressants and have thus become the preferred choice. In general, initial response rates for all antidepressant medications hover around 50% (Hollon et al., 2005.)

Psychosocial Treatment Approaches Dating from Freud's era, depression has been treated with a variety of psychosocial methods. For instance, marital therapy has been used in cases where marital functioning and depression appear to be entangled. Brief dynamic therapy and behavioral therapy have also shown some evidence of efficacy (Depression Guideline Panel, 1993). For example, two fairly recent behaviorally based treatments have reported some success in treating depression (e.g., Dimidjian, et al., 2006; Jacobson et al., 1996). However, we emphasize cognitive therapy and interpersonal therapy because they currently dominate psychosocial approaches for the treatment of depression, and both have demonstrated considerable and consistent efficacy in the treatment of the depression.

COGNITIVE THERAPY Before discussing cognitive therapy, several caveats are in order. First, there are a number of different approaches to modifying dysfunction that fall within the domain of cognitive therapy. Our focus is on cognitive therapy as developed by Beck (e.g., Beck, Rush, Shaw & Emery, 1979), largely because the research literature has tended to evaluate this particular version of cognitive therapy the most extensively, and because it was the first psychotherapy approach to focus explicitly on the modification of cognitive factors. Second, while at initial glance it might appear that the development of cognitive treatment methods would follow from theory and research on the cognitive factors in depression, it was in fact the early success of cognitive therapy that stimulated much of the theory and research on cognitive processes. Lastly, even though the goal of these approaches is the modification of cognitive factors that are presumed to play an important role in both the onset and maintenance of depressed states, most cognitive approaches also make considerable use of behavioral methods to help achieve these ends. Hence, cognitive and cognitive-behavioral therapy are terms that can be reasonably used interchangeably.

The goal of cognitive therapy in the treatment of depression (and in other disordered states) is to teach individuals to recognize and modify beliefs and cognitions that are dysfunctional (Beck et al., 1979). To do so, cognitive therapists make use of *collaborative empiricism* which entails working together with the patient to test the validity, and where possible, modify negative thinking processes that are embedded in the patient's meaning system. Thus, the goal is to first help patients recognize the thoughts that may be maintaining depression, and then to test the validity of these thoughts. Cognitive therapists use a variety of methods, but tend to rely heavily on *Socratic questioning* and *behavioral experiments* to achieve these goals. Socratic questioning takes the form of asking questions such as "What is the evidence for this belief?"; "Are there other ways to view the situation?"; and if the belief is accurate, "What is the meaning of this?" Initially these methods should help the patient minimize distress in a particular situation, but can also be employed in other situations and after therapy has ended to deal with future stressful situations. Behavioral methods entail experiments designed to help the patient test the validity of the belief. For example, if a depressed individual thought that "No one wants to hang out with me," he might devise a behavioral experiment to test this belief. In one possible scenario, the client could ask five friends/acquaintances to accompany him to dinner or coffee. During this process, he would gather evidence that either supported or refuted his original dysfunctional belief.

What is the empirical evidence for the efficacy of cognitive therapy? Cognitive therapy is among the most extensively tested treatments for depression and is widely recognized as one of the most effective psychosocial treatments available (Hollon, Haman, & Brown, 2002). Well controlled studies have suggested that cognitive therapy produces outcomes that are roughly equivalent to psychophar-macological interventions (Hollon et al., 2002). Data also suggest that cognitive therapy may substantially reduce the rate of relapse (the return of the treated episode) and recurrence (the appearance of a new episode) (Hollon et al., 2005). For these reasons, cognitive therapy is listed as an empirically supported treatment for depression (as well as other disorders) (Ingram, Scott, & Hayes, 2000; see also Stewart & Chambliss, this volume.)

Some data suggest that combining cognitive therapy with medication may enhance the positive response rates (Conti, Plutchik, Wild, & Karasu, 1986), but such conclusions are not without qualification. For example, superior efficacy for combined approaches may only be obtained for cases of depression that are more severe, complex, or have a high degree of comorbidity. Alternatively, combined therapy and medication may enhance responsiveness for those individuals who are not responsive to either modality alone. In this latter regard, practice guidelines typically call for the addition of a different approach if symptoms are not reduced within six to eight weeks (American Psychiatric Association, 2000). Thus, it appears that in some cases medication may enhance the effects of cognitive therapy, but this is far from a universal conclusion in all cases of depression. Data show that positive effects for medication (e.g., approximately a 50% response rate) are obtained fairly quickly and then tail off, with substantial relapse rates if antidepressants are withdrawn. However, cognitive therapy, both alone or combined with medication, is associated with substantially less relapse than medication alone (Hollon et al., 2005), suggesting that cognitive therapy is the key factor in preventing future depressive episodes.

INTERPERSONAL PSYCHOTHERAPY Interpersonal approaches can trace their origin to more analytic approaches to treatment seen in the work of Adolph Meyer and Harry Stack Sullivan (Klerman & Weissman, 1993) and explicitly rely on interpersonal theories of personality proposed by these early theories. Interpersonal difficulties in the areas of grief, role disputes, role transitions, or interpersonal deficits are considered to constitute the core problems in depression. Despite these factors, interpersonal therapy also explicitly considers depression to be a medical problem, and assigns a "sick role" to the patient to remove guilt about the diagnosis of depression. Whereas cognitive therapy provides a fairly structured set of therapeutic methods, interpersonal therapy is typically unstructured.

After an assessment of depressive symptoms, patients are asked to describe in detail the nature of their interpersonal relationships and difficulties, which provides a basis for the therapist to focus on one or two of the major areas of interpersonal functioning (e.g., grief, role disputes, role transitions, or interpersonal deficits). If grief is the focus, the therapist attempts to help the patient mourn in a healthy way and, when appropriate, to develop new relationships. Role transitions (e.g., the loss of a job) are dealt with by helping the patient to cope and acquire new skills that will facilitate a positive transition. When a role dispute is the focus of treatment (e.g., difficulties in a close relationship such as marriage), the therapist works with the patient to try to resolve the dispute. Such resolutions can take the form of renegotiating the nature of the relationship, or might take the form of dissolution of the relationship. In this latter case, grief at the loss of the relationship may also become a focus of therapy. Finally, if interpersonal deficits are the focal point of treatment, the therapist helps the patient develop more effective social skills through role playing and related methods.

A reasonably large body of data supports the efficacy of interpersonal therapy for depression. An initial study reported by Weissman et al. (1979) found that interpersonal therapy was equivalent in efficacy to medication, specifically amitriptyline. Data have also suggested that the combination of psychopharmacological approaches and interpersonal therapy is effective, with some evidence to suggest that the combination is better than either treatment alone (DiMasico et al., 1979). Interpersonal therapy was also found to be as effective as psychopharmacological treatment in a large scale study conducted by the National Institute of Mental Health (Elkin, Gibbons et al., 1995; Elkin, Shea et al., 1989). This study also found that interpersonal therapy was superior to cognitive therapy, although it has subsequently become clear that cognitive therapy at some of the sites in this study was not practiced optimally (Hollon, 1999) and was thus not well-represented in the study. Given its demonstrated efficacy in these studies, IPT is also considered to be an empirically supported treatment for depression.

Summary

In this chapter, we began with a basic overview of the major classes of mood disorders, with a primary focus on unipolar depression. We noted the *DSM-IV-TR* required symptoms, the general course of mood disorder, and issues in defining the idea of depression. We also explored epidemiological data, gender differences, and cultural issues. Some epidemiological studies estimate lifetime prevalence rates of depression to be as high as 25%, although these figures may depend on the way depression is defined, and in what culture depression is assessed. About twice as many women suffer from unipolar depression as men, though there are few gender differences in bipolar disorders. Cultural issues explore how depression can be manifested and conceptualized differently in various cultures, and while *DSM*-inspired notions of depression rely heavily on Western society, depression may be thought of very differently in other cultures.

After this general introduction, we examined some of the theoretical models of depression, as well as corresponding research findings. Diathesis-stress conceptualizations focus on the interaction between internal and external sources in the development of depression, and although not universally the case, most theories of depression reflect such perspectives to some degree. We next noted the major theoretical viewpoints. Biomedical models focus on genetics, biological evidence, and progressions in affective neuroscience. Genetic perspectives look to family studies, twin studies, and adoption studies, which show familial clusters of mood disorders as evidence for genetic contributions to depression. In the area of biological approaches to depression, several pathophysiological processes have been noted, such as serotonin and norepinephrine dysregulation, high levels of cortisol, and sleep disturbances. Affective neuroscience, which focuses on neural processes linked to emotion, has suggested abnormalities of the prefrontal cortex, the anterior cingulate cortex, the hippocampus, and the amygdala. Each of these perspectives has provided important insights into the nature of depression, but our understanding of biomedical processes is still far from complete.

The other major classification of models presented were the psychosocial approaches to depression. Despite differences in emphasis, the common theme among cognitive models is that negative cognitive processes play an important role in the cause and course of depression. Empirical studies affirm a number of aspects of these cognitive models. Interpersonal approaches also represent a psychosocial view of depression, but focus on interactional patterns as key features in depression. As with cognitive models, interpersonal approaches vary, but tend to converge on the idea that troubled interaction patterns may both cause and maintain depression.

Lastly, we examined various forms of treatment and prevention for mood disorders. In the area of prevention, research has made some strides in demonstrating that prevention may help reduce depressive symptoms in high risk groups. In particular, children and adolescents seem to benefit most from prevention programs, although much of this work is in the very early stages. Paralleling the two major areas of depression theory and research, the main forms of treatment consist of biologically based treatment and psychosocial interventions. Biologically based treatment entails the use of pharmacotherapy, with the three main types of antidepressant medications consisting of MAOIs, tricyclics, and SSRIs. All of these can be effective for certain groups of people, although SSRIs are prescribed most often because of both their efficacy and their limited side effects. Major psychosocial interventions include cognitive therapy and interpersonal psychotherapy. Cognitive therapy aims to help individuals recognize and modify their dysfunctional beliefs. Socratic questioning and behavioral experiments are two techniques that cognitive therapists employ. Data have repeatedly shown the efficacy of such approaches. Interpersonal psychotherapy focuses on the areas of grief, role disputes, role transitions, or interpersonal deficits as the core issues that are addressed in therapy. As with cognitive therapy, a considerable body of research supports the efficacy of this psychosocial intervention.

As should be clear from the information we have provided, significant strides have been made in understanding the core factors involved in depression, as well as mechanisms that may be involved in its onset and course. As significant as these strides have been, however, much is still not known about the essential features of depression. We thus end this chapter with a theme that has occurred throughout our review of the theory and research on depression. Most depression theorists and researchers believe that there are a number of different types of depression, and although these all result in a similar symptom constellation, they may have very different causes, courses, and correlates. This heterogeneity has significant implications not only for theory and research on depression, but also for prevention and treatment efforts; prevention programs and treatment tailored to the causal factors in different kinds of depressive disorders may dramatically improve positive outcomes. From a more general perspective, this heterogeneity illustrates a concept that is important to keep in mind in any exploration of depression. Mood disorders are dynamic constructs whose understanding will hinge upon definitions and cultural contexts. The key to unlocking the secrets of depression may therefore lie in cataloging the different subtypes of the disorders that we call depression, and then examining the biological and psychological factors that contribute to their various causes and courses.

References

Abramson, L. Y., & Alloy, L. B. (2006). Cognitive vulnerability to depression: Current status and developmental origins. In T. E. Joiner, J. S. Brown, & J. Kistner (Eds), *The interpersonal, cognitive, and social nature of depression* (pp. 83–100). Mahwah, NJ: Erlbaum.

Abramson, L. Y., Metalsky, G. I., & Alloy, L. B. (1989). Hopelessness depression: A theory-based subtype of depression. *Psychological Review, 96*, 358–372.

Abramson, L. Y., Seligman, M. E. P., & Teasdale, J. (1978). Learned helplessness in humans: Critique and reformulation. *Journal of Abnormal Psychology, 87*, 49–74.

Albee, G. W. (2000). Critique of psychotherapy in American society. In C. R. Snyder & R. E. Ingram (Eds.), *Handbook of psychological change: Psychotherapy processes and practices for the 21st century* (pp. 689–706). New York: Wiley.

Alloy, L. B., & Abramson, L. Y. (1999). The Temple-Wisconsin Cognitive Vulnerability to Depression Project: Conceptual background, design, and methods. *Journal of Cognitive Psychotherapy, 13*, 227–262.

American Psychiatric Association. (2000). *Diagnostic and statistical manual of mental disorders (4th ed., rev.)*. Washington, D.C.: Author.

Barnard, P. J., & Teasdale, J. D. (1991). Interacting cognitive subsystems: A systemic approach to cognitive-affective interaction and change. *Cognition and Emotion, 5*, 1–39.

Beck, A. T. (1963). Thinking and depression: I. Idiosyncratic content and cognitive distortions. *Archives of General Psychiatry, 9*, 324–333.

Beck, A. T. (1967). *Depression: Causes and treatment*. Philadelphia: University of Pennsylvania Press.

Beck, A. T. (1976). *Cognitive therapy and the emotional disorders*. New York: International Universities Press.

Beck, A. T. (1987). Cognitive model of depression. *Journal of Cognitive Psychotherapy, 1*, 2–27.

Beck, A. T. (2002). Cognitive models of depression. In R. L. Leahy & T. E. Dowd (Eds.), *Clinical advances in cognitive psychotherapy: Theory and application* (pp. 29–61). New York: Springer.

Beck, A. T., Rush, A. J., Shaw, B. F., & Emery, G. (1979). *Cognitive therapy of depression*. New York: Guilford.

Blackburn, I. M., Bishop, S., Glen, A. I. M., Whalley, L. J., & Christie, J. E. (1981). The pharmacotherapy. Each alone and in combination. *British Journal of Psychiatry, 139*, 181–189.

Blatt, S. J. (1974). Level of object representation in anaclitic and introjective depression. *Psychoanalytic Study of the Child, 29*, 107–157.

Blatt, S. J., & Homann, E. (1992). Parent-child interaction in the etiology of dependent and self-critical depression. *Clinical Psychology Review, 12*, 47–91.

Brems, C. (1995). Women and depression: A comprehensive analysis. In E. E. Beckham & W. R. Leber (Eds.), *Handbook of depression* (2nd ed., pp. 539–566). New York: Guilford.

Buysse, D. J., Germain, A., Nofzinger, E. A., & Kupfer, D. J. (2006). Mood disorders and sleep. In D. J. Stein, D. J. Kupfer, & A. F. Schatzberg (Eds.), *Textbook of mood disorders* (pp. 717–737). Arlington, VA: American Psychiatric Publishing.

Carver, C. S. (1979). A cybernenetic model of self-attention processes. *Journal of Personality and Social Psychology, 37*, 1186–1195.

Conti, H. R., Plutchik, R., Wild, K. V., & Karasu, T. B. (1986). Combined psychotherapy and pharmacotherapy for depression. *Archives of General Psychiatry, 43*, 471–479.

Coyne, J. C. (1976). Toward an interactional description of depression. *Psychiatry, 39*, 28–40.

Coyne, J. C. (1999). Thinking interactionally about depression: A radical restatement. In T. E. Joiner & J. C. Coyne (Eds.), *The interactional nature of depression* (pp. 365–392). Washington, D.C.: American Psychological Association.

Davidson, R. J. (1993). Cerebral asymmetry and emotion: Conceptual and methodological conundrums. *Cognition and Emotion, 7*, 115–138.

Davidson, R. J., Pizzagalli, D., & Nitschke, J. B. (2002). The representation and regulation of emotion in depression: Perspectives from affective neuroscience. In I. H. Gotlib & C. L. Hammen (Eds.), *Handbook of depression* (3rd ed., pp. 219–244). New York: Guilford.

Delgado, P. L., & Moreno, F. A. (2006). Neurochemistry of mood disorders. In D. J. Stein, D. J. Kupfer, & A. F. Schatzberg (Eds.) *Textbook of mood disorders* (pp. 101–117). Arlington, VA: American Psychiatric Publishing.

Depression Guideline Panel (1993). *Depression in primary care: Vol. 2. Treatment of major depression* (Clinical Practice Guideline No. 5, AHCPR Publication No. 9300551). Rockville, MD: Department of Health and Human Services, Public Health Service, Agency for Health Care Policy and Research.

Dill, J. C., & Anderson, C. A. (1999). Loneliness, shyness and depression: The etiology and interrelationships of everyday problems in living. In T. E. Joiner & J. C. Coyne (Eds.), *The interactional nature of depression* (pp. 93–126). Washington, D.C.: American Psychological Association.

DiMascio, A., Weissman, M. M., Prusoff, B. A., Neu, C., Zwilling, M., & Klerman, G. L. (1979). Differential symptom reduction by drugs and psychotherapy in acute depression. *Archives of General Psychiatry, 36*, 1450–1456.

Dimidjian, S., Hollon, S., Dobson, K. S., Schmaling, K. B., Kohlenberg, R., Addis, M. E., et al. (2006). Randomized trial of behavioral activation, cognitive therapy, and antidepressant dedication in the acute treatment of adults with major depression. *Journal of Consulting and Clinical Psychology, 74*, 658–670.

Dorzab, J., Baker, M., Winokur, G., & Cadoret, R. J. (1971). Depressive disease: Clinical course. *Diseases of the Nervous System, 32*, 269–273.

Dougherty, D., & Rauch, S. L. (1997). Neuroimaging and neurobiological models of depression. *Harvard Review of Psychiatry, 5*, 138–159.

Drevets, W. C. (1998). Functional neuroimagining studies of depression: The anatomy of melancholia. *Annual Review of Medicine, 49*, 341–361.

Drevets, W. C. (2001). Neuroimagining and neuropathological studies of depression: Implications for the cognitive-emotional features of mood disorders. *Current Opinion in Neurobiology, 11*, 240–249.

Drevets, W. C., Price, J. L., Simpson, J. R. J., Todd, R. D., Reich, T., Vannier, M. et al. (1997). Subgenial prefrontal cortex abnormalities in mood disorders. *Nature, 386*, 824–827.

Duval, S., & Wicklund, R. (1972). *A theory of objective self-awareness*. New York: Academic Press.

Elkin, I., Gibbons, R., Shea, M. T., Sotsky, S., Watkins, J., Pilkonis, P., & Hedeker, D. (1995). Initial severity and differential treatment outcome in the National Institute of Mental Health Treatment of Depression Collaborative Research Program. *Journal of Consulting and Clinical Psychology, 63*, 841–847.

Elkin, I., Shea, M. T., Watkins, J., Imber, S., Sotsky, S., Collins, J., et al. (1989). National Institute of Mental Health Treatment of Depression Collaborative Research Program: General effectiveness of treatments. *Archives of General Psychiatry, 46*, 971–982.

Ellis, A. (1996). *Better, deeper and more enduring brief therapy: The rational emotive behavior therapy approach*. New York: Brunner/Mazel.

Enns, M., & Cox, B. (1997). Personality dimensions and depression: Review and commentary. *Canadian Journal of Psychiatry, 42*, 274–284.

Faraone, S. V., Tsuang, T., & Tsuang, D. (1999). *Genetics of mental disorders: A guide for students, clinicians, and researchers*. New York: Guilford.

Fava, G. A., Rafanelli, C., Grandi, S., Conti, S., & Belluardo, P. (1998). Prevention of recurrent depression with cognitive-behavioral therapy. *Archives of General Psychiatry, 55*, 816–820.

Flett, G. L., Vredenburg, K., & Krames, L. (1997). The continuity of depression in clinical and no clinical samples. *Psychological Bulletin, 121*, 395–416.

Flores, B. & Schatzberg, A. F. (2006). Psychotic depression. In D. J. Stein, D. J. Kupfer, & A. F. Schatzberg (Eds.), *Textbook of mood disorders* (pp. 561–571). Arlington, VA: American Psychiatric Publishing.

Foley, D. L., Neale, M., & Kendler, K. (1996). A longitudinal study of stressful life events. *Psychiatric Medicine, 26*, 1239–1252.

Frewen, P. A., & Dozois, D. J. A. (2006). Self-worth appraisal of life events and Beck's congruency model of depression vulnerability. *Journal of Cognitive Psychotherapy, 20*, 231–240.

Garber, J., & Flynn, C. (2001). Predictors of depressive cognitions in young adolescents. *Cognitive Therapy and Research, 4*, 353–376.

Garber, J., & Hollon, S. (1991). What can specificity designs say about causality in psychopathology research? *Psychological Bulletin, 110*, 129–136.

Gitlin, M. J. (2002). Pharmacological treatment of depression. In I. H. Gotlib & C. L. Hammen (Eds.), *Handbook of depression* (3rd ed., pp. 360–382). New York: Guilford.

Goodwin, R. D., Jacob, F., Bittner, A., & Wittchen, H. (2006). Epidemiology of mood disorders. In D. J. Stein, D. J. Kupfer, & A. F. Schatzberg (Eds.) *Textbook of mood disorders*. Arlington: American Psychiatric Publishing.

Goodwin, F. K., & Jamison, K. R. (1990). *Manic-depressive illness*. New York: Oxford University Press.

Gotlib, I. H., & Hammen, C. L. (1992). *Psychological aspects of depression: Toward a cognitive-interpersonal integration*. Chichester, UK: Wiley.

Hammen, C. (1991). The generation of stress in the course of unipolar depression. *Journal of Abnormal Psychology, 100*, 555–561.

Hammen, C. (1999). The emergence of an interpersonal approach to depression. In T. E. Joiner & J. C. Coyne (Eds.), *The interactional nature of depression* (pp. 21–36). Washington, D.C.: American Psychological Association.

Hammen, C. L. (2001). Vulnerability to depression in adulthood. In R. E. Ingram, & J. M. Price (Eds.), *Vulnerability to psychopathology: Risk across the lifespan* (pp. 226–257). New York: Guilford.

Hollon, S. D. (1999). Allegiance effects in treatment research: A commentary. *Clinical Psychology: Science and Practice, 6,* 107–112.

Hollon, S. D., Haman, K. L., & Brown, L. L. (2002). Cognitive-behavioral treatment of depression. In I. H. Gotlib & C. L. Hammen (Eds.), *Handbook of depression* (3rd ed., pp. 383–403). New York: Guilford.

Hollon, S. D., Jarrett, R. B., Nierenberg, A. A., Thase, M. E., Trivedi, M., & Rush, A. J. (2005). Psychotherapy and medication in the treatment of adult and geriatric depression: Which monotherapy or combined treatment? *Journal of Clinical Psychiatry, 66,* 455–468.

Ingram, R. E. (1984). Toward an information processing analysis of depression. *Cognitive Therapy and Research, 8,* 443–478.

Ingram, R. E. (2001). Developing perspectives on the cognitive-developmental origins of depression: Back is the future. *Cognitive Therapy and Research, 25,* 497–504.

Ingram, R. E., Miranda, J., & Segal, Z. (1998). *Cognitive vulnerability to depression.* New York: Guilford.

Ingram, R. E., Miranda, J., & Segal, Z. V. (2005). Cognitive vulnerability to depression: Theory, research and future directions. In L. B. Alloy & J. Riskind (Eds.), *Cognitive vulnerability to emotional disorders.* New York: Erlbaum.

Ingram, R. E., Odom, M., & Mitchusson, L. (2004). Secondary prevention of depression: Risk, vulnerability and intervention. In D. J. A. Dozois & K. S. Dobson (Eds.), *The prevention of anxiety and depression: Theory, research, and practice.* Washington, D.C.: American Psychological Association.

Ingram, R. E., & Price, J. (2001). (Eds.). *Vulnerability to Psychopathology: Risk across the Lifespan.* New York: Guilford.

Ingram, R. E., Scott, W., & Hayes, A. (2000). Empirically validated treatment: A critical analysis. In C. R. Snyder & R. E. Ingram, R. E. (Eds.). *Handbook of psychological change: Psychotherapy processes and practices for the 21st century.* New York: Wiley.

Irwin, M. (2002). Psychoneuroimmunology of depression: Clinical implications. *Brain, Behavior, and Immunity, 16,* 1–16.

Jacobson, N. S., Dobson, K. S., Truax, P. A., Addis, M. E., Koerner, K., Gollan, J. K., Gortner, E., & Prince, S. E. (1996). A component analysis of cognitive-behavioral treatment for depression. *Journal of Consulting and Clinical Psychology, 64,* 295–304.

Joiner, T. E. (2002). Depression in it's interpersonal context. In I. H. Gotlib & C. L. Hammen (Eds.), *Handbook of depression* (3rd ed., pp. 295–313). New York: Guilford.

Joiner, T. E., & Coyne, J. C. (1999) (Eds.). *The interactional nature of depression.* Washington, D.C.: American Psychological Association.

Keller, M. B., Shapiro, R. W., Lavori, P. W., & Wolfe, N. (1982). Relapse in RDC major depressive disorders: Analysis with the life table. *Archives of General Psychiatry, 39,* 911–915.

Kendall, P. C., Hollon, S. D., Beck, A. T., Hammen, C. L., & Ingram, R. E. (1987). Issues and recommendations regarding use of the Beck Depression Inventory. *Cognitive Therapy and Research, 11,* 289–299.

Kendell, R. E. (1975). *The role of diagnosis in psychiatry.* Oxford: Blackwell.

Kendler K., & Gardner, C. O. (1998). Twins studies of adult psychiatric and substance dependence disorders. *Psychological Medicine, 28,* 625–633.

Kendler, K., Neale, M., Kessler, R., Heath, A., & Eaves, L. (1992). Major depression and generalized anxiety disorder. *Archives of General Psychiatry, 49,* 716–722.

Kessler, R. C. (2002). Epidemiology of depression. In I. H. Gotlib & C. L. Hammen (Eds.), *Handbook of depression* (3rd ed., pp. 23–42). New York: Guilford.

Kessler, R. C., Berglund, P., Demler, O., Jin, R., Koretz, D., Merikangas, K. R., et al. (2003). The epidemiology of major depressive disorder: Results from the National Comorbidity Survey Replication (NCS-R). *Journal of the American Medical Association, 289,* 3095–3105.

Kessler, R. C., Demier, O., Frank, R. G., Olfson, M., Pincus, H. A., Walters, E. E., et al. (2005) Prevalence and treatment of mental disorders, 1990 to 2003. *New England Journal of Medicine, 352,* 2515–2523.

Keyes, C. L. M. & Goodman, S. H. (2006). (Eds.) *Women and depression: A handbook for the social, behavioral, and biomedical sciences.* New York: Cambridge University Press.

Klerman, G. L., & Weissman, M. M. (1993). *New applications of interpersonal psychotherapy.* Washington, D.C.: American Psychiatric Association.

Korf, J., & van Praag, H. H. (1971). Retarded depressions and the dopamine hypothesis. *Psychopharmacologia, 19,* 199–203.

Kornstein, S. G., & Sloan, D. M. E. (2006). Depression and gender. In D. J. Stein, D. J. Kupfer, & A. F. Schatzberg (Eds.) *Textbook of mood disorders* (pp. 687–698). Arlington, VA: American Psychiatric Publishing.

Lewinsohn, P. (1985). A behavioral approach to depression. In J. C. Coyne (Ed.) *Essential papers in depression.* New York: New York University Press.

Lewinsohn, P., & Amenson, C. (1978). Some relations between pleasant and unpleasant mood-related events and depression. *Journal of Abnormal Psychology, 87,* 644–654.

Lindsay, J. E., & Scott, W. D. (2005). Dysphoria and self-esteem following an achievement event: Predictive validity of goal orientation and personality style theories of vulnerability. *Cognitive Therapy and Research, 29,* 769–785.

Luyten, P., Corveleyn, J., & Blatt, S. J. (2005). The convergence among psychodynamic and cognitive-behavioral theories of depression: A critical review of empirical research. In J. Corveleyn, P. Luyten, & S. J. Blatt (Eds). *The theory and treatment of depression: Towards a dynamic interactionism model.* (pp. 95–135). Leuven, Belgium: Leuven University Press.

Maes, M., & Meltzer, H. Y. (1995). The serotonin hypothesis of major depression. In F. E. Bloom & D. J. Kupfer (Eds.), *Psychopharmacology: The fourth generation of progress* (pp. 933–944). New York: Raven Press.

Malhi, G. S., Moore, J., & McGuffin, P. (2000). The genetics of major depression. *Current Psychiatry Reports, 2,* 165–169.

Mallon, L., Broman, J. E., Hetta, J. (2000). Relationship between insomnia, depression and mortality: A 12-year follow-up of older adults in the community. *International Psychogeriatrics, 12,* 295–306.

Mayberg, H. (2006). Brain imagining. In D. J. Stein, D. J. Kupfer, & A. F. Schatzberg (Eds.), *Textbook of mood disorders* (pp. 219–234). Arlington, VA: American Psychiatric Publishing.

Mazure, C. M. (1998). Life stressors as risk factors in depression. *Clinical Psychology: Science and Practice, 5,* 291–313.

Meehl, P. E. (1962). Schizotaxia, schizotypy, schizophrenia. *American Psychologist, 17,* 827–838.

McGuffin, P., Katz, R., & Rutherford, J. (1991). Nature, nurture, and depression: A twin study. *Psychological Medicine, 21,* 329–335.

Monroe, S. M. & Hadjiyannakis, K. (2002). The social environment and depression: Focusing on severe life stress. In I. H. Gotlib & C. L. Hammen (Eds.), *Handbook of depression* (3rd ed., pp. 314–341). New York: Guilford.

Monroe, S. M. & Harkness, K. L. (2005). Life stress, the "kindling" hypothesis, and the recurrence of depression: Considerations from a life stress perspective. *Psychological Review, 112,* 417–445.

Monroe, S. M., & Simons, A. D. (1991). Diathesis-stress theories in the context of life stress research: Implications for the depressive disorders. *Psychological Bulletin,110,* 406–425.

Munoz, R., Le, H., Clarke, G., & Jaycox, L. (2002). Preventing the onset of major depression. In I. H. Gotlib & C. L. Hammen (Eds.), *Handbook of depression* (3rd ed., pp. 343–359). New York: Guilford.

Nolen-Hoeksema, S. (2002). Gender differences in depression. In I. H. Gotlib & C. L. Hammen (Eds.), *Handbook of depression* (3rd ed., pp. 492–509). New York: Guilford.

Nurcombe, B. (1992). The evolution and validity of the diagnosis of major depression in childhood and adolescence. In D. Cicchetti & S. L. Toth (Eds.), *Developmental perspectives on depression.* Rochester, NY: University of Rochester Press.

Pinel, J. P. J. (2000). *Biopsychology.* Needman Heights, MA: Pearson Education.

Potter, W. Z., Paich, R. A., Rudorfer, M. V. & Krishnan, R. R. (2006). Tricyclics, teracyclics, and monoamine oxidase inhibitors. In D. J. Stein, D. J. Kupfer, & A. F. Schatzberg (Eds.), *Textbook of mood disorders* (pp. 251–262). Arlington, VA: American Psychiatric Publishing.

Rajowska, G. (2006). Anatomical pathology. In D. J. Stein, D. J. Kupfer, & A. F. Schatzberg (Eds.), *Textbook of mood disorders* (pp. 179–195). Arlington, VA: American Psychiatric Publishing.

Rapaport, M., & Judd, L. L. (1998). Minor depressive disorder and subsyndromal depressive symptoms: Functional impairment and response to treatment. *Journal of Affective Disorders, 48,* 227–232.

Rosenthal, J. Z. & Rosenthal, N. E. (2006). Seasonal affective disorder. In D. J. Stein, D. J. Kupfer, & A. F. Schatzberg (Eds.) *Textbook of mood disorders* (pp. 527–546). Arlington, VA: American Psychiatric Publishing.

Ressler, K. J., & Nemeroff, C. B. (1999). Role of norepinephrine in the pathophysiology and treatment of mood disorders. *Biological Psychiatry, 46,* 1219–1233.

Rush, A. J., Beck, A. T., Kovacs, M., & Hollon, S. D. (1977). Comparative efficacy of cognitive therapy and pharmacotherapy in the treatment of depressed outpatients. *Cognitive Therapy and Research, 1,* 17–38.

Saz, P. & Dewey, M. (2001). Depression, depressive symptoms and mortality in persons aged 65 and over living in the community: A systematic review of the literature. *International Journal of Geriatric Psychiatry, 16,* 622–630.

Scher, C. D., Ingram, R. E., & Segal, Z. V. (2005). Cognitive reactivity and vulnerability: Empirical evaluation of construct activation and cognitive diathesis in unipolar depression. *Clinical Psychology Review, 25,* 487–510.

Schildkraut, J. J. (1965). The catecholamine hypothesis of affective disorders: A review of supporting evidence. *American Journal of Psychiatry, 122,* 509–522.

Segal, Z. V., Gemar, M., & Williams, S. (1999). Differential cognitive response to a mood challenge following successful cognitive therapy or pharmacotherapy for unipolar depression. *Journal of Abnormal Psychology, 108,* 3–10.

Segal, Z. V. & Ingram, R. E. (1994). Mood priming and construct activation in tests of cognitive vulnerability to unipolar depression. *Clinical Psychology Review, 14,* 663–695.

Segal, Z. V., (1988). Appraisal of the self-schema construct in cognitive models of depression. *Psychological Bulletin, 103,* 147–162.

Segal, Z. V., Kennedy, S., Gemar, M., Hood, K., Pedersen, R., & Buis, T. (2006). Cognitive reactivity to sad mood provocation and the prediction of depressive relapse. *Archives of General Psychiatry, 63,* 749–755.

Seidman, S. N. (2006). Psychoneuroendocrinology of mood disorders. In D. J. Stein, D. J. Kupfer, & A. F. Schatzberg (Eds.) *Textbook of mood disorders* (pp. 117–130). Arlington: American Psychiatric Publishing.

Sheline, Y. I, Gado, M. H., & Kraemer, H. C. (2003). Untreated depression and hippocampal volume loss. *American Journal of Psychiatry, 161,* 1309–1310.

Siegle, G. J., & Ingram, R. E. (1996). The big picture. *Contemporary Psychology, 41,* 163–164.

Siegle, G. J., Steinhauer, S. R., Thase, M. E., Stenger, A., & Carter, C. S. (2002). Can't shake that feeling: Event-related fMRI assessment of sustained amygdala activity in response to emotional information in depressed individuals. *Biological Psychiatry, 51,* 693–707.

Simon, G. E. (2003). Social and economic burden of mood disorders. *Biological Psychiatry, 54,* 208–215.

Seligman, M. E. P. (1975). *Helplessness: On depression, development, and death.* San Francisco: Freeman.

Sobczak, S., Riedel, W. J., Booij, I., Aan., M., Deutz, N. E. P., & Honig, A. (2002) Cognition following acute tryptophan depletion: Difference between first-degree relatives of bipolar disorder patients and matched healthy control volunteers. *Psychological Medicine, 32,* 503–515.

Stader, S. R., & Hokanson, J. E. (1998). Psychosocial antecedents of depressive symptoms: An evaluation using daily experiences methodology. *Journal of Abnormal Psychology, 107,* 17–26.

Sullivan, P. F., Neale, M. C., & Kendler, K. S. (2000). Genetic epidemiology of major depression: Review and meta-analysis. *American Journal of Psychiatry, 157,* 1552–1562.

Teasdale, J. D. (1993). Emotion and two kinds of meaning: Cognitive therapy and applied cognitive science. *Behaviour Research and Therapy, 31*, 339–354.

Teasdale, J. D. (1999). Multi-level theories of cognition-emotion relations. In T. Dalgleish & M. Power (Eds.), *Handbook of cognition and emotion* (pp. 665–681). Chichester, UK: Wiley

Teasdale, J. D., & Barnard, P. J. (1993). *Affect, cognition, and change.* Hillsdale, NJ: Erlbaum.

Tennant, C. (2001). Work-related stress and depressive disorders. *Journal of Psychosomatic Research, 51*, 697–704.

Thase, M. E., Jindal, R., & Howland, R. H. (2002). Biological aspects of depression. In I. H. Gotlib & C. L. Hammen (Eds.), *Handbook of depression* (3rd ed., pp. 192–218). New York: Guilford.

Trull, T. J., Widiger, T. A., & Guthrie, P. (1990). Categorical versus dimensional status of borderline personality disorder. *Journal of Abnormal Psychology, 99*, 40–48.

Tsai, J. L., & Chentsova-Dutton, Y. (2002). Understanding depression across cultures. In I. H. Gotlib & C. L. Hammen (Eds.), *Handbook of Depression* (3rd ed., pp. 467–491). New York: Guilford.

Wallace, J., Schneider, T., & McGuffin, P. (2002). In I. H. Gotlib & C. L. Hammen (Eds.), *Handbook of depression* (3rd ed., pp. 169–191). New York: Guilford.

Weissman, M., Prusoff, B. A., DiMascio, A., Neu, C., Goklaney, M., & Klerman, G. (1979). The efficacy of drugs and psychotherapy in the treatment of acute depressive episodes. *American Journal of Psychiatry, 136*, 555–558.

Whisman, M. A. (2001). The association between depression and marital dissatisfaction. In S. R. H. Beach (Ed). *Marital and family processes in depression: A scientific foundation for clinical practice* (pp. 3–24). Washington, D.C.: American Psychological Association.

Zuroff, D. C., & Fitzpatrick, D. K. (1995). Depressive personality styles: Implications for adult attachment. *Personality and Individual Differences, 18*, 253–365.

10
Schizophrenia

Elaine Walker, Annie Bollini, Karen Hochman,
Lisa Kestler, and Vijay A. Mittal

Schizophrenia is among the most debilitating of mental illnesses. It is typically diagnosed between 20 and 25 years of age, a stage of life when most people gain independence from parents, develop intimate romantic relationships, plan educational pursuits, and begin work or career endeavors (DeLisi, 1992). Because the clinical onset usually occurs during this pivotal time, the illness can have a profoundly negative impact on the individual's opportunities for attaining social and occupational success, and the consequences can be devastating for the patient's life course, as well as for family members. Further, the illness knows no national boundaries. Across cultures, estimates of the lifetime prevalence of schizophrenia range around 1% (1 per 100 people) (Arajarvi et al., 2005; Keith, Regier, & Rae, 1991, Kulhara, & Chakrabarti, 2001; Torrey, 1987), although the prognosis may differ among countries (Kulhara & Chakrabarti, 2001).

The origins of this devastating mental disorder have continued to elude researchers, despite many decades of scientific research. To date, no single factor has been found to characterize all patients with the illness. This holds for potential etiological factors, as well as clinical phenomena. Schizophrenia patients vary in symptom profiles, developmental histories, family backgrounds, cognitive functions, and even brain morphology and neurochemistry. Although this has led some to express dismay at our chances of ever finding the cause of schizophrenia, there is reason to be optimistic. Research efforts have succeeded in revealing numerous pieces of what is now recognized as a complex puzzle of etiological processes.

The consensus in the field, based on findings from various lines of research, is that (1) schizophrenia is a brain disease; (2) its etiology involves the interplay between genetic and environmental factors; (3) multiple developmental pathways eventually lead to disease onset; and (4) brain maturational processes play a role in the etiological process. In this chapter, we will provide an overview of the current state of our knowledge about schizophrenia. We will begin with a discussion of the history and phenomenology of the disorder, and then proceed to a description of some of the key findings that have shed light on the illness.

History and Phenomenology

Written descriptions of patients experiencing psychotic symptoms have been recorded since antiquity. However, because psychotic symptoms can be a manifestation of a variety of disorders, it is unclear whether schizophrenia, as such, is an ancient or relatively new phenomenon. In the mid- to late 19th century, European psychiatrists were investigating the etiology, classification, and prognoses of various types of psychosis. At that time, the most common cause of psychosis was tertiary syphilis, although researchers were unaware that there was any link between psychosis and syphilis. The psychological symptoms of tertiary syphilis frequently overlap with symptoms of what we now call schizophrenia. The cause of syphilis was eventually traced to an infection with the spirochete, *treponema pallidum*, and antibiotics were found to be effective for prevention and treatment of the disorder. This important discovery served to illustrate how a psychological syndrome can be produced by an infectious agent. It also sensitized researchers to the fact that similar syndromes might be the result of different causes.

Emil Kraepelin (1856–1926) was the medical director of the famous Heidelberg Clinic. He was the first to differentiate schizophrenia, which he referred to as "dementia praecox" (or dementia of the young) from manic-depressive psychosis (Kraepelin, 1913/1919). He also lumped together "hebephrenia," "paranoia," and "catatonia" (previously thought to be distinct disorders), and classified all of them as variants of dementia praecox. He based this classification on their similarities in age of onset, and the clinical feature of poor prognosis. Kraepelin did not believe that any one symptom was diagnostic of dementia praecox, but instead focused on the total clinical picture and changes in symptoms over time. If a psychotic patient deteriorated over an extended period of time (months/years), the condition was assumed to be dementia praecox.

Many contemporary mental health professionals continue to expect negative outcomes in those afflicted with schizophrenia, and this expectation infuses the mental health profession with an unfortunate sense of therapeutic nihilism. Yet, while it is true that the majority of patients manifest a chronic course that entails lifelong disability, this bleak scenario is not always the case (Carpenter & Buchanan, 1994). The story of Dr. John Nash, professor and mathematician at Princeton, as told in the movie, *A Beautiful Mind*, illustrates this point quite well. Dr. Nash was able to function at a very high level in his academic field, despite his struggle with schizophrenia.

The term *schizophrenia* was introduced at the beginning of the 20th century by Eugen Bleuler (1857–1939), a Swiss psychiatrist and the medical director of a mental hospital in Zurich (Howells, 1991, pp. xii, 95). The word is derived from two Greek words: *schizo*, which means to tear or to split, and *phren*, which has several meanings: In ancient times, the word *phren*, meant "the intellect" or "the mind." The word *phren* also referred to the lungs and the diaphragm, which were believed to be the seat of emotions. Thus, the word *schizophrenia* literally means the splitting or tearing of the patient's mind and emotional stability.

Bleuler classified the symptoms of schizophrenia into fundamental and accessory symptoms. The fundamental symptoms of schizophrenia are often reported in textbooks as the four As, although, in fact, there are six As and one D (Bleuler, 1911/1950). The fundamental symptoms are listed in Table 10.1. According to Bleuler, these symptoms are present in all patients, at all stages of the illness, and are *diagnostic* of schizophrenia.

Table 10.1 Bleuler's fundamental symptoms of schizophrenia

Disturbances of association (loose, illogical thought processes).
Disturbances of affect (indifference, apathy, or inappropriateness).
Ambivalence (conflicting thoughts, emotions, or impulses which are present
    simultaneously or in rapid succession).
Autism (detachment from social life with inner preoccupation).
Abulia (lack of drive or motivation).
Dementia (irreversible change in personality).

Table 10.2 The Schneiderian "first rank symptoms"

Thought echoing or audible thoughts (patients hear their thoughts out loud).
Thought broadcasting (patients believe that others can hear their thoughts out loud).
Thought intrusion (patients feel that some of their thoughts are from outside; that is, not originating in patients'
own minds).
Thought withdrawal (patients believe that the cause of having lost track of a thought is that someone is taking
their thoughts away).
Somatic hallucinations (unusual, unexplained sensations in one's body).
Passivity feelings (patients believe that their thoughts, feelings, or actions are controlled by another or others).
Delusional perception (a sudden, fixed, false belief about a particular everyday occurrence or perception.

Bleuler's "accessory symptoms" of schizophrenia included delusions, hallucinations, movement disturbances, somatic symptoms, and manic and melancholic states. In contrast to fundamental symptoms, he believed that these accessory symptoms were not present in all schizophrenia patients, and often occurred in other illnesses. For these reasons, the accessory symptoms were not assumed to be as diagnostic of schizophrenia.

Further refinements in the diagnostic criteria for schizophrenia were proposed by Kurt Schneider in the mid-20th century. Like Bleuler, Kurt Schneider thought that certain key symptoms were diagnostic of schizophrenia (Schneider, 1959). In his classification, he referred to these diagnostic symptoms as "first rank symptoms" (see Table 10.2). He believed that, after medical causes of psychosis were ruled out, one could make the diagnosis of schizophrenia if one or more first rank symptoms were present. Schneider's descriptions of the symptoms were more detailed and specific than were Bleuler's fundamental symptoms. Subsequent diagnostic criteria for schizophrenia have been heavily influenced by Schneider's approach.

In subsequent years, investigators began to make a distinction between "positive" and "negative" symptoms of schizophrenia (Harvey & Walker, 1987). The positive symptoms are those that involve an excess of ideas, sensory experiences, or behavior. Hallucinations, delusions, and bizarre behaviors fall in this category. Most of the first rank symptoms described by Schneider are also considered to be positive symptoms. Negative symptoms, in contrast, involve a decrease in behavior, such as blunted or flat affect, anhedonia, and lack of motivation. These symptoms were highlighted by Bleuler.

During the middle of the 20th century, different diagnostic criteria for schizophrenia became popular in different parts of the world. The "Kraepelinian" tradition, with its longitudinal requirements for diagnosis, identified patients with poorer long-term prognosis. In contrast, the Bleulerian and Schneiderian diagnostic systems allowed for a wider range of psychotic patients to be diagnosed with schizophrenia. Thus the patients diagnosed with these two systems tended to have a better prognosis than those diagnosed in the more stringent Kraepelinian tradition. Because of these discrepancies, the use of multiple diagnostic systems had a detrimental effect on research progress; research findings from countries using different diagnostic criteria were not comparable, thus limiting the generalizability of the results.

The next generation of diagnostic systems evolved with the intent of achieving uniformity in diagnostic criteria and improving diagnostic reliability. Among these were the Feighner or St. Louis diagnostic criteria (Feighner, Robins, & Guze, 1972), and the Research Diagnostic Criteria developed by Robert Spitzer and his colleagues (Spitzer et al., 1978). These two approaches to the diagnosis of schizophrenia strongly influenced modern day diagnostic systems, most notably, the *Diagnostic and Statistical Manual of Mental Disorders* (*DSM*) (American Psychiatric Association, 2000).

The *DSM* is now the most widely used system for diagnosing schizophrenia and other mental disorders. The most recent version of the *DSM* is the *DSM-IV-TR* (2000). Using *DSM-IV-TR* criteria, schizophrenia can be diagnosed when signs and symptoms of the disorder have been present for six months or more (including prodromal and residual phases). The characteristic symptom criteria for schizophrenia include the following; (1) hallucinations; (2) delusions; (3) disorganized speech (e g., frequent derailment or incoherence); (4) grossly disorganized or catatonic behavior; and (5) negative symptoms (i.e. affective flattening, alogia or avolition).

At least two or more of these psychotic symptoms must be present for at least one month (or less if successfully treated). Only one of the symptoms is necessary if the delusions are bizarre, or the hallucinated voices consist of a running commentary or of two voices conversing (both of these are derived from Schneider's first rank symptoms in Table 10.2). In addition to the clinical symptoms, there must be social/occupational dysfunction. Further, significant mood disorder, such as depression or manic symptoms, must not be present (this excludes individuals who meet criteria for major depressive disorder with psychotic symptoms and bipolar disorder with psychotic symptoms). Finally, general medical conditions or substance abuse that might lead to psychotic symptoms must be ruled out.

The four subtypes of schizophrenia described in *DSM-IV-TR* are *paranoid, disorganized, catatonic, and undifferentiated* (Table 10.3). The paranoid type is characterized by a preoccupation with delusions or hallucinations, but there is no disorganized speech, disorganized or catatonic behavior, or flat or inappropriate affect. This subtype has the best prognosis. In the disorganized type, all of the following are prominent: disorganized speech, disorganized behavior, and flat or inappropriate affect, but the criteria for the catatonic subtype are not met. In terms of the course of illness this subtype is considered to have the worst prognosis. The catatonic type involves a clinical syndrome that is dominated by at least two of the following: motoric immobility, excessive, purposeless motor activity (catatonic excitement); extreme negativism (purposeless resistance to movement or all instructions); mutism (absence of speech); peculiar voluntary movements (voluntary assumption of bizarre or unusual postures), stereotyped movements (repetitive, nonfunctional, yet voluntary); prominent mannerisms (repetitive gestures or expressions); prominent facial grimacing, echolalia (repetition of another person's words or phrases); or echopraxia (repetition of another person's actions). Finally, the undifferentiated subtype is diagnosed when the patient does not meet criteria for the previous subtypes, yet does meet the general criteria for schizophrenia. The inclusion of this subtype in the *DSM-IV-TR* serves to remind

Table 10.3 Subtypes of schizophrenia

Subtype	Prognosis
Paranoid	*Good*
Well organized delusional beliefs, frequently reflecting persecutory or grandiose beliefs	
Frequent auditory hallucinations	
Little or no negative (e.g., flat affect) or disorganized symptomatology	
Disorganized	*Poor*
Flat and inappropriate emotional expressions	
Severely disorganized speech and behavior	
Delusional ideas, hallucinations, and behavior characterized by fragmentation (i.e., not following a sequential course)	
Catatonic	*Poorest*
Highly irregular movements or actions (e.g., extreme excitement, bizarre postures or facial grimaces, complete immobility)	
Echoing of words spoken by others, imitations of others movements	
Undifferentiated*	—
Display of schizophrenic symptomatology in a pattern that does not fit other categories	

*Because the undifferentiated category is a bin for cases that don't fit within the other subtypes, it serves as a reminder that these labels are artificially constructed categories, rather than distinct diagnostic entities.

us that these are constructed categories, not distinct diagnostic entities with "natural" boundaries. Nonetheless they are useful in clinical settings to convey predominant symptoms.

Two other diagnostic categories in the schizophrenia spectrum are worth noting. One is a category for individuals who have met criteria for schizophrenia in the past, but no longer do. This is referred to as the "residual type." This diagnosis is applied when there is a prominence of negative symptoms or two or more attenuated characteristic symptoms, but no prominent delusions, hallucinations, catatonic symptoms, or disorganized behavior or speech. The other category, schizophreniform disorder, is for individuals whose symptoms do not meet the six-month criterion. This diagnosis is frequently made as a prelude to the diagnosis of schizophrenia, when the patient presents for treatment early in the course of the disorder. Some individuals who fall into this category, however, will recover completely and not suffer further episodes of psychosis.

It is important to emphasize that, despite advances in diagnosis; the diagnostic boundaries of schizophrenia are still quite unclear (Wolff, 1991). Moreover, the boundaries between schizophrenia and mood disorders are sometimes obscure. Many individuals who meet criteria for schizophrenia show marked signs of depression or manic tendencies. These symptoms are sometimes present before the onset of schizophrenia, and frequently occur in combination with marked psychotic symptoms. As a result, the *DSM-IV-TR* includes a diagnostic category called *schizoaffective disorder*. This disorder can be conceived of, conceptually, as a hybrid between the mood disorders (bipolar disorder or major depression with psychotic features) and schizophrenia. The two subtypes of schizoaffective disorder are the depressive subtype (i.e., if the mood disturbance includes only depressive episodes) and the bipolar subtype (i.e., where the symptoms of the disorder have included either a manic or a mixed episode). Interestingly, the prognosis for patients with schizoaffective disorder is, on average, somewhere between that of schizophrenia and the mood disorders.

Cognitive and Emotional Aspects of Schizophrenia

Among the most well-established aspects of schizophrenia are the cognitive impairments that accompany the illness. Schizophrenia patients manifest performance deficits on a broad range of cognitive tasks, from simple to complex (Bozikas, Kosmidis, Kiosseoglou, & Karavatos, 2006; Green, Kern, Braff, & Mintz, 2000). One of the most basic is the deficit in the very earliest stages of visual information processing. Using a laboratory procedure called backward masking, researchers have shown that compared to both healthy individuals and psychiatric controls, schizophrenia patients are slower in the initial processing of stimuli (Green et al., 1999; Green, Nuechterlein, Breitmeyer, & Mintz, 2006). Among the higher level cognitive functions, schizophrenia patients show deficits in verbal and spatial memory, abstract reasoning, psychomotor speed, and planning (Caspi et al., 2003; Kuperberg & Heckers, 2000).

There are also deficits in thinking about social phenomena. Studies of social-cognitive abilities in schizophrenia patients have consistently shown that patients are impaired in their ability to comprehend and solve social problems (Niendam et al., 2006; Penn, Corrigan, Bentall, Racenstein, & Newman, 1997). Deficits in social cognition may be partially due to limitations in more basic cognitive processes, such as memory and reasoning. However, basic cognitive impairments do not account completely for the more pervasive and persistent social-cognitive dysfunction observed in schizophrenia.

One of the diagnostic criteria for schizophrenia is blunted or inappropriate affect. It is not surprising therefore, that patients show abnormalities in the expression of emotion in both their faces and verbal communications. These abnormalities include less positive and more negative emotion, as well as emotional expressions that seem inconsistent with the social context (Brozgold, Borod, Martin, Pick, Alpert, & Welkowitz, 1998; Tremeau et al., 2005). Further, schizophrenia patients are less accurate than normal comparison subjects in their ability to label facial expressions of emotion (Bigelow et al., 2006; Martin, Baudouin, Tiberghien, & Franck, 2005; Penn, Combs, Ritchie, Francis, Cassisi, Morris et al., 2000; Walker et al., 1981). Patients with more severe impairments in their abilities to recognize and express emotion also have more problems in social adjustment.

The Origins of Schizophrenia

Psychosocial Theories

In the early part of the 20th century, psychosocial theories of schizophrenia dominated the literature. For example, Sigmund Freud, the father of psychoanalysis, believed that psychological processes resulted in the development of psychotic symptoms (Howells, 1991). In 1948, Frieda Fromm-Reichmann proposed a theory of schizophrenia which postulated that the disorder arose in response to rearing by a 'schizophrenogenic mother' (Fromm-Reichmann, 1948). This hypothesis has fallen into disfavor because of lack of support from empirical research, but while it was popular it caused considerable suffering for families. The theory added to the stigma and burden of family members seeking treatment for their ill family members. Subsequently, family interaction models of the etiology of schizophrenia were offered by various theorists (Howells, 1991). Again, these contributed relatively little to our understanding of the etiology of schizophrenia, although they did eventually serve to highlight the importance of considering the role of the family in providing support for the recovering patient.

Biological Theories

Kraepelin, Bleuler, and other early writers on schizophrenia did not offer specific theories about the origins of schizophrenia. They did suggest, however, that there might be a biological basis for at least some cases of the illness. Likewise, contemporary ideas about the origins of schizophrenia focus on biological vulnerabilities that are assumed to be present at birth. Researchers have identified two sources of constitutional vulnerability: genetic factors and prenatal or obstetric factors. Both appear to have implications for prenatal and postnatal brain development.

The Genetics of Schizophrenia One of the most well-established findings in schizophrenia research is that a vulnerability to the illness can be inherited (Gottesman, 1991). Behavior genetic studies utilizing twin, adoption, and family history methods have all yielded evidence that the risk for schizophrenia is elevated in individuals who have a biological relative with the disorder; the closer the level of genetic relatedness, the greater the likelihood the relative will also suffer from schizophrenia.

In a review of family, twin, and adoption studies conducted from 1916 to 1989, Irving (1991) outlined the compelling evidence for the role of genetic factors in schizophrenia. Monozygotic (MZ) twins, who essentially share 100% of their genes, have the highest concordance rate for schizophrenia. Among monozygotic cotwins of patients with schizophrenia, 25 to 50% will develop the illness. Dizygotic (DZ) twins and other siblings share, on average, only about half of their genes. About 10 to 15% of the DZ cotwins of patients are also diagnosed with the illness. Further, as genetic relatedness of the relative to the patient becomes more distant, such as from first degree (parents and siblings) to second degree relatives (grandparents, half siblings, aunts, and uncles), the relative's lifetime risk for schizophrenia is reduced.

Adoption studies have provided evidence that the tendency for schizophrenia to run in families is primarily due to genetic factors, rather than the environmental stressor of growing up in close proximity to a mentally ill family member. In a seminal adoption study, Heston (1966) examined the rates of schizophrenia in adoptees with and without a biological parent who was diagnosed with the illness. He found higher rates of schizophrenia, and other mental illnesses, in the biological offspring of parents with schizophrenia, when compared to adoptees with no mental illness in biological parents.

Similarly, in a Danish sample, Kety (1988) examined the rates of mental illness in the relatives of adoptees with and without schizophrenia. He found that the biological relatives of adoptees who suffered from schizophrenia had a significantly higher rate of the disorder than did the adoptive relatives who reared them. Also, the rate of schizophrenia in the biological relatives of adoptees with schizophrenia was higher than in the relatives (biological or adoptive) of healthy adoptees. These adoption studies provide ample evidence for a significant genetic component in the etiology of schizophrenia.

More recent findings from an adoption study indicate that the genetic influences often act in concert with environmental factors. Tienari and colleagues (Tienari, Wynne, Moring, & Lahti, 1994) conducted an adoption study in Finland, and found that the rate of psychosis and other severe disorders was significantly higher than in the matched control adoptees. However, the difference between the groups was only detected in adoptive families that were rated as dysfunctional. The genetic vulnerability was mainly expressed in association with a disruptive adoptive environment, and was not detected in adoptees reared in a healthy, possibly protective, family environment. These findings, which highlight a genetic vulnerability interacting with environmental events, are consistent with the prevailing diathesis-stress models of etiology.

Taken together, the findings from behavioral genetic studies of schizophrenia lead to the conclusion that the disorder involves multiple genes, rather than a single gene (Gottesman, 1991). This conclusion is based on several observations, most notably the fact that the pattern of familial transmission does not conform to what would be expected from a single genetic locus, or even a small number of genes. Consistent with this assumption, attempts to identify a genetic locus that accounts for a significant proportion of cases of schizophrenia have not met with success. Instead, researchers using molecular genetic techniques have identified several genes that may account for a small proportion of cases. Candidate gene analyses and linkage studies have provided evidence for the involvement of some specific genes, such as the serotonin type 2a receptor (5-HT2a) gene and the dopamine D3 receptor gene, and several chromosomal regions (i.e., regions on chromosomes 6, 8, 13, and 22) (Mowry & Nancarrow, 2001). But the picture is quite complex; for example, because viral infection may play a role in the pathophysiology of schizophrenia, genes associated with the immune process are also likely candidates. While this is only one direction in gene research, it serves as an illustrative example of the complexities and seemingly endless possibilities that genetic researchers face when interpreting results.

One of the most noteworthy genetic discoveries is a line of research concerning genetic abnormalities that affect dopamine (DA) activity. The catecho-O-methyltransferase (COMT) gene creates the enzyme that breaks down DA. While a majority of people inherit two copies, approximately one in 4,000 children are born with one copy of the COMT gene: this is referred to as 22q11 deletion or velocardiofacial syndrome. The 22q11 deletion occurs in about .025% of the general population, involves a microdeletion on chromosome 22q112, and is often accompanied by a physical syndrome that includes structural anomalies of the face, head, and heart. People with schizophrenia show an 80-fold increased prevalence of 22q11 deletion compared to the general population (Karayiorgou, Morris, & Morrow, 1995) and roughly 30% of 22q11 deletion patients manifest schizophrenia (Murphy, Jones, & Owen, 1999). Furthermore, the rate of 22q11 deletion may be higher in patients with an earlier onset of schizophrenia (Bassett et al., 1998; Karayiorgou et al., 1995).

There are some ongoing controversies, and concomitant shifting of paradigms, concerning the genetics of schizophrenia. One of the controversies concerns the specificity of the genetic liability for schizophrenia. Early behavioral genetic studies led to the conclusion that there were separable genetic liabilities for schizophrenia and the major affective disorders, namely, bipolar disorder and psychotic depression. But more recent evidence indicates that this is not the case. Using quantitative genetic techniques with large twin samples, researchers have shown that there is significant overlap in the genes that contribute to schizophrenia, schizoaffective disorder and manic syndromes (Cardno, Rijsdijk, Sham, Murray, & McGuffin, 2002; Fanous & Kendler, 2005). Other studies have yielded similar results, leading many in the field to conclude that genetic vulnerability does not conform to the diagnostic boundaries listed in *DSM* and other taxonomies (e.g., Potash et al., 2001). Rather, it appears that there is a genetic vulnerability to psychosis in general, and that the expression of this vulnerability can take the form of schizophrenia *or* an affective psychosis, depending on other genetic and acquired risk factors.

The second major controversy in the field concerns the magnitude and extent of the genetic vulnerability for schizophrenia. In other words, what is the relative importance of inherited vulnerability *versus* external factors that affect a developing individual? As mentioned above, we now know that the environment begins to have an impact before birth; prenatal events are linked with risk for schizophrenia, and some of these events are discussed below. Thus, in order to index environmental events that contribute to nongenetic constitutional vulnerability, we must include both the prenatal and postnatal periods. However, researchers are not in a position to estimate the relative magnitude of the inherited and environmental contributors to the etiology of schizophrenia at this point. We do not yet know whether genetic vulnerability is present in all cases of the illness.. Some cases of schizophrenia may be solely attributable to environmental risk factors.

Further, we do not know whether the genetic predisposition to schizophrenia is always expressed, though there is substantive evidence to indicate that it is not. It is well established that the concordance rate for schizophrenia in MZ twins is nowhere near 100%, suggesting that some genetically vulnerable individuals do not develop the illness. However, the genetic liability for schizophrenia may result from a mutation that occurs in only the affected member of discordant MZ pairs. But findings from studies of discordant MZ twins indicate that the rate of schizophrenia is similar, and elevated, in the offspring of both the affected *and* nonaffected cotwins (Gottesman & Bertelsen, 1989; Kringlen & Cramer, 1989). In other words, the offspring of the normal MZ twin have a rate of schizophrenia similar to the offspring of the ill cotwin, even though the former was not raised by a schizophrenic parent. This provides support for the notion that some individuals possess a genetic vulnerability for schizophrenia that they pass on to their offspring, despite the fact that they are never diagnosed with the illness. Thus, unexpressed genetic vulnerabilities for schizophrenia may be common in the general population. The presence of individuals who have an unexpressed genetic vulnerability to schizophrenia makes the work of genetic researchers much more difficult. At the same time, the evidence of unexpressed genotypes for schizophrenia leads us to inquire about factors that trigger the expression of illness in vulnerable individuals, and the hope that this knowledge may, some day, lead to effective preventative interventions.

Prenatal and Perinatal Factors In addition to the support it provides for hereditary influences on schizophrenia, the behavior genetic literature clearly illustrates the relevance of environmental factors. Identifying these factors is a primary focus of many investigators, and the prenatal period has received greater attention in recent years. There is extensive evidence that obstetrical complications (OCs) have an adverse impact on the developing fetal brain, and may contribute to vulnerability for schizophrenia. Birth cohort studies have shown that schizophrenia patients are more likely to have a history of exposure to OCs (Buka, Tsuang, & Lipsitt, 1993; Dalman, Allebeck, Cullberg, Grunewald, & Koester, 1999; McNeil, 1988; Takagai et al., 2006). Included among these are prenatal conditions, such as toxemia and preeclampsia, and labor and delivery complications. A review of the OC literature by Cannon (1997) concluded that, among the different types of OCs, the labor and delivery complications often associated with fetal hypoxia (oxygen deprivation) were the most strongly linked with later schizophrenia. In the National Collaborative Perinatal Project, which involved over 9,000 children followed from birth through adulthood, the odds of developing adult onset schizophrenia increased linearly with an increasing number of hypoxia-related OCs (Cannon, 1998; Cannon, Hollister, Bearden, & Hadley, 1997; Zornberg, Buka, & Tsuang, 2000).

Another prenatal event that has been linked with increased risk for schizophrenia is maternal viral infection. The risk rate for schizophrenia is elevated for individuals born shortly after a flu epidemic (Barr, Mednick, & Munk-Jorgensen, 1990; Brown, Cohen, Harkavy-Friedman, & Babulas, 2004; Limosin, Rouillon, Payan, Cohen, & Strub, 2003; Murray, Jones, O'Callaghan, & Takei, 1992), or after being prenatally exposed to rubella (Brown et al., 2001). The critical period of exposure appears to be between the fourth and sixth months of pregnancy. The findings from research on prenatal maternal infection might be connected to the "season-of-birth" effect in schizophrenia. Several studies have found that a disproportionate number of schizophrenic patients are born during the winter months (Bradbury & Miller, 1985; Narita et al., 2000; Torrey, Miller, Rawlings, & Yolken, 1997). This timing may reflect seasonal exposure to viral infections, which are most common in late fall and early winter. Thus the fetus would have been exposed to the infection during the second trimester. The second trimester is an important time for brain development, and disruptions during this stage may lead to developmental abnormalities.

Studies of rodents and nonhuman primates have shown that prenatal maternal stress can interfere with fetal brain development, and is associated with elevated glucocorticoid release and hippocampal abnormalities in the offspring (Coe et al., 2003; Smythe, McCormick, Rochford, & Meaney, 1994; Weinstock, 1996). Along the same lines, in humans, there is evidence that stressful events during pregnancy are associated with greater risk for schizophrenia and other psychiatric disorders in adult offspring. Researchers have found higher rates of schizophrenia in the offspring of women whose spouses had died during their pregnancies (Huttunen, 1989), and in women who were exposed to a military invasion during their pregnancies (van Os & Selten, 1998). It is likely that prenatal stress triggers the release of maternal stress hormones, which have been found to disturb fetal neurodevelopment and subsequent functioning of the hypothalamic-pituitary-adrenal axis, which, in turn influences behavior and cognition (Welberg & Seckl, 2001).

One of the chief questions confronting researchers is whether OCs act independently to increase risk for schizophrenia or have their effect in conjunction with a genetic vulnerability. One possibility is that the genetic vulnerability for schizophrenia involves an increased sensitivity to prenatal factors that interfere with fetal neurodevelopment (Cannon, 1997, 1998; Preti, 2005; Walshe et al., 2005). It is also plausible that obstetrical events act independently of genetic vulnerabilities, although such effects would likely entail complex interactions among factors. For example, in order to produce the neurodevelopmental abnormalities that confer risk for schizophrenia, it may be necessary for a specific OC to occur during a critical period of cellular migration or in conjunction with other factors such as maternal fever or immune response. These possibilities are currently the focus of research.

Biological Indicators of Vulnerability

Having identified two likely sources of vulnerability for schizophrenia, genetic and obstetrical factors, we now turn to the *nature* of vulnerability. Where does the weakness lie? Since the turn of the 20th century, writers in the field of psychopathology had suspected that schizophrenia involved some abnormality in the brain (Bleuler, 1965). This assumption was based, in part, on the severity of the symptoms and the deteriorating clinical course. However, it was not until the advent of neuro-imaging techniques that solid, empirical data were gathered to support this assumption.

Abnormalities in Brain Structure

The first reports were based on computerized axial tomography (CAT) scans, and showed that affected individuals had enlarged brain ventricles, especially increased volume of the lateral ventricles (Dennert & Andreasen, 1983). As new techniques for brain scanning were developed, these findings were replicated, and additional abnormalities were detected (Henn & Braus, 1999). Magnetic resonance imaging (MRI) revealed decreased frontal, temporal, and whole brain volume among people with schizophrenia (Lawrie & Abukmeil, 1998). More fine grained analyses demonstrated reductions in the size of structures such as the thalamus and hippocampus. In fact, of all the regions studied, the hippocampus is one that has most consistently been identified as distinguishing people with schizophrenia from healthy controls (Schmajuk, 2001).

A landmark study of monozygotic (MZ) twins discordant for schizophrenia was the first to demonstrate that these brain abnormalities were not solely attributable to genetic factors (Suddath, Christison, Torrey, Casanova & Weinberger, 1990). When compared to their healthy identical cotwins, twins with schizophrenia were found to have smaller temporal lobe volumes, with the hippocampal region showing the most dramatic difference between the affected and nonaffected cotwins. Subsequent studies have confirmed smaller brain volumes among affected twins than among their healthy identical cotwins (Baare, van Oel, Pol, Schnack, Durston, Sitskoorn, et al., 2001). These studies lend support to the hypothesis that the brain abnormalities observed in schizophrenia are at least partially due to factors that interfere with prenatal brain development.

Despite the plethora of research findings indicating the presence of abnormalities in the brains of patients with schizophrenia, no specific abnormality has yet been shown to be pathognomonic. In other words, there is no evidence that a specific morphological abnormality is unique to schizophrenia or characterizes all schizophrenia patients. The structural brain abnormalities observed in schizophrenia are, therefore, gross manifestations of the occurrence of a deviation in neurodevelopment that has implications for the functioning of neurocircuitry.

Neurotransmitters

The idea that schizophrenia involves an abnormality in neurotransmission has a long history. Initial neurotransmitter theories focused on epinephrine and norepinephrine. Subsequent approaches have hypothesized that serotonin, glutamate, or GABA abnormalities are involved in schizophrenia. But, compared to other neurotransmitters, dopamine has played a more enduring role in theorizing about the biochemical basis of schizophrenia. In this section we will review the major neurotransmitter theories of schizophrenia, with an emphasis on dopamine.

In the early 1950s, investigators began to suspect that dopamine might be playing a central role in schizophrenia. Dopamine is widely distributed in the brain and is one of the neurotransmitters that enables communication in the circuits that link subcortical with cortical brain regions (Jentsch, Roth, & Taylor, 2001). Since the 1950s, support for this idea has waxed and waned. Since the mid-1990s, however, there has been a resurgence of interest in dopamine, largely because research findings have offered a new perspective.

The initial support for the role of dopamine in schizophrenia was based on two indirect pieces of evidence (Carlsson, 1988): (1) drugs that reduce dopamine activity also serve to diminish psychotic symptoms, and (2) drugs that heighten dopamine activity exacerbate or trigger psychotic episodes. It was eventually shown that standard antipsychotic drugs had their effect by blocking dopamine receptors, especially the "D2" subtype that is prevalent in subcortical regions of the brain. The newer antipsychotic drugs, or "atypical" antipsychotics, have the advantage of causing fewer motor side effects. Nonetheless, they also act on the dopamine system by blocking various subtypes of dopamine receptors.

The relationship between DA and psychotic symptomology can be demonstrated by studies examining compounds such as levodopa that are used to treat Parkinson's disease by increasing DA transmission. For example, motor abnormalities associated with Parkinson's disease (i.e., hypokinesias; slow jerking movements, rigidity) are related to low levels of dopamine characteristic of the disease. However, patients with Parkinson's disease, who are being treated with dopamine agonists (i.e., levodopa induced elevated striatal DA) show drug-induced dyskinesias (Hoff, van den Plas, Wagemans, & van Hilten, 2001), and in extreme cases, psychotic symptomatology (Papapetropoulos & Mash, 2005). In a similar vein, other amphetamines such as cocaine, increase dopamine activity, and can cause both hyperkinesias and psychotic symptoms (Weiner, Rabinstein, Levin, Weiner, & Shulman, 2001). The interplay between DA and movement can also be seen in research examining genetics and drug responsivity in schizophrenia. For example, schizophrenia patients with the type *3 or *4 alleles of the CYP2D6 gene related to poor metabolization of neuroleptic drugs show a heightened rate of dyskinesias (Ellingrod, Schultz, & Arndt, 2002).

Early studies of dopamine in schizophrenia sought to determine whether there was evidence of excess neurotransmitter in schizophrenia patients. But concentrations of dopamine and its metabolites were generally found to not be elevated in body fluids from schizophrenia patients. When investigators examined dopamine receptors, however, there was some evidence of increased densities. Both postmortem and functional MRI studies of patients' brains yielded evidence that the number of dopamine D2 receptors tends to be greater in patients than normal controls (Kestler, Walker, & Vega, 2001). Controversy has surrounded this literature, because antipsychotic drugs can change dopamine receptor density. Nonetheless, even studies of never-medicated patients with schizophrenia have shown elevations in dopamine receptors (Kestler et al., 2001).

Other abnormalities in dopamine transmission have also been found. It appears, for example, that dopamine synthesis and release may be more pronounced in the brains of people with schizophrenia than among normals (Lindstrom et al., 1999). When schizophrenia patients and normal controls are given amphetamine, a drug that enhances dopamine release, the patients show more augmented dopamine release (Abi-Dargham et al., 1998; Soares & Innis, 1999).

Glutamate, an excitatory neurotransmitter, also may play an important role in the neurochemistry of schizophrenia. Glutamatergic neurons are part of the pathways that connect the hippocampus, prefrontal cortex, and thalamus, all regions that have been implicated in schizophrenia. There is evidence of diminished activity at glutamatergic receptors among schizophrenia patients in these brain regions (Carlsson, Hansson, Waters, & Carlsson, 1999; Goff & Coyle, 2001; Tsai & Coyle, 2002). One of the chief receptors for glutamate in the brain is the N-methyl-D-aspartic acid (NMDA) subtype of receptor. Blockade of NMDA receptors produces the symptomatic manifestations of schizophrenia in normal subjects, including negative symptoms and cognitive impairments. For example, administration of NMDA receptor antagonists, such as phencyclidine (PCP) and ketamine, induces a broad range of schizophrenic-like symptomatology in humans, and these findings have contributed to a hypoglutamatergic hypothesis of schizophrenia. Conversely, drugs that indirectly enhance NMDA receptor function can reduce negative symptoms and improve cognitive functioning in schizophrenia patients. It is important to note that the idea of dysfunction of glutamatergic transmission is not inconsistent with the dopamine hypothesis of schizophrenia, because there are reciprocal connections between forebrain dopamine projections and systems that use glutamate. Thus dysregulation of one system would be expected to alter neurotransmission in the other.

In addition, there is evidence that GABA, an inhibitory neurotransmitter, may have excessive inhibitory effects in psychotic disorders (Squires & Saederup, 1991). On the other hand, some studies of postmortem brain tissue from schizophrenia patients have shown that the uptake and the release of GABA is reduced (Lewis, Pierri, Volk, Melchitzky, & Woo, 1999), and that there are abnormalities in the interconnections among GABA neurons (Benes & Berretta, 2001). More specifically, there is evidence of a loss of cortical GABA interneurons. Current theories about the role of GABA in schizophrenia assume that it is important because cortical processes require an optimal balance between GABA inhibition and glutamatergic excitation.

The true picture of the neurochemical abnormalities in schizophrenia may be more complex than we would like to assume. All neurotransmitter systems interact in intricate ways at multiple levels in the brain's circuitry (Carlsson, Waters et al., 2001). Consequently, an alteration in the synthesis, reuptake or receptor density, or affinity for any one of the neurotransmitter systems would be expected to have implications for one or more of the other neurotransmitter systems. Further, because neural circuits involve multiple segments that rely on different transmitters, it is easy to imagine how an abnormality in even one specific subgroup of receptors could result in the dysfunction of all the brain regions linked by a particular brain circuit.

Course and Prognosis

Assuming that genetic and obstetrical factors confer the vulnerability for schizophrenia, the diathesis must be present at birth. Yet, schizophrenia is typically diagnosed in late adolescence or early adulthood, with the average age of diagnosis in males about four years earlier than for females (Riecher-Rossler & Hafner, 2000). This raises intriguing questions about the developmental course prior to the clinical onset.

Premorbid Development

There is compelling evidence that there are signs of schizophrenia long before the illness is diagnosed. Most of these signs are subtle and do not reach the severity of clinical disorder. Nonetheless, when compared to children with healthy adult outcomes, children who later develop schizophrenia manifest deficits in multiple domains. In some of these domains, the deficits are apparent as early as infancy.

In the area of cognitive functioning, children who later develop schizophrenia tend to perform below their healthy siblings and classmates. These cognitive deficits are reflected in lower scores on measures of intelligence and achievement, and poorer grades in school (Aylward, Walker, & Bettes, 1984; Jones, Rodgers, Murray, & Marmot, 1994). Preschizophrenic children also show abnormalities in social behavior. They are less responsive in social situations, show less positive emotion (Walker, Grimes, Davis, & Smith, 1993; Walker & Lewine, 1990), and have poorer social adjustment than children with healthy adult outcomes (Done, Crow, Johnstone, & Sacker, 1994). In our studies of the childhood home movies of schizophrenia patients, we found that the preschizophrenic children showed more negative facial expression of emotion than did their siblings as early as the first year of life, indicating that the vulnerability for schizophrenia is subtly manifested in the earliest interpersonal interactions (Walker, Grimes et al., 1993).

Vulnerability to schizophrenia is also apparent in motor functions. When compared to their siblings with healthy adult outcomes, preschizophrenic children show more delays and abnormalities in motor development, including deficits in the acquisition of early motor milestones such as bimanual manipulation and walking (Walker, Savoi, & Davis, 1994). Deficits in motor function extend throughout the premorbid period (Walker, Lewis, Loewy, & Paylo, 1999), and persist after the onset of the clinical illness (McNeil, Cantor-Graae, & Weinberger, 2000). Furthermore, abnormal gesture behavior has been observed in both premorbid (Mittal et al., 2006) and unmedicated individuals with schizophrenia (Troisi, Spalletta, & Pasini, 1998). These data imply that the movement abnormalities recognized in schizophrenia are likely to have complex interactions with language and motor planning centers.

It is important to note that neuromotor abnormalities are not pathognomonic for schizophrenia, in that they are observed in children at risk for a variety of disorders, including learning disabilities, and conduct and mood disorders. But they are one of several important clues pointing to the involvement of brain dysfunction in schizophrenia. Further, although medication-induced movement abnormalities, such as tardive dyskinesia, involve characteristic motor signs, these are not to be confused with involuntary movements which have been demonstrated to be present in drug free groups such as at-risk infants (Walker, 1994), at-risk adolescents (Walker, Lewis, et al., 1999), and never medically treated schizophrenia patients (Khot & Wyatt, 1991).

Despite the subtle signs of abnormality that have been identified in children at risk for schizophrenia, most of these children do not manifest diagnosable mental disorders in childhood. Thus, while their parents may recall some irregularities in their development, most preschizophrenic children were not viewed as clinically disturbed. But the picture often changes in adolescence. Many adolescents who go on to develop schizophrenia show a pattern of escalating adjustment problems (Walker & Baum, 1998). They show a gradual increase in feelings of depression, social withdrawal, irritability, and noncompliance. This developmental pattern is not unique to schizophrenia; adolescence is also the critical period for the expression of the first signs of mood disorders, substance abuse, and some other mental disorders. As a result, researchers view adolescence as a critical period for the emergence of various kinds of behavioral dysfunction (Corcoran et al., 2003; Walker, 2002).

Among the behavioral risk indicators sometimes observed in preschizophrenic adolescents are subclinical signs of psychotic symptoms. These signs are also the defining features of a *DSM* Axis II disorder; namely, *schizotypal personality disorder* (SPD). The diagnostic criteria for SPD include social anxiety or withdrawal, affective abnormalities, eccentric behavior, unusual ideas (e g., persistent belief in ESP, aliens, extrasensory phenomena, etc.), and unusual sensory experiences (e g., repeated experiences with confusing noises with peoples' voices, or seeing objects move, etc.). Although the individual's unusual ideas and perceptions are not severe or persistent enough to meet criteria for delusions or hallucinations, they are recurring and atypical of the person's cultural context. An extensive body of research demonstrates genetic and developmental links between schizophrenia and SPD. The genetic link between SPD and schizophrenia has been documented in twin and family history studies (Kendler, McGuire, Gruenberg, & Walsh, 1995b; Kendler, Neale, & Walsh, 1995; Raine & Mednick, 1995). The developmental transition from schizotypal signs to schizophrenia in young adulthood has been followed in several recent longitudinal studies, with researchers reporting that 20 to 40% of schizotypal youth eventually show an Axis I schizophrenia spectrum disorder (Miller et al., 2002; Yung et al., 1998). Other young adults with SPD either go on to develop other adjustment problems, or have a complete remission of symptoms. Given the high rate of progression to schizophrenia, researchers are now attempting to determine whether schizotypal youth who will eventually manifest schizophrenia can be identified prior to the onset of the illness.

Recent investigations have revealed that adolescents with SPD manifest some of the same functional abnormalities observed in patients with schizophrenia. For example, SPD youth show motor abnormalities (Mittal et al., 2006; Neumann & Walker, 2003; Walker, Lewis et al., 1999), cognitive deficits (Diforio, Kestler, & Walker, 2000; Harvey, Reichenberg, Romero, Granholm, & Siever, 2006), and an increase in cortisol, a stress hormone that is elevated in several psychiatric disorders (Mitropoulou et al., 2004; Weinstein, Diforio, Schiffman, Walker, & Bonsall, 1999). These new findings may eventually aid in the identification of SPD adolescents who are at greatest risk for developing schizophrenia.

The Illness Onset

The onset of the first-episode of schizophrenia may be sudden or gradual. But as mentioned above, it is usually preceded by escalating adjustment problems, a period referred to as the *prodromal* phase (Lencz, Smith, Auther, Correll, & Cornblatt, 2003; Lieberman et al., 2001). There is some evidence that longer untreated psychotic episodes may be harmful for schizophrenia patients and may result in a worse course of illness (Davidson & McGlashan, 1997; Harris et al., 2004; Perkins et al., 2004).

However, this conclusion is controversial, and some researchers suggest that the relation between longer duration of untreated psychosis and worse prognosis may be a product of poorer premorbid functioning and an insidious onset (Larsen et al., 2001).

People with schizophrenia vary in their course of illness and prognosis. Being male, having a gradual onset, an early age of onset, poor premorbid functioning, and a family history of schizophrenia are all associated with poorer prognosis (Gottesman, 1991). In addition, some environmental factors contribute to a worse outcome. For example, schizophrenia patients who live in homes where family members express more negative emotion are more likely than those with supportive families to have more frequent relapses (Butzlaff & Hooley, 1998; Rosenfarb, Bellack, & Aziz, 2006). Also, exposure to stress can exacerbate schizophrenia symptoms. Researchers have found an increase in the number of stressful events in the months immediately preceding a schizophrenia relapse (Horan et al., 2005; Ventura, Neuchterlein, Hardesty, & Gitlin, 1992). Finally, there is a rapidly accumulating body of research indicating that cannabis use is associated with an increase in risk for psychotic disorders, earlier onset of disorder in vulnerable individuals, and exacerbation of psychotic symptoms (Rey, Martin, & Krabman, 2004).

As outlined, the prognosis for many schizophrenia patients is poor. Only 20 to 30% are able to lead somewhat normal lives, meaning they can live independently and maintain a job (Grebb & Cancro, 1989). The majority experiences a more debilitating course, with 20 to 30% manifesting continued moderate symptoms, and over half experiencing significant impairment for the rest of their lives. Further, patients with schizophrenia often suffer from other comorbid (i.e., co-occurring) conditions. For example, the rate of substance abuse among schizophrenia patients is very high, with as many as 47% in the community and 90% in prison settings meeting lifetime *DSM-IV-TR* criteria for substance abuse or dependence (Regier et al., 1990).

Suicide is the leading cause of death among people with schizophrenia. It has been estimated that 25 to 50% of schizophrenia patients attempt suicide and 4 to 13% successfully commit suicide (Meltzer, 2001). Risk factors associated with suicide in this population include more severe depressive symptoms, being male, having an earlier onset, and suffering recent traumatic events (Schwartz & Cohen, 2001).

The Treatment of Schizophrenia

Researchers have not yet identified any biological or psychological cures for schizophrenia. However, significant progress has been made in treatments that greatly improve the prognosis of the illness. As a result of this research progress, the quality of life for individuals with schizophrenia is dramatically better than it was at the turn of the 21st century.

The first issue to be addressed in the evaluation and treatment of schizophrenia is safety. The risk of self-harm and potential for violence must be assessed (McGirr et al., 2006; Siris, 2001). A medical examination is typically conducted in order to rule out other illnesses that can cause or exacerbate psychotic symptoms. This examination includes a review of the medical history, a physical examination, and laboratory tests. Many patients with schizophrenia have untreated or undertreated medical conditions such as nutritional deficiencies and infections that are a result of their psychological or socioeconomic limitations (Goff, Heckers, & Freudenreich, 2001).

If a patient is not at acute risk to self or others, the next consideration becomes the type of treatment that would be most beneficial. There are several factors to consider. These include the person's living situation (many patients with schizophrenia are homeless), level of insight, willingness to accept treatment, past treatment history, financial resources, including health insurance, and family and other available social support. To increase chances of success, the patient with schizophrenia should be encouraged to talk openly about his or her treatment preferences, beliefs about medication, and concerns about side effects or changes.

The treatment of schizophrenia can be divided into three phases: the acute, stabilization, and maintenance phases (Sadock & Sadock, 2000). In the acute phase, the goal of treatment is to reduce the severity of symptoms. This phase is usually four to eight weeks in duration. In the stabilization phase, the goal is to consolidate treatment gains. This usually takes about six months. Finally, during the maintenance phase, the symptoms are in remission (partial or complete). At this point, the goal of treatment is to prevent relapse and improve functioning.

Antipsychotic Medication

The mainstay of the biological treatment of schizophrenia is antipsychotic. First developed in the 1950s these medications had an enormous impact on the lives of people afflicted with schizophrenia. Their psychotic symptoms improved and many were able to leave psychiatric hospitals (deinstitutionalization). The first effective biological treatment for schizophrenia, chlorpromazine (Thorazine), was the first in a line of medications now referred to as the "typical" antipsychotics or "neuroleptics." All of these medications act by blocking activity in the dopamine systems. The typical antipsychotic medications are classified as high, medium, and low potency, and differ from each other in side-effect profiles (see Table 10.4). *High potency* neuroleptics tend to carry a higher risk of extrapyramidal side-effects (e.g., motor abnormalities), and are prescribed in low dosages. Some examples of high potency agents are: Prolixin (fluphenazine), Stelazine (trifluoperazine), and Haldol (haloperidol). *Low potency* neuroleptics are prescribed in higher milligram doses and have lower risk of motor side effects, but a higher risk of inducing seizures, antihistaminic effects (including sedation and weight gain), anticholinergic effects (including cognitive dulling, dry mouth, blurry vision, urinary hesitancy, and constipation), and antiadrenergic effects (including postural hypotension and sexual dysfunction). Examples of low potency neuroleptics include Thorazine (chlorpromazine), and Mellaril (thioridazine). *Medium potency* agents tend to have side-effects intermediate between the low and high potency drugs. Examples of these include: Trilafon (perphenazine), and Loxapac (loxapine).

In the 1990s a new generation of antipsychotic medications became available for therapeutic use in Europe and North America. The new class of medication is commonly referred to as "the atypical" or "second generation" antipsychotics. Medications in this class share a lower risk of both the early occurring and the late emerging (or tardive) movement disorders. The atypical antipsychotics include: Risperdal (risperidone), Zyprexa (olanzapine), Seroquel (quetiapine), Geodon (ziprazadone), Abilify (aripiprazole) and Clozaril (clozapine). The individual medications differ significantly from one another

Table 10.4 Selected antipsychotic drugs

Drug	Route of administration	Usual daily oral dose	Sedation	Autonomic	Extrapyramidal Adverse effects
chlorpromazine	Oral, IM	200–600	+++	+++	++
fluphenazine	Oral, IM, depot	2–20	+	+	+++
trifluoperazine	Oral, IM	5–30	++	+	+++
perphenazine	Oral, IM	8–64	++	+	+++
haloperidol	Oral, IM, depot	5–20	+	+	+++
loxapine	Oral, IM	20–100	++	+	++
olanzapine	Oral	7.5–25	+	++	0?
quetiapine	Oral	150–750	++	++	0?
risperidone	Oral	2–16	+	++	+
clozapine	Oral	150–900	+++	+++	0?

Source: Kaplan and Sadock (2000, p. 1204)

in the neurotransmitter receptors that they occupy. Although all block dopamine neurotransmission to some extent, they vary in the extent to which they affect serotonin, glutamate, and other neuro-transmitters. These atypical antipsychotics have become first-line in the treatment of schizophrenia. The efficacy of the atypical antipsychotics for the treatment of positive symptoms is at least equivalent to that of the typical antipsychotics, and some studies suggest that they are more effective for negative symptoms and the cognitive impairments associated with the disorder (Forster, Buckley, & Phelps, 1999; Kaplan & Sadock, 2000). Of practical/clinical significance, however, is the substantial risk of developing a "metabolic syndrome" related to the use of this class of medicines. Recent research has revealed that the atypical antipsychotics may carry an elevated risk of substantial weight gain, new onset or worsening diabetes mellitus, and lipid abnormalities (Newcomer, 2005).

Antipsychotic medications are usually administered orally. For patients who are not compliant with oral medication, injectible, long-lasting (depot) antipsychotic medication may be administered (usually every two to four weeks). Three depot neuroleptics are commercially available in the United States. Two are first generation or "typical" antipsychotics: Prolixin (fluphenazine decanoate), and Haldol (haloperidol decanoate). The third is a second generation or "atypical" agent, Risperdal Consta (risperidone). Benefits of depot neuroleptics include the ease of use for the patient, and the fact that compliance is easily monitored by the clinician. The risks are similar to the risks of all of the "typical antipsychotics." The only additional risk is that of localized pain or swelling at the injection site.

Drug-induced movement disorders can be divided into early and late emerging syndromes (Kaplan & Sadock, 2000, table 12.8–3, p. 1207). Early emerging motor symptoms include pseudo-parkinsonism, bradykinesias (decreased movement), rigidity, and dystonic reactions (sudden onset of sustained intense, uncontrollable muscle contraction commonly occurring in the facial and neck muscles). Tardive dyskinesia is a late emerging syndrome that includes irregular choreiform (twist-ing, or wormlike) movements that usually involve the facial muscles, but can involve any voluntary muscle group. It is fortunate that the rate of tardive dyskinesia has declined since the introduction of atypical neuroleptics. It is important to note the these drug-induced movement abnormalities are a distinct and separate entity from the spontaneous movement abnormalities noted earlier, which occur as a natural correlate of schizophrenia.

Mention should also be made of the neuroleptic malignant syndrome (NMS). This is a rare, idi-opathic, life-threatening complication of neuroleptic medication. It is characterized by mental status changes (delirium), immobility, rigidity, tremulousness, staring, fever, sweating, and autonomic insta-bility (labile blood pressure and tachycardia). Laboratory investigations often reveal an elevated white blood cell count (in the absence of infection), and an elevated Creatine Phosphokinase (CPK) level. Treatment involves discontinuation of neuroleptic medication, supportive medical treatment, a pe-ripheral muscle relaxant, and bromocriptine (a D2 receptor agonist) (Rosebush & Mazurek, 2001).

Antipsychotic Medication for Prodromal Populations Several reports indicate that antipsychotics may be effective in reducing the progression of prodromal syndromes into Axis I psychotic disorders. Prodromal signs are typically defined as subclinical psychotic symptoms. Many prodromal patients meet criteria for schizotypal personality disorder. An early study suggested that a low-dose conventional antipsychotic may prevent onset of schizophrenia (Falloon, 1992). Subsequent studies indicate that atypical antipsychotics have the same potential. In one study, prodromal young adults were randomly assigned to either low-dose risperidone with cognitive therapy or to usual care alone (McGorry et al., 2002). After six months, the rate of conversion to psychosis was 9.7% for risperidone and cognitive treatment, and 35.7% for usual care ($p \leq .05$). For risperidone compliant patients, protection against progression extended for six months after cessation of drug treatment. In another study, the authors conducted a double-blind, randomized, placebo-controlled trial with sixty patients who met prodromal criteria (Wood et al., 2003). Olanzapine or placebo was administered for eight weeks. Although both groups showed a decline in scores from the Scale of Prodromal Symptoms, analyses revealed that the olanzapine–placebo difference was marginally significant by week 6 and *significant* at week 8. Movement symptoms were low; however, olanzapine patients gained significantly more weight.

However, it is important to acknowledge that we do not yet know the effects of these medications on prodromal adolescents. The increased use of psychotropic medication with children presents a valuable opportunity to study a population of youth less likely to meet the restrictive inclusion criteria of preventive clinical trials, but more likely to represent youth who are currently being seen in actual clinical practice. Thus, it behooves us to conduct naturalistic prospective studies aimed at elucidating the developmental course of symptoms in these children and adolescents (Simeon, Milin, & Walker, 2002). As our knowledge of the effects of psychotropic medication on adolescent growth and development increases, we will be in a better position to weigh any adverse effects against potential benefits, both short-term and long-term (Jensen et al., 1999).

Psychosocial Treatments of Schizophrenia

Although antipsychotic medication is the crucial first step in the treatment of schizophrenia, there is substantial evidence that psychosocial interventions can also be beneficial for both the patient and the family. It is unfortunate that such treatments are not always available because of limited mental health resources. Nonetheless, it is generally agreed that the optimal treatment approach is one that integrates pharmacologic and psychosocial interventions.

Research supports the use of family therapy, which includes psychoeducational and behavioral components, in treatment programs for schizophrenia (Bustillo, Lauriello, Horan, & Keith, 2001). Family therapy has been shown to reduce the risk of relapse, reduce family burden, and improve family members' knowledge of and coping with schizophrenia.

Comprehensive programs for supporting the patient's transition back into the community have been effective in enhancing recovery and reducing relapse. One such program, called Assertive Community Treatment (ACT), was originally developed in the 1970s by researchers in Madison, Wisconsin (Bustillo et al., 2001; Kaplan & Sadock, 2000; Udechuko et al., 2005). ACT is a comprehensive treatment approach for the seriously mentally ill living in the community. Patients are assigned to a multidisciplinary team (nurse, case manager, general physician, and psychiatrist) that has a fixed caseload and a high staff/patient ratio (1:12). The team delivers all services to the patient when and where he or she needs it, and is available to the patient at all times. Services include home delivery of medication, monitoring of physical and mental health status, in vivo social skills training, and frequent contact with family members. Studies suggest that ACT can reduce time spent in hospital, improve housing stability, and increase patient and family satisfaction.

Social skills training seeks to improve the overall functioning of patients by teaching the skills necessary to improve performance of activities of daily living, employment related skills, and interaction with others. Research indicates that social skills training can improve social competence in the laboratory and in the clinic (Bustillo et al., 2001; Penn & Mueser, 1996). However, it remains unclear to what extent this improvement in social competence translates into better functioning in the community.

The rate of competitive employment for the severely mentally ill has been estimated at less than 20% (Lehman, 1995), thus vocational rehabilitation has been a major focus of many treatment programs. Vocational rehabilitation programs have a positive influence on work-related activities, although they have not yet been shown to have a substantial impact on patients' abilities to obtain employment in the community (Lehman, 1995). Some evidence suggests that supported employment programs produce better results than traditional vocational rehabilitation programs as measured by patients' ability to obtain competitive, independent employment. Nonetheless job retention remains a significant problem (Lehman et al., 2002), and little evidence supports the contention that employment improves self-esteem or quality of life (Bustillo et al., 2001).

Finally, cognitive behavior therapy for schizophrenia draws on the tenets of cognitive therapy that were originally developed by Beck and Ellis (Beck, 1976; Ellis, 1986). The theory is that normal psychological processes can help maintain or reduce specific psychotic symptoms. Cognitive-behavioral therapy (CBT) for psychosis challenges the notion of a discontinuity between psychotic and normal thinking. The normal cognitive mechanisms that are already being used in the nonpsychotic aspects of the patient's thinking can be used to help the psychotic individuals deal directly with their symptoms (Kingdon & Turkington, 2005). Individual CBT emphasizes a collaborative relationship between patient and therapist. The therapist and patient jointly examine the patient's specific symptoms. The choice of target symptoms is based on the patient's preference or severity of the problems created by the psychotic symptom in question. Psychotic beliefs are never directly confronted, although specific psychotic symptoms such as hallucinations, delusions, and related problems are targeted for intervention (Dickerson, 2000). The few published randomized controlled trials available for review suggest that CBT is at least somewhat effective in reducing hallucinations and delusions in medication-resistant patients and as a complement to pharmacotherapy in acute psychosis (Bustillo et al., 2001; Wykes et al., 2005). A recent meta-analysis examining 14 studies including 1,484 patients concluded that, compared to other adjunctive therapies (supplementing medication), CBT was more effective; this finding was significantly more robust for acute patients in comparison to those suffering from chronic schizophrenia (Zimmermann, Favrod, Trieu, & Pomini, 2005). However, the authors note that many moderating factors still need to be evaluated, including the therapeutic alliance, as well as the extent of neurocognitive deficits (Zimmermann et al., 2005).

Summary

This chapter has reviewed a broad range of scientific research on the nature and origins of schizophrenia. Spanning over a century, the efforts of investigators have yielded, piece by piece, a clearer view of the illness. The puzzle is not solved, but we can certainly claim progress toward a solution. The picture that has emerged is best described in the framework of the *diathesis-stress* model that has dominated the field for several decades.

Figure 10.1 illustrates a contemporary version of the diathesis-stress model. This particular model postulates that constitutional vulnerability (i.e., the *diathesis*) emanates from both inherited and acquired constitutional factors. The inherited factors are genetically determined characteristics of the brain that influence its structure and function. Acquired vulnerabilities arise mainly from prenatal events that compromise fetal neurodevelopment.

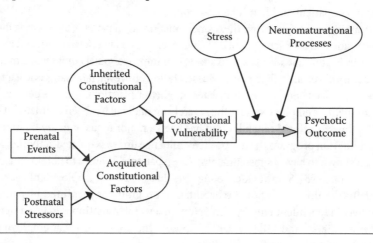

Figure 10.1

Whether the constitutional vulnerability is a consequence of genetic factors, or environmental factors, or a combination of both, the model assumes that vulnerability is, in most cases, congenital. But the assumption that vulnerability is present at birth does not imply that it will be clinically expressed at any point in the life span. Rather, the model posits that two sets of factors determine the postnatal course of the vulnerable individual. First, external stressors influence the expression of the vulnerability. Although this is a long-standing assumption among theorists, it is important to clarify it. Empirical research has provided evidence that episodes of schizophrenia follow periods of increased life stress (Ventura, Neuchterlein, Hardesty, & Gitlin, 1992). Nonetheless, there is no evidence that individuals affected by schizophrenia experience more stress than nonschizophrenic persons, but rather that they are more sensitive to stress when it occurs. This assumption is the essence of the model; the interaction between vulnerability and stress is critical. In addition, the model assumes that neuromaturation is a key element. In particular, adolescence/early adulthood appears to be a critical period for the expression of the vulnerability for schizophrenia. Thus some aspects(s) of brain maturational processes during the postpubertal period are likely playing an important role in triggering the clinical expression of latent liabilities (Corcoran et al., 2003; Walker, 2004).

In summary, although we have not found all the pieces of the puzzle, we have made significant progress in moving toward a comprehensive account of the etiology of schizophrenia. Among the mental disorders, schizophrenia remains a clear illustration of the complex interactions taking place between the individual and the environment. In the coming years, we can expect research to yield important information about the precise nature of the brain vulnerabilities associated with schizophrenia, and the mechanisms involved in the interaction of congenital vulnerability with subsequent life stress and neuromaturation. Genetic data and research into gene expression will provide insight into etiology, as well as further our understanding of the role of neurotransmitter abnormalities in schizophrenia. Longitudinal studies conducted during the prodromal period hold strong promise to elucidate the complicated interactions between development (e.g., hormones, neural maturation), and latent constitutional vulnerabilities. Furthermore, research during this period holds strong potential to inform the next generation of psychosocial and pharmacological preventive interventions.

References

Abi-Dargham, A., Gil, R., Krystal, J., Baldwin, R. M., Seibyl, J. P., Bowers, M., et al. (1998). Increased striatal dopamine transmission in schizophrenia: Confirmation in a second cohort. *American Journal of Psychiatry, 155*(6), 761–767.

American Psychiatric Association. (2000). *Diagnostic and statistical manual of mental disorders* (4th ed., rev.). Washington, D.C.: Author.

Arajarvi, R., Suvisaari, J., Suokas, J., Schreck, M., Haukka, J., Hintikka, J., et al. (2005, October). Prevalence and diagnosis of schizophrenia based on register, case record and interview data in an isolated Finnish birth cohort born 1940–1969. *Social Psychiatry and Psychiatric Epidemiology, 40*(10), 808–816.

Aylward, E., Walker, E., & Bettes, B. (1984). Intelligence in schizophrenia: Meta-analysis of the research. *Schizophrenia Bulletin, 10,* 430–459.

Baare, W. F., van Oel, C. J., Pol H. E., Schnack, H. G., Durston, S., Sitskoorn, M. M., et al. (2001). Volumes of brain structures in twins discordant for schizophrenia. *Archives of General Psychiatry, 58*(1), 33–40.

Beck, A. T. (1976). *Cognitive therapy and the emotional disorders.* Oxford, UK: International Universities Press.

Barr, C. E., Mednick, S. A., & Munk-Jorgensen, P. (1990). Exposure to influenza epidemics during gestation and adult schizophrenia: A 40-year study. *Archives of General Psychiatry, 47,* 869–874.

Bassett, A. S., Hodgkinson, K., Chow, E. W., Correia, S., Scutt, L. E., & Weksberg, R. (1998). 22q11 deletion syndrome in adults with schizophrenia. *American Journal of Medical Genetics, 81*(4), 328–337.

Benes, F. M., & Berretta, S. (2001). GABAergic interneurons: Implications for understanding schizophrenia and bipolar disorder. *Neuropsychopharmacology, 25*(1), 1–27.

Bigelow, N. O., Paradiso, S., Adolphs, R., Moser, D. J., Arndt, S., Heberlein, A., et al. (2006, April). Perception of socially relevant stimuli in schizophrenia. *Schizophrenia Research, 83*(2–3), 257–267.

Bleuler, E. (1950). *Group of schizophrenias* (J. Zinkin, Trans.). New York: International Universities Press. (Original work published in 1911)

Bleuler, M. (1965). Conception of schizophrenia within the last fifty years and today. *International Journal of Psychiatry, 1*(4), 501–523.

Bozikas, V. P., Kosmidis, M. H., Kiosseoglou, G., & Karavatos, A. (2006). Neuropsychological profile of cognitively impaired patients with schizophrenia. *Comprehensive Psychiatry, 47*(2), 136–143.

Bradbury, T. N., & Miller, G. A. (1985). Season of birth in schizophrenia: A review of evidence, methodology, and etiology *Psychological Bulletin, 98,* 569–594.

Brown, A. S., Begg, M. D., Gravenstein, S., Schaefer, C. A., Wyatt, R. J., Bresnahan, M., et al. (2004). Serologic evidence o prenatal influenza in the etiology of schizophrenia. *Archives of General Psychiatry, 61*(8), 774–780.

Brown, A. S., Cohen, P., Harkavy-Friedman, J., & Babulas, V. (2001). Prenatal rubella, premorbid abnormalities, and adul schizophrenia. *Biological Psychiatry, 49,* 473–486.

Brozgold, A.Z., Borod, J.C., Martin, C.C., Pick, L.H., Alpert, M., & Welkowitz, J. (1998). Social functioning and facial emotiona expression in neurological and psychiatric disorders. *Applied Neuropsychology, 5*(1), 15–23.

Buka, S. L., Tsuang, M. T., & Lipsitt, L. P. (1993). Pregnancy/delivery complications and psychiatric diagnosis: A prospectiv study. *Archives of General Psychiatry, 50,* 151–156.

Bustillo, J. R., Lauriello, J., Horan, W. P., & Keith. S. J. (2001). The psychosocial treatment of schizophrenia: An update. *Th American Journal of Psychiatry, 158* (2), 163–175.

Butzlaff, R. L., & Hooley, J. M. (1998). Expressed emotion and psychiatric relapse. *Archives of General Psychiatry, 55*(6, 547–552.

Cannon, T. D. (1997). On the nature and mechanisms of obstetric influences in schizophrenia: A review and synthesis c epidemiologic studies. *International Review of Psychiatry, 9,* 387–397.

Cannon, T. D. (1998). Genetic and perinatal influences in the etiology of schizophrenia: A neurodevelopmental model. I M. F. Lenzenweger & R. H. Dworkin (Eds.), *Origins and development of schizophrenia* (pp. 67–92). Washington, D.C American Psychological Association.

Cannon, T. D., Hollister, J. M., Bearden, C. E., & Hadley, T. (1997). A prospective cohort study of genetic and perinatal influ ences in schizophrenia. *Schizophrenia Research, 24,* 248.

Cardno, A.G., Rijsdijk, F. V., Sham, P. C., Murray, R. M., & McGuffin, P. (2002). A twin study of genetic relationships betwee1 psychotic symptoms. *American Journal of Psychiatry, 159*(4), 539–545.

Carlsson A. (1988). The current status of the dopamine hypothesis of schizophrenia. *Neuropsychopharmacology, 1*(3) 179–86.

Carlsson, A., Hansson, L. O., Waters, N., & Carlsson, M. L. (1997). Neurotransmitter aberrations in schizophrenia: New per spectives and therapeutic implications. *Life Sciences, 61*(2), 75–94.

Carlsson, A., Hansson, L. O., Waters, N., & Carlsson, M. L. (1999). A glutamatergic deficiency model of schizophrenia. *Britisl Journal of Psychiatry, 37,* 2–6.

Carlsson, A., Waters, N., Holm-Waters, S., Tedroff, J., Nilsson, M., & Carlsson, M. L. (2001). Interactions between monoamines glutamate, and GABA in schizophrenia: New evidence. *Annual Review of Pharmacology & Toxicology, 41,* 237–260.

Carpenter, W. T., & Buchanan, R. W. (1994). Schizophrenia. *New England Journal of Medicine, 330*(10), 681–690.

Caspi, A., Reichenberg, A., Weiser, M., Rabinowitz, J., Kaplan, Z. E., Knobler, H., et al. (2003, December). Cognitive per formance in schizophrenia patients assessed before and following the first psychotic episode. *Schizophrenia Research 65*(2–3), 87–94.

Coe, C. L., Kramer, M., Czeh, B., et al. (2003). Prenatal stress diminishes neurogenesis in the dentate gyrus of juvenile rhesu monkeys. *Biological Psychiatry, 54*(10), 1025–1034.

Corcoran, C., Walker, E. F., Huot, R., Mittal, V. A., Tessner, K., Kestler, K., et al. (2003). The stress cascade and schizophrenia Etiology and onset. *Schizophrenia Bulletin, 29*(4), 671–692.

Dalman, C., Allebeck, P., Cullberg, J., Grunewald, C., & Koester, M. (1999). Obstetric complications and the risk of schizophreni¿ A longitudinal study of a national birth cohort. *Archives of General Psychiatry, 56*(3), 234–240.

Davidson, L., & McGlashan, T. H. (1997). The varied outcomes of schizophrenia. *Canadian Journal of Psychiatry, 42,* 34–43.

De Lisi, L. E. (1992). The significance of age of onset for schizophrenia. *Schizophrenia Bulletin, 18,* 209–215.

Dennert, J. W., & Andreasen N. C. (1983). CT scanning and schizophrenia: A review. *Psychiatric Developments, 1*(1) 105–122.

Dickerson, F. B. (2000). Cognitive behavioral psychotherapy for schizophrenia: A review of recent empirical studies. *Schizo phrenia Research, 43,* 71–90.

Diforio, D., Kestler, L., & Walker, E. (2000). Executive functions in adolescents with schizotypal personality disorder. *Schizo phrenia Research, 42,* 125–134.

Done, D. J., Crow, T. J., Johnstone, E. C., & Sacker, A. (1994). Childhood antecedents of schizophrenia and affective illnes¿ Social adjustment at ages 7 and 11. *British Medical Journal, 309*(6956), 699–703.

Ellingrod V. L., Schultz, S. K., & Arndt, S. (2002). Abnormal movements and tardive dyskinesia in smokers and nonsmoke1 with schizophrenia genotyped for cytochrome P450 2D6. *Pharmacotherapy, 22*(11), 1416–1419.

Ellis, A. (1986). Rational-emotive therapy and cognitive-behavioral therapy: Similarities and differences. In A. Ellis and F Grieger (Eds.), *Handbook of rational-emotive therapy* (Vol. 2, pp. 31–45). New York: Springer.

Falloon, I. R. H., (1992). Early intervention for first episodes of schizophrenia: A preliminary exploration. *Psychiatry, 5! 4–15.

Feighner, J. P., Robins, E., & Guze, S. B. (1972). Diagnostic criteria for use in psychiatric research. *Archives of General Psychiatr; 26,* 57–63.

Fish, B., Marcus, J., Hans, S. L., Auerbach, J. G., & Purdue, S. (1992) Infants at risk for schizophrenia: Sequelae of a geneti neurointegrative defect. *Archives of General Psychiatry, 49,* 221–235.

Forster, P. L., Buckley, R., & Phelps, M.A. (1999). Phenomenology and treatment of psychotic disorders in the psychiatr: emergency service. *Psychiatric Clinics of North America, 22*(4), 735–754.

Fromm-Reichmann, F. (1948). Notes on the treatment of schizophrenia by psychoanalytic psychotherapy. *Psychiatry, 1 263.*

Goff, D. C., & Coyle, J. T. (2001). The emerging role of glutamate in the pathophysiology and treatment of schizophrenia. *American Journal of Psychiatry, 158*(9), 1367–1377.

Goff, D. C., Heckers, S., & Freudenreich, O. (2001). Advances in the pathophysiology and treatment of psychiatric disorders: Implications for internal medicine. *Medical Clinics of North America, 85*(3), 663–689.

Gottesman, I. (1991). *Schizophrenia genesis: The origins of madness.* New York: W. H. Freeman.

Gottesman, I. I., & Bertelsen, A. (1989). Confirming unexpressed genotypes for schizophrenia: Risks in the offspring of Fischer's Danish identical and fraternal discordant twins. *Archives of General Psychiatry, 46*(10), 867–872.

Grebb, J. A., & Cancro, R. (1989). Schizophrenia: Clinical features. In J. I. Kaplan & B. J. Sadock (Eds.), *Synopsis of psychiatry: Behavioral sciences, clinical psychiatry* (5th ed., pp. 757–777). Baltimore: Williams & Wilkins.

Green, M. F., Kern, R. S., Braff, D. L., & Mintz, J. (2000). Neurocognitive deficits and functional outcome in schizophrenia: Are we measuring the "right stuff"? *Schizophrenia Bulletin, 26*(1), 119–136.

Green, M. F., Nuechterlein, K. H., Breitmeyer, B., & Mintz, J. (1999). Backward masking in unmedicated schizophrenic patients in psychotic remission: Possible reflection of aberrant cortical oscillation. *American Journal of Psychiatry, 156*(9), 1367–1373.

Green, M. F., Nuechterlein, K. H., Breitmeyer, B., & Mintz, J. (2006). Forward and backward visual masking in unaffected siblings of schizophrenic patients. *Biological Psychiatry, 59*(5), 446–451.

Harris, M. G., Henry, L. P., Harrigan, S. M., Purcell, R., Schwartz, O. S., Farrelly, S. E., et al. (2005). The relationship between duration of untreated psychosis and outcome: An eight-year prospective study. *Schizophrenia Research, 79*(1), 85–93.

Harvey, P. D., Reichenberg, A., Romero, M., Granholm, E., & Siever, L. J. (2006). Dual-task information processing in schizotypal personality disorder: Evidence of impaired processing capacity. *Neuropsychology, 20*(4), 453–460.

Harvey, P. D., & Walker, E. F. (Eds.). (1987). *Positive and negative symptoms of psychosis: Description, research, and future directions.* Hillsdale, NJ: Erlbaum.

Henn, F. A., & Braus, D. F. (1999). Structural neuro-imaging in schizophrenia. An integrative view of neuromorphology. *European Archives of Psychiatry & Clinical Neuroscience, 249* (Suppl. 4), 48–56.

Heston, L. L. (1966). Psychiatric disorders in foster home reared children of schizophrenic mothers. *British Journal of Psychiatry, 112,* 819–825.

Hoff, J. I., van den Plas, A. A., Wagemans, E. A., & van Hilten, J. J. (2001). Accelerometric assessment of levodopa-induced dyskinesias in Parkinson's disease. *Movement Disorders, 16*(1), 58–61.

Howells, J. G. (1991*). The concept of schizophrenia: Historical perspectives.* Washington, D.C.: American Psychiatric Press.

Huttunen, M. (1989). Maternal stress during pregnancy and the behavior of the offspring. In S. Doxiadis & S. Stewart (Eds.), *Early influences shaping the individual. NATO Advanced Science Institute Series: Life Sciences* (Vol. 160). New York: Plenum.

Ito, C. (2005). *Molecular genetics and transcriptome analysis of schizophrenia.* Mary V. Lang (Ed.),

Jentsch, J. D., Roth, R. H., & Taylor, J. R. (2000). Role for dopamine in the behavioral functions of the prefrontal corticostriatal system: Implications for mental disorders and psychotropic drug action. *Progress in Brain Research, 126,* 433–453.

Jones, P., Rodgers, B., Murray, R., & Marmot, M. (1994). Child developmental risk factors for adult schizophrenia in the British 1946 birth cohort. *Lancet, 344,* 1398–1402.

Karayiorgou, M., Morris, M. A., & Morrow, B. (1995). Schizophrenia susceptibility associated with interstitial deletions of chromosome 22q11. *Proceedings of the National Academy of Science 92,* 7612–7616.

Keith, S. J., Regier, D. A., & Rae, D. S. (1991). Schizophrenic disorders. In L. N. Robins & D. A. Regier (Eds.), *Psychiatric disorders in America: The Epidemiologic Catchment Area study* (pp. 33–52). New York: Free Press.

Kendler, K. S., McGuire, M., Gruenberg, A. M., & Walsh, D. (1995b). Schizotypal symptoms and signs in the Roscommon Family Study: Their factor structure and familial relationship with psychotic and affective disorders. *Archives of General Psychiatry, 52,* 296–303.

Kendler, K. S., Neale, M. C., & Walsh, D. (1995a). Evaluating the spectrum concept of schizophrenia in the Roscommon Family Study. *American Journal of Psychiatry, 152,* 749–754.

Kestler, L. P., Walker, E., & Vega, E. M. (2001). Dopamine receptors in the brains of schizophrenia patients: A meta-analysis of the findings. *Behavioural Pharmacology, 12*(5), 355–371.

Kety, S. S. (1988). Schizophrenic illness in the families of schizophrenic adoptees: Findings from the Danish national sample. *Schizophrenia Bulletin, 14,* 217–222.

Khot, V., & Wyatt, R. J. (1991). Not all that moves is tardive dyskinesia. *American Journal of Psychiatry, 148,* 661–666.

Kingdon, D. G., & Turkington, D. (2005). *Cognitive therapy of schizophrenia.* J. B. Persons (series editor). New York: Guilford.

Kraepelin E. (1919). *Dementia praecox and paraphrenia* (8th ed., R. M. Barclay, Trans.). Edinburgh: Livingstone Press. (Original work, *Psychiatrie,* from vol. 3, part 2, published 1913)

Kringlen, E., & Cramer, G. (1989). Offspring of monozygotic twins discordant for schizophrenia. *Archives of General Psychiatry, 46,* 873–877.

Kulhara, P., & Chakrabarti, S. (2001). Culture and schizophrenia and other psychotic disorders. *Psychiatric Clinics of North America, 24*(3), 449–464.

Kuperberg, G., & Heckers, S. (2000). Schizophrenia and cognitive function. *Current Opinion in Neurobiology, 10*(2), 205–210.

Lane, H.-Y., Liu, Y.-C., Huang, C.-L., Chang, Y.-C., Wu, P.-L., Lu, C.-T., et al. (2006). Risperidone-related weight gain: Genetic and nongenetic predictors. *Journal of Clinical Psychopharmacology, 26*(2), 128–134.

Larsen, T. K., Friis, S., Haahr, U., Joa, I., Johannessen, J. O., Melle, I., et al. (2001). Early detection and intervention in first-episode schizophrenia: A critical review. *Acta Psychiatrica Scandinavica, 103*(5), 323–334.

Lawrie, S. M., & Abukmeil, S. S. (1998). Brain abnormality in schizophrenia: A systematic and quantitative review of volumetric magnetic resonance imaging studies. *British Journal of Psychiatry, 172,* 110–120.

Lehman, A. F. (1995). Vocational rehabilitation in schizophrenia. *Schizophrenia Bulletin, 21*(4), 64–56.

Lehman, A. F., Goldberg, R., Dixon, L., McNary, S., Postrado, L., Hackman, A., et al. (2002). Improving employment outcomes for persons with severe mental illnesses. *Archives of General Psychiatry, 59*(2), 165–172.

Lencz, T., Smith, C. W., Auther, A. M., Correll, C. U., & Cornblatt, B. A. (2003). The assessment of "prodromal schizophrenia": Unresolved issues and future directions. *Schizophrenia Bulletin, 29*(4), 717–728.

Lewis, D. A., Pierri, J. N., Volk, D. W., Melchitzky, D. S., & Woo, T. U. (1999). Altered GABA neurotransmission and prefrontal cortical dysfunction in schizophrenia. *Biological Psychiatry, 46*(5), 616–626.

Lieberman, J. A., Perkins, D., Belger, A., Chakos, M., Jarskog, F., Boteva, K., et al. (2001). The early stages of schizophrenia: Speculations on pathogenesis, pathophysiology, and therapeutic approaches. *Biological Psychiatry, 50*(11), 884–897.

Lima, A. R., Soares-Weiser, K., Bacaltchuk, J., & Barnes, T. R. (2002). Benzodiazepines for neuroleptic-induced acute akithisia. *Cochrane Database System Review*, (1):CD001950.

Limosin, F., Rouillon, F., Payan, C., Cohen, J., & Strub, N. (2003). Prenatal exposure to influenza as a risk factor for adult schizophrenia. *Acta Psychiatrica Scandinavica 107*(5), 331–335.

Lindstrom, L. H., Gefvert, O., Hagberg, G., Lundberg, T., Bergstrom, M., Hartvig, P., et al. (1999). Increased dopamine synthesis rate in medial prefrontal cortex and striatum in schizophrenia indicated by L-(beta-11C) DOPA and PET. *Biological Psychiatry, 46*(5), 681–688.

Martin, F., Baudouin, J.-Y., Tiberghien, G., & Franck, N. (2005). Processing emotional expression and facial identity in schizophrenia. *Psychiatry Research, 134*(1), 43–53.

McGirr, A., Tousignant, M., Routhier, D., Pouliot, L., Chawky, N., Margolese, H., et al. (2006). Risk factors for completed suicide in schizophrenia and other chronic psychotic disorders: A case-control study. *Schizophrenia Research, 84*(1), 132–143.

McGorry, P. D., Yung, A. F., Phillips, L. J., Yuen, H. P., Francey, S., & Cosgrave E. M. (2002). Randomized controlled trial of interventions designed to reduce the risk of progression to first-episode psychosis in a clinical sample with subthreshold symptoms. *Archives of General Psychiatry, 59*, 921–928.

McNeil, T. F. (1988). Obstetric factors and perinatal injuries. In M. T. Tsuang & J. C. Simpson (Eds.), *Handbook of schizophrenia: Nosology, epidemiology and genetics* (Vol. 3, pp. 319–343). Amsterdam: Elsevier Science.

McNeil, T. F., Cantor-Graae, E., & Weinberger, D. R. (2000). Relationship of obstetric complications and differences in size of brain structures in monozygotic twin pairs discordant for schizophrenia. *American Journal of Psychiatry, 157*(2), 203–212.

Meltzer, H. J. (2001). Treatment of suicidality in schizophrenia. In H. Hendin & J. J. Mann (Eds.), *The clinical science of suicide prevention. Annals of the New York Academy of Sciences* (Vol. 932, pp. 44–60). New York: New York Academy of Sciences.

Miller, T. J., McGlashan, T. H., Rosen, J. L., Somjee, L., Markovich, P. J., Stein, K., et al. (2002). Prospective diagnosis of the initial prodrome for schizophrenia based on the Structured Interview for Prodromal Syndromes: Preliminary evidence of interrater reliability and predictive validity. *American Journal of Psychiatry, 159*(5), 863–865.

Mitropoulou, V., Goodman, M., Sevy, S., Elman, I., New, A. S., Iskander, E. G., et al. (2004). Effects of acute metabolic stress on the dopaminergic and pituitary-adrenal axis activity in patients with schizotypal personality disorder. *Schizophrenia Research, 70*(1), 27–31.

Mittal, V. A., Tessner K., Sabuwalla Z., McMillan, A., Trottman, H., & Walker, E. F. (2006). Gesture behavior in unmedicated schizotypal adolescents. *Journal of Abnormal Psychology, 115*(2), 351–358.

Mowry, B. J., & Nancarrow, D. J. (2001). Molecular genetics of schizophrenia. *Clinical & Experimental Pharmacology & Physiology, 28*, 66–69.

Murphy K. C., Jones, L. A., & Owen, M. J. (1999). High rates of schizophrenia in adults with velo-cardio-facial syndrome. *Archives of General Psychiatry, 56*, 940–945.

Murray, R. M., Jones, P. B., O'Callaghan, E., & Takei, N. (1992). Genes, viruses and neurodevelopmental schizophrenia. *Journal of Psychiatric Research, 26*, 225–235.

Narita, K., Sasaki, T., Akaho, R., Okazaki, Y., Kusumi, I., Kato, T., et al. (2000). Human leukocyte antigen and season of birth in Japanese patients with schizophrenia. *American Journal of Psychiatry 157*(7), 1173–1175.

Newcomer, J. W. (2005). Second-generation (atypical) antipsychotics and metabolic effects: A comprehensive literature review. *CNS Drugs, 19* (Suppl. 1), 1–93.

Neumann, C., Walker, E., Lewine, R., & Baum, K. (1996). Childhood behavior and adult neuropsychological dysfunction in schizophrenia. *Neuropsychiatry, Neuropsychology and Behavioral Neurology, 9*, 221–229.

Neumann, C. S., & Walker, E. F. (2003). Neuromotor functioning in adolescents with schizotypal personality disorder: Associations with symptoms and neurocognition. *Schizophrenia Bulletin, 29*(2), 285–298.

Niendam, T. A., Bearden, C. E., Johnson, J. K., McKinley, M., Loewy, R., O'Brien, M., et al. (2006). Neurocognitive performance and functional disability in the psychosis prodrome. *Schizophrenia Research, 84*(1), 100–111.

Norton, N., Williams, H. J., & Owen, M. J. (2006). An update on the genetics of schizophrenia. *Current Opinion in Psychiatry, 19*(2), 158–164.

Nurnberger, J. (2006). Meeting Report for molecular psychiatry, 2005. *Psychiatric Genetics, 16*(3), 89–90.

Papapetropoulos S., & Mash D. C. (2005). Psychotic symptoms in Parkinson's disease: From description to etiology. *Journal of Neurology, 252*(7), 753–764.

Penn, D. L., Corrigan, P. W., Bentall, R. P., Racenstein, J. M., & Newman, L. (1997). Social cognition in schizophrenia. *Psychological Bulletin, 121*(1), 114–132.

Penn, D. L., & Mueser, K. T. (1996). Research update on the psychosocial treatment of schizophrenia. *American Journal of Psychiatry, 153*(5), 607–617.

Perkins, D. O., Lieberman, J. A., Gu, H., Tohen, M., McEvoy, J., Green, A. I., et al. (2004). Predictors of antipsychotic treatment response in patients with first-episode schizophrenia, schizoaffective and schizophreniform disorders. *British Journal of Psychiatry, 185*(1), 18–24.

Potash, J. B., Willour, V. L., Chiu, Y. F., Simpson, S. G., MacKinnon, D. F., Pearlson, G. D., et al. (2001). The familial aggregation of psychotic symptoms in bipolar disorder pedigrees. *American Journal of Psychiatry, 158*(8), 1258–1264.

Preti, A. (2005). Obstetric complications, genetics and schizophrenia. *European Psychiatry, 20*(4), 354.

Raine, A., & Mednick, S. (Eds.). (1995). *Schizotypal personality disorder*. London: Cambridge University Press.

Regier, D. A., Farmer, M. E., Rae, D. S., Locke, B. Z., Keith, S. J., Judd, L. L., et al. (1990). Comorbility of mental disorders with alcohol and other drug abuse. Results from the Epidemiologic Catchment Area (ECA) Study. *Journal of the American Medical Association, 264*, 2511–2518.

Rey, J. M., Martin, A., & Krabman, P. (2004). Is the party over? Cannabis and juvenile psychiatric disorder: the past 10 years. *Journal of the American Academy of Child & Adolescent Psychiatry, 43*(10), 1194–1205.

Riecher-Rossler, A., & Hafner, H. Gender aspects in schizophrenia: Bridging the border between social and biological psychiatry. *Acta Psychiatrica Scandinavica, 102*(407) (Suppl.), 58–62.

Roffman, J. L., Weiss, A. P., Goff, D. C., Rauch, S. L., & Weinberger, D. R. (2006). Neuro-imaging-genetic paradigms: A new approach to investigate the pathophysiology and treatment of cognitive deficits in schizophrenia. *Harvard Review of Psychiatry, 14*(2), 78–91.

Rosebush, P.I., & Mazurek, M.F. (2001). Identification and treatment of neuroleptic malignant syndrome. *Child and Adolescent Psychopharmacology News, 6*(3), 4.

Rosenfarb, I. S., Bellack, A. S., & Aziz, N. (2006). Family interactions and the course of schizophrenia in African American and white patients. *Journal of Abnormal Psychology, 115*(1), 112–120.

Sadock, B. J., & Sadock, V. A. (Eds.). (2000). *Kaplan & Sadock's comprehensive textbook of psychiatry* (7th ed., Vol. 1). New York: Lippincott Williams & Wilkins.

Schmajuk, N. A. (2001). Hippocampal dysfunction in schizophrenia. *Hippocampus, 11*(5), 599–613.

Schmidt-Kastner, R., van Os, J., Steinbusch, H. W., & Schmitz, C. (2006). Gene regulation by hypoxia and the neurodevelopmental origin of schizophrenia. *Schizophrenia Research,84*(2–3), 253–271.

Schneider, K. (1959). *Clinical psychopathology*. New York: Grune & Stratton.

Schwarz, M. J., Kronig, H., Riedel, M., Dehning, S., Douhet, A., Spellmann, I., et al. (2006). IL-2 and IL-4 polymorphisms as candidate genes in schizophrenia. *European Archives of Psychiatry and Clinical Neuroscience, 256*(2), 72–76.

Schwartz, R. C., & Cohen, B. N. (2001). Risk factors for suicidality among clients with schizophrenia. *Journal of Counseling & Development, 79*(3), 314–319.

Simeon, J., Milin, R., & Walker, S. (2002). A retrospective chart review of risperidone use in treatment-resistant children and adolescents with psychiatric disorders. *Progress in Neuropsychopharmacology and Biological Psychiatry, 26*(2), 267–275.

Siris, S.G. (2001). Suicide and schizophrenia. *Journal of Psychopharmacology, 1*(2), 127–135.

Smythe, J. W., McCormick, C. M., Rochford, J., & Meaney, M. J. (1994). The interaction between prenatal stress and neonatal handling on nociceptive response latencies in male and female rats. *Physiology and Behavior, 55*, 971–974.

Soares, J. C., & Innis, R. B. (1999). Neurochemical brain imaging investigations of schizophrenia. *Biological Psychiatry, 46*(5), 600–615.

Spitzer, R. L., Endicott, J., & Robins, E. (1978). *Research diagnostic criteria (RDC) for a selected group of functional disorders*. New York: Biometrics Research.

Squires, R. F., & Saederup, E. (1991). A review of evidence for GABergic redominance/glutamatergic deficit as a common etiological factor in both schizophrenia and affective psychoses: More support for a continuum hypothesis of "functional" psychosis. *Neurochemical Research, 16*(10), 1099–1111.

Suddath, R. L., Christison, G. W., Torrey, E. F., Casanova, M. F., & Weinberger, D. R. (1990). Anatomical abnormalities in the brains of monozygotic twins discordant for schizophrenia. *New England Journal of Medicine, 322*(12), 789–794.

Sullivan, P. F., Owen, M. J., O'Donovan, M. C., & Freedman, R. (2006). J. A. Lieberman, T. Scott Stroup, & D. O. Perkins (Eds.), *Genetics*.

Susser, E. S., & Brown, A. S. (Eds.). (1999). *Prenatal exposures in schizophrenia: Progress in psychiatry*. Washington, D.C.: American Psychiatric Press.

Takagai, S., Kawai, M., Tsuchiya, K. J., Mori, N., Toulopoulou, T., & Takei, N. (2006). Increased rate of birth complications and small head size at birth in winter-born male patients with schizophrenia. *Schizophrenia Research, 83*(2–3), 303–305.

Tienari, P., Wynne, L. C., Moring, J., & Lahti, I. (1994). The Finnish adoptive family study of schizophrenia: Implications for family research. *British Journal of Psychiatry, 164*(Suppl. 23), 20–26.

Torrey, E. F. (1987). Prevalence studies in schizophrenia. *British Journal of Psychiatry, 150*, 598–608.

Torrey, E. F., Bowler, A. E., & Taylor, E. H. (1994). *Schizophrenia and manic-depressive disorder: The biological roots of mental illness as revealed by the landmark study of identical twins*. New York: Basic Books.

Torrey, E. F., Miller, J., Rawlings, R., & Yolken, R. H. (1997). Seasonality of births in schizophrenia and bipolar disorder: A review of the literature. *Schizophrenia Research, 28*, 1–38.

Tremeau, F., Malaspina, D., Duval, F., Correa, H., Hager-Budny, M., Coin-Bariou, L., et al. (2005). Facial expressiveness in patients with schizophrenia compared to depressed patients and nonpatient comparison subjects. *American Journal of Psychiatry, 162*(1), 92–101.

Troisi, A., Spalletta, G., & Pasini, A. (1998). Non-verbal behavior deficits in schizophrenia: An ethological study of drug-free patients. *Acta Psychiatrica Scandinavica, 97*, 109–115.

Tsai, G., & Coyle, J. T. (2002). Glutamatergic mechanisms in schizophrenia. *Annual Review of Pharmacology & Toxicology, 42*, 165–179.

Udechuku, A., Olver, J., Hallam, K., Blyth, F., Leslie, M., Nasso, M., et al. (2005). Assertive community treatment of the mentally ill: Service model and effectiveness. *Australasian Psychiatry 13*(2), 129–134.

van Os, J., & Selten, J. (1998). Prenatal exposure to maternal stress and subsequent schizophrenia: The May 1940 invasion of The Netherlands. *British Journal of Psychiatry, 172*, 324–326.

Ventura, J., Nuechterlein, K. H., Hardesty, J. P., & Gitlin, M. (1992). Life events and schizophrenic relapse after withdrawal of medication. *British Journal of Psychiatry, 161*, 615–620.

Walder, D., Walker, E., & Lewine, R.J. (2000). The relations among cortisol release, cognitive function and symptom severity in psychotic patients. *Biological Psychiatry, 48,* 1121–1132.

Walker, E. (1994). Developmentally moderated expressions of the neuropathology underlying schizophrenia. *Schizophrenia Bulletin, 20,* 453–480.

Walker, E. (2002) Adolescent neurodevelopment and psychopathology. *Current Directions in Psychological Science, 11,* 24–28.

Walker, E., & Baum, K. (1998). Developmental changes in the behavioral expression of the vulnerability for schizophrenia. In M. Lenzenweger & R. Dworkin (Eds.), *Origins and development of schizophrenia: Advances in experimental psychopathology* (pp. 469–491). Washington, D.C.: American Psychological Association.

Walker E., & Diforio, D. (1997). Schizophrenia: A neural diathesis-stress model. *Psychological Review, 104,* 1–19.

Walker, E., Grimes, K., Davis, D., & Smith, A. (1993). Childhood precursors of schizophrenia: Facial expressions of emotion. *American Journal of Psychiatry, 150,* 1654–1660.

Walker, E., & Lewine, R. J. (1990). Prediction of adult-onset schizophrenia from childhood home movies of the patients. *American Journal of Psychiatry, 147,* 1052–1056.

Walker, E., Lewine, R. J., & Neumann, C. (1996). Childhood behavioral characteristics and adult brain morphology in schizophrenia patients. *Schizophrenia Research, 22,* 93–101.

Walker, E., Lewis, N., Loewy, R., & Palyo, S. (1999a). Motor dysfunction and risk for schizophrenia. *Development and Psychopathology, 11,* 509–523.

Walker, E., Lewis, N., Loewy, R., Paylo, S. (1999b) Motor functions and psychopathology. [Special issue]. *Development and Psychopathology, 11,* 509–523.

Walker, E., Savoie, T., & Davis, D. (1994). Neuromotor precursors of schizophrenia. *Schizophrenia Bulletin, 20,* 441–452.

Walker, E., Walder, D., & Reynolds, F. (2001). Developmental changes in cortisol secretion in normal and at-risk youth. *Development and Psychopathology, 13,* 719–730.

Walshe, M., McDonald, C., Taylor, M., Zhao, J., Sham, P., Grech, A., et al. (2005). Obstetric complications in patients with schizophrenia and their unaffected siblings. *European Psychiatry, 20(1),* 28–34.

Weiner, W. J., Rabinstein, A., Levin, B., Weiner, C., & Shulman, L. (2001). Cocaine-induced persistent dyskinesias. *Neurology, 56(7),* 964–965.

Weinstein, D., Diforio, D., Schiffman, J., Walker, E., & Bonsall, B. (1999). Minor physical anomalies, dermatoglyphic asymmetries and cortisol levels in adolescents with schizotypal personality disorder. *American Journal of Psychiatry, 156,* 617–623.

Weinstock, M. (1996). Does prenatal stress impair coping and regulation of hypothalamic-pituitary-adrenal axis? *Neuroscience and Biobehavioral Reviews, 21,* 1–10.

Welberg, L. A., & Seckl, J. R. (2001). Prenatal stress, glucocorticoids and the programming of the brain. *Journal of Neuroendocrinology, 2,* 113–28.

Wood, G. E., Young, L. T., Reagan, L. P., Chen, B., & McEwen, B. S. (2004). Stress-induced structural remodeling in hippocampus: Prevention by lithium treatment. *Proceedings of the National Academy of Sciences U.S.A., 101(11),* 3973–3978.

Woods, S. W., Breier, A., Zipursky, R. B., Perkins, D. O., Addington, J., Miller, T. J., Hawkins, K. A., Marquez, E., Linborg, S. R., Tohen, M., & McGlashan, T. H. (2003). Randomized trial of olanzapine versus placebo in the symptomatic acute treatment of the schizophrenic prodrome. *Biological Psychiatry, 54(4),* 453–464.

Wykes, T., Hayward, P., Thomas, N., Green, N., Surguladze, S., Fannon, D., et al. (2005). What are the effects of group cognitive behaviour therapy for voices? A randomised control trial. *Schizophrenia Research, 77(2-3),* 201–210.

Yung, A. R., Phillips, L. J., McGorry, P. D., Hallgren, M. A., McFarlane, C. A., Jackson, H. J., et al. (1998). Prediction of psychosis: A step towards indicated prevention of schizophrenia. *British Journal of Psychiatry, 172*(Suppl. 33), 14–20.

Zhao, X., Li, H., Shi, Y., Tang, R., Chen, W., Liu, J., et al. (2006). Significant association between the genetic variations in the 5' end of the N-Methyl-D-Aspartate receptor subunit gene GRIN1 and schizophrenia. *Biological Psychiatry, 59*(8) 747–753.

Zimmermann, G., Favrod, J., Trieu, V., & Pomini, V. (2005). The effect of cognitive behavioral treatment on the positive symptoms of schizophrenia spectrum disorders: A meta-analysis. *Schizophrenia Research 77*(1), 1–9.

Zornberg, G. L., Buka, S. L., & Tsuang, M. T. (2000). Hypoxic-ischemia-related fetal/neonatal complications and risk of schizophrenia and other nonaffective psychoses: A 19-year longitudinal study. *American Journal of Psychiatry 157*(2), 196–202.

11
Personality Disorders

Jennifer Ruth Lowe and Thomas A. Widiger

In 1980, the American Psychiatric Association published the third edition of the *Diagnostic and Statistical Manual of Mental Disorders* (*DSM-III*), introducing a multiaxial classification system. Axis II of this new manual was devoted primarily to personality dysfunction, due to the considerable prevalence of maladaptive personality traits in general clinical practice and the substantial impact of these traits on the course and treatment of other mental disorders (Frances, 1980). In this chapter, we begin by discussing issues in the diagnosis of personality disorders as defined in the fourth, text revision, edition of the diagnostic manual (i.e., *DSM-IV-TR*; American Psychiatric Association, 2000). We also include an alternative model for the diagnosis and classification of maladaptive personality functioning, the Five-Factor Model (FFM; Costa & McCrae, 1992).

DSM-IV-TR includes 10 individual personality disorders, organized into three clusters: (1) paranoid, schizoid, and schizotypal (the odd-eccentric cluster); (2) antisocial, borderline, histrionic, and narcissistic (dramatic-emotional-erratic cluster); and (3) avoidant, dependent, and obsessive-compulsive (anxious-fearful cluster). We present what is currently known about five of the more heavily researched personality disorders (i.e., antisocial, borderline, narcissistic, schizotypal, and dependent), as well as how each of them can be understood from the perspective of the FFM. Space limitations prohibit detailed coverage of all of the *DSM-IV-TR* personality disorders, but some information concerning the others is provided in the general discussion.

Personality Disorder

Virtually all people with psychological problems have a characteristic manner of thinking, feeling, behaving, and relating to others that is present prior to the onset of an Axis I disorder. For many of these people, these personality traits are so maladaptive that they constitute a personality disorder. A personality disorder is defined in *DSM-IV-TR* as "an enduring pattern of inner experience and behavior that deviates markedly from the expectations of the individual's culture, is pervasive and inflexible, has an onset in adolescence or early adulthood, is stable over time, and leads to distress or impairment" (APA, 2000, p. 686).

The prevalence of personality disorders within clinical settings is estimated to be well above 50% (Mattia & Zimmerman, 2001). As many as 60% of inpatients within some clinical settings are diagnosed with borderline personality disorder (American Psychiatric Association, 2000; Gunderson, 2001). Antisocial personality disorder may be diagnosed in up to 50% of inmates within a correctional setting (Derefinko & Widiger, in press). The prevalence of personality disorder though is generally underestimated in clinical practice (Zimmerman & Mattia, 1999) due to a lack of time to provide systematic or comprehensive evaluations of personality functioning (Widiger & Coker, 2002) and perhaps a reluctance to diagnose them because insurance companies may consider personality disorders untreatable (Zimmerman & Mattia, 1999).

It is estimated that 10 to 15% of the general population meet criteria for one of the 10 *DSM-IV-TR* personality disorders (Mattia & Zimmerman, 2001; Torgesen, 2005a). Table 11.1 provides prevalence data reported by the best available studies to date for estimating the prevalence of individual personality disorders within the community. These prevalence estimates are generally close to those provided in *DSM-IV-TR*.

A common misconception concerning personality disorders is that they are untreatable. This is not the case. Personality disorders are among the most difficult of disorders to treat because they involve well-established behaviors that can be integral to a client's self-image (Stone, 1993). Nevertheless, personality dysfunction is often the focus of treatment (Beck, Freeman et al., 1990; Gunderson & Gabbard, 2000; Markovitz, 2001; Young, Klosko, & Weishaar, 2003) and psychosocial and pharmacologic treatments can produce clinically and socially meaningful changes (Perry, Banon, Ianni, 1999; Sanislow & McGlashan, 1998). The development of an ideal or fully healthy personality structure is unlikely to occur, but given the considerable social, public health, and personal costs associated with some of the personality disorders, such as the antisocial and borderline, even moderate improvements to personality functioning can be clinically and socially significant.

DSM-IV-TR provides diagnostic criterion sets to help guide a clinician toward a correct diagnosis and an additional section devoted to differential diagnosis that indicates "how to differentiate [the] disorder from other disorders that have similar presenting characteristics" (APA, 2000, p. 10). The intention of this information is to help the clinician determine which particular mental disorder is present, the identification of which would hopefully indicate the presence of a specific pathology and suggest a specific treatment (Frances, First, & Pincus, 1995). It is evident, however, that *DSM-IV-TR* routinely fails in this goal, despite the best efforts of the leading clinicians and researchers who have authored the manual. Quite a few reviews have well documented this concern (e.g., Bornstein, 1998; Clark, in press; Livesley, 2003; Widiger & Trull, 1998). Several studies have further demonstrated that much of the personality disorder diagnostic co-occurrence is readily explained if they are understood as maladaptive variants of general personality structure (Lynam & Widiger, 2001; O'Connor, 2005).

Diagnostic co-occurrence is so common and so extensive (see Table 11.2) that most personality disorder researchers believe that a dimensional description provides a clearer and more accurate picture of personality dysfunction (Cloninger, 2000; Livesley, 2003; Oldham & Skodol, 2000; Widiger, 2000). In 1999, a *DSM* Research Planning Conference was held under joint sponsorship of the American Psychiatric Association and the National Institute of Mental Health, the purpose of which was to set research priorities that would optimally inform the authors of future editions of the diagnostic manual. The Nomenclature Work Group of this conference recommended that efforts toward a dimensional model of classification be developed for the personality disorders. "If a dimensional system of personality performs well and is acceptable to clinicians, it might then be appropriate to explore dimensional approaches in other domains" (Rounsaville et al., 2002, p. 13). This conference was followed by a series of international conferences, each covering a particular domain of the diagnostic manual. The first of this series was devoted to setting a research agenda that would be most effective in leading the field toward a dimensional classification of personality disorder (Widiger, Simonsen, Krueger, Livesley, & Verheul, 2005).

One approach to converting the *DSM* personality disorder nomenclature to a dimensional model is to integrate it with the five-factor model (FFM) of general personality structure. Five broad domains of personality functioning have been identified empirically through the study of the languages of a

Table 11.1 Epidemiology of personality disorders

	Sample	N	DSM	PRN	SZD	STP	ATS	BDL	HST	NCS	AVD	DPD	OCP
Drake et al. (1988)	Men	369	DSM-III	1.1	4.1	2.4	0.8	0.5	3.8	3.5	1.6	10.3	0.5
Coryell et al. (1989)	R-HN	185	DSM-II	0.5	1.6	2.2	1.6	1.1	1.6	0.0	1.6	0.5	3.2
Maier et al. (1992)	Comm	452	DSM-III-R	1.8	0.4	0.7	0.2	1.1	1.3	0.0	1.1	1.5	2.2
Black et al. (1993)	R-HN	127	DSM-III	1.6	0.0	3.9	0.0	5.5	3.9	0.0	3.2	2.4	7.9
Black et al. (1993)	R-OCD	120	DSM-III	1.7	0.0	2.5	0.8	0.8	2.5	0.0	0.8	0.8	10.8
Molden et al. (1994)	HN	302	DSM-III-R	0.0	0.0	0.7	2.6	2.0	0.3	0.0	0.7	1.0	0.7
Samuels et al. (1994)	Comm	762	DSM-III	0.0	0.0	0.1	1.5	0.4	2.1	0.0	0.0	0.1	1.7
Klein et al. (1995)	R-DP	258	DSM-III-R	1.7	0.9	0.0	2.2	1.7	1.7	3.9	5.2	0.4	2.6
Lenzenweger (1997)	Stdts	1646	DSM-III-R	0.4	0.4	0.0	0.8	0.0	1.9	1.2	0.4	0.4	0.0
Torgersen et al. (2001)	Comm	2053	DSM-III-R	2.4	1.7	0.6	0.7	0.7	2.0	0.8	5.0	1.5	2.0
Samuels et al. (2002)	Comm	742	DSM-IV-TR	0.7	0.7	1.8	4.5	1.2	0.4	0.1	1.4	0.3	1.2
Median				1.1	0.4	0.7	0.8	1.1	1.9	0.0	1.6	0.8	2.2
DSM-IV-TR estimates				.5–2.5	uncm	3.0	2.0	2.0	2–3	<1	.5–1	—	1.0

Note: N=number of persons in study; *DSM*=Edition of *Diagnostic and Statistical Manual* that was used; PRN=paranoid; SZD=schizoid; STP=schizotypal; ATS=antisocial; BDL=borderline; HST=histrionic; NCS=narcissistic; AVD=avoidant; DPD=dependent; OCP=obsessive-compulsive; R-HN=relatives of hyper-normal (persons without history of mental disorder); R-OCD=relatives of persons with obsessive-compulsive anxiety disorder; R-DP=relatives of persons with depression; Stdts=students; Comm=community; uncm=uncommon.

TABLE 11.2   *DSM-III-R* personality disorder diagnostic co-occurrence aggregated across six research sites

	PRN	SZD	SZT	ATS	BDL	HST	NCS	AVD	DPD	OCP
Paranoid (PRN)		8	19	15	41	28	26	44	23	21
Schizoid (SZD)	38		39	8	22	8	22	55	11	20
Schizotypal (SZT)	43	32		19	44	17	26	68	34	19
Antisocial (ATS)	30	8	15		59	39	40	25	19	9
Borderline (BDL)	31	6	16	23		30	19	39	36	12
Histrionic (HST)	29	2	7	17	41		40	21	28	13
Narcissistic (NCS)	41	12	18	25	38	60		32	24	21
Avoidant (AVD)	33	15	22	11	39	16	15		43	16
Dependent (DPD)	26	3	16	16	48	24	14	57		15
Obsessive-Compulsive (OCP)	31	10	11	4	25	21	19	37	27	

Note. Sites used *DSM-III-R* criterion sets. Data obtained for purposes of informing the development of the *DSM-IV-TR* personality disorder diagnostic criteria (Widiger & Trull, 1998). Read table as follows: 8% of persons diagnosed with paranoid personality disorder met *DSM*-III-R criteria for schizoid; 38% of persons diagnosed with schizoid personality disorder met *DSM-III-R* criteria for paranoid.

number of different cultures (Ashton & Lee, 2001). Language can be understood as a sedimentary deposit of the observations of persons over the thousands of years of the language's development and transformation. The most important domains of personality functioning would be those with the greatest number of terms to describe and differentiate their various manifestations and nuances, and the structure of personality would be evident in the empirical relationship among the trait terms (Goldberg, 1993). Such lexical analyses of languages have typically identified five fundamental dimensions of personality: neuroticism (or negative affectivity) versus emotional stability, introversion versus extraversion, conscientiousness (constraint) versus disinhibition, antagonism versus agreeableness, and closedness versus openness to experience. Each of these five broad domains can be differentiated further in terms of underlying facets. For example, the facets of antagonism versus agreeableness include suspiciousness versus trusting gullibility, callous tough-mindedness versus tender-mindedness, confidence and arrogance versus modesty and meekness, exploitation versus altruism and sacrifice, oppositional and aggressive versus compliant, and deception and manipulation versus straightforwardness and honesty (Costa & McCrae, 1992).

Each of the *DSM-IV-TR* personality disorders can be readily understood as maladaptive and extreme variants of these personality dimensions (Widiger, Trull, Clarkin, Sanderson, & Costa, 2002). Lynam and Widiger (2001) surveyed 120 personality disorder researchers and asked them to describe a prototypic case with respect to the 30 facets of the FFM. Between 25 and 30 experts provided ratings for each disorder. Table 11.3 lists the 30 facets of the FFM (both poles of each domain and facet are provided to facilitate their clinical understanding), along with a summary of the researchers' ratings. For example, from the perspective of the FFM, the obsessive-compulsive is primarily a disorder of maladaptively extreme conscientiousness, including the facets of deliberation (rumination), self-discipline, achievement-striving (workaholism), dutifulness (overconscientiousness, scrupulousness about matters of ethics and morality), order (preoccupation with details), and competence (perfectionism). The FFM description also goes beyond the *DSM-IV-TR* criteria by including high anxiousness, low impulsiveness, low excitement seeking, and closed mindedness to feelings, values, ideas, and actions.

The researchers' FFM descriptions converged well with an earlier description of the *DSM-IV-TR* personality disorders provided by Widiger et al. (2002) that was based on a coding of the *DSM-IV-TR* diagnostic criterion sets. Intraclass correlations ranged from .54 for the narcissistic to .83 for the avoidant. The relatively lower convergent validity coefficients for the narcissistic, schizoid, and histrionic

TABLE 11.3   *DSM-IV-TR* personality disorders from the perspective of the five-factor model of general personality structure

	PRN	SZD	SZT	ATS	BDL	HST	NCS	AVD	DPD	OCP
Neuroticism (vs. emotional stability)										
Anxiousness (vs unconcerned)			H	L	H			H	H	H
Angry hostility (vs dispassionate)	H			H	H		H			
Depressiveness (vs optimistic)					H					
Self-Consciousness (vs shameless)			H	L		L	L	H	H	
Impulsivity (vs restrained)				H	H	H			L	L
Vulnerability (vs fearless)				L	H			H	H	
Extraversion (vs. introversion)										
Warmth (vs coldness)	L	L	L				L			
Gregariousness (vs withdrawal)	L	L	L	H		H		L		
Assertiveness (vs submissiveness)		L		H			H	L	L	
Activity (vs passivity)		L		H		H				
Excitement-seeking (vs dullness)		L		H		H	H	L		L
Positive emotionality (vs anhedonia)		L	L			H		L		
Openness (vs. closedness)										
Fantasy (vs concrete)						H				
Aesthetics (vs disinterest)										
Feelings (vs alexithymia)		L			H	H	L			L
Actions (vs routine)	L	L		H	H	H	H	L		L
Ideas (vs closed-minded)			H							L
Values (vs dogmatic)	L									L
Agreeableness (vs. antagonism)										
Trust (vs mistrust)	L			L	L	H	L		H	
Straightforwardness (vs deception)	L			L			L			
Altruism (vs exploitation)	L			L			L			
Compliance (vs opposition, aggression)	L			L	L		L		H	
Modesty (vs arrogance)				L			L	H	H	
Tender-mindedness (vs. tough-minded)	L			L			L			
Conscientiousness (vs. disinhibition)										
Competence (vs laxness)					L					H
Order (vs disordered)			L							H
Dutifulness (vs irresponsibility)				L						H
Achievement-striving (vs lackadaisical)										H
Self-discipline (vs negligence)				L			L			H
Deliberation (vs rashness)				L	L	L				H

Note. PRN=paranoid, SZD=schizoid, SZT=schizotypal, ATS=antisocial, BDL=borderline, HST=histrionic, NCS=narcissistic, AVD=avoidant, DPD=dependent, and OCP=obsessive-compulsive. H=mean score was 4.0 or above and L=mean score was 2.0 or below in Lynam and Widiger (2001).

personality disorders were attributable to the fact that the Widiger et al. descriptions were confined to features explicitly included within the *DSM-IV-TR* criterion sets (e.g., the researchers described histrionic persons as being very low in self-consciousness and high in impulsivity, traits that are not included within the *DSM-IV-TR* criterion set). Lynam and Widiger concluded that the researchers' expert consensus FFM profiles may provide a more complete, fuller description of these personality disorders than is provided by *DSM-IV-TR*. Samuel and Widiger (2004) subsequently replicated Lynam and Widiger, but this time surveying clinical psychologists within private practice. The convergent validity of their FFM descriptions with the researchers' descriptions ranged from .90 (dependent) to .97 (antisocial). Most importantly, over 100 studies have now been conducted on the relationship of the FFM to the *DSM-IV-TR* personality disorders and the findings have well supported the belief that the *DSM-IV-TR* personality disorders are maladaptive variants of the domains and facets of general personality structure (Clark, in press; Livesley, 2001; Mullins-Sweatt & Widiger, 2006; Saulsman & Page, 2004; Widiger & Trull, in press).

Five Personality Disorders and Their Five-Factor Formulations

We now turn our attention to five *DSM-IV-TR* personality disorders: antisocial, narcissistic, borderline, schizotypal, and dependent. We describe for each of them what is known about their etiology, pathology, differential diagnosis, comorbidity, course, and treatment. We also indicate how each of them can be understood from the perspective of the FFM of general personality functioning and how this conceptualization can also help to address one or more issues that have been problematic for that personality disorder.

Antisocial Personality Disorder

Antisocial personality disorder (ASPD) has been included within every edition of the APA diagnostic manual. One might even characterize ASPD as the prototypic personality disorder because the term *psychopath* originally referred to all cases of personality disorder (Schneider, 1923). The term *psychopathy* now refers to a more severe variant of ASPD (Derefinko & Widiger, in press). Much of the current research on ASPD is being conducted with regard to this more severe variant, as assessed, for instance, by the Psychopathy Checklist-Revised (PCL-R; Hare, 2003).

Definition *DSM-IV-TR* defines ASPD as a pervasive pattern of disregard for and violation of the rights of others (2000). Its primary diagnostic criteria include criminal activity, deceitfulness, impulsivity, recklessness, aggressiveness, irresponsibility, and indifference to the mistreatment of others. *DSM-IV-TR* overlaps substantially with PCL-R psychopathy. The primary differences are the inclusion of glib charm, arrogance, lack of empathy, and shallow affect within the PCL-R, and the requirement within *DSM-IV-TR* for the evidence of conduct disorder within childhood (Widiger, 2005b).

Etiology and Pathology Twin, family, and adoption studies have provided substantial support for a genetic contribution to the etiology of the criminal, delinquent tendencies of persons meeting criteria for ASPD, accounting for approximately 50% of the variance in antisocial behavior (Waldman & Rhee, 2006). Exactly what is inherited in ASPD, however, is not known. It could be impulsivity, an antagonistic callousness, or an abnormally low anxiousness, or all of these dispositions combined.

Numerous environmental factors have also been implicated in the etiology of antisocial behavior. Shared, or common, environmental influences account for 15 to 20% of variation in criminality or delinquency (Rhee & Waldman, 2002). Not surprisingly, shared environmental factors such as low family income, inner city residence, poor parental supervision, single-parent households, rearing by antisocial parents, delinquent siblings, parental conflict, harsh discipline, neglect, large family size, and young mother have all been implicated as risk factors for antisocial behavior (Farrington, 2006). The effects of these factors are not limited to learning. For instance, neglect and physical abuse can generate several possible avenues to the development of antisocial and aggressive behavior, such as desensitization to pain, impulsive coping styles, and early contact with the justice system (Sutker &

Allain, 2001). Nonshared environmental influences are also substantial contributors. Factors specific to the individual appear to account for fully 30% of antisocial behavior (Moffitt, 2005). In short, this is the remaining variance not accounted for by genetic (50%) or shared environmental (20%) influences. Nonshared environmental factors may include delinquent peers, individual social and academic experiences, or sexual, physical abuse.

The interactive effects of genetic and environmental influences are difficult to tease apart, and likely create confusion about what these estimates mean in terms of causation. For example, the individual who is genetically predisposed to antisocial behavior will subsequently elicit environmental factors associated with criminal outcomes, such as peer problems, academic difficulty, and harsh discipline from parents. In addition, antisocial individuals receive their genes from antisocial parents who also exhibit delinquent and irresponsible behavior, thus creating an immediate home environment that is likely to model instability and criminality. Studies that explicitly address these issues have found though that environmental factors continue to play a large part in etiology of antisocial behavior beyond genetic factors alone. For instance, after controlling for the genetic component of physical maltreatment, Jaffee, Caspi, Moffitt, and Taylor (2004) found that the environmental etiological effect of physical maltreatment remained.

Considerable research effort has been focused on the pathology of antisocial behavior. This extensive research base indicates that many deficits are involved in antisocial behavior, leading to a very complex picture of pathology. Historically, the antisocial individual was said to suffer from a "superego lacunae" or deficits of the conscience, later modified in Cleckley's (1941) and Hare's (2003) descriptions of "semantic dementia," or a deficient processing of feelings and emotion. Laboratory research is now providing support for this theoretical model in studies assessing the psychopath's autonomic reaction to emotional words and fearful images (e.g., Patrick, Cuthbert, & Lang, 1994).

Many psychophysiological deficits have also been associated with psychopathy. Lykken's (1957) classical conditioning paradigm demonstrated that psychopathic inmates had abnormally low physiological responses (reduced skin conductance) to a conditioned stimulus paired with electric shock, indicating that the psychopath may not develop the expected anticipatory arousal from threat of physical punishment. Interestingly, while low skin conductance has been associated with crimes of evasion (e.g., white collar crimes and customs offenses), it has not been found to be associated with other criminal activity, such as violent offenses (Raine, 1993).

Additional autonomic arousal assessments include low resting heart rate levels and startle response deficits (Derefinko & Widiger, in press). There is also the suggestion that persons with ASPD may have abnormally low levels of anxiousness. Some distress-proneness (FFM anxiousness or neuroticism) and attentional self-regulation (FFM constraint or conscientiousness) may be necessary in order to develop an adequate sense of guilt or conscience. Normal levels of neuroticism will promote the internalization of a conscience by associating wrongdoing or misbehavior with distress and anxiety, and the temperament of self-regulation will help modulate impulses into socially acceptable channels (Fowles & Kochanska, 2000).

Cognitive functioning deficits have been implicated in the pathology of antisocial behavior. The psychopath's notorious failure to accurately anticipate negative consequences has often suggested a psychopathic cognitive deficit (Hiatt & Newman, 2006). Existing literature indicates that the psychopath experiences stable deficits in the cognitive domains of attention and response modulation. According to this theory, psychopaths continue to engage in positively reinforcing behaviors even when they become substantially maladaptive (Newman & Lorenz, 2003).

Differential Diagnosis ASPD is most closely associated with narcissistic personality traits, the differentiation of which will be discussed later in this chapter. At times, ASPD will be difficult to differentiate from a substance dependence disorder because many persons with ASPD develop a substance-related disorder, and many persons with substance dependence engage in antisocial acts. However, the requirement that conduct disorder be present prior to the age of 15 will usually assure the onset of ASPD prior to the onset of a substance-related disorder. If both were evident prior to the age of 15, then it is likely that both disorders are now present and both diagnoses should be given. Often, ASPD and substance-dependence will interact, exacerbating each other's development (Sutker & Allain, 2001).

Epidemiology The National Institute of Mental Health Epidemiologic Catchment Area (ECA) study estimated that 3% of males and 1% of females meet *DSM* criteria for ASPD (Robins, Tipp, & Przybeck, 1991). Subsequent studies have replicated this rate, but it has also been suggested that the ECA finding may have underestimated the prevalence in males, due to a failure to consider the full range of ASPD features. Other estimates have been as high as 6% in males (Kessler et al., 1994). Within prison and forensic settings, the rate of ASPD has been estimated to be 50% (Hare, 2003; Robins et al., 1991). However, the ASPD criteria may inflate the prevalence within such settings due to the emphasis on overt acts of criminality, delinquency, and irresponsibility (Sutker & Allain, 2001). More specific criteria for psychopathy provided by the PCL-R obtain a more conservative estimate of 20 to 30% of male prisoners meeting criteria for ASPD (Hare, 2003), by placing relatively less emphasis on the history of criminal behavior and more emphasis on personality traits associated with this criminal history (e.g., callousness and arrogance).

ASPD is much more common in men than in women (Corbitt & Widiger, 1995; Robins et al., 1991). A sociobiological explanation for the differential sex prevalence is the presence of a genetic advantage for social irresponsibility, infidelity, superficial charm, and deceit in males that contributes to a higher likelihood of developing features of ASPD (i.e., males with these traits are more likely to have offspring than males without these traits) (Sutker & Allain, 2001).

Course ASPD is the only personality disorder for which much is known about childhood antecedents because it is well documented that persons diagnosed with childhood onset conduct disorder have a substantial risk of meeting the *DSM-IV-TR* criteria for ASPD as adults (American Psychiatric Association, 2000). There are also compelling data to indicate that ASPD is a relatively chronic disorder, although as the person reaches middle to older age research suggests that the frequency of criminal acts appears to decrease. Nevertheless, the core personality traits may remain largely stable (Harper & Hare, 1994).

Five-Factor Model Reformulation ASPD can be understood primarily as excessive, maladaptively low conscientiousness and high antagonism (see Table 11.3). Specifically, these individuals would be described as aimless, unreliable, lax, negligent, and hedonistic (low in the facets of self-discipline and deliberation), as well as manipulative, exploitative, aggressive, and ruthless (low in straightforwardness, altruism, compliance, and tender-mindedness). Additional facets of the FFM seen in prototypic cases of ASPD include low anxiousness, low self-consciousness (glib charm), low vulnerability (fearlessness), high impulsivity, high angry hostility, and high gregariousness (Lynam & Widiger, 2001).

An ongoing issue surrounding the APA diagnosis of ASPD has been the failure to include all of the personality traits of psychopathy identified originally by Cleckley (1941), emphasizing instead those traits that could most easily be identified by objectively observed behaviors (e.g., irresponsible and/or illegal acts). An advantage of the FFM conceptualization of psychopathy is that it includes all of the traits that are common to both ASPD and the PCL-R, including deception, exploitation, aggression, irresponsibility, negligence, rashness, angry hostility, impulsivity, excitement-seeking, and assertiveness (see Table 11.3). However, the FFM also includes many of the traits that are unique to the PCL-R, including glib charm (low self-consciousness), arrogance, and lack of empathy (tough-minded callousness). In addition, the FFM includes as well traits of psychopathy emphasized originally by Cleckely (1941) but not included in either the *DSM-IV-TR* or the PCL-R (low anxiousness and fearlessness). Considerable evidence supports the FFM conceptualization of ASPD (Lynam & Widiger, in press). Miller and his colleagues have shown that the extent to which an individual's FFM profile matches the FFM profile for a prototypic case of psychopathy (see Table 11.3) can itself be used as a quantitative indication of the likelihood that a person would be diagnosed as psychopathic (Miller & Lynam, 2003).

An FFM conceptualization of ASPD also provides some clarity in regards to the often discussed but poorly understood concept of the "successful psychopath" (Hall & Benning, 2005). Systematic research has been confined largely to the study of the "unsuccessful" psychopath, which typically means the incarcerated criminal (Sutker & Allain, 2001). However, there is considerable social and theoretical interest in understanding the psychopath who is equally exploitative, callous, and ruthless, but either manages never to get arrested or convicted, or who pursues a white-collar career that only flirts with the edges of the legal system (Hall & Benning, 2005). From the perspective of the FFM, these persons would share many of the traits of the prototypic psychopath (i.e., low anxiousness, high fearlessness, high in assertiveness and gregariousness, and high in the exploitativeness, deceptiveness, and callousness of antagonism), but would be high rather than low in the facets of conscientiousness. Such persons would be even more dangerous than most of the incarcerated psychopaths because they would share the disposition to engage in behavior harmful to others, but would also possess the traits (deliberation, competence, and self-discipline) that would contribute to a more "successful" criminal career. A potential case illustration of such a "successful" psychopath is provided by the infamous serial killer, Theodore Bundy (Samuel & Widiger, 2006).

Researchers have for many years been attempting to identify the single, core pathology of psychopathy, and a variety of compelling but inconsistent models have been proposed. These alternative conceptualizations can be integrated and their inconsistencies addressed by the FFM (Lynam & Widiger, in press). Their apparent inconsistency may reflect that each alternative model of pathology is focusing on a different facet and at times even a different domain of the FFM. Lykken (1957), and Patrick et al. (1994) have argued that the primary deficit of psychopathy lies in poor fear conditioning and electrodermal hypoarousal, a focus of research that places particular emphasis on low neuroticism (i.e., low anxiousness or low vulnerability). Others have argued that a lack of response modulation is the primary deficit, an inability to refrain from acting on first impulse (Newman & Lorenz, 2003), represented in the FFM domain of conscientiousness by the facet of deliberation. Cleckley (1941) and Hare (2003) described the core of psychopathy as a "semantic dementia," referring to a deficit in processing affective language. This can be understood in terms of the antagonism facet of callous tough-mindedness. In sum, the personality profile for the prototypic psychopath involves a constellation of personality traits that together provides a quite virulent and at times even lethal mix (i.e., high antagonism, low conscientiousness, low vulnerability, low anxiousness, high assertiveness, high gregariousness, and high excitement-seeking). Researchers are perhaps approaching this constellation like the blind men from Indostan, each interpreting the elephant upon which they are laying their hands in a much different manner, depending upon which component is the focus of their attention (Lynam & Widiger, in press).

Treatment ASPD is considered to be the most difficult personality disorder to treat (Gunderson & Gabbard, 2000; Stone, 1993). Individuals with ASPD can be seductively charming and declare a commitment to change, but they often lack sufficient motivation. Their declarations of wanting to change might even be dishonest. They often fail to see the costs associated with antisocial acts (e.g., imprisonment and lack of meaningful interpersonal relationships), and may stay in treatment only as required by an external source, such as a parole. Residential programs that provide a carefully controlled environment of structure and supervision, combined with peer confrontation, have been recommended (Gunderson & Gabbard, 2000). However, it is unknown what benefits may be sustained after the ASPD individual leaves this environment. When in inpatient treatment, individuals with ASPD may manipulate and exploit staff and fellow patients. Studies have indicated that outpatient therapy is not likely to be successful, although the extent to which persons with ASPD are entirely unresponsive to treatment may have been somewhat exaggerated (Salekin, 2002).

Therapists of individuals with ASPD should bear in mind that they may have considerable negative feelings toward clients with extensive histories of aggressive, exploitative, and abusive behaviors (Gunderson & Gabbard, 2000). Rather than attempt to develop a sense of conscience in these individuals, therapeutic techniques should perhaps be focused on rational and utilitarian arguments against repeating past mistakes. These approaches would focus on the tangible, material value of prosocial behavior (Beck et al., 1990; Young et al., 2003). Some research has indicated that impulsive aggression might be treated with lithium, though its effect on other ASPD symptoms remains to be seen (Markovitz, 2001).

Narcissistic Personality Disorder

This personality disorder was first included within the APA diagnostic manual in *DSM-III* (American Psychiatric Association, 1980). Its inclusion "was suggested by an increasing psychoanalytic literature and by the isolation of narcissism as a personality factor in a variety of psychological studies" (Frances, 1980, p. 1053). However, it is still not included within the World Health Organization's (WHO) International Classification of Diseases (ICD-10; WHO, 1992) despite its presence since 1980 within *DSM-III* because it has been perceived internationally as largely an American concept.

Definition Narcissistic personality disorder (NPD) is defined in *DSM-IV-TR* as a pervasive pattern of grandiosity (in fantasy or behavior), need for admiration or adulation, and lack of empathy. Its primary diagnostic criteria include a grandiose sense of self-importance, preoccupation with success, power, brilliance, or beauty, the belief that one is special and can only be understood by high status individuals, a demand for excessive admiration, a strong sense of entitlement, an exploitation of others, a lack of empathy, and arrogance (2000).

Etiology and Pathology There has been little systematic research on the etiology of narcissism. Two twin studies have supported heritability for narcissistic personality traits (Jang, Livesley, Vernon, & Jackson, 1996; Torgersen et al., 2000), although given the trait complexity of narcissism (Fossatti et al., 2005; Morf & Rhodewalt, 2000; Raskin & Terry, 1988; Ronningstam, 2005), it is not entirely clear what precisely is being inherited. The predominant models for the etiology of narcissism have been largely social learning or psychodynamic (Auerbach, 1993; Ronningstam, 2005). One model proposes that narcissism develops through an excessive idealization by parental figures, which is then incorporated by the child into his or her self-image (Millon et al., 1996). Narcissism may also develop through unempathic, neglectful, inconsistent, or even devaluing parental figures who have failed to adequately mirror a child's natural need for idealization (Kohut, 1977). The child may find that the attention, interest, and perceived love of a parent are contingent largely on achievements or successes. They may fail to perceive the parents as valuing or loving them for their own sake, but may instead recognize that the love and attention are largely conditional on successful accomplishments. They might then develop the belief that their own feelings of self-worth are dependent upon a continued recognition of such achievements, status, or success by others. The character armor of arrogant self-confidence then masks a vulnerability and at times rage over the feeling of having been so neglected, and perhaps even mistreated and denigrated, as a child.

Conflicts and deficits with respect to self-esteem are central to the pathology of the disorder (Kernberg, 1998; Stone, 1993; Ronninstam, 2005), and there is considerable empirical support for this pathology in studies published within the general personality literature (Morf & Rhodewalt, 2000). Narcissistic persons must continually seek and obtain signs and symbols of recognition to compensate for conscious or perhaps even unconscious feelings of inadequacy. Narcissism is not simply arrogant self-confidence as it is more highly correlated with unstable self-esteem rather than a consistently high self-confidence. Their feelings of insecurity will at times be evident but may also be masked by a disdainful indifference to criticism or even by overt expressions of anger and rage (Baumeister, Smart, & Boden, 1996). Narcissistic persons may at times claim that it is not narcissism if they are in fact brilliant, talented, and successful. However, the pathology would still be evident by the excessive need for the recognition of their achievements. They are uncomfortable when they are not being adequately appreciated for their accomplishments and they may in fact feel grossly insulted or enraged when they feel unjustly slighted (Stone, 1993).

Differential Diagnosis Narcissistic personality disorder overlaps substantially with psychopathy. Kernberg (1998) in fact considers the antisocial and narcissistic personality disorders to lie along a common continuum of psychopathology. Both disorders include a disposition to dominate, humiliate, and manipulate others. Stone (1993) goes so far as to suggest that "all psychopathic persons are at the same time narcissistic persons" (Stone, 1993, p. 292). Hart and Hare (1998) suggest that "psychopathy can be viewed as a higher-order construct with two distinct, albeit related facets, one of which is very similar to the clinical concept of narcissism" (p. 429).

To help differentiate the narcissistic and antisocial personality disorders, it has been suggested that "narcissists are usually more grandiose, while ASPD patients are exploitative, have a superficial value system, and are involved in recurrent antisocial activities" (Ronningstam, 1999, p. 681). It is also suggested that "exploitiveness in antisocial patients is probably more likely to be consciously and actively related to materialistic or sexual gain, while exploitive behavior in narcissistic patients is more passive, serving to enhance self-image by attaining praise or power" (Ronningstam, 1999, p. 681). Kernberg (1998) suggests "the way to differentiate…narcissistic personality disorder from an antisocial personality disorder proper is the absence in the latter of the capacity for feeling guilt and remorse" (pp. 42–43). Narcissistic persons will feel guilty and remorseful when confronted with the negative effects of their exploitative use of others, whereas antisocial persons will not. These speculations are compelling and have perhaps been beneficial in clinical practice, but they have not yet been empirically evaluated.

Epidemiology NPD is among the least frequently diagnosed personality disorders within clinical settings (Gunderson, Ronningstam, & Smith, 1991), with estimates of prevalence as low as 2% (American Psychiatric Association, 2000). A curious finding is that many community studies that have used a semistructured interview have not even been able to identify one single case (see Table 11.1), despite the substantial amount of research on maladaptive narcissistic personality traits within normal community and college samples (Morf & Rhodewalt, 2000; Ronningstam, 2005). It may be that the *DSM-IV-TR* diagnostic criteria do not fully capture the essential features of NPD (Gunderson et al., 1991). *DSM-IV-TR* NPD is diagnosed more frequently in males (2000), consistent with the finding within general personality research that men tend to be, on average, more arrogant than women (Costa, Terracciano, & McCrae, 2001).

Course Little is known empirically about the course of narcissism or NPD through the lifespan. Clinical experience suggests that this disorder does not abate with age and may even become more evident into middle or older age (Kernberg, 1998). Persons with this disorder might be seemingly well adjusted and even successful as young adults, having experienced substantial achievements in education, career, and perhaps even within relationships (Ronningstam, 2005). However, their relationships with their colleagues, peers, and intimates might become strained over time as their lack of consideration for and even exploitative use of others becomes cumulatively evident. Successes might also become more infrequent as their inability to accurately perceive or address criticism and setback contributes to a mounting number of failures. Persons with this disorder may at times not recognize their pathology until they have had a substantial number of setbacks, or they have finally recognized that the excessive importance they have given to achievement, success, and status has led to an emptiness and loneliness in their older age (Stone, 1993). As a result, midlife and late-life transitions may be particularly difficult for persons with this disorder.

Five-Factor Model Reformulation One of the facets of FFM antagonism is arrogance, the central trait of NPD (American Psychiatric Association, 2000; Millon et al., 1996). An advantage of the FFM dimensional classification of personality disorder though is the ability to distinguish between arrogant persons who are high versus low in neuroticism. A longstanding concern within the clinical literature on narcissism is the distinction between narcissistic persons who are consistently self-confident, arrogant, and conceited (what Ronningstam, 2005, describes as the "arrogant narcissist") versus the narcissistic person who is quite insecure and self-conscious (the "shy narcissist"; Ronningstam, 2005). The dimensional perspective of the FFM would not create subtypes of a diagnostic category to address the considerable variation that does occur, but would simply describe the extent to which a person high in arrogance is also low in the anxiousness, self-consciousness, and vulnerability facets of neuroticism. Further distinctions would be provided by the extent to which the person is low in extraversion (the shy narcissist) versus high in extraversion (the outgoing, interpersonally engaging narcissist), or high in conscientiousness (the narcissist who is relatively successful in school, college, and career).

Treatment Persons rarely seek treatment for their narcissism. Individuals with NPD enter treatment seeking assistance for another mental disorder, such as substance abuse (secondary to career stress), mood disorder (secondary to career setback), or even something quite specific, such as test anxiety. One may at times have narcissistic persons seeking treatment for a growing sense of discontent and futility with their lives (Ronningstam, 2005). Once an individual with NPD is in treatment, he or she will have difficulty perceiving the relationship as collaborative and will likely attempt to dominate, impress or devalue the therapist. They can idealize their therapists (to affirm that he or she is indeed of sufficient status or quality) but they may also devalue them to affirm that they are of greater intelligence, capacity, or quality, to reject the insights that they have failed to identify themselves, and to indicate that they warrant or deserve an even better therapist. How best to respond is often unclear as the establishment and maintenance of rapport will be an early and ongoing issue. It may at times be preferable to simply accept the praise or criticism, particularly when exploration will likely be unsuccessful, whereas at other times it is preferable to confront and discuss the motivation for the devaluation (or the idealization).

The optimal response to a narcissist's idealization has been a significant controversy within the psychoanalytic literature (Gabbard, 2000a). Kohut (1977) had generally recommended a provision of empathy and a reflection (or mirroring) of positive regard and self-esteem, whereas Kernberg (1998) generally recommended active confrontation of idealization as early idealization would inevitably be followed by devaluation. Cognitive-behavior approaches to NPD emphasize increasing awareness of the impact of narcissistic behaviors and statements on interpersonal relationships (Beck et al., 1990; Young et al., 2003). The idealization and devaluation can be responsive to role playing and rational introspection, an intellectual approach that may itself be valued by some persons with NPD. However, therapists must be careful not to become embroiled within intellectual conflicts and competitions. Narcissistic persons can be acutely aware of the self-esteem conflicts of their therapist, and it is best for the therapist to model a comfortable indifference to losing disputes or conflicts.

Borderline Personality Disorder

Borderline personality disorder (BPD) was a new addition to *DSM-III* (1980; Spitzer, Endicott, & Gibbon, 1979). Since that time it has become the single most frequently diagnosed (Gunderson, 2001) and studied (Blashfield & Intoccia, 2000) personality disorder.

Definition BPD is a pervasive pattern of impulsivity and instability in interpersonal relationships, affect, and self-image (American Psychiatric Association, 2000). Its primary diagnostic criteria include frantic efforts to avoid abandonment, unstable and intense relationships, impulsivity (e.g., substance abuse, binge eating, or sexual promiscuity), recurrent suicidal thoughts and gestures, self-mutilation, and episodes of rage and anger.

Etiology and Pathology There are studies supportive of BPD as a disorder with a distinct genetic disposition but many studies have also suggested a shared genetic association with mood and impulse control disorders (Torgersen, 2005b). There is also substantial empirical support for a childhood history of physical or sexual abuse, parental conflict, loss, and neglect (Silk, Wolf, Ben-Ami, & Poortinga, 2005). Past traumatic events are present in many (if not most) cases of BPD, contributing to the comorbidity with posttraumatic stress and dissociative disorders (Gunderson, 2001; Hefferman & Cloitre, 2000). BPD is perhaps best understood as an interaction of an emotionally unstable temperament with a cumulative and evolving series of intensely pathogenic relationships (Gunderson, 2001; Widiger, 2005c).

The pathogenic mechanisms of BPD are addressed in numerous theories. Most concern issues of abandonment, separation, or exploitative abuse. Persons with BPD will often describe quite intense, disturbed, or abusive relationships with the significant persons of their past life (Gunderson, 2001). The development of malevolent perceptions and expectations of others is not surprising (Ornduff, 2000). These malevolent expectations and lingering feelings of bitterness and rage, along with an impairment in the ability to regulate affect (Linehan, 1993), may contribute to the perpetuation of intense, hostile, and unstable relationships.

Differential Diagnosis Most persons with BPD develop quite a number of Axis I mental disorders, including mood, dissociative, eating, substance use, and anxiety disorders (Pfohl, 2005). It can be difficult to differentiate BPD from these disorders if the assessment is confined to current symptoms (Gunderson, 2001). The diagnostic criteria for BPD require that the symptoms be evident since adolescence, which should differentiate BPD from Axis I disorder in all cases other than a chronic mood disorder. If a chronic mood disorder is present, then the additional features of transient, stress-related paranoid ideation, dissociative experiences, impulsivity, and anger dyscontrol of BPD should be emphasized in the diagnosis (Gunderson, 2001).

Epidemiology It is estimated that 1 to 2% of the general population would meet the *DSM-IV-TR* criteria for BPD (see Table 11.1). BPD is the most prevalent personality disorder within most clinical settings (although perhaps not the most prevalent in community settings; see Table 11.1). Approximately 15% of all inpatients (51% of inpatients with a personality disorder) and 8% of all outpatients (27% of outpatients with a personality disorder) will meet criteria for borderline personality disorder. Approximately 75% of persons with BPD will be female (Corbitt & Widiger, 1995; Gunderson, 2001).

Course Individuals with BPD are likely to have been emotionally unstable, impulsive, and hostile as children but there is in fact little longitudinal research on the childhood antecedents of BPD (Gunderson, 2001; Silk et al., 2005). As adolescents, their intense affectivity and impulsivity may contribute to involvement with rebellious groups, along with a variety of Axis I disorders, including eating, substance, and mood disorders. BPD is at times diagnosed in children and adolescents but considerable caution should be used when doing so, as some of the symptoms of BPD (e.g., identity disturbance, hostility, and unstable relationships) could be confused with a normal adolescent rebellion or identity crisis (Ad-Dab'bagh & Greenfield, 2001; Gunderson, 2001).

As adults, persons with BPD may be repeatedly hospitalized, due to their affect and impulse dyscontrol, psychoticlike and dissociative symptomatology, and suicide attempts (Gunderson, 2001). The risk of suicide is increased with a comorbid mood disorder and substance-related disorder. It is estimated that 3 to 10% of persons with BPD will have committed suicide by the age of 30 (Gunderson, 2001). Intimate relationships tend to be very unstable and explosive, and employment history is generally poor (Stone, 2001). As the person reaches the age of 30, affective lability and impulsivity may begin to diminish. These symptoms may lessen earlier if the person becomes involved with a supportive and patient sexual partner (Stone, 2001). Some, however, may obtain stability by abandoning the effort to obtain a relationship, opting instead for a lonelier but less volatile life. Occurrence of a severe stressor, however, can result in a brief psychotic, dissociative, or mood disorder episode.

A controversy within the research literature is the rate of remission of BPD. Two longitudinal studies currently provide quite high estimates for remission (Skodol et al., 2005; Zanarini, Frankenburg, Hennen, Reich, & Silk, 2005). However, a considerable portion of these findings may have simply represented diagnostic errors (Widiger, 2005a). Gunderson et al. (2003) provided details concerning the recent history for many of the 18 borderlines described as experiencing sudden, dramatic remissions within the first six months of the onset of the Collaborative Longitudinal Study of Personality Disorder (Skodol et al., 2005). For one of the participants, the symptoms were attributed to the use of a stimulant for weight reduction during the year prior to the beginning of the study: "the most dramatic improvement following a treatment intervention occurred when a subject discontinued a psychostimulant she had used the year prior to baseline for purposes of weight loss…. Discontinuation was followed by a dramatic reduction of her depression, panic, abandonment fears, and self-destructiveness" (Gunderson et al., 2003, p. 116). Five of the 18 remissions "had the dramatic reduction of BPD criteria at the same time as the remission of a coexisting Axis I disorder" (Gunderson et al., 2003, p. 114). "In these five cases, the remission of the Axis I disorder was judged to be the most likely cause for the sudden BPD improvement" (p. 114). The remission for the rest of the cases involved gaining relief from severely stressful situations they were in at the time of the baseline assessment.

Warner et al. (2004), using data from the CLPS project, considered the role of FFM personality traits in accounting for the symptoms of BPD over time. They first indicated that BPD features as diagnosed according to *DSM-IV-TR* do change over time but that there appears to be common latent variables underlying the personality traits and BPD symptoms. Most importantly, "the results indicate that there is a specific temporal relationship between traits and disorder whereby changes in the [FFM] personality traits hypothesized to underlie personality disorders lead to subsequent changes in the disorder [but] this relationship does not seem to hold in the opposite direction, which supports the contention that personality disorders stem from particular constellations of personality traits" (Warner et al., 2004, pp. 222–223).

Five-Factor Model Reformulation BPD is primarily composed of excessively high neuroticism. In particular, these individuals are at the very highest range of anxiousness, angry hostility, depressiveness, impulsiveness, and vulnerability (see Table 11.3). Borderline clients will also likely be low in the agreeableness facets of trust and compliance, and low on the conscientiousness facet of competence.

Describing persons with BPD as being high in neuroticism may not convey well the severity of this personality disorder as the term *neuroticism* refers to the normal range of the domain. Persons diagnosed with BPD will be at the very highest levels within the population for angry hostility (e.g., episodes of rage), vulnerability (frantic efforts to avoid abandonment), depressiveness (suicidal ideation), and anxiousness (panicked reactions to stress). Empirical support for the FFM conceptualization of BPD is provided in studies by Clarkin, Hull, Cantor, and Sanderson (1993) and Wilberg, Urnes, Friis, Pederson, and Karterud (1999). Coker and Widiger (2004) averaged 22 correlations between measures of the FFM domains and borderline personality disorder reported in 13 studies. The median correlations were .47 (neuroticism), .00 (extraversion), .00 (openness), .26 (antagonism), and –.21 (conscientiousness), consistent with expectations (Lynam & Widiger, 2001; Widiger et al., 2002). A median correlation of only .47 with neuroticism might appear to be lower than what should be obtained. However, it is useful to compare this correlation with the convergent validity of alternative measures of borderline personality disorder. Widiger and Coker (2002) reported a median convergent validity coefficient for borderline personality disorder of .53 across 45 studies. In other words, FFM neuroticism is correlated with borderline personality disorder almost as high as any two borderline measures correlated with one another.

Morey and Zanarini (2000) provided FFM data on 290 persons who met diagnostic criteria for BPD. They reported that the FFM did account well for BPD symptoms, particularly the domain of neuroticism. They concluded their paper by stating that "the FFM could indicate a temperamental vulnerability to a disorder that is then triggered by developmental events (such as childhood neglect or abuse), resulting in functional levels that may be quite variable in response to situational elements even while the underlying traits remain relatively stable" (Morey & Zanarini, 2000, p. 737).

Trull, Widiger, Lynam, and Costa (2003) replicated and extended the findings of Morey and Zanarini (2000). They developed an FFM borderline index by correlating each participant's FFM profile as assessed by the NEO Personality Inventory-Revised (NEO PI-R; Costa & McCrae, 1992) with the prototypic FFM trait profile provided by Lynam and Widiger (2001). The correlation of each participant's actual FFM trait profile with the profile of a prototypic case was then used as a numerical index of the extent to which the participant had a borderline personality disorder from the perspective of the FFM. They reported that this FFM borderline index correlated as highly with self-report measures of BPD as the latter correlated with one another, including the borderline scales of the Personality Assessment Inventory (PAI; Morey, 1991), the Personality Diagnostic Questionnaire-4 (PDQ-4; Bagby & Farvolden, 2004), the Minnesota Multiphasic Personality Inventory (Colligan, Morey, & Offord, 1994), and the Schedule for Nonadaptive and Adaptive Personality (SNAP; Clark et al., in press). For example, the FFM borderline index correlated .77 with the PAI borderline scale, .68 with the SNAP, and .68 with the PDQ-4. The PDQ-4 correlated .61 with the SNAP, and the PAI correlated .70 with the SNAP.

The FFM conceptualization of BPD is helpful in explaining its substantial prevalence within clinical settings and its excessive diagnostic comorbidity. Persons with BPD are likely to meet *DSM-IV-TR* criteria for at least one other personality disorder, particularly histrionic, dependent, antisocial, schizotypal, and passive-aggressive (see Table 11.2). Neuroticism, as a characteristic level of emotional instability (i.e., vulnerability to stress, impulse dyscontrol, anxiousness, depressiveness, and other components of negative affectivity) will be almost ubiquitous within clinical populations. A diagnostic category defined primarily by and including essentially all of the facets of neuroticism should be highly prevalent within clinical settings. In addition, all of the other *DSM-IV-TR* personality disorders include at least some components of neuroticism, and the variants in symptomatology accounted for by neuroticism explain much of the comorbidity of BPD with other personality disorders (Lynam & Widiger, 2001).

Treatment Clients with BPD form relationships with therapists that are similar to their other significant relationships; that is, the therapeutic relationship can often be tremendously unstable, intense, and volatile. Ongoing consultation with colleagues is recommended to address the therapist's negative reactions toward the client (e.g., distancing, rejecting, or abandoning the patient in response to feelings of anger or frustration) as well as positive reactions (e.g., fantasies of being the therapist who in fact rescues or cures the patient, or romantic, sexual feelings in response to a seductive patient). Sessions should emphasize the building of a strong therapeutic alliance, monitoring self-destructive and suicidal behaviors, validation of suffering and abusive experience (but also helping the client take responsibility for actions), promotion of self-reflection rather than impulsive action, and setting limits on self-destructive behavior (Gunderson, 2001). The tendency of borderline patients to engage in "splitting" (polarization of an emotional response) should also be carefully monitored and addressed (e.g., devaluation of prior therapists, coupled with idealization of current therapist). The American Psychiatric Association (2001) has published practice guidelines for the psychotherapeutic and pharmacologic treatment of persons with BPD. Because borderline patients can present with significant suicide risk, a thorough evaluation of the potential for suicidal ideation and activity should have the initial priority. Also, many patients with BPD will have comorbid Axis I disorders, some of which might take priority (e.g., major depressive disorder, substance dependence, or dissociative disorder).

Dialectical behavior therapy (DBT; Linehan, 1993) has been shown empirically to be a particularly effective treatment of BPD (Lynch, Trost, Salsman, & Linehan, in press). The APA (2001) concluded that psychodynamic psychotherapy has obtained empirical support for the treatment of BPD that is equal to DBT, but this conclusion has been disputed (Sanderson, Swenson, & Bohus, 2002). The dialectical component of DBT was derived largely from Zen Buddhist principles of overcoming suffering through acceptance. Mastery of conflict is achieved in part through no longer struggling or fighting adversity; pain is overcome when it is accepted as an inevitable, fundamental part of life. This principle is taught in part through the meditative technique of mindfulness, in which one attempts to empty one's mind of all thoughts, but accepts whenever and wherever the mind naturally travels. DBT initially focuses on reducing self-harm and para-suicidal behaviors that are disruptive to treatment. Contracts are at times used in which time with the therapist is limited secondary to treatment disruptive behavior. This can even go so far as to include suspension of treatment secondary to suicidal behavior. After mastery of treatment disruptive behavior, DBT teaches coping skills focused on emotional control and interpersonal relatedness. Individuals in DBT attend regular sessions with an individual therapist and discuss problems in applying the new skills. These sessions are augmented with a didactic skills-training group.

Schizotypal Personality Disorder

Schizotypal personality disorder (STPD) was a new addition to *DSM-III* (American Psychiatric Association, 1980). It was developed through the process of constructing borderline personality disorder, both of which were gleaned from a broad clinical and research literature discussing cases of "borderline schizophrenia," "borderline personality," "latent schizophrenia," and similar constructs (Spitzer et al., 1979).

Definition STPD is characterized by a pervasive pattern of social and interpersonal deficits marked by an acute discomfort with close relationships, eccentricities of behavior, and cognitive-perceptual aberrations. Its diagnostic criterion set was developed originally from studies of biological relatives of persons diagnosed with schizophrenia (Spitzer et al., 1979). Diagnostic criteria for STPD include odd beliefs, magical thinking, social withdrawal, unusual perceptual experiences, odd speech, inappropriate or constricted affect, social anxiety, and social withdrawal.

Etiology and Pathology STPD is not included within the personality disorder section of the ICD-10, classified instead as a form of schizophrenia (WHO, 1992). There is compelling empirical support for a genetic association of STPD with schizophrenia (Fanous, Gardner, Walsh, & Kendler, 2001; Jang & Vernon, 2001) which is not surprising given that the diagnostic criteria were obtained from the observations of biological relatives of persons with schizophrenia (Miller, Useda, Trull, Burr, & Minks-Brown, 2001; Siever & Davis, 2004).

A predominant model for the psychopathology of STPD is deficits or defects in the attention and selection processes that organize a person's cognitive-perceptual evaluation of and relatedness to his or her environment (Raine, 2006). These deficits may lead to discomfort within social situations, misperceptions and suspicions, and a coping strategy of social isolation. Correlates of central nervous system dysfunction seen in persons with schizophrenia have been observed in STPD laboratory studies, including performance on tests of visual and auditory attention (e.g., backward masking and sensory gating tests) and smooth pursuit eye movement (Parnas, Licht, & Bovet, 2005). This dysfunction may be the result of dysregulation along dopaminergic pathways, which could be serving to modulate the expression of an underlying schizotypal genotype.

Differential Diagnosis An initial concern for many clinicians when confronted with a person with STPD is whether the more appropriate diagnosis might be schizophrenia. Persons with more severe variants of STPD can closely resemble persons within the prodromal (or residual) phase of schizophrenia (American Psychiatric Association, 1987). A differentiation of the two conditions can be guided in part by age of onset and whether there is a recent deterioration in functioning. Persons with STPD will have evidenced their social anxiety, social withdrawal, magical thinking, odd behavior, and perceptual aberrations well into childhood, and will not typically be characterized by any recent deterioration in functioning. Longitudinal follow-up would provide the conclusive differentiation, as a prodomal phase of schizophrenia will eventually be followed by an active psychotic episode.

The more problematic differential diagnoses for STPD will often be other personality disorders, particularly the schizoid and avoidant. The schizoid personality disorder shares the feature of social withdrawal, but is distinguished from the schizotypal by the absence of social anxiety and the cognitive-perceptual aberrations. Central to schizoid personality disorder is an anhedonia that provides the temperament basis for the social withdrawal (Coker & Widiger, 2004). Just as STPD might represent subsyndromal positive symptoms of schizophrenia (e.g., cognitive-perceptual aberrations and magical thinking), the schizoid may represent subsyndromal negative symptoms (social and physical anhedonia). Avoidant personality disorder also shares the feature of social withdrawal, as well as social anxiety, but the social anxiety of STPD does not diminish with familiarity and the anxiety of the avoidant is concerned primarily with the initiation of a relationship (American Psychiatric Association, 2000). STPD is also a more severe disorder that includes the cognitive and perceptual aberrations that are not seen in persons with avoidant personality disorder.

The close relationship of STPD to the phenomenology, genetics, and pathology of schizophrenia has suggested that it should in fact be classified in future editions of the diagnostic manual as a variant of schizophrenia rather than a personality disorder (First et al., 2002). However, contrary to this proposal are the arguments that schizophrenia itself may have polygenetic determinants (not all of which will be evident in persons with schizotypia), STPD is much more comorbid with other personality disorders than with psychotic disorders, and schizotypal symptomatology appears to be evident within the general population but with no apparent relationship to schizophrenia (Raine, 2006).

Epidemiology STPD may occur in as much as 3% of the general population although most studies with semistructured interviews have suggested a somewhat lower percent (see Table 11.1). STPD might occur somewhat more often in males (Parnas et al., 2005; Raine, 2006). Common Axis I disorders are major depressive disorder and generalized social phobia (Miller et al., 2001).

Course There is insufficient research to describe the childhood precursors of adult STPD. There are though studies on infant and childhood neurodevelopmental abnormalities of persons with STPD (Parnas et al., 2004; Raine, 2006). They would be expected to appear peculiar and odd to their peers, and may have been teased or ostracized. Achievement in school might be impaired, and they may have been heavily involved in esoteric fantasies and peculiar interests. As adults, they may drift toward esoteric, fringe groups that support their magical thinking and aberrant beliefs. These activities can provide structure for some persons with STPD, but they can also contribute to a further loosening and deterioration if there is an encouragement of aberrant experiences. The symptomatology of STPD does not appear to remit with age (Miller et al., 2001; Raine, 2006). The course appears to be relatively stable, with some proportion of schizotypal persons remaining marginally employed, withdrawn, and transient throughout their lives. Some persons meeting *DSM-IV-TR* criteria for STPD do eventually go on to develop schizophrenia (Walker, Kestler, Bollini, & Hochman, 2004). However, the vast majority of cases do not (Raine, 2006). Schizotypal symptomatology, as measured in scales assessing cognitive-perceptual abberrations, magical thinking, and social and physical anhedonia, have been studied longitudinally in a number of community samples, and the findings to date do not suggest any meaningful likelihood of the development of schizophrenia (Gooding, Tallent, & Matts, 2005).

Five-Factor Model Reformulation The FFM conceptualization of STPD does consider it to be a disorder of personality, including introversion (social withdrawal) and the anxiousness facet of neuroticism. Key to STPD are the magical ideation, cognitive-perceptual aberrations, and eccentric behaviors, which are considered within the FFM of personality disorder to be maladaptive variants of openness to ideas, fantasies, and actions (Widiger et al., 2002), as supported in a number of empirical studies (Ross, Lutz, & Bailey, 2002; Trull, Widiger, & Burr, 2001; Wiggins & Pincus, 1989).

The relationship of FFM general personality structure to maladaptive personality functioning has not been as strong for openness as it has been for the other domains of the FFM (Widiger & Simonsen, 2005). This may be due in part to a limitation of the NEO PI-R (Costa & McCrae, 1992) assessment of openness. Haigler and Widiger (2001) reported insignificant correlations of NEO PI-R (Costa & McCrae, 1992) openness with three measures of schizotypal personality disorder (i.e., PDQ-4, MMPI-2, and SNAP). They revised NEO PI-R openness items by inserting words to indicate that the behavior described within the item was excessive, extreme, or maladaptive. The content of the items was not otherwise altered. This experimentally revised openness scale then obtained significant correlations with all three measures of STPD. Haigler and Widiger (2001) concluded that their findings "offer further support for the hypothesis that personality disorders are maladaptive variants of normal personality traits by indicating that correlations of NEO PI-R [Openness with schizotypal symptomatology] would ... be obtained by simply altering existing NEO PI-R ... items that describe desirable, adaptive behaviors or traits into items that describe undesirable, maladaptive variants of the same traits" (p. 356). Their findings also suggest though a limitation of the NEO PI-R as a measure of maladaptive personality functioning. An alternative conceptualization of this domain is unconventionality (Watson, 2006), and scales to assess this unconventionality might provide a more effective measure.

The FFM conceptualization of STPD is helpful in providing a more differentiated and specific description of persons meeting *DSM-IV-TR* criteria for the avoidant, schizoid, and schizotypal personality disorders. The disorders are comorbid because all three concern extreme levels of introversion (Lynam & Widiger, 2001) but they can be differentiated with respect to other domains of the FFM. Avoidant persons will be characterized by high levels of self-consciousness, vulnerability, and anxiousness, and persons with STPD by high levels of openness (or unconventionality). It should be emphasized, however, that most cases of persons diagnosed with the avoidant, schizoid, or schizotypal personality disorder will not represent prototypic cases, and they will then be more accurately described simply by a dimensional profile of the extent to which they are relatively high in neuroticism, introversion, and unconventionality (Widiger & Trull, in press).

Treatment Persons with STPD may seek treatment for anxiousness, perceptual disturbances, or depression. Treatment of STPD should be cognitive, behavioral, supportive, or pharmacologic, as they will often find the intimacy and emotionality of reflective, exploratory psychotherapy to be too stressful and they have the potential for psychotic decompensation (Stone, 1993).

Persons with STPD will often fail to consider their social isolation and aberrant cognitions and perceptions to be particularly problematic or maladaptive. They may consider themselves to be simply eccentric, creative, or nonconformist. Rapport can be difficult to develop, as increasing familiarity and intimacy may only increase their level of discomfort and anxiety (Millon et al., 1996). They are unlikely to be responsive to informality or playful humor. The sessions should be well-structured to avoid loose and tangential ideation.

Practical advice is usually helpful and often necessary (Beck et al., 1990). The therapist should serve as the patient's counselor or guide to more adaptive decisions with respect to everyday problems (e.g., finding an apartment, interviewing for a job, and personal appearance). Persons with STPD should also receive social skills training directed at their awkward and odd behavior, mannerisms, dress, and speech. Specific, concrete discussions on what to expect and do in various social situations (e.g., formal meetings, casual encounters, and dates) should be provided (Stone, 1993).

Most of the systematic empirical research on the treatment of STPD has been confined to pharmacologic interventions. Low doses of neuroleptic medications (e.g., thiothixene) have shown some effectiveness in the treatment of schizotypal symptoms, particularly the perceptual aberrations and social anxiousness (Markovitz, 2001). Group therapy has also been recommended for persons with STPD but only when the group is highly structured and supportive (Millon et al., 1996). The emotional intensity and intimacy of unstructured groups will usually be too stressful. Schizotypal patients with predominant paranoid symptoms may even have difficulty in highly structured groups.

Dependent Personality Disorder

A diagnosis of dependent personality (DPD) was, technically speaking, a new addition to *DSM-III* (1980) in that it had not been included within the prior edition of the diagnostic manual. However, a diagnosis of passive-dependent personality trait disturbance was included within the first edition of the APA diagnostic manual.

Definition DPD involves a pervasive and excessive need to be taken care of that leads to submissiveness, clinging, and fears of separation (American Psychiatric Press, 2000; Bornstein, 1998; Pincus & Wilson, 2001). Its primary diagnostic criteria include extreme difficulty making decisions without others' input, need for others to assume responsibility for most aspects of daily life, extreme difficulty disagreeing with others, inability to initiate projects due to lack of self-confidence, and going to excessive lengths to obtain the approval of others.

Etiology and Pathology Insecure interpersonal attachment is considered to be central to the etiology and pathology of DPD (Bornstein, 2005; Pincus & Wilson, 2001; Stone, 1993), although there is actually limited empirical research concerning the etiology and pathology of DPD. Insecure attachment and helplessness may be generated through a parent–child relationship, perhaps by a clinging parent or a continued infantilization during a time in which individuation and separation normally occur (Gabbard, 2000a; Thompson & Zuroff, 1998). However, the combination of an anxious or inhibited temperament with inconsistent or overprotective parenting may also generate and exacerbate dependent personality traits (Bornstein, 2005; O'Neill & Kendler, 1998). Unable to generate feelings of security and confidence for themselves, dependent persons may rely on a parental figure for constant reassurance of their worth. Eventually, persons with DPD may come to believe that their self-worth is defined by their importance to another person (Beck et al., 1990).

Differential Diagnosis Excessively dependent behavior may be seen in persons who have developed debilitating mental and physical conditions, such as agoraphobia, schizophrenia, severe injuries, or dementia. However, a diagnosis of DPD requires the presence of the dependent traits since late childhood or adolescence (American Psychiatric Association, 2000). One can diagnose the presence of a personality disorder at any age during a person's lifetime, but if (for example) a DPD diagnosis is given to a person at the age of 75, this presumes that the dependent behavior was evident since the age of approximately 18 (i.e., predates the onset of a comorbid physical disorder secondary to aging).

Differences in personality due to differing cultural norms should not be confused with the presence of a personality disorder (Bornstein, 2005; Millon & Grossman, 2005). Cultural groups will differ greatly in the degree of importance attached to deferent behavior, politeness, and passivity. The diagnosis of DPD requires that the dependent behavior result in clinically significant functional impairment or distress.

Epidemiology DPD is one of the more prevalent personality disorders and is estimated to occur in 5 to 30% of patients and 2 to 4% of the general community (Mattia & Zimmerman, 2001). Studies have indicated that dependent personality traits are a risk factor for the development of depression in response to interpersonal loss (Blatt, 2004; Bornstein, 2005; Zuroff, Mongrain, & Santor, 2004).

Course To the extent that independent responsibility and initiative are required, job functioning will be impaired or unsatisfactory. Individuals with DPD are prone to mood disorders throughout life, particularly major depression and dysthymia, and to anxiety disorders, particularly agoraphobia, social phobia, and panic disorder (Bornstein, 2005). However, the severity of the symptomatology will tend to lessen with age, particularly if the person has obtained a reliable, empathic partner.

The self-esteem of a person with DPD is said to depend substantially on the maintenance of a supportive and nurturant relationship (Blatt, 2004; Bornstein, 2005), yet these intense needs for reassurance can have the paradoxical effect of driving the needed person away. The dependent person's worst fears are then realized (i.e., he or she is abandoned and alone), and his or her sense of self-worth, meaning, or value is then furthere injured, perhaps even crushed by the rejection (Shahar, Joiner, Zuroff, & Blatt, 2004). The dependent person might then indiscriminately select a readily available but unreliable, undependable, and perhaps even abusive person simply to be with someone. This partner would again reaffirm the worst fears through the abuse, derogation, and denigration (i.e., conveying to the dependent person that he or she is indeed undesirable and unlovable, and that the relationship is again tenuous). In other words, a combination of evocative, reactive, and then proactive transactions with the environment are the means by which a dependent personality style can lead to depression.

Research on the relationship of dependency to depression, however, is not without fundamental concerns (Coyne, Thompson, & Whiffen, 2004). An important focus of future research will be a further articulation of the precise process or mechanism through which this association occurs. In theory, dependent personality traits contribute to the instability of intimate and supportive relationships through the expression of excessive needs for reassurance or a premorbid emotional instability and pathogenic cognitions that contribute to intense feelings of helplessness and neediness. However, it is also possible that the emotional instability and pathologic attitudes are themselves the result of unstable interpersonal relationships. Dependency is a personality disposition that is seen much more often in women than in men (Bornstein, 1996). A provocative reformulation of dependency in women is that the apparent feelings of insecurity may say less about the women than the persons with whom the women are involved. "Men and women may differ in what they seek from relationships, but they may also differ in what they provide to each other" (Coyne & Whiffen, 1995, p. 368). In other words, "women might appear (and be) less dependent if they weren't involved with such undependable men" (Widiger & Anderson, 2003, p. 63).

Five-Factor Model Reformulation Dependent personality is characterized in terms of the FFM by maladaptively high levels of agreeableness (meek, gullible, and compliant) and the neuroticism facets of anxiousness, self-consciousness, and vulnerability (see Table 11.3). McCrae and Costa (1987) had stated that extremely high scores on the NEO PI-R agreeableness may describe a "dependent and fawning" (p. 88) person, and researchers have verified an association between the FFM domain of agreeableness and dependent personality disorder symptoms (Costa & McCrae, 1990; Dyce & O'Connor, 1998; Hyer et al., 1994). Some studies have not confirmed the association (Bornstein & Cecero, 2000) but this again appears to be due to the finding that the most commonly used measure of the FFM, the NEO-PI-R, does not adequately assess maladaptively high levels of agreeableness (Haigler & Widiger, 2001).

A controversial issue in the diagnosis of DPD is its differential sex prevalence (Widiger, in press). DPD is diagnosed much more frequently in females (American Psychiatric Association, 2000) and some have argued that this may reflect a masculine bias toward what constitutes a personality disorder (Kaplan, 1983) or a failure of males to acknowledge the presence of dependency needs (Bornstein, 1995). One difficulty in resolving this issue is the absence of any gold standard or even theoretical basis for hypothesizing, let alone determining, whether there should in fact be a differential sex prevalence rate. Understanding the *DSM-IV-TR* personality disorders from the perspective of the FFM, however, does provide a theoretical basis for gender difference expectations (Corbitt & Widiger, 1995). Researchers have consistently found that women tend to score higher than men on the domains of agreeableness and neuroticism (Costa & McCrae, 1992; Feingold, 1994). Costa, Terracciano, and McCrae (2001) found these differences to be consistent across 26 cultures, ranging from very traditional (Pakistan) to modern (The Netherlands). Thus, to the extent that DPD is a maladaptive variant of FFM agreeableness and neuroticism, one should then expect to obtain a differential sex prevalence rate. This is not to suggest, however, that no gender bias operates in clinical assessments. Gender stereotyping could occur in clinical settings, due in part to the relationship of DPD to common gender differences.

Studies have indicated that some self-report inventories are providing gender biased assessments of DPD (Lindsay, Sankis, & Widiger, 2000). The MCMI-III (Millon et al., 1997) and the MMPI-2 (Colligan et al., 1994) are personality disorder inventories that include gender-related items that are keyed in the direction of adaptive rather than maladaptive functioning. An item need not assess for dysfunction to contribute to a valid assessment of personality disorders. For example, items assessing for gregariousness can identify histrionic persons, items assessing for confidence can identify narcissistic persons, and items assessing conscientiousness can identify obsessive-compulsive persons (Millon et al., 1997). Items keyed in the direction of adaptive rather than maladaptive functioning can be helpful in countering the tendency of some respondents to deny or minimize personality disorder symptoms. However, these items will not be useful in differentiating abnormal from normal personality functioning and they are likely to contribute to an overdiagnosis of personality disorders in normal or minimally dysfunctional populations, such as seen in student counseling centers, child custody disputes, and personnel selection (Boyle & Le Dean, 2000; Lampel, 1999).

Treatment There are no empirically validated treatments for DPD. Treatment recommendations are based essentially on anecdotal clinical experience. Persons with DPD will often be in treatment for one or more Axis I disorders, particularly a mood (depressive) or an anxiety disorder. These individuals will tend to be very agreeable, compliant, and grateful, at times to excess (Bornstein, 2005). Many individuals with DPD will find that the therapeutic relationship itself satisfies their need for support and concern and may then desist from seeking a partner. The therapist can be perceived as the caring partner who will always be there. The dependent client might then even fear successful treatment, because termination may shortly follow (Gabbard, 2000). Thus, the client may remain excessively compliant and agreeable, in order to be a patient that the therapist would continue to treat. Therapists should be careful not to unwittingly encourage this submissiveness, nor to reject the client in order to be rid of their clinging dependency.

An important component of treatment will often be a thorough exploration of the need for support and its root causes. Cognitive-behavioral techniques can be useful to address feelings of inadequacy and helplessness and to provide training in assertiveness and problem-solving techniques (Beck et al., 1990; Young et al., 2003). Group therapy may be useful for persons with DPD, providing interpersonal feedback and modeling autonomous behavior. DPD is not known to respond to pharmacotherapy.

Conclusions

Maladaptive personality traits can be the focus of clinical treatment and will often impair or impede the treatment of other mental disorders. Chart reviews of practitioners suggest that they are not being diagnosed as frequently as they in fact occur, perhaps because it can be difficult to obtain coverage for their treatment. This is regrettable because some maladaptive personality traits (e.g., borderline and antisocial) have substantial social and public health care costs.

The five-factor model offers a compelling alternative to the categorical diagnosis of personality disorders as provided in *DSM-IV-TR*. Advantages of understanding personality disorders in terms of this dimensional model are the provision of more specific descriptions of individual patients (including adaptive as well as maladaptive personality functioning), the avoidance of arbitrary categorical distinctions, and the ability to bring to bear the extensive amount of research on the heritability, temperament, development, and course of general personality functioning to an understanding of personality disorders.

References

Ad-Dab'bagh, Y., & Greenfield, B. (2001). Multiple complex developmental disorder: The "multiple and complex" evolution of the "childhood borderline syndrome" construct. *Journal of American Academic Child and Adolescent Psychiatry, 40,* 954–964.

American Psychiatric Association. (1980). *Diagnostic and statistical manual of mental disorders* (3rd ed.). Washington, D.C.: Author.

American Psychiatric Association. (1987). *Diagnostic and statistical manual of mental disorders* (3rd ed., rev.). Washington, D.C.: Author.

American Psychiatric Association. (2000). *Diagnostic and statistical manual of mental disorders* (4th ed., rev.). Washington, D.C.: Author.

American Psychiatric Association. (2001). *Practice guidelines for the treatment of patients with borderline personality disorder.* Washington, D.C.: Author.

Ashton, M. C., & Lee, K. (2001). A theoretical basis for the major dimensions of personality. *European Journal of Personality, 15,* 327–353.

Auerbach, J. S. (1993). The origins of narcissism and narcissistic personality disorder: A theoretical and empirical reformulation. In J. M. Masling & R. F. Bornstein (Eds.), *Psychoanalytic perspectives on psychopathology* (pp. 43–110). Washington, D.C.: American Psychological Association.

Bagby, R. M., & Farvolden, P. (2004). The Personality Diagnostic Questionnaire-4 (PDQ-4). In M. J., Hilsenroth, D. L. Segal, & M. Hersen (Eds.), *Comprehensive handbook of psychological assessment: Vol. 2. Personality assessment* (pp. 122–133). New York: Wiley.

Baumeister, R. F., Smart, L., & Boden, J. M. (1996). Relation of threatened egoism to violence and aggression: the dark side of high self-esteem. *Psychological Review, 103,* 5–33.

Beck, A. T., Freeman, A., et al. (1990). *Cognitive therapy of personality disorders.* New York: Guilford.

Black, D. W., Noyes, R., Pfohl, B., Goldstein, R. B., & Blum, N. (1993). Personality disorder in obsessive-compulsive volunteers, well comparison subjects, and their first degree relatives. *American Journal of Psychiatry, 150*, 1226–1232.

Blashfield, R. K., & Intoccia, V. (2000). Growth of the literature on the topic of personality disorders. *American Journal of Psychiatry, 157,* 472–473.

Blatt, S. J. (2004). *Experiences of depression: Theoretical, clinical, and research perspectives.* Washington, D.C.: American Psychological Association.

Bornstein, R. F. (1995). Sex differences in objective and projective dependency tests: A meta-analytic review. *Assessment, 2,* 319–331.

Bornstein, R. F. (1998). Reconceptualizing personality disorder diagnoses in the *DSM-V*: The discriminant validity challenge. *Clinical Psychology: Science and Practice, 5,* 333–343.

Bornstein, R. F. (2005). *The dependent patient. A practitioner's guide.* Washington, D.C.: American Psychological Association.

Bornstein, R. F., & Cecero, J. J. (2000). Deconstructing dependency in a five-factor world: A meta-analytic review. *Journal of Personality Assessment, 74,* 324–343.

Boyle, G. J., & Le Dean, L. (2000). Discriminant validity of the Illness Behavior Questionnaire and Millon Clinical Multiaxial Inventory-III in a heterogeneous sample of psychiatric outpatients. *Journal of Clinical Psychology, 56,* 779–791.

Clark, L. A. (in press). Assessment and diagnosis of personality disorder. Perennial issues and an emerging reconceptualization. *Annual Review of Psychology.*

Clark, L. A., Simms, L. J., Wu, K. D., & Casillas, A. (in press). *Manual for the Schedule for Nonadaptive and Adaptive Personality (SNAP-2).* Minneapolis, MN: University of Minnesota Press.

Clarkin, J. F., Hull, J. W., Cantor, J., & Sanderson, C. (1993). Borderline personality disorder and personality traits: A comparison of SCID-II BPD and NEO-PI. *Psychological Assessment, 5,* 472–476.

Cleckley, H. (1941). *The mask of sanity.* St. Louis, MO: Mosby.

Cloninger, C. R. (2000). A practical way to diagnose personality disorders: A proposal. *Journal of Personality Disorders, 14,* 99–108.

Coker, L. A., & Widiger, T. A. (2004). Personality disorders. In J. Maddux & B. Winstead (Eds.), *Psychopathology: Foundation for a contemporary understanding* (pp. 201–227). New York: Erlbaum.

Colligan, R. C., Morey, L. C., & Offord, K. P. (1994). MMPI/MMPI-2 personality disorder scales. Contemporary norms for adults and adolescents. *Journal of Clinical Psychology, 50,* 168–200.

Corbitt, E. M., & Widiger, T. A. (1995). Sex differences among the personality disorders: An exploration of the data. *Clinical Psychology: Science and Practice, 2,* 225–238.

Coryell, W. H., & Zimmerman, M. (1989). Personality disorder in the families of depressed, schizophrenic, and never-ill probands. *American Journal of Psychiatry, 146,* 496–502.

Costa, P. T. Jr., & McCrae, R. R. (1990). Personality disorders and the five-factor model of personality. *Journal of Personality Disorders, 4,* 362–371.

Costa, P. T., Jr. & McCrae, R. R. (1992). *Revised NEO Personality Inventory (NEO-PI-R) and NEO Five Factor Inventory (NEO-FFI) Professional Manual.* Odessa, FL: Psychological Assessment Resources.

Costa, P. T., Jr., Terracciano, A., & McCrae, R. R. (2001). Gender differences in personality traits across cultures: Robust and surprising findings. *Journal of Personality and Social Psychology, 81,* 322–331.

Coyne, J. C., Thompson, R., & Whiffen, V. (2004). Is the promissary note of personality as vulnerability to depression in default? Reply to Zuroff, Mongrain, and Santor (2004). *Psychological Bulletin, 130,* 512–517.

Coyne, J. C., & Whiffen, V. E. (1995). Issues in personality as diathesis for depression: The case of sociotropy dependency and autonomy self-criticism. *Psychological Bulletin, 118,* 358–378.

Derefinko, K. J., & Widiger, T. A. (in press). Antisocial personality disorder. In S. H. Fatemi & P. Clayton (Eds.), *The medical basis of psychiatry* (3rd ed.). Totowa, NJ: Humana Press.

Drake, R. E., Adler, D. A., & Vaillant, G. E. (1988). Antecedents of personality disorders in a community sample of men. *Journal of Personality Disorders, 2,* 60–68.

Dyce, J. A., & O'Connor, B. P. (1998). Personality disorders and the five-factor model: A test of facet-level predictions. *Journal of Personality Disorders, 12,* 31–45.

Fanous, A., Gardner, C., Walsh, D., & Kendler, K. (2001). Relationship between positive and negative symptoms of schizophrenia and schizotypal symptoms in nonpsychotic relatives. *Archives of General Psychiatry, 58,* 669–673.

Farrington, D. P. (2006). Family background and psychopathy. In C. J. Patrick (Ed.), *Handbook of psychopathy* (pp. 229–250). New York: Guilford.

Feingold, A. (1994). Gender differences in personality: A meta-analysis. *Psychological Bulletin, 116,* 429–456.

First, M. B., Bell, C. B., Cuthbert, B., Krystal, J. H., Malison, R., Offord, D. R., et al. (2002). Personality disorders and relational disorders: A research agenda for addressing crucial gaps in DSM. In D. J. Kupfer, M. B. First, & D. A. Regier (Eds.), *A research agenda for DSM-V* (pp. 123–199) Washington, D.C.: American Psychiatric Association.

Fossati, A., Beauchaine, T. P., Grazioli, F., Carretta, I., Cortinovis, F., & Maffei, C. (2005). A latent structure analysis of *Diagnostic and statistical manual of mental disorders*, fourth edition, narcissistic personality disorder criteria. *Comprehensive Psychiatry, 46,* 361–367.

Fowles, D. C., & Kochanska, G. (2000). Temperament as a moderator of pathways to conscience in children: the contribution of electrodermal activity. *Psychophysiology, 37,* 788–795.

Frances, A. J. (1980). The *DSM-III* personality disorders section: a commentary. *American Journal of Psychiatry, 137,* 1050–1054.

Frances, A. J., First, M. B., & Pincus, H. A. (1995). *DSM-IV guidebook.* Washington, D.C.: American Psychiatric Press.

Gabbard, G. O. (2000a) *Psychodynamic psychiatry in clinical practice* (3rd ed). Washington, D.C.: American Psychiatric Press.

Gabbard, G. O. (2000b). Psychodynamic psychotherapy of borderline personality disorder: A contemporary approach. *Bulletin of the Menninger Clinic, 65,* 41–57.

Goldberg, L. R. (1993). The structure of phenotypic personality traits. *American Psychologist, 48,* 26–34.

Gooding, D. C., Tallent, K. A., & Matts, C. W. (2005). Clinical status of at-risk individuals 5 years later: Further validation of the psychometric high-risk strategy. *Journal of Abnormal Psychology, 114,* 170–175.

Gunderson, J. G. (2001). *Borderline personality disorder: A clinical guide.* Washington, D.C.: American Psychiatric Press.

Gunderson, J. G., Bender, D., Sanislow, C., Yen, S., Rettew, J. B., Dolan Sewell, R., Dyck, I., Morey, L. C., McGlashan, T. H., Shea, M. T., & Skodol, A. E. (2003). Plausibility and possible determinants of sudden "remissions" in borderline patients. *Psychiatry, 66,* 111–119.

Gunderson, J. G., & Gabbard, G. O. (Eds.). (2000). *Psychotherapy for personality disorders.* Washington, D.C.: American Psychiatric Press.

Gunderson, J. G., Ronningstam, E., & Smith, L. E. (1991). Narcissistic personality disorder: A review of data on *DSM-III-R* descriptions. *Journal of Personality Disorder, 5,* 167–177.

Haigler, E. D., & Widiger, T. A. (2001). Experimental manipulation of NEO-PI-R items. *Journal of Personality Assessment, 77,* 339–358.

Hall, J. R., & Benning, S. D. (2005). The "successful" psychopath: adaptive and subclinical manifestations of psychopathy in the general population. In C. Patrick (Ed.), *Handbook of psychopathy* (pp. 459–478). New York: Guilford.

Hare, R. D. (2003). *Hare Psychopathy Checklist Revised (PCL-R): Technical manual.* North Tonawanda, NY: Multi-Health Systems.

Hart, S. D., & Hare, R. D. (1989). Discriminant validity of the Psychopathy Checklist in a forensic psychiatric population. *Psychological Assessment, 1,* 211–218.

Harpur, T. J., & Hare, R. D. (1994). Assessment of psychopathy as a function of age. *Journal of Abnormal Psychology, 103,* 604–609.

Hefferman, K., & Cloitre, M. (2000). A comparison of posttraumatic stress disorder with and without borderline personality disorder among women with a history of childhood sexual abuse: Etiological and clinical characteristics. *Journal of Nervous and Mental Disorder, 188,* 589–595.

Hiatt, K. D., & Newman, J. P. (2006). Understanding psychopathy: The cognitive side. In C. J. Patrick (Ed.), *Handbook of psychopathy* (pp. 156–171). New York: Guilford.

Hyer, L., Brawell, L., Albrecht, B., Boyd, S., Boudewyns, P., & Talbert, S. (1994). Relationship of NEO-PI to personality styles and severity of trauma in chronic PTSD victims. *Journal of Clinical Psychology, 50,* 699–707.

Jaffee, S. R., Caspi, A., Moffitt, T. E., & Taylor, A. (2004). Physical maltreatment victim to antisocial child: Evidence of an environmentally mediated process. *Journal of Abnormal Psychology, 113,* 44–55.

Jang, K. L., Livesley, W. J., Vernon, P. A., & Jackson, D. N. (1996). Heritability of personality disorder traits: A twin study. *Acta Psychiatrica Scandinavica, 94,* 438–444.

Jang, K. L., & Vernon, P. A. (2001) Genetics. In W.J. Livesley (Ed.), *Handbook of personality disorders* (pp. 177–195). New York: Guilford.

Kaplan, M. (1983). A woman's view of *DSM-III. American Psychologist, 38,* 786–792.

Kernberg, O. F. (1998). Pathological narcissism and narcissistic personality disorder: Theoretical background and diagnostic classification. In E. F. Ronningstam (Ed.), *Disorders of narcissism: Diagnostic, clinical, and empirical implications* (pp. 29–52). Washington, D.C.: American Psychiatric Press.

Kessler, R. C., McGonagle, K. A., Zhao, S., et al. (1994). Lifetime and 12-month prevalence of *DSM-III-R* psychiatric disorders in the United States: Results from the national comorbidity survey. *Archives of General Psychiatry, 51,* 8–19.

Klein, D. N., Riso, L. P., Donaldson, S. K., Schwartz, J. E., Anderson, R. L., Oiumette, P. C., et al. (1995). Family study of early-onset dysthymia: Mood and personality disorders in relatives of outpatients with dysthymia and episodic major depressive and normal controls. *Archives of General Psychiatry, 52,* 487–496.

Kohut H (1977). *The restoration of the self.* New York: International Universities Press.

Lampel, A. K. (1999). Use of the Millon Clinical Multiaxial Inventory-III in evaluating child custody litigants. *American Journal of Forensic Psychology, 17,* 19–31.

Lenzenweger, M. F., Loranger, A. W., Korfine, L., & Neff, C. (1997). Detecting personality disorders in a nonclinical population. *Archives of General Psychiatry, 54,* 345–351.

Lindsay, K. A., Sankis, L. M., & Widiger, T. A. (2000). Gender bias in self-report personality disorder inventories. *Journal of Personality Disorders, 14,* 218–232.

Linehan, M. M. (1993). *Cognitive-behavioral treatment of borderline personality disorder.* New York: Guilford.

Livesley, W. J. (2001). Conceptual and taxonomic issues. In W. J. Livesley (Ed.), *Handbook of personality disorders: Theory, research, and treatment* (pp. 3–38). New York: Guilford.

Livesley, W. J. (2003). Diagnostic dilemmas in classifying personality disorder. In K. A. Phillips, M. B. First, & H. A. Pincus (Eds.), *Advancing DSM-: Dilemmas in psychiatric diagnosis* (pp. 153–190). Washington, D.C.: American Psychiatric Publishing.

Lykken, D. T. (1957). A study of anxiety in the sociopathic personality. *Journal of Abnormal and Clinical Psychology, 55,* 6–10.

Lynam, D. R., & Widiger, T.A. (2001). Using the five-factor model to represent the personality disorders. *Journal of Abnormal Psychology, 110,* 401–412.

Lynam, D. R., & Widiger, T. A. (in press). Using a general model of personality to identify the basic elements of psychopathy. *Journal of Personality Disorders.*

Lynch, T. R., Trost, W. T., Salsman, N., & Linehan, M. M. (in press). Dialectical behavior therapy for borderline personality disorder. *Annual Review of Clinical Psychology.*

Maier, W., Lichtermann, D., Klinger, T., & Heun, R. (1992). Prevalences of personality disorders (*DSM-III-R*) in the community. *Journal of Personality Disorders, 6*, 187–196.

Markovitz, P. (2001). Pharmacotherapy. In W. J. Livesley (Ed.), *Handbook of personality disorders* (pp. 475–493). New York: Guilford.

Mattia, J. I., & Zimmerman, M. (2001). Epidemiology. In W. J. Livesley (Ed.), *Handbook of personality disorders* (pp. 107–123). New York: Guilford.

McCrae, R. R., & Costa, P.T., Jr. (1987). Validation of the five-factor model of personality across instruments and observers. *Journal of Personality and Social Psychology, 52*, 81–90.

Miller, J. D., & Lynam, D. R. (2003). Psychopathy and the five-factor model of personality: A replication and extension. *Journal of Personality Assessment, 81*, 168–178.

Miller, M. B., Useda, J. D., Trull, T. J., Burr, R. M., & Minks-Brown, C. (2001). Paranoid, schizoid, and schizotypal personality disorders. In H. E. Adams & P. B. Sutker (Eds.), *Comprehensive handbook of psychopathology* (3rd ed., pp. 535–558). New York: Plenum.

Millon, T., Davis, R. D., Millon, C.M., Wenger, A., Van Zullen, M. H., Fuchs, M., et al. (1996). *Disorders of personality: DSM-IV and beyond* (2nd. ed.). New York: Wiley

Millon, T., & Grossman, S. D. (2005). Sociocultural factors. In J. M. Oldham, A. E. Skodol, & D. S. Bender (Eds.), *Textbook of personality disorders* (pp. 223–235). Washington, D.C.: American Psychiatric Publishing.

Millon, T., Millon, C., & Davis, R. (1997). *MCMI-III manual* (2nd ed.). Minneapolis, MN: National Computer Systems.

Moffitt, T. E. (2005). The new look of behavioral genetics in developmental psychopathology: Gene-environment interplay in antisocial behaviors. *Psychological Bulletin, 131*, 533–554.

Moldin, S. O., Rice, J. P., Erlenmeyer-Kimling, L., & Squires-Wheeler, E. (1994). Latent structure of *DSM-III-R* Axis II psychopathology in a normal sample. *Journal of Abnormal Psychology, 103*, 259–266.

Morey, L. C. (1991). *The Personality Assessment Inventory professional manual*. Odessa, FL: Psychological Assessment Resources.

Morey, L. C., & Zanarini, M. C. (2000). Borderline personality: traits and disorder. *Journal of Abnormal Psychology, 109*, 733–737.

Morf, C. C., & Rhodewalt, F. (2001). Unraveling the paradoxes of narcissism: A dynamic self-regulatory processing model. *Psychological Inquiry, 12*, 177–196.

Mullins-Sweatt, S. N., & Widiger, T. A. (2006). The five-factor model of personality disorder: A translation across science and practice. In R. Krueger & J. Tackett (Eds.), *Personality and psychopathology: Building bridges* (pp. 39–70). New York: Guilford.

Newman, J. P., & Lorenz, A. R. (2003). Response modulation and emotion processing: Implications for psychopathy and other dysregulatory psychopathology. In R. J. Davidson, K. Scherer, & H. H. Goldsmith (Eds.), *Handbook of affective sciences* (pp. 1043–1067). New York: Oxford University Press.

O'Connor, B. P. (2005). A search for consensus on the dimensional structure of personality disorders. *Journal of Clinical Psychology, 61*, 323–345.

Oldham, J. M., & Skodol, A. E. (2000). Charting the future of Axis II. *Journal of Personality Disorders, 14*, 17–29.

O'Neill, F. A., & Kendler, K. S. (1998). Longitudinal study of interpersonal dependency in female twins. *British Journal of Psychiatry, 172*, 154–158.

Ornduff, S. R. (2000). Childhood maltreatment and malevolence: Quantitative research findings. *Clinical Psychology Review, 20*, 991–1018.

Ozer, D. J., & Reise, S. P. (1994). Personality assessment. *Annual Review of Psychology, 45*, 357–388.

Parnas, J., Licht, D., & Bovet, P. (2005). Cluster A personality disorders: A review. In M. Maj, H. S. Akiskal, J. E. Mezzich, & A. Okasha (Eds.), *Personality disorders* (pp. 1–74). NewYork: Wiley.

Patrick, C. J., Cuthbert, B. N,, & Lang, P. J. (1994). Emotion in the criminal psychopath: Startle reflex modulation. *Journal of Abnormal Psychology, 103*, 523–534.

Perry, J. C., Banon, E., & Ianni, F. (1999). Effectiveness of psychotherapy for personality disorders. *American Journal of Psychiatry, 156*, 1312–1321.

Pfohl, B. (2005). Comorbidity and borderline personality disorder. In M. Zanarini (Ed.), *Borderline personality disorder* (pp. 135–153). Washington, D.C.: American Psychiatric Press.

Pincus, A. L., & Wilson, K. R. (2001). Interpersonal variability in dependent personality. *Journal of Personality, 69*, 223–252.

Raine, A. (1993). *The psychopathology of crime: Criminal Behavior as a clinical disorder*. San Diego: Academic Press.

Raine, A. (2006). Schizotypal personality: Neurodevelopmental and psychosocial trajectories. *Annual Review of Clinical Psychology, 2*, 291–326.

Raskin, R., & Terry, H. (1988). A principal-components analysis of the Narcissistic Personality Inventory and further evidence of its construct validity. *Journal of Personality and Social Psychology, 54*, 890–902.

Rhee, S. H., & Waldman, I. D. (2002). Genetic and environmental influences on antisocial behavior: A meta-analysis of twin and adoption studies. *Psychological Bulletin, 128*, 490–529.

Robins, L. N., Tipp, J., & Przybeck, T. (1991). Antisocial personality. In L. N. Robins & D. A. Regier (Eds.), *Psychiatric disorders in America* (pp. 258–290). New York: Free Press.

Ronningstam, E. (1999). Narcissistic personality disorder. In T. Millon, P. H. Blaney, & R. D. Davis (Eds.), *Oxford textbook of psychopathology* (pp. 674–693). New York: Oxford University Press.

Ronningstam, E. (2005). Narcissistic personality disorder: A review. In M. Maj, H. S. Akiskal, J. E. Mezzich, & A. Okasha (Eds.), *Personality disorders* (pp. 278–327). New York: Wiley.

Ross, S. R., Lutz, C. J., & Bailey, S. E. (2002). Positive and negative symptoms of schizotypy and the five-factor model: A domain and facet level analysis. *Journal of Personality Assessment, 79*, 53–72.

Rounsaville, B. J., Alarcon, R. D., Andrews, G., Jackson, J. S., Kendell, R. E., & Kendler, K. (2002). Basic nomenclature issues for *DSM-V*. In D. J. Kupfer, M. B. First, & D. E. Regier (Eds.), *A research agenda for DSM-V* (pp. 1–29). Washington, D.C.: American Psychiatric Press.

Salekin, R. T. (2002). Psychopathy and therapeutic pessimism: Clinical lore or clinical reality? *Clinical Psychology Review, 22,* 79–112.

Samuel, D. B., & Widiger, T. A. (2004). Clinicians' personality descriptions of prototypic personality disorders. *Journal of Personality Disorders, 18,* 286–308.

Samuel, D. B., & Widiger, T. A. (2006). Clinicians' judgments of clinical utility: A comparison of the *DSM-IV* and five factor models. *Journal of Abnormal Psychology, 115,* 298–308.

Samuels, J. F., Nestadt, G., & Romanoski, A. J. (1994). *DSM-III* personality disorders in the community. *American Journal of Psychiatry, 151,* 1055–1062.

Sanderson, C. J., Swenson, C., & Bohus, S. (2002). A critique of the American Psychiatric Practice guidelines for the treatment of patients with borderline personality disorder. *Journal of Personality Disorders, 16,* 122–129.

Sanislow, C. A., & McGlashan, T. H. (1998). Treatment outcome of personality disorders. *Canadian Journal of Psychiatry, 43,* 237–250.

Saulsman, L. M., & Page, A. C. (2004). The five-factor model and personality disorder empirical literature: a meta-analytic review. *Clinical Psychology Review, 23,* 1055–1085.

Schneider, K. (1923). *Psychopathic personalities.* Springfield, IL: Charles C. Thomas.

Shahar, G., Joiner, T. E., Zuroff, D. C., & Blatt, S. J. (2004). Personality, interpersonal behavior, and depression: Co-existence of stress-specific moderating and mediating effects. *Personality and Individual Differences, 36,* 1583–1596.

Siever, L. J. & Davis, K. L. (2004). The pathophysiology of schizophrenia disorders: Perspectives from the spectrum. *American Journal of Psychiatry, 161,* 398–403.

Silk, K. R., Wolf, T. L., Ben-Ami, D., & Poortinga, E. W. (2005). Environmental factors in the etiology of borderline personality disorder. In M. Zanarini (Ed.). *Borderline personality disorder* (pp. 41–62). Washington, D.C.: American Psychiatric Press.

Skodol, A. E., Gunderson, J. G., Shea, M. T., McGlashan, T. H., Morey, L. C., Sanislow, C. A., et al. (2005). The Collaborative Longitudinal Personality Disorders Study (CLPS): Overview and implications. *Journal of Personality Disorders, 19,* 487–504.

Spitzer, R., Endicott, J., & Gibbon, M. (1979). Crossing the border into borderline personality and borderline schizophrenia. *Archives of General Psychiatry, 36,* 17–24.

Stone, M. H. (1993). *Abnormalities of personality: Within and beyond the realm of treatment.* New York: W.W. Norton.

Stone, M. H. (2001). Natural history and long-term outcome. In W. J. Livesley (Ed.), *Handbook of personality disorders* (pp. 259–273). New York: Guilford.

Sutker, P. B., & Allain, A. N. (2001). Antisocial personality disorder. In P. B. Sutker & H. E. Adams (Eds.), *Comprehensive textbook of psychopathology* (3rd ed., pp. 445–490). New York: Plenum.

Thompson, S., & Zuroff, D.C. (1998). Dependent and self-critical mothers' responses to adolescent autonomy and competence. *Personality and Individual Differences, 24,* 311–324.

Torgersen, S. (2005a). Epidemiology. In J. M. Oldham, A. E. Skodol, & D. S. Bender (Eds.), *Textbook of personality disorders* (pp. 129–141). Washington, D.C.: American Psychiatric Publishing.

Torgersen, S. (2005b). Genetics of borderline personality disorder. In M. Zanarini (Ed.), *Borderline personality disorder* (pp. 127–134). Washington, D.C.: American Psychiatric Press.

Torgersen, S., Kringlen, E., & Cramer, V. (2001). The prevalence of personality disorders in a community sample. *Archives of General Psychiatry, 58,* 590–596.

Torgersen, S., Lygren, S., Oien, P. A., Skre, I., Onstad, S., Edvardson, E., et al. (2000). A twin study of personality disorders. *Comprehensive Psychiatry, 41,* 416–425.

Trull, T. J., Widiger, T. A., & Burr, R. (2001). A structured interview for the assessment of the five-factor model of personality: 2. Facet-level relations to the Axis II personality disorders. *Journal of Personality, 69,* 175–198.

Trull, T. J., Widiger, T. A., Lynam, D. R., & Costa, P. T. (2003). Borderline personality disorder from the perspective of general personality functioning. *Journal of Abnormal Psychology, 112,* 193–202.

Waldman, I. D., & Rhee, S. H. (2006). Genetic and environmental influences on psychopathy and antisocial behavior. In C. J. Patrick (Ed.), *Handbook of psychopathy* (pp. 205–228). New York: Guilford.

Walker, E., Kestler, L., Bollini, A., & Hochman, K. M. (2004). Schizophrenia: Etiology and course. *Annual Review of Psychology, 55,* 401–430.

Warner, M. B., Morey, L. C., Finch, J. F., Gunderson, J. G., Skodol, A. E., Sanislow, C. A., et al. (2004). The longitudinal relationship of personality traits and disorders. *Journal of Abnormal Psychology, 113,* 217–227.

Watson, D. (2006, October). Toward an integrated model of normal and abnormal personality. In D. Watson (Chair), *Integrating personality and psychopathology research.* Symposium conducted at the 21st annual meeting of the Society of Research in Psychopathology, San Diego, CA.

Widiger, T. A. (2000). Personality disorders in the 21st century. *Journal of Personality Disorders, 14,* 3–16.

Widiger, T. A. (2005a). CIC, CLPS, and MSAD. *Journal of Personality Disorders, 19,* 586–593.

Widiger, T. A. (2005b). Psychopathy and *DSM-IV* psychopathology. In C. Patrick (Ed.), *Handbook of psychopathy* (pp. 156–171). New York: Guilford.

Widiger, T. A. (2005c). A temperament model of borderline personality disorder. In M. Zanarini (Ed.), *Borderline personality disorder* (pp. 63–81). Washington, D.C.: American Psychiatric Press.

Widiger, T. A. (in press). DSM's approach to gender: history and controversies. In K. A. Phillips & M. B. First (Eds.), *A sex research agenda for DSM-V.* Washington, D.C.: American Psychiatric Publishing.

Widiger, T. A., & Anderson, K. G., (2003). Personality and depression in women. *Journal of Affective Disorders, 74*, 59–66.

Widiger, T. A., & Coker, L. A. (2002). Assessing personality disorders. In J. N. Butcher (Ed.), *Clinical personality assessment. Practical approaches* (2nd ed., pp. 407–434). New York: Oxford University Press.

Widiger, T. A., & Simonsen, E. (2005). Alternative dimensional models of personality disorder: Finding a common ground. *Journal of Personality Disorders, 19*, 110–130.

Widiger, T. A., Simonsen, E., Krueger, R., Livesley, J., & Verheul, R. (2005). Personality disorder research agenda for the *DSM-V*. *Journal of Personality Disorders, 19*, 317–340.

Widiger, T. A., & Trull, T. J. (1998). Performance characteristics of the *DSM-III-R* personality disorder criteria sets. In T. A. Widiger, A. J. Frances, H. A. Pincus, R. Ross, M. B. First, W. W. Davis, & M. Klein (Eds.), *DSM-IV sourcebook* (Vol. 4, pp. 357–373). Washington, D.C.: American Psychiatric Press.

Widiger, T. A., & Trull, T. J. (in press). Plate tectonics in the classification of personality disorder: Shifting to a dimensional model. *American Psychologist*.

Widiger, T. A., Trull, T. J., Clarkin, J. F., Sanderson, C., & Costa, P. T., Jr. (2002). A description of the *DSM-IV* personality disorders with the five-factor model of personality. In P. T. Costa, Jr. & T. A. Widiger (Eds.), *Personality disorders and the five-factor model of personality* (pp. 89–99). Washington, D.C.: American Psychological Association.

Wiggins, J. S., & Pincus, H. A. (1989). Conceptions of personality disorder and dimensions of personality. *Psychological Assessment, 1*, 305–316.

Wilberg, T., Urnes, O., Friis, S., Pederson, G., & Karterud, S. (1999). Borderline and avoidant personality disorders and the five-factor model of personality: A comparison between *DSM-IV* diagnoses and NEO-PI-R. *Journal of Personality Disorders, 13*, 226–240.

World Health Organization (1992). *The ICD-10 classification of mental and behavioural disorders: Clinical descriptions and diagnostic guidelines*. Geneva, Switzerland: Author.

Young, J. E., Klosko, J. S., & Weishaar, M. E. (2003). *Schema therapy: A practitioner's guide*. New York: Guilford.

Zanarini, M. C., Frankenburg, F. R., Hennen, R., Reich, D. B., & Silk, K. R. (2005). The McLean Study of Adult Development (MSAD): Overview and implications of the first six years of prospective follow-up. *Journal of Personality Disorders, 19*, 505–523.

Zimmerman, M., & Mattia, J. I. (1999). Differences between clinical and research practices in diagnosing borderline personality disorder. *American Journal of Psychiatry, 156*, 1570–1574.

Zuroff, D. C., Mongrain, M., & Santor, D. A. (2004). Conceptualizing and measuring personality vulnerability to depression: Comment on Coyne and Whiffen (1995). *Psychological Bulletin, 130*, 489–511.

12
Eating Disorders

Janet Polivy, C. Peter Herman, and Michele Boivin

Until the 1960s and 1970s, few people had heard of anorexia nervosa (AN), but it soon began to be reported with increasing frequency in Western societies. Young females from middle- and upper-class families were voluntarily starving themselves and losing weight to the point of emaciation and sometimes death. A decade later, a new eating disorder was recognized; in bulimia nervosa (BN),[1] young women alternate between starving and eating prodigious amounts of food, often followed by purging. Although these eating disorders have flourished recently in Westernized societies during periods of relative affluence and enhanced social opportunities for women (Bemporad, 1996, 1997), voluntary self-starvation and periods of binge eating and purging have been reported throughout history. Eating disorders that would be recognizable today as anorexia nervosa and bulimia nervosa have existed since ancient times (Bemporad, 1997). Eating disorder not otherwise specified (or EDNOS, which will not be discussed in this chapter, because it is not a clear diagnostic category) and binge eating disorder (BED) were added in the *Diagnostic and Statistical Manual of Mental Disorders* (*DSM–IV*; American Psychiatric Association, 1994).

Whether the various eating disorders are fundamentally different is debatable (e.g., Fairburn, Cooper, & Shafran, 2003; Joiner, Vohs, & Heatherton, 2000); core symptoms (e.g., preoccupation with food, disturbed body perception, and inadequate sexual behavior) do not differ between AN and BN patients. Bulimic eating disorders appear to exist on a continuum of clinical severity, from BED (least severe), through nonpurging-type BN (intermediate severity), to purging-type BN (most severe) (Hay & Fairburn, 1998). The spectrum hypothesis considers all eating disorders as different manifestations of a single disorder or syndrome (VanderHam, Meulman, VanStrien, & vanEngeland, 1997). In this chapter, we will discuss the major eating disorders, using the *DSM* to describe the primary features of AN, BN, and the newer BED (about which substantially less is known). We will then review the prevalence and prognosis of eating disorders and provide an overview of the main hypotheses concerning what causes them to occur in a given individual. Finally, we will discuss the principal treatments for eating disorders.

Diagnostic Criteria and Core Pathological Features of Eating Disorders

The *DSM–IV-TR* (American Psychiatric Association, 2000) is the most widely accepted set of criteria for psychological/ psychiatric disorders in North America. The symptoms of eating disorders were compiled by a panel of experts who treat these problems, and the symptoms were then sent to others in the field for comments and corrections. In this version of the DSM, all symptoms are supposed to be empirically supported and to reflect a consensus among those who treat and study the disorders. For eating disorders, this is a difficult proposition, as we shall see. Not all criteria for the disorder are easy to define (e.g., exactly what behaviors constitute binge eating?); the criteria as listed have some ambiguities. Moreover, there are controversies concerning just how universal some symptoms are (e.g., amenorrhea). Finally, many psychologists object to the medicalization of abnormal behavior implied by a diagnosis. Despite these debates about the utility of the *DSM*, many researchers use the *DSM* criteria for eating disorders to facilitate communication across research settings, to ensure that all are studying the same phenomena. For clinicians treating the problems, diagnostic criteria can point to symptoms that need to be treated and methods of treating them, and also can allow for assessment of successful change. For these reasons, we will use the criteria for eating disorders as set out in the *DSM,* but we will point out where these criteria have been questioned.

The *DSM–IV* diagnostic criteria for AN are refusal to maintain body weight at or above a minimum of 85% of normal weight for age and height, accompanied by an intense fear of fatness, disturbed experience of one's body weight or shape, and amenorrhea (for at least three consecutive menstrual cycles). In addition, bulimic-type anorexia includes regular episodes of binge eating or purging, but restrictor-type anorexia entails only starving (and both types may involve compulsive exercising). Although amenorrhea has been an important criterion for AN for some time, women with AN and women with all the features of AN except amenorrhoea are otherwise indistinguishable, leading some to question the utility of amenorrhea as a diagnostic criterion (Cachelin & Maher, 1998; Garfinkel et al., 1996).

Usually, the early (preadolescent) onset of an eating disorder predicts a better outcome. Extremely early onset of AN seems to occur more frequently in boys than in girls. There is a risk of permanent side effects, such as short stature, if those with early-onset AN experience lengthy or chronic malnutrition (Theander, 1996).

The *DSM–IV* describes BN as recurrent episodes of binge eating (i.e., eating more food than most people would eat in a similar time period and situation and feeling out of control of one's eating during the episode) accompanied by compensatory behaviors (such as purging, exercising, or fasting) to prevent a corresponding weight gain. These behaviors must occur at least twice a week for at least three months. It has been argued (Grilo, 2006) that the core symptom of BN is that the individual's self-evaluation relies excessively on body weight and shape. If any of these symptoms occur in the context of an episode of AN, then AN becomes the primary diagnosis. The purging type of BN features self-induced vomiting or laxative, diuretic, or enema abuse; nonpurging BN involves fasting, exercising, or other (nonpurging) means of compensating for binge eating (American Psychiatric Association, 1994). Impulsive behaviors such as sexual promiscuity, suicide attempts, drug abuse, and stealing or shoplifting are common among people with BN (e.g., Goldner, Geller, Birmingham, & Remick, 2000; Matsunaga, Kiriike et al., 2000).

Both AN and BN often emerge during late adolescence, with a female-to-male ratio between 10:1 and 15:1 (Bramon-Bosch, Troop, & Treasure, 2000; Braun, Sunday, Huang, & Halmi, 1999). Although the disorders are more prevalent in females, the nature of the disorders is the same in the two sexes. For individuals with eating disorder, a negative body image and a variety of psychological problems appear to emerge during puberty (e.g., Polivy & Herman, 2002, for a review). Even before the onset of their disorder, adolescents with BN report various problems such as weight-related concerns, attitudes of withdrawal and social isolation, and deterioration of body-image, self-image, and relationships with siblings and peers. The prevalence of these problems among adolescents with BN suggests that early psychological distress may precede the onset of an eating disorder (Corcos et al., 2000).

Binge eating disorder (BED) is described by *DSM–IV* (in the research appendix) as similar to BN in that it entails recurrent binge eating episodes accompanied by subjective feelings of lack of control over one's eating. The difference between BN and BED is that the purging and compensatory behaviors that occur regularly in BN are infrequent in BED (APA, 1994). The binge eating typically begins in late adolescence or the early 20s and frequently follows dieting and weight loss. Typically, individuals with BED are overweight and do not exhibit the chronic weight and shape concerns that characterize people with AN and BN. Eating disorder not otherwise specified (EDNOS) is a catchall category for syndromes that do not quite fit the diagnostic criteria for the other eating disorders (e.g., binge eating occurring with some regularity, but less than twice a week) (American Psychiatric Association, 1994).

Despite the primacy of binge eating as a diagnostic feature of BN, BED, and bulimic-type AN, attempts to define binge eating have been unsatisfactory, and there is considerable variability in what sorts of eating episodes individuals label as binges (Johnson, Carr-Nangle, Nangle, Antony, & Zayfert, 1997). What, for instance, is a larger than normal amount of food? Commonly noted triggers for binge eating include negative affect or stress, the presence of attractive fattening food, abstinence violation (i.e., having already eaten something fattening or diet-breaking), ingestion of alcohol, and being alone (Polivy & Herman, 1993). Examination of videotaped eating episodes indicates that feelings of loss of control and violation of dietary strictures are critical in leading people to construe a particular episode as a binge (Johnson, Boutelle, Torgrud, Davig, & Turner, 2000). Laxative abuse among women with eating disorders is an indicator of greater psychopathology, irrespective of other features such as eating disorder diagnostic category, age, body weight, impulsive behaviors, or personality features (Pryor, Wiederman, & McGilley, 1996).

Incidence and Prevalence of Eating Disorders

Since the 1950s, the incidence of AN in females aged 15 to 24 has increased markedly; it is currently estimated at 8.1 per 100,000 population per year (or .008%, with BN even higher at 11.4 per 100,000, or .011%) (Hoek, 1993, 2002), and some estimate that the number is as high as 19.2 (or .019%) (Rooney, McClelland, Crisp, & Sedgwick, 1995). Of course, this increase may represent a combination of a true increase in incidence as well as increased recognition of cases that formerly would not have been acknowledged (Wakeling, 1996). Nevertheless, these incidence figures may well be significant underestimates; the disorders still often escape detection or diagnosis (Rooney et al., 1995) because dieting and the pursuit of thinness are so ubiquitous and socially acceptable in Western culture, and because of the secretive nature of the disorder (Grilo, 2006). Indeed, more recent studies find incidence rates as high as 300 per 100,000 (.30%) for females and 20 per 100,000 (.02%) for males (Striegel-Moore, Garvin, Dohm, & Rosenheck, 1999). In a recent national study, 5% of the 700 women sampled reported binge eating within the past 30 days, 29% reported intense dieting or fasting in the past three months, 43% claimed that their weight and shape were very important or more important than anything else, and 1.5% of the women met criteria for nonpurging BN (Vogeltanz-Holm et al., 2000). Some of these reports, however, may be unreliable because of changes in diagnostic and referral practices (Fombonne, 1996). Changing diagnostic and referral practices make it virtually impossible to know the true rate of increase in the incidence of eating disorders. More ominously, however, the prevalence of partial or subclinical eating disorders is at least twice that of full-syndrome eating disorders (Shisslak, Crago, & Estes, 1995). Longitudinal studies also provide evidence of progression from less to more severe disturbances in eating behavior in a small number of individuals; some normal dieters become pathological dieters, who in turn progress to partial-or full-syndrome eating disorders (Shisslak et al., 1995). Of course, we do not claim that this is the normal course of events; but some evidence suggests that eating disorders often begin with the normal dieting found in a majority of young females (Polivy & Herman, 1987).

Concomitant Psychological Problems

As many as 80% of eating disorder patients exhibit one or more other psychiatric disorders at some point, with major depression being the most common diagnosis (Grilo, 2006). People with eating disorders often engage in obsessive-compulsive behaviors such as calorie counting, body preoccupation, ruminations about food, ritualism, perfectionism, and meticulousness (Kaye, 1997). The lifetime prevalence of obsessive-compulsive disorder has been estimated to be 30% among people with eating disorders (e.g., Hudson, Pope, & Jonas, 1983) but only 2.5 to 3% among the general population. Obsessive-compulsive disorders are three times more common among people with AN than among people with BN (Hudson et al., 1983).

Several other disorders are frequently found in conjunction with eating disorders. Alcohol abuse is commonly found in BN, and anxiety disorders and depression are prevalent in both AN and BN (e.g., Dansky, Brewerton, & Kilpatrick, 2000; Hudson et al., 1983). A follow-up of a large sample of AN patients found that 10 years later, 51% still met criteria for an Axis I psychiatric disorder (especially anxiety disorder), and 23% met the criteria for a personality disorder (most often avoidant-dependent and obsessive-compulsive) (Herpertz-Dahlman et al., 2001).

Axis II personality disorders are frequently observed among people with eating disorders (e.g., Wilfley et al., 2000; Wonderlich, 1995; Wonderlich & Mitchell, 2001). Obsessive-compulsive personality disorder, like obsessive-compulsive disorder, is common in AN. Disorders related to impulsive personality, as well as borderline personality disorders, are more often present in BN and BED (e.g., Wonderlich & Mitchell, 2001). Because malnutrition can exaggerate symptoms of personality disorders, Matsunaga, Kaye, and colleagues (2000) studied individuals who had recovered from eating disorders for at least a year to be certain that the measurement of personality disorders was not distorted by malnutrition and eating disorder symptomatology. They found that 25% of their participants met the criteria for at least one personality disorder.

Prognosis for Eating Disorders

Eating disorders are serious problems. Mortality-rate estimates range from just over 5% (Casper & Jabine, 1996; Herzog, Greenwood, Dorer et al., 2000; Sullivan, 1995) to 8.3% (Steinhausen, Seidel, & Metzke, 2000). A recent longitudinal study confirmed the mortality rate in AN of over 5% per decade (Birmingham, Su, Hlynsky, et al., 2005). Nevertheless, approximately 50 to 60% of patients have a good outcome, with significant reduction of symptoms five years after beginning treatment (Casper & Jabine, 1996; Herpertz-Dahlman et al., 2001; Steinhausen et al., 2000). Unfortunately, about one-third of patients continue to meet diagnostic criteria five years or more after initial treatment (Fairburn, Cooper, Doll, Norman, & O'Connor, 2000; Keel, Mitchell, Miller, Davis, & Crow, 1999). A history of substance-use problems and a longer duration of the disorder at presentation are predictors of worse outcome (Keel et al., 1999). The long-term prognosis for bulimics is generally poor, with about one-third of those assessed remitting each year, but another one-third relapsing each year over five years; those with BED are likely to improve on their own, with only 18% still meeting diagnostic criteria after five years (Fairburn et al., 2000).

Causal Theories of Eating Disorders

Eating disorders are not uniform conditions; there is no single cause or even invariable symptom. The *DSM* definition (using terms such as *refusal* to maintain one's weight, and *fear of fatness*) strongly implies that eating disorders have a psychological foundation, though biological/genetic formulations have been offered. The actual etiology of eating disorders is not really understood as yet, but there seem to be multiple causes and pathways (Grilo, 2006).

Hilde Bruch, one of the first modern theorists to discuss eating disorders, described AN as "a complex condition determined by many simultaneously interacting factors" (1975, p. 159). She was the first to point out that these patients use eating to fulfill a variety of nonnutritional needs. Moreover, despite the characteristic preoccupation with food and eating accompanying eating disorders, patients are "unable to recognize hunger or distinguish it from other states of bodily tension or emotional arousal" (p. 160). Bruch posited that patients interpret all tension states as a "need to eat" instead of identifying the correct source (Bruch, 1975).

Fairburn (e.g., Fairburn, Welch, Doll, Davies, & O'Connor, 1997) hypothesizes that there are two broad classes of risk factors for eating disorders: those enhancing the general risk for psychiatric disorder and those that specifically increase the risk for dieting and eating problems. With respect to exposure to most potential risk factors, BN patients resemble patients with other psychiatric disorders more than they resemble people without diagnosable psychological problems. BN patients, however, show a distinctive pattern of exposure to factors likely to elevate the risk of dieting and negative self-evaluation, supporting the hypothesis that BN is the result of exposure to both general risk factors for psychiatric disorder and specific risk factors for dieting.

The addiction model (Davis & Claridge, 1998; Wilson, 1991) posits an addictive process operating in eating disorders. Conditioned physiological responses to food produce anticipatory secretion of insulin (Booth, 1988; Woods & Brief, 1988), which causes both craving and overeating, if only through increased tolerance to food (e.g., Booth, 1988; Wilson, 1991; Woods & Brief, 1988). Some argue that self-starvation accompanied by excessive exercising reflects an addiction to the body's endogenous opioids (Davis & Claridge, 1998), citing both high scores by AN and BN patients on the Addiction Scale of the Eysenck Personality Questionnaire and correlations between the addiction scale and weight preoccupation and excessive exercising. Wilson, however, dismisses the addiction model for three reasons. First, evidence for an addictive personality is lacking. Second, the model does not address the core clinical characteristics of eating disorders (e.g., the role of dietary restraint and abnormal attitudes about the importance of body shape) or the identified concomitant psychopathology (e.g., extremely low self-esteem, interpersonal distrust, and feelings of ineffectiveness). Third, it fails to account for psychobiological connections between dieting and eating disorders. Wilson notes that bulimic behavior does not meet the criteria for an addictive disorder (i.e., tolerance, physical dependence, or craving), and therefore he sees the addiction model as a conceptual dead end (Wilson, 1991).

Cognitive theories of eating disorders emphasize the biases in people's beliefs, expectancies, and information processing pertaining to body size and eating. Some research has supported predictions derived from these cognitive theories (Williamson, Muller, Reas, & Thaw, 1999). As we shall discuss later, these theories dominate current treatment strategies. Information-processing biases, such as a focus on food and weight to the exclusion of other information, may explain several psychopathological features of AN and BN, including denial, resistance to treatment, and misinterpretation of therapeutic interventions.

Personality factors are also thought to contribute to susceptibility to eating disorders. Some assessment instruments such as the Eating Disorders Inventory (EDI; Garner, Olmsted, & Polivy, 1983) were specifically designed to measure underlying personality dispositions theoretically linked to eating disorders. Investigations using this scale have found that personality factors such as perfectionism, feelings of ineffectiveness (or low self-esteem), reduced interoceptive awareness (or sensitivity to internal signals such as hunger and satiety), and interpersonal distrust are characteristic of those with eating disorders (e.g., Garner, Olmsted, Polivy, & Garfinkel, 1984; Leon, Fulkerson, Perry, & Early-Zald, 1995). Strober (1980) found evidence of obsessive personality traits, extraversion, and need for social approval before the development of the disorder in anorexic adolescents who had returned to normal weight.

A recent investigation took the innovative step of simply asking the patients what caused the emergence of their eating disorder (Nevonen & Broberg, 2000). Interpersonal and weight-related problems were the most commonly reported causes, and dieting or dieting plus purging was the most commonly reported response to these stresses. Thus, interpersonal and weight-related distress, together with dieting behavior, are what people see as responsible for the emergence of their eating disorders. Self-report—in response to oral or written questions—is one of the main sources of data in research on eating disorders; unfortunately, self-report is notoriously unreliable (Nisbett & Wilson, 1977). Eating disorder researchers by and large are too eager to take patients' self-descriptions at face value, if only because such descriptions are easy to elicit. It is not likely that people with eating disorders would be able to identify the source of their disorder with such ease when the research of several decades has not been able to do so. A full understanding of the causes of eating disorders will require more work and more sophisticated research designs than are currently being used.

Sociocultural models suggest that the idealization of thinness and unremitting portrayals of slim role models in the media contribute to widespread body dissatisfaction, which in some susceptible individuals produces pathological dieting and ultimately eating disorders (e.g., Heatherton & Polivy, 1992; Stice, 2001; Striegel-Moore, 1993). Some research (Mills, Polivy, Herman, & Tiggemann, 2002) suggests that exposure to idealized models may promote dieting not by causing body dissatisfaction but rather by inspiring young women to work toward a fantasized, thinner future self. The sociobiological position posits that eating disorders and the societal pursuit of thinness reflect sexual competition among women (Abed, 1998). Thinness may either enhance women's reproductive prospects by making them more attractive to males or, in a contrary version, delay reproduction (by impairing fertility through emaciation) until a more propitious time.

Speculation about the cause(s) of eating disorders has thus gone through many phases over the last three decades, variously favoring biological, familial, and psychosocial factors, which are hypothesized to interact in complex ways to produce the disorders (Ward, Tiller, Treasure, & Russell, 2000). For at least the last decade, the biopsychosocial model, positing an interplay between the organism, its past behavior, and its environment (biological, psychological, and environmental variables) has been the primary explanatory model of eating disorders (e.g., Schlundt & Johnson, 1990). For example, in binge eating, environmental (e.g., situational influences, sociorelationship systems), behavioral (e.g., previous eating or dieting, ongoing activity), cognitive (e.g., knowledge of dieting, expectations, body image), emotional (e.g., mood, psychopathology), and physiological (e.g., blood levels of nutrients, hormones, neurochemicals) antecedents affect behaviors such as binge eating, purging, and dieting, which then themselves have consequences for behavior, cognition, emotion, and physiology.

Risk Factors for Eating Disorders

Current theories of eating disorders—what causes them, why they afflict women, and why there has been such an increase in recent times—thus range widely. The basic question of what goes wrong to produce AN and BN has been addressed at the broad level of sociocultural influences, at the narrow level of familial effects, and at the even narrower level of individual risk factors related to personality, cognition, or physiology (e.g., Leung, Geller, & Katzman, 1996; Polivy & Herman, 2002; Polivy, Herman, Mills, & Wheeler, 2003). One might expect that the research on specific risk factors would be derived from one or another of the causal theories, but such is not the case. The voluminous literature on risk factors is to a great extent independent of and uninformed by the causal theories outlined previously. Whereas some self-report questionnaires (such as the EDI) are based on theoretical models (such as Bruch, 1975), research on risk factors for eating disorders seems to be, for the most part, atheoretical. Many studies in this area merely report correlations among self-report inventories and make no attempt to tie the particular measures chosen to any particular theory of how eating disorders develop. In part, this situation no doubt reflects the difficulty of measuring preclinical pathological processes with paper-and-pencil self-report devices, as well as the problem of operationalizing theoretical constructs. Despite these drawbacks, literally thousands of studies have attempted to specify the risk factors for eating disorders, and numerous chapters and books have addressed these questions. It is crucial to remember, however, that the risk-factor approach is essentially correlational, and that risk factors are really just variables associated with eating disorders, usually in an unspecified fashion. While the reader would no doubt like us to provide an in-depth review of these risk factors here, space limitations permit only a brief overview of prominent research trends examining risk factors associated with eating disorders.

Sociocultural Factors

For several decades, an unrealistically thin body shape has been the cultural ideal for women in Western society. To attain this physique, women have become increasingly likely to diet or exercise (e.g., Polivy & Herman, 1987; Stice, 2001), but are unlikely to succeed in this quest. This societal obsession with a slim female body has been blamed for women's widespread dissatisfaction with their bodies and a concomitant rise in the prevalence of eating disorders (Stice, 2001). These sociocultural pressures have long been targeted as causes (or at least contributors) to eating disorders (e.g., Grilo, 2006; Striegel-Moore, 1993). Girls who participate in sports or professions that emphasize having a slim body such as gymnastics or ballet seem to be more at risk than usual, supporting the view that the sociocultural emphasis on slimness contributes to the disorder (Davison, Earnest, & Birch, 2002). The chief promoters of this sociocultural pressure to be thin are the media, sex-role expectations, and particular economic, racial, and ethnic contexts.

Peer and Media Influences To no one's surprise, it has been shown that adolescents watch more television, read more magazines, and in general appear to attend more to the media than any other age group, and are thus bombarded with messages about thinness and dieting (Polivy & Herman, 2002; Polivy et al., 2003). These messages are directed primarily at girls, who are presented with thin, attractive models, an insistence that thinness will bring success and happiness in all spheres of life (no matter how unrelated to appearance), and a blatant derogation of fat or even normal-weight physiques (Polivy & Herman, 2002; Polivy et al., 2003). Many studies have demonstrated an increase in depression and negative self-image in young women following exposure to thin media images (Dittmar, 2005; Pinhas, Toner, Ali, Garfinkel, & Stuckless, 1999), and those with greater eating disorder symptomatology tend to expose themselves to larger doses of these media images than do most women their age (Stice & Shaw, 1994).

Recent data, however, suggest that it would be premature to blame the media for the increase in eating disorder. Mills et al. (2002) found that looking at pictures of thin models actually made chronic dieters feel thinner and better about themselves, possibly by inspiring them to fantasize about emulating the models. This outcome should not be so surprising—after all, why would women voluntarily buy and read fashion magazines if looking at them induced depression and self-derogation? More to the point, eating disorders have been reliably documented for centuries—of course, without the benefit of 20th-century media exposure. Media idealization of an unrealistically thin female shape may be a contributor to the increased prevalence of eating disorder, but it is clearly not the primary cause. After all, this "cause" is so prevalent in our culture that if it were as important as is sometimes claimed, we would be hard-pressed to explain why fewer than 10% of young women have eating disorders.

Gender "Why women?" and "Why now?" are the two most frequently asked questions about the recent increase in the prevalence of eating disorders (e.g., Polivy et al., 2003; Striegel-Moore, 1993). Around the time that eating disorders began to proliferate, the social role of women was undergoing drastic changes. Instead of enacting the role of homemaker and mother, women were expected to fulfill the "superwoman ideal," requiring them to be smart, beautiful, have a successful career, and still maintain a perfect house, perfect children, and a perfect relationship with the perfect man. The stress of trying to be all things to all people may drive some young women to focus on one thing that they think they can control, their weight. The societal preference for thin female shapes may provide a goal that seems more attainable than becoming a superwoman, or perhaps even a means of becoming a superwoman. This role change may help to explain "Why women?" and "Why now?"

In addition, the pressure to be thin makes women dissatisfied with their bodies. When dissatisfied with their bodies, men tend to turn to healthy eating (Nowak, 1998) and exercise, but women turn to dieting (Drewnowski, Kurth, & Krahn, 1995). Dieting, however, is more likely to produce eating disorder symptomatology than sustained weight loss (e.g., Polivy & Herman, 1993; Stice, 2001). The thin ideal thus produces body dissatisfaction in women, which elicits dieting, which encourages pathological eating. But if this were the whole story, all female adolescents who are unable to achieve thinness (or at least all who diet) would be eating disordered, which is clearly not the case. Therefore we must look further for an explanation.

Binge eating disorder (BED) is radically different from AN and BN in sex distribution, with only a 3:1 ratio of women to men compared to 10:1 and 15:1 for AN and BN, suggesting possible etiological differences for this disorder (Grilo, 2006).

Race, Ethnicity, and Social Class Until around the mid-1980s, eating disorders were restricted primarily to Western, middle- and upper-class, white adolescent females. Now, however, they have penetrated all social classes, races, and even some non-Western venues such as Japan. Although the prevalence is still lower in most nonwhite groups and nonindustrial countries (Polivy et al., 2003), black women in the United States are as likely as are white women to display eating disorder symptoms (Mulholland & Mintz, 2001). In addition, they are quickly becoming comparable to their white counterparts with respect to body-image dissatisfaction (Grant et al., 1999), vomiting, and abuse of laxatives or diuretics, and they are more likely to report binge eating (Striegel-Moore et al., 2000). Among the several potential explanations for the globalization of eating disorders, the most obvious is the influence of the media (Nasser, 1997).

Young minority-group females who are heavier, better educated, and who identify more closely with white, middle-class values have an increased risk of eating disorder. Assimilation into white culture thus carries with it an associated risk of developing eating disorders (Cachelin, Veisel, Barzegarnazari, & Streigel-Moore, 2000). After acculturation, nonwhite women appear to have eating attitudes similar to those of Western whites, although some studies do not find this (e.g., Ogden & Elder, 1998). Black women in predominantly black cultures, however, still seem much less likely to develop eating disorders, with a recent study in Curaçao finding no cases at all in the majority black population (Hoek, van Harten, Hermans et al., 2005).

The expression of eating disorders among nonwhite groups differs in some ways from what is found with white women. Minority women with eating problems are usually truly overweight, whereas white women with disordered eating may only feel overweight, but actually be normal weight (Striegel-Moore et al., 2000). Body dissatisfaction and fear of fatness occur less frequently, if at all, among nonwhite groups, but black adolescents are more likely to binge and use laxatives than are whites, who are more likely to restrict their eating (Striegel-Moore et al., 2000). Black adolescent girls may experience less pressure to conform to the thin ideal plaguing white girls and seem less inclined to derive their self-esteem, identity, and perception of self-control from their weight and appearance (Polivy et al., 2003). When eating disorder symptoms do occur among nonwhites, however, they seem to be related to the same risk factors and precipitants—including low family connectedness, perfectionism, emotional distress, body dissatisfaction, and sometimes serious depression and anxiety (e.g., Davis & Katzman, 1999)—as they are among whites. Mixed race women (in Curaçao) who experienced the identity challenge of being of mixed race and trying to fit into the wealthier white subculture and distance themselves from the black majority, were also particularly likely to develop eating disorders (Katzman, Hermans, Van Hoeken, & Hoek, 2004).

Familial Influences

If societal values and pressures can have enough impact on an individual to constitute a risk factor for the development of an eating disorder, how much more influential are familial interactions? The family can be a source of cultural transmission of pathological values or a stressor on its own (through miscommunication, lack of emotional support, or internal conflict). It can also be a protective factor.

Family influences, such as how the family mediates cultural ideas about thinness and how family members convey these messages to each other, have been implicated as causes of eating disorders (Haworth-Hoeppner, 2000; Laliberte, Boland, & Leichner, 1999; Strober, Freeman, Lampert, Diamond, & Kaye, 2000; Strober & Katz, 1988). A critical family environment, coercive parental control, and a dominating discourse on weight in the household appear to increase the risk of eating disorders (Haworth-Hoeppner, 2000). Even during treatment, family influences are important. For example, mothers' expressed emotion (especially critical comments) predicted an adverse outcome for eating disorder patients (Vanfurth et al., 1996).

Both mothers and fathers contribute to the development of eating disorders. For example, AN patients complain that their mothers do not care about them. Mothers who themselves have an eating disorder transmit pathological behaviors to their daughters by the time the girls are 5 years old. Even when the mothers do not have eating disorders, mothers of daughters with eating disorder symptoms find their daughters less attractive and more in need of weight loss than do mothers whose daughters are asymptomatic. Mothers' comments about weight and shape convey their attitudes and behaviors to their daughters. Daughters of mothers who diet are more likely to do so themselves, and to use more extreme weight-loss techniques if mothers encourage them to or are dissatisfied with their own bodies (Polivy & Herman, 2002; Polivy et al., 2003). Moreover, if either parent is inaccurate in estimating their daughter's body esteem, the daughter is more likely to have greater body dissatisfaction (Geller et al., 2003).

Critical comments and expression of negative emotions by either parent predict both the development of AN and a worse outcome for AN patients. Mothers' complaints about a lack of family cohesion also foretell daughters' increased eating pathology two years later. High parental expectations for achievement that ignore the daughter's needs and goals have also been detected in girls with eating disorders; these extrinsic goals force these girls to struggle to please others at the expense of their own autonomy. Parents of both AN and BN patients appear to discourage autonomy, negating their daughters' needs and self-expression. The patients feel that their parents are overcontrolling in an affectionless manner. The fact that these sorts of parent–adolescent conflicts over autonomy and identity tend to be more intense among girls than among boys may help to explain why eating disorders are so much more common among females than among males (Polivy et al., 2003).

Individual Factors

If sociocultural influences on pathogenesis were very powerful, AN and BN would presumably be more common than they are. In addition, the numerous clear descriptions of AN from at least the middle of the 19th century and possibly earlier suggest that factors other than our current culture cause the disorders. Moreover, although there is some evidence that the disorders may afflict more than one offspring in a family, if the family were responsible for the development of an eating disorder, we would expect to see greater concurrence among the female offspring in a family. Thus, whereas culture and family contribute to the development of eating disorders, they are not sufficient to explain the appearance of a disorder in a given person. In light of the causal models discussed earlier, perhaps we may find the missing piece of the puzzle in factors specific to the individual, such as biological, identity, personality, or cognitive determinants.

Genetic and Physiological Factors The reasonably stereotypic and reliable clinical presentation of AN and BN, with a consistent sex distribution and age of onset, suggests a biological substrate for the disorders. Twin studies, family studies, and recent molecular-genetic findings point to a potential genetic factor (e.g., Klump, & Gobrogge, 2005), especially for AN. Females with a first-degree relative who has an eating disorder are two to three times more likely to develop one themselves (Polivy et al., 2003). Recent research has attempted to link specific genes to specific eating disorders, suggesting that AN may be linked to a different gene from the one that influences BN (Grilo, 2006: Tozzi & Bulik, 2003).

A genetic predisposition to eating disorder may operate through faults in neurotransmitters, of which serotonin is the most frequently studied, possibly because it inhibits feeding, stimulus reactivity, and sexual activity. A disturbance of serotonergic activity is consistent with descriptions of anorectic patients as constrained, perfectionistic, and needing order even after weight restoration (Kaye, Weltzin, & Hsu, 1993). Moreover, anorexics who have returned to normal weight still have elevated levels of brain serotonin metabolites. Women who develop AN might have intrinsic vulnerabilities for perfectionistic, anxious, and obsessional behavior as a result of elevated serotonin levels, and these tendencies could become increasingly dysfunctional as a result of stress or other psychosocial stimuli (Kaye et al., 1993). Most recently, research has begun to examine genetic contributions to these personality traits (perfectionism, obsessiveness, rigidity, fearfulness) thought to underlie and contribute to the disorders, finding these temperamental differences in the families of patients (Grilo, 2006). New molecular genetics findings support these temperamental effects, and find differences in the underlying biological vulnerabilities of AN and BN patients (Collier & Treasure, 2004).

Patients with BN show signs of serotonin dysregulation and this may contribute to their symptoms, including binge eating (Steiger et al., 2001; Wolfe, Metzger, & Jimerson, 1997). Serotonin may be associated with impulsivity, which may relate to the binge eating behavior and other impulsive behaviors exhibited by BN patients (Steiger et al., 2001). Because the evidence for the influence of elevated serotonin on eating disorders is strictly correlational, it is not possible to conclude that elevated serotonin causes eating disorder. Indeed, it may instead be a consequence of the disorder.

Hormonal changes associated with puberty may also increase susceptibility to eating disorder. Puberty in females is accompanied by increased body fat and a drastically different body shape—the curves that develop in pubescent girls definitely subvert the thin ideal to which girls aspire. This new, curvy shape may give rise to the increased body dissatisfaction and accompanying dieting that become normative in adolescent females and that are themselves potential risk factors for eating disorders (e.g., Polivy et al., 2003; Striegel-Moore, 1993). At the same time, hormonal development pushes girls into heterosexual interactions, which girls appear to find more stressful than do boys (Striegel-Moore, 1993). Those who undergo early puberty seem to be particularly at risk for developing an eating disorder.

Finally, developmental physical factors such as premature birth or birth trauma, being born between April and June, early childhood eating or digestive problems, having a high premorbid BMI, and experiencing childhood sexual or physical abuse or neglect all seem to increase the risk of developing an eating disorder (Touyz, Polivy, & Hay, 2008).

Self-Esteem and Identity Among dieters who do not have eating disorders, depression scores are elevated and self-esteem scores are reduced; these scores are even more extreme among those with eating disorders (e.g., Polivy & Herman, 2002; Polivy et al., 2003), as they are in certain other psychological syndromes. Negative emotions are linked to disruptive eating behaviors, in a cyclic or spiral pattern (e.g., Polivy et al., 2003). Negative self-evaluation is possibly the most ubiquitous risk factor among eating disorder patients (Fairburn, Cooper, Doll, & Welch, 1999; Grilo, 2006); feelings of ineffectiveness and lack of a strong sense of self were recognized as hallmarks of eating disorders as early as the 1970s (e.g., Bruch, 1975). The lower self-esteem among those with eating disorders also seems to be connected to a lack of a cohesive identity and distrust of one's body's ability to function on its own, both of which appear to be distinctively related to eating disorders.

The low self-esteem of those with eating disorders may reflect negative life experiences such as sexual or emotional abuse, which may also interfere with formation of a stable identity. Constructing an identity based on eating, weight, and shape may mask more basic problems with one's sense of self and create a sense of control that is otherwise lacking (Polivy & Herman, 2002; Polivy & Herman, in press). Threats to a precarious identity may exacerbate eating problems. For example, chronic dieters (restrained eaters), who resemble eating disorder patients in many ways, have been studied in the laboratory to learn about processes in eating disorder. Restrained eaters exposed to false feedback (from an inaccurate scale) indicating that they have gained weight react by overeating (McFarlane, Polivy, & Herman, 1998). Similarly, when allowed to eat after reporting about ways in which they have failed to meet their life goals, restrained eaters responded by overeating (Wheeler, Polivy, & Herman, 2002). Threats to one's identity seem to elicit disordered eating behavior (Polivy & Herman, in press).

Body Dissatisfaction and Dieting The negative self-perception and low self-esteem characterizing eating disorders crystallize in negative feelings about one's body and an investment in improving it as a means of self-redemption (Polivy & Herman, 2002, 2007). Body dissatisfaction is a diagnostic criterion for eating disorder, according to the *DSM–IV* (1994). Stice's dual-pathway model (e.g., Stice, 2001) posits that it is the thin ideal that produces body image dissatisfaction, which then produces dieting, and eventually eating disorder symptomatology. Adolescent girls do have greater body dissatisfaction than do boys or older women, and those who place more emphasis on their bodies and are more dissatisfied with them tend to exhibit greater eating pathology (Dittmar, 2005; Polivy et al., 2003). Moreover, dieting has been implicated as a cause of binge eating and is thought to be a primary contributor to the "dieting disorders," as eating disorders are often called (Polivy & Herman, 2002). But if all the girls who embraced the thin ideal, dieted, and were dissatisfied with their bodies became eating disordered, much of the adolescent female population would be incapacitated! Thus, although most models of eating disorder include a role for body dissatisfaction and dieting, it is clear that these risk factors must interact with other factors such as extremely low self-esteem and identity deficiencies, other personality factors, and the familial and cultural issues discussed earlier.

Personality Factors Those with eating disorders exhibit a consistent pattern of personality traits before, during, and after the disordered eating phase. Converging evidence from clinical reports, psychometric studies, and family or collateral sources presents the premorbid (i.e., before the onset of the disorder) personality of AN patients as perfectionistic, obsessive, socially inhibited, compliant, and emotionally restrained or fearful (e.g., Grilo, 2006; Wonderlich, 1995). Bulimics are not only compliant and perfectionistic, but also tend to be impulsive, emotional, lacking in interoceptive awareness, and extraverted (e.g., Lilenfeld et al., 2000; Steiger et al., 2001). Perfectionism and negative self-evaluation characterize AN and BN patients before, during, and after recovery from the disorder (Fairburn et al., 1999). Negative affect, behavioral inhibition, and obsessiveness also continue after recovery from AN (Kaye, Gendall, & Strober, 1998). Moreover, perfectionism, ineffectiveness, and interpersonal distrust are found in family members of eating disorder patients who do not themselves show symptoms of eating disorders (Lilenfeld et al., 2000). There are thus a number of personality traits linked to eating disorders. Although the evidence is correlational, the persistence of such traits before and after the disorder and their presence in nondisordered family members suggest that they could interact with adverse familial and social experiences and render an individual more likely to develop an eating disorder (e.g., Lilenfeld et al., 2000; Strober & Humphrey, 1987).

Cognitive Factors People with eating disorders display several cognitive aberrations such as obsessive thoughts, distortions of attention and memory (reflecting a focus on food, weight, and shape), and rigid, all-or-nothing thinking (Polivy & Herman, 2002). Obsessing about weight and shape, and using these characteristics to determine one's self-worth, are central (and defining) features of eating disorders. The tendency to see the world through weight and shape schemata, which affect attention and memory, reflects an obsessive preoccupation with these issues. Experimental techniques such as the Stroop color-naming task demonstrate biased attention to weight and shape in eating disorder patients. All-or-nothing, black-and-white thinking makes them see themselves as failures if they eat so much as one bite of a "forbidden" food, and may promote binges in BN patients (Polivy & Herman, 2002). The prominent role of cognitive features in eating disorder has encouraged the use of cognitive therapies (see later) to normalize the cognitions that are presumed to underlie the eating disorder.

Combining Risk Factors

Because risk factor research is of necessity correlational, it cannot determine cause and effect. Furthermore, no single risk factor alone is capable of producing an eating disorder, and it would be simplistic to suppose that a disorder as complex as eating disorders would have a single cause. In 1987, Johnson and Connors proposed a biopsychosocial model of eating disorder development. This model posits that biological predispositions (from genetic, hormonal, and pubertal influences), family factors, and cultural pressures to be thin and to fulfill a demanding social role interact to produce an identity-conflicted, vulnerable dieter. Those dieters with low self-esteem and affective instability are most susceptible to an eating disordered identity, particularly in response to stress or failure. Striegel-Moore (1993) has suggested that the number of simultaneous life challenges faced by an individual is related to her susceptibility to eating disorder. Girls who mature early and begin dating at the same time report more disturbed attitudes about eating and shape. Striegel-Moore also posits that early maturation is a source of adjustment difficulties, which, along with body dissatisfaction, dieting, and conflict with parents is sufficiently stressful to increase risk for an eating disorder. A related theory proposes that the many transitions that occur in adolescence (e.g., moving to junior high or high school, puberty, dating, disruptions in friendships, increased academic and sex role demands) and the restructuring of personality and behavior demanded by these transitions may overwhelm an adolescent who is already vulnerable because of familial or personal problems (e.g., Smolak & Levine, 1996).

The combination of (1) the contextual background of sociocultural expectations to look and act a certain way; (2) familial interaction patterns that negate the individual's attempts to achieve autonomy; (3) individual vulnerabilities based on genetics and personality, self-esteem, and identity deficit; and (4) the stresses required by transitional adjustments offers a potential starting point for identifying individuals most likely to develop an eating disorder. Although these combinatory models attempt to incorporate the complexity of eating disorders and the many identified risk factors, they have not yet provided predictive power sufficient to identify individuals most likely to succumb to the pressures and develop eating disorders (e.g., Jacobi, Haywood, de Zwaan et al., 2004, for a review).

Treatment of Eating Disorders

Although the causes of eating disorders remain obscure, clinicians must nevertheless treat them. Here we review the basic rationale and techniques of the major therapies used in the treatment of eating disorder. We start with treatments targeting the most focal eating disorder symptoms and then discuss treatments that modify symptoms indirectly, by altering other internal or external processes. Next, we review the empirical literature on therapeutic efficacy. Finally, we discuss the factors contributing to relapse.

Cognitive-Behavioral Therapy

The most widely used and presumably most effective therapeutic technique for treating eating disorders continues to be cognitive-behavior therapy. The basic ideas underlying this therapy were initially described by Beck and his colleagues, who applied them to depression (see Beck, Rush, Shaw, & Emery, 1979, for a review). Soon thereafter, it was modified and extended to the treatment of the eating disorders. In 1981, Fairburn was the first to outline a cognitive-behavioral approach to the management of BN, and in 1982 Garner and Bemis applied cognitive behavior therapy to AN. Inevitably, this treatment has now been proposed for use with BED (e.g., Wilson & Fairburn, 2000). Although identifying, modifying, and replacing maladaptive thoughts and behaviors are central to therapy in all of these cases, the distinctive symptomatology of each disorder means that treatment must be adapted accordingly, although Fairburn and colleagues have argued recently that treatment should be "transdiagnostic" as the eating disorders share more characteristics than they differ on (Fairburn, Cooper, & Shaffran, 2003).

Cognitive-Behavior Therapy for AN The rationale for the use of cognitive-behavior therapy for AN is that irrational and recalcitrant beliefs about the importance of body weight and shape support relentlessly pursued maladaptive behavior (especially weight loss). That these patients also suffer from deficiencies of identity and self-worth makes treatment even more difficult. Cognitive-behavior therapy for AN focuses both on specific symptoms and on underlying difficulties. According to Vitousek (1995), this therapy for AN targets four main areas. The first is the ego-syntonic nature of the disorder (i.e., seeing the disorder as positive or desirable); because individuals with AN prize slenderness, they must first acknowledge that the pursuit of slimness has a negative impact on their lives. Vitousek proposes asking the client to list both the positive and negative aspects of her anorexia; in turn, "each claimed advantage and disadvantage is cast as a hypothesis that can be examined for its validity and adaptiveness" (1995, p. 326), an exercise effectively constituting the first steps toward modifying cognitions. The second focus involves setting behavioral goals for normalized eating and weight gain and implementing cognitive coping strategies to deal with these changes. For instance, the myth that certain "forbidden" foods cause drastic weight gain may be debunked by having patients try these foods in controlled exposures. The third, related focus of treatment is modifying beliefs about weight and food. Clients are taught to challenge their self-defeating thoughts by learning to examine them rationally and replace them with more realistic possibilities (e.g., "there are no forbidden foods per se; it is excess caloric intake that leads to weight gain"). Once these most urgent aspects of the disorder have been addressed, treatment can then focus on the underlying self-concept issues that may be maintaining the disorder; ideally, other more attainable and adaptive goals may be identified to replace slenderness as the basis of identity.

In contrast to this traditional approach incorporating general issues such as self-esteem, Fairburn, Shafran, and Cooper (1998) have proposed a more focused cognitive-behavioral program for AN, targeting the patient's need for control and the attempt to attain this control through dieting. Treatment involves helping the client to achieve success and fulfillment from pursuits unrelated to weight and shape. They suggest that this streamlined treatment should be used first and broadened only if other issues prove to be obstacles to change (Fairburn et al., 1998).

Cognitive-Behavior Therapy for BN Because BN is less ego-syntonic (i.e., acceptable to one's self-image) than is AN—the binge–purge cycle is often extremely distressing to the individual—cognitive behavior therapy for BN has a narrower focus, typically limited to eating behavior and thoughts about food, weight, and shape. Thus, as in AN, BN clients are taught to establish a normalized eating pattern consisting of regularly scheduled meals. (Skipping meals is avoided to prevent the extreme hunger that may foster a binge.) In addition, clients work on the reduction or elimination of bingeing and purging (through behavioral contracts with the therapist) and the development of coping techniques to prevent binges and associated compensatory behaviors. They are taught to identify the usual precipitants to bingeing (often with the help of a daily food diary), and to use distraction techniques (alternatives to binges such as taking a walk, calling a supportive friend, or delaying eating) or coping mechanisms (such as self-talk). Compensatory behaviors after lapses—such as purging, laxative use, excessive exercise or dietary restraint—are discouraged, in an attempt to break the binge–purge cycle; this technique is akin to the behavioral technique of exposure with response prevention. Finally, as with AN, excessive concern with body weight and shape is challenged through cognitive restructuring (e.g., Wilson, 1996, 1999).

Cognitive-Behavior Therapy for BED Because BED involves bingeing without purging or any other form of compensatory behavior, individuals with BED are more often overweight than are those with BN. Thus, behavioral weight-loss strategies (e.g., an exercise plan) may be required, and the individual's societally induced prejudices against overweight must be eliminated in addition to merely challenging the importance of slenderness. It has been suggested (Wilson & Fairburn, 2000) that "the treatment of choice [for BED] would appear to be cognitive behavioral self-help"(p. 352). Indeed, no difference in outcome between therapist-led versus self-help format cognitive-behavior therapy has been found, and there were significant improvements over wait-list controls in the latter, suggesting that it may be a cost-effective, accessible alternative for patients with BED (Loeb, Wilson, Gilbert, & Labouvie, 2000).

It should be noted that these descriptions of cognitive-behavior therapy for eating disorders reflect either how it is carried out in experimental tests or in the ideal clinical setting, neither of which necessarily corresponds to clinical reality. Individual clinicians often tailor the technique as they see fit for individual clients, or they may combine cognitive-behavior therapy with other treatment strategies in an eclectic treatment plan.

Nutritional Counseling and Psychoeducation

As its name implies, nutritional or dietary counseling involves educating the patient about normal caloric needs and physiological processes. Kahm (1994) explained that while people with eating disorders may have a wealth of knowledge regarding the calorie content of most foods, this knowledge is usually used to achieve drastic weight loss rather than to maintain a healthy body. In fact, Beumont and Touyz (1995) suggested that failing to address nutritional issues in eating disorders "is as ridiculous as prohibiting the discussion of drinking behavior with patients with alcohol related disease"(p. 306). They also stated that this therapy is intended to change attitudes about food and eating, and then eating behavior, by arming people with accurate knowledge.

Psychoeducation provides accurate nutritional information, but also educates patients about the nature of their disorder. Olmsted and Kaplan (1995) advocated addressing four main topics beyond dietary information: the complex etiology of eating disorders, the often serious medical consequences of severe food restriction or continual bingeing and vomiting, the sociocultural idealization of the thin female body, and cognitive and behavioral strategies that one may use to modify eating problems. Although nutritional counseling and psychoeducation are rarely used as stand-alone therapies, Olmsted and Kaplan claimed that educational information is incorporated in up to 75% of studies of treatment for BN.

Motivational Interviewing

Because CBT involves modifying problematic thoughts and behaviors related to eating disorder pathology, it is often considered an "action-oriented" approach; that is, individuals participating in

CBT are asked to take action, often within the first several weeks of initiating treatment, to challenge their beliefs and change their eating disordered behavior. However, individuals with eating disorders often harbor a great deal of ambivalence about overcoming their symptoms, and as a result, may be reluctant to engage in action-oriented treatment. Motivational Interviewing (MI; Miller & Rollnick, 2002), is an approach to treatment that acknowledges fluctuations in motivation and readiness for change; as opposed to persuading an individual to change and highlighting the problematic aspects of symptoms, the therapist's task is to collaboratively explore and resolve ambivalence. MI is based on the transtheoretical model (TTM) of change (Prochaska & DiClemente, 1992), which describes the process of behavioral change with reference to five "stages": precontemplation (denial of problem existence), contemplation (acknowledgment of problem and plan to change in next six months), preparation (intending to change within the next month and preparing to take action), action (initiating behavioral change), and maintenance (sustaining change). Although the theory is reviewed extensively elsewhere (Prochaska & DiClemente 1992 for a review), TTM posits that these stages are universal, nonlinear, and cyclical: that is, individuals are presumed to possess fluctuating insight into and motivation to change problem behaviors, and may relapse often before achieving sustained behavioral modification.

Research has now begun on the use of motivational interviewing, or motivational enhancement therapy (MET), with individuals who have eating disorders (Wilson & Schlam, 2004 for a review; Killick & Allen, 1997 for BN; Treasure & Ward, 1997 for AN). A handful of small-N studies suggest its potential utility with this population. Feld, Woodside, Kaplan, Olmsted, and Carter (2000) described the use of a four session, group-based MET program conducted prior to the initiation of CBT, during which individuals (N = 19) were encouraged to examine the costs and benefits of their eating disorder and its consistency with their values, among other topics. Results showed that compared with patients' own baseline levels, group participation resulted in increased motivation, confidence, and readiness to change (but did not affect eating disorder symptoms). Similarly, individuals with refractory anorexia (N = 8) who participated in an MET program for five hours a day, twice a week over six months displayed increased motivation for change, representing a shift from "early" to "late" contemplation (George, Thornton, Touyz, Waller, & Beumont, 2004). However, these studies did not employ control groups, did not examine the effect of participating in MET on subsequent outcome during CBT or other action-based treatment, and may have tested patients who represented a self-selected subset at an already more advanced stage of change than other individuals with treatment-refractory symptoms.

It is important to note that MET is not intended as a standalone treatment approach, but rather as a potentially useful precursor or adjunct to other more action-oriented approaches. Because MET maintains a focus on an individual's readiness for change, actual symptom change is not an intended outcome of this intervention. Therefore, successful outcomes following MET presume that the individual will move on to implement the changes she has decided are appropriate. Further, although MET finds a natural niche among individuals whose symptoms are recalcitrant, its applicability does have limits. For instance, if an individual is medically compromised due to severe or very rapid weight loss (Killick & Allen, 1997), respect for her ambivalence will necessarily be weighed against the potential consequences of inaction.

Interpersonal Therapy

In contrast to psychoeducation and cognitive-behavioral therapy, which are entirely focused on weight-related behaviors and, in the latter case, cognitions, interpersonal therapy does not touch on these issues in the treatment of eating disorders. Instead, it targets maladaptive personal relationships and relational styles because difficulties in these areas are seen as contributing to the development and maintenance of eating disorders (Birchall, 1999). Thus, the fundamental task of the interpersonal therapist is to identify one of Birchall's "problem areas—Grief, Role Transitions, Interpersonal Role

Disputes (or) Interpersonal Deficits" (p. 315), and to work to improve the client's functioning in that area. Improved interpersonal relationships might reduce eating disorder symptoms in a number of ways. Enhanced control in relationships may generalize to enhanced control of eating in BN or BED. Furthermore, interpersonal therapy may reduce or eliminate common interpersonal triggers to binge-ing. For example, depressed mood and interpersonal stress may be alleviated, and more frequent, positive social interactions may reduce boredom. Decreasing interpersonal stress may also improve anorectic behavior by providing a greater sense of control in areas of one's life other than eating. Despite the fact that CBT is considered the gold standard treatment for eating disorders, some authors (e.g., Tantleff-Dunn, Gokee-LaRose, & Peterson, 2004) view IPT as a viable alternative first-line treatment due to its conceptual similarities with etiological theories of the development of these disorders.

Dialectical Behavior Therapy

Dialectical behavior therapy (DBT; Linehan, 1993) was developed to treat borderline personality disorder and is now being considered in the treatment of eating disorder symptoms that have been refractory to first-line treatments (such as CBT). DBT encourages commitment to and enactment of behavioral change while validating individuals' emotions and treatment ambivalence, with a specific focus on building skills in emotional recognition and regulation. McCabe and Marcus (2002) suggest that DBT has the potential to be effective in the treatment of anorexia nervosa through its concep-tualization of eating disorder symptoms as maladaptive emotional avoidance or regulation strategies that can be improved by increasing commitment to change and building the requisite skills to do so; although clinical experience suggests this may be the case, further empirical evidence is required to support this conclusion. Safer, Telch and Agras (2001) found that patients with BN showed significantly fewer binge/purge episodes following 20 weeks of DBT as compared to those in the wait-list condi-tion, though no other significant improvements were noted. Similarly, DBT appears to be effective in reducing binge eating among individuals with BED (e.g., Telch, Agras, & Linehan, 2000, 2001), but ineffective in producing similar gains on other indices of recovery (such as weight, mood, and affect regulation). Given these preliminary findings, it appears that DBT may be a useful option for those with treatment refractory symptoms, in particular among individuals for whom affect dysregulation is prominent (i.e., those with comorbid borderline personality disorder; e.g., Palmer et al., 2003).

Family Therapy

Family therapy focuses on interpersonal relationships, emphasizing the importance of stresses within the family as a whole rather than on individuals. It postulates that change by one member affects every other member in turn (Minuchin, Rosman, & Baker, 1978; Thode, 1990). The eating disorder patient is seen in conjunction with her parents and siblings (or with her spouse and children, as the case may be), and the goal becomes that of reducing family stressors and miscommunications to bring about a reduction in eating disorder symptoms. Thus, family therapy places responsibility for recovery on both the patient and her relatives. Geist, Heinmaa, Stephens, Davis, and Katzman's (2000) description of treatment provides a good example of the specific content of family therapy: (1) recruiting parents to actively engage in managing the patient's weight gain and eating; (2) ameliorating maladaptive communication within the family and particularly between the parents; and (3) elucidating the difference between normal methods of coping with family conflict and the symptoms the patient is currently exhibiting.

Psychoanalytic Therapy

Psychoanalytic or psychodynamic therapy may encompass a wide variety of specific techniques or foci. Herzog (1995) defines it broadly as "all long-term therapies that explicitly use the relationship between the patient and therapist as the primary treatment tool and that attend to transference and countertransference reactions" (p. 330). This therapy assumes that eating disorder symptoms are merely the overt pathological manifestations of underlying conflicts that the client has been unable to resolve adaptively. The psychoanalyst's task is to determine the unique meanings of these symptoms for each client. Many theorists suggest that establishing a strong therapeutic alliance is the first (and perhaps most crucial) step (Gonzalez, 1988; Herzog, 1995). Establishing such an alliance may be particularly difficult and take longer in AN, because the patient will perceive the therapist as someone who wants her to give up her ego-syntonic dietary restriction. Once trust has developed, the psychoanalyst establishes a neutral stance toward the patient, who then free associates: "the hope is that the patients will project upon this 'blank screen' their characteristic thoughts and behaviors (transference)" (Johnson, 1995, p. 351). Much of therapy is then devoted to analyzing these transference reactions in the context of a thorough developmental history. Another strategy used in identifying the roots of the eating disorder is the analysis of dreams to determine their symbolic meaning. The countertransference relationship also constitutes an important source of information about the client; therapists interpret their own reactions to the client to further elucidate the quality of the client's interpersonal relationships. A nonjudgmental relationship between the therapist and client is said to serve a further purpose, providing the patient with an opportunity to relate appropriately on an interpersonal level, allowing the patient to resolve dependent or otherwise pathological relations with others (Herzog, 1995).

Contemporary psychoanalytic writers acknowledge that psychoanalysis may not be appropriate for all eating disorder patients. Herzog (1995) maintains that the treatment is appropriate for those patients presenting with character pathology; both Herzog and Johnson recommend psychoanalysis for prior-treatment nonresponders (i.e., for those patients whose symptoms linger after a course of cognitive or interpersonal therapy). Finally, Gonzalez (1988) cautions against using psychoanalysis for suicidal patients or for those whose extremely low weight makes hospitalization necessary; in these cases, the long-term focus of psychoanalysis would leave the patient at immediate risk of harm.

Pharmacotherapy

Pharmacotherapy departs significantly from other treatments by postulating some sort of organic cause for the disorder—or at least that the symptoms can be controlled pharmacologically—and attempting to treat symptoms accordingly, with drugs. By far the most common drugs are tricyclic antidepressants and selective serotonin reuptake inhibitors (SSRIs). Their use is based on the fact that depressive symptoms are prominent in both AN and BN and that some symptoms of both of these disorders resemble the clinical features of other disorders that respond favorably to these medications (e.g., Kruger & Kennedy, 2000; Mayer & Walsh, 1998). Other drugs that have been tried include antipsychotics (to treat the delusionlike obsessions with weight and shape), anxiolytics (to target the anxiety associated with eating disordered behavior and weight restoration in AN), mood stabilizers such as lithium (which may promote weight gain in AN and regulate affective lability in BN), and antiserotonergics (assumed to increase food intake and lead to weight gain in AN as it does in general medical usage; Carter et al., 2003 (for BED); Kruger & Kennedy, 2000, for a review).

Efficacy of Treatment

With a few exceptions (such as pharmacotherapy for AN), the efficacy of most of these treatments has been empirically validated; that is, they have been shown to lead to statistically significant improvements when compared to placebo or wait-list controls. We are left with the more interesting and useful question of which treatments are relatively more useful in treating eating disorders.

Treatment Recommendations for AN Because of its low prevalence and its additional medical complications, there are significantly fewer controlled treatment trials for AN than there are for BN and

BED. Furthermore, very few studies directly compare various forms of treatment for AN, making differences in efficacy somewhat difficult to gauge. Despite these limitations, there is a tenuous consensus that family therapy is the first-line treatment for most cases of AN (e.g., Wilson, 1999). On the basis of three available controlled trials of family therapy with AN, Russell, Dare, Eisler, and Le Grange (1992) concluded that family therapy is effective for anorectics with early onset (before age 18). It may be particularly effective for adolescents because they tend to express greater denial and less desire for help (Fisher, Schneider, Burns, Symons, & Mandel, 2001), making family involvement potentially more important. Most researchers (Kruger & Kennedy, 2000; Mayer & Walsh, 1998) recommend against the use of drugs in the acute treatment of AN, but some (e.g., Kaye et al., 1998) are now postulating a place for SSRIs in the maintenance of treatment gains. Psychoanalysis for AN has not been well studied, but Herzog (1995) stated that patients often require a minimum of 1 to 2 years of psychoanalysis, and maybe as much as 8 to 10 years for improvement to take place. A recently published long-term outcome study (Steinhausen et al., 2000) found that 80% of surviving AN patients recovered at 11-year follow-up regardless of the type of therapy received. In light of this finding, it is difficult to make a case for the use of long-term psychoanalysis in the treatment of AN. Further research is required to determine the efficacy of cognitive-behavior therapy for AN. Inpatient treatment of anorexia, which often involves a variety of therapeutic strategies (including medical monitoring, pharmacotherapy, nutritional supplementation, or normalization of eating for weight restoration, and group-based psychosocial programming) is an option for those individuals with very low body weight or intractable symptoms. Results of a prospective study (Ro, Martinsen, Hoffart, & Rosenvinge, 2004), which followed 24 patients who had completed a 23-week inpatient treatment program, showed that long-term outcome was poor (with 58% of patients showing no significant improvement), and that all observed improvements occurred during the acute treatment phase, with no significant improvements noted from discharge to follow-up. This speaks not only to the treatment resistance of this disorder (particularly among the subset of individuals whose symptoms become severe enough to warrant hospital admission), but also to the need for a long-term approach to treatment that focuses on maintenance of gains and relapse prevention (see below).

Treatment Recommendations for BN Cognitive-behavior therapy is often considered the treatment of choice for BN (e.g., Wilson, 1996, 1999); it leads to reduction or remission of bingeing and purging in 50% of patients and improvements in dietary restraint, attitudes toward shape and weight, and associated psychopathology (Wilson, 1996). However, interpersonal therapy may be a suitable alternative; most studies comparing the two find them to be equally effective by the end of treatment and at follow-up, although cognitive-behavior therapy is faster-acting in the beginning (Birchall, 1999; Fairburn, Norman et al., 1995).

The efficacy of these first-line treatments is still somewhat limited (recall that only 50% of BN patients cease or significantly decrease binge eating and purging), so it is important to be aware of viable alternatives. Antidepressants are superior to placebos in reducing bingeing and purging (e.g., Goldstein, Wilson, Thompson, Potvin, & Rampey, 1995). On the other hand, a review of six controlled studies (Wilson, 1996) found cognitive-behavior therapy on its own to be superior to antidepressant drugs alone; moreover, cognitive-behavior therapy plus drugs was better than drugs alone, but no more effective than therapy alone or cognitive-behavior therapy plus placebo. Pharmacotherapy thus may not be a viable second choice if psychotherapy fails.

Family therapy for BN has not been well studied, though Dare and Eisler (2000) reported encouraging preliminary findings for their multifamily treatment program for adolescents with BN. Similarly, outcome data for psychodynamic treatment of BN are scarce, leading Johnson (1995) to recommend this approach only for those patients who do not respond to briefer forms of therapy.

Treatment Recommendations for BED Since 2003, there has been a dramatic increase in research on the treatment of BED, focusing primarily on cognitive-behavior therapy, interpersonal therapy, pharmacotherapy, and, given the disproportionate number of obese individuals with BED (45% among the obese vs. 2 to 3% in the general population; Carter & Pindynck, 2003), weight-loss treatments. Cognitive-behavior therapy seems to be effective in reducing the behavioral and psychological features of BED (i.e., binge eating episodes and psychological distress), but not in reducing obesity (e.g., Grilo, Masheb & Wilson, 2005; Loeb et al., 2000; Wilson & Fairburn, 2000). Interpersonal therapy has been shown to be as effective as cognitive-behavior therapy in reducing binges (and as ineffective at producing weight loss), and the rate of improvement for BED (unlike AN) is equal in both therapies (Tasca, Ritchie, Conrad, Balfour, Gayton et al., 2006; Wilfley, Welch, Stein, Spurrell, Cohen et al., 2002; Wilson & Fairburn, 2000). In contrast, certain modes of pharmacotherapy have shown some promise in reducing not only binges but also weight. Many drugs, from appetite suppressants to antidepressants, and more recently, anticonvulsants, have demonstrated efficacy in reducing binge eating (e.g., Shapira, Goldsmith, & McElroy, 2000, for appetite suppressants; McElroy, Hudson et al., 2003; McElroy et al., 2000 for antidepressants; McElroy, Shapira et al., 2004, for anticonvulsants). Although tricyclic antidepressants are not effective for weight loss, SSRIs are well tolerated and do appear to produce weight loss among patients with BED (Appolinaro et al., 2003; Hudson, Carter & Pope, 1996), as does the augmentation of CBT with obesity medications (such as orlistat, a lipase inhibitor; Grilo et al., 2005). An important caveat is that this weight loss is modest at best (e.g., responder status was defined as a 5% weight loss from baseline by Grilo et al., 2005) and often does not seem to be maintained (e.g., Devlin, Goldfein, Carino, & Wolk, 2000). There now appears to be preliminary evidence supporting the use of anticonvulsants in the treatment of BED. Initial trials of the anticonvulsants topiramate (McElroy et al., 2004; McElroy, Arnold, et al., 2003) and zonisamide (McElroy, Kotwal, Hudson, Nelson, & Keck, 2004) resulted in significant decreases in binge eating episodes and body weight; however, these medications also appear to be associated with a high discontinuation rate as a result of adverse events and nonadherence (McElroy, Kotwal, et al., 2004), and we are not aware of any studies to date that have compared anticonvulsants to other pharmacotherapies or psychotherapies. Bellini and Merli (2004) conducted a review of pharmacotherapy studies for BN and BED, and concluded that SSRIs should be considered the first line treatment choice due to their acceptability, patients' ability to tolerate them, and their overall efficacy (though they note that long term outcomes are still lacking). Anticonvulsants such as topiramate should be considered for SSRI nonresponders, for individuals with co-occurring bipolar disorder (due to their putative mood stabilizing effects), and for individuals whose obesity poses a threat of medical morbidity (Carter & Pindynck, 2003; Marx, Kotwal, McElroy, & Malhorta, 2003). Although obesity medications have shown preliminary evidence of utility as an augmentation to CBT, further research is required to determine their utility as a monotherapy for BED. Finally, behavioral weight-loss therapy has been suggested in the treatment of BED. One study found that although this was superior to weight-loss treatment in reducing binges in the short term (12 weeks), the difference disappeared at follow-up (Agras et al., 1994). Research suggests that neither cognitive-behavior therapy (Agras et al., 1994; de Zwaan, Mitchell, Crosby, Mussell, Raymond et al., 2005) nor desipramine, a tricyclic antidepressant (Agras et al., 1994) added to the efficacy of the behavioral weight-loss programs in decreasing weight, binge eating, and other psychopathology in the long-term. Interestingly, de Zwaan et al. (2005) found that the Very-Low-Calorie Diet program was equal to CBT and pharmacotherapy in reducing binge eating. Levine, Marcus, and Moulton (1996) found that 81% of women given an exercise-and-diet program were abstinent from bingeing at posttreatment, a significant improvement over those in a delayed-treatment control condition. This finding suggests that incorporating exercise in treatment for BED may assist in the remission of binge eating.

Conclusions about Treatment of Eating Disorders

Despite our poor understanding of the development of eating disorders, research into their treatment has made some progress. However, controlled trials comparing treatments may not reflect clinical reality, where therapists may sample from the available therapies and tailor treatments to specific clients. For instance, individual cognitive-behavior therapy might be paired with administration of drugs to help patients with BN, or interpersonal and family therapy might be bolstered with psychoeducation in the treatment of AN. These so-called multifaceted treatments (see Lansky & Levitt, 1992, for a review) may provide the best form of care, because the components of one therapy may enhance the effects of another or provide additional benefits beyond those available in the empirically established first-line treatment. Still, individually tailored treatments are difficult to evaluate systematically; although such tailoring makes some sense, it also makes it difficult for researchers to evaluate treatment efficacy.

Relapse

Defining relapse is difficult. A search of the literature on relapse in eating disorders yields a heterogeneous group of studies, none of which adequately define *relapse*. Theoretically, relapse signifies a return to disordered functioning following a period of symptom amelioration. Pike (1998) attempted to define relapse relative to initial treatment response, remission, and recovery. An initial satisfactory response for AN (before which relapse cannot occur) is operationalized as increasing body mass index (BMI) to at least 20, consuming significantly more calories (although not necessarily normalized eating), reducing fears about weight gain, a resumption of menses, and medical stabilization. Thus, complete symptom alleviation is not necessary for relapse to occur. According to Pike, relapse involves weight dropping to a BMI below 18.5, restrictive eating or bingeing with compensatory behavior, a return to overvaluing weight and shape, loss of menses, and in some cases a return of associated medical problems.

Unfortunately, many of the studies of relapse do not adopt a stringent operational definition. We will discuss relapse in all three forms of eating disorder as indexed by a return of disordered eating or a significant decline in functioning following some period of improvement.

Relapse in AN

Studies of relapse in AN place the risk at approximately 30% within 15 months after treatment, though a recent study followed 40 patients for one year and found that 31 (77.5%) were readmitted in that time (e.g., Herzog et al., 1999; Strober, Freeman, & Morrell, 1997). AN patients seem particularly vulnerable to relapse soon after regaining weight and being discharged from the hospital and may need more attention then (Fennig & Roe, 2002).

Various factors have been found to predict relapse in AN, including later age of onset (Pike, 1998), duration of illness of longer than 6 years (Howard et al., 1999), increased duration of eating pathology before treatment (Herzog, Keller, Strober, Yeh, & Pai, 1992), amenorrhea lasting longer than 2.5 years, and a low BMI at hospitalization (Howard et al., 1999; Pike, 1998).

Personality and attitudinal variables also predict relapse. Greater obsessiveness before treatment predicts more severe dieting, higher eating disorder scores, and more frequent hospitalizations at two-year follow-up (Zubieta, Demitrack, Fenick, & Krahn, 1995), at which time obsessionality is associated with lower weight and increased eating disorder symptomatology. It is unclear, however, whether obsessionality increases the risk of relapse or of a more negative course overall. In addition, a compulsive drive to exercise following discharge from treatment after initial improvement predicts relapse (Strober et al., 1997). Persistent anorexic attitudes (i.e., overvaluing weight and shape) and low desired weight (despite some weight restoration) predict relapse within one year of treatment termination (Pike, 1998); behavioral changes without corresponding cognitive changes increase the risk of relapse into anorexic symptoms.

Comorbidity (i.e., having more than one psychological problem) may pose an additional risk for relapse. A 10-year follow-up of anorexics discharged from hospital treatment found that those with a diagnosable eating disorder at follow-up had more and worse comorbid psychopathology, whereas those who"had no eating disorder at follow-up displayed essentially no general psychopathology" (Schork, Eckert, & Halmi, 1994, p. 113). However, Pike (1998) cautioned that the directionality of this relation is questionable; it is possible that more severe or longer-lasting eating disorder symptoms lead to other psychopathology rather than the reverse.

Few other prospective predictors of relapse have been identified. However, one recent study (Cockell, Zaitsoff, & Geller, 2004) obtained a retrospective account of self-reported factors that helped or hindered maintenance of treatment gains from 32 patients who had completed a 15-week inpatient treatment program at six months postdischarge. Factors identified as supporting maintenance were: (1) maintaining connections with professionals (for expertise and monitoring) and nonprofessionals (for support and understanding); (2) application of the nutritional knowledge (what constitutes a normal meal, meal planning, etc.) and psychological skills (self-monitoring and emotional expression) learned in treatment; and (3) focusing beyond the eating disorder (such as on fulfilling higher order values). Factors that were believed to hinder maintenance included (1) loss of structure and specialized support; (2) self-defeating beliefs (e.g., need for control); and (3) daily hassles that they had been protected from while in treatment. Another 7.5-year follow-up study found no significant predictors of relapse after recovery (Herzog et al., 1999). Similarly, although Strober et al. (1997) identified some predictors of postdischarge relapse following partial recovery, they were unable to identify any significant predictors of relapse following full recovery. This finding highlights an important practical distinction. Although AN is associated with a high rate (83%) of partial recovery, the rate of full recovery is much lower (33%; Herzog et al., 1999). Relapse may be more likely and more easily predicted following partial recovery, but it would be worthwhile to explore relapse following complete recovery.

Relapse in BN

Relapse rates for BN, as for AN, are typically around 30% (Herzog et al, 1999; Olmsted, Kaplan, & Rockert, 1994). Again, most relapses occur fairly quickly, usually within six months (Olmsted et al., 1994). Keller, Herzog, Lavori, Bradburn, and Mahoney (1992) found a cumulative probability of relapse of 63%, with 50% of those achieving complete recovery eventually relapsing into another episode of full-blown BN.

Contrary to AN, younger age was among the strongest predictors of relapse in BN (Olmsted et al., 1994). Higher vomiting frequency both before and following treatment was also associated with increased risk, indicating that severity of the disorder determines how intractable it is. Personality and attitudinal variables that have been shown to predict relapse in BN include impulsivity (Miller, 2000), obsessionality (Zubieta et al., 1995), poor body image (Freeman, Beach, Davis, & Solyom, 1985; Keller et al., 1992), more disordered attitudes toward eating before treatment, and greater interpersonal distrust following treatment (Olmsted et al., 1994). Factors that appear to decrease the risk of relapse include a reduced fear of maturity (Miller, 2000) and having a good support system (Keller et al., 1992).

Negative affect appears to play a significant role in relapse in BN. Bulimics who experience stressful situations (and anxiety, nervousness, and depression) are more likely to relapse after gaining control of their eating behavior than are those who do not (Mitchell, Davis & Goff, 1985). Because negative affect triggers disinhibited eating, it is not surprising that it too has been shown to trigger relapse among recovering bulimics. Fluvoxamine, an antidepressant, reduces the risk of relapse among BN patients, at least in the short term (Fichter, Krueger, Rief, Holland, & Doehne, 1996). Learning how to deal with negative affect is clearly a key to relapse prevention.

Relapse in BED

Current estimates of relapse rates in BED are somewhat more optimistic than are those observed in AN and BN. The only longitudinal study of BED to assess relapse rates (Fichter, Quadflieg, & Gnutzmann, 1998) found that at six years posttreatment, most participants did not have a diagnosable eating disorder, although approximately 15% had shifted to another diagnostic category (7.4% to BN and 7.4% to EDNOS), and approximately 6% met the criteria for BED once again.

Possibly because research into BED is relatively more recent, much of the currently available studies of BED assess predictors of negative treatment outcome rather than predictors of relapse. These two categories may eventually be shown to overlap. As is the case with both AN and BN, the severity of the disorder appears to be a prime determinant of negative outcome in BED: the more frequent bingeing is at treatment intake, the more frequent it is following treatment (Peterson et al., 2000). Negative affect also predicts poorer treatment outcome for BED (Eldredge & Agras, 1997). With respect to relapse, Safer, Lively, Telch, and Agras (2002) found that the two strongest predictors of setbacks following a successful course of DBT were earlier onset of binge eating (i.e., at or prior to age 16), and greater (cognitive) dietary restraint. Although BN and BED are distinct clinical syndromes, relapse factors in BN may well be fruitful guides to the further studying of relapse factors in BED.

The fact that treatment for eating disorders has proceeded virtually independently of research on the causes of eating disorders should give us pause. Do we have to understand a problem to treat it, or can we simply tinker with different treatments until we find one (or some combination) that works, without necessarily understanding what caused the problem in the first place? If we did understand what caused the problem, would our treatments necessarily improve? Is it likely that we could therapeutically reverse the original causes? These are questions that pertain to all of psychopathology, but they are particularly salient in the domain of eating disorders. Moreover, they are not rhetorical questions. We really do not know how important the connection is between cause and treatment.

Even if treatment is not dependent on understanding causes, the question of what causes eating disorders remains important. Most of the interventions for eating disorders are therapeutic rather than preventative; that is, we tend to focus our efforts on treating eating disorders rather than preventing them from arising in the first place. An effective public health effort—stopping eating disorders before they get started—probably would be more valuable than effective therapy; but preventative interventions require a better understanding of what causes the disorder. Some efforts have been made in this area, but with limited success. For example, a program that provided girls as young as 10 or 11 with information on healthy eating and attitudes toward one's body changed only attitudes, not behavior (Smolak, Levine, & Schermer, 1998). Similarly, adolescents who participated in an eight-week eating disorder prevention program seemed to have improved both attitudes and behaviors immediately following the program. Within six months, however, they had not only reverted to their former behaviors but had become even more restrained in their eating than when they started. This result led the authors to conclude that prevention programs might do more harm than good! (Carter, Stewart, Dunn, & Fairburn, 1997).

Whether our interest in understanding what causes eating disorders is practical or just a matter of scientific curiosity, we must acknowledge that (1) we have not come a long way since the mid-1970s toward a better understanding of why and how these disorders develop, and (2) the obstacles to making explanatory progress are significant. The most obvious obstacle is that the vast majority of studies examine correlates (or recollected precursors) of established eating disorders. This sort of research is inevitably inconclusive about causation. Path-analytic strategies attempt to extract causal patterns from correlational data (e.g., Stice, 2001). There are severe limits, however, to the persuasiveness of such analyses. True experimentation is not likely to occur, and if it did, it would quickly be halted on ethical grounds. For example, it is difficult to get permission to study the bingeing of a BN patient in the lab. Although such patients binge all the time, it is regarded as unethical for researchers to actively induce a binge. Prospective research is more compelling than is retrospective research; but it too is correlational and therefore unsatisfying. Perhaps researchers will simply have to get used to the idea that they may never have a genuine understanding of eating disorders.

Of course, although many of us would be most pleased with a tight, experimentally based analysis of eating disorders, there are other satisfactions to be had. Decades ago, Hilde Bruch (1975, 1978) provided us with an account of eating disorders, based on her vast clinical experience and insight. The empirical research that has been conducted since Bruch first presented her elegant formulations has done little to undermine her analysis. Indeed, it may be argued that the empirical research enterprise has done little more than add some confirmation to her views, much as paleontology has been a footnote to Darwin. The reader who wants a clear understanding of eating disorders would be well-advised to skip the journal articles and go directly to Bruch, or if not to her, to her patients. As one of them concluded, "The main thing I've learned is that the worry about dieting, the worry about being skinny or fat, is just a smokescreen. This is not the real illness. The real illness has to do with the way you feel about yourself" (Bruch, 1978, p. 127).

Note

1. Bulimia comes from the Greek word bulimos meaning "ox hunger." Bulimics thus act as if they are "as hungry as an ox."

References

Abed, R. T. (1998). The sexual competition hypothesis for eating disorders. *British Journal of Medical Psychology, 71,* 525–547.

Agras, W. S., Telch, C. F., Arnow, B., Eldredge, K., Wilfley, D. E., Raeburn, S. D., et al. (1994). Weight loss, cognitive-behavioral, and desipramine treatments in binge eating disorder: An additive design. *Behavior Therapy, 25,* 225–238.

American Psychiatric Association. (1994). *Diagnostic and statistical manual of mental disorders* (4th ed.). Washington, D.C.: Author.

Appolinario, J. C., Bacaltchuk, J., Sichieri, R., Claudino, A. M., Godoy-Matos, A., & Morgan, C., et al. (2003). A randomized, double-blind, placebo-controlled study of sibutramine in the treatment of binge-eating disorder. *Archives of General Psychiatry, 60*(11), 1109–1116.

Beck, A. T., Rush, A. J., Shaw, B. F., & Emery, G. (1979). *Cognitive therapy of depression.* New York: Guilford.

Bellini, M., & Merli, M. (2004). Current drug treatment of patients with bulimia nervosa and binge-eating disorder: Selective serotonin reuptake inhibitors versus mood stabilizers. *International Journal of Psychiatry in Clinical Practice, 8*(4), 235–243.

Bemporad, J. R. (1996). Self-starvation through the ages: Reflections on the pre-history of anorexia nervosa. *International Journal of Eating Disorders, 19,* 217–237.

Bemporad, J. R. (1997). Cultural and historical aspects of eating disorders. *Theoretical Medicine, 18,* 401–420.

Beumont, P. J. V., & Touyz, S. W. (1995). The nutritional management of anorexia and bulimia nervosa. In K. D. Brownell & C. G. Fairburn (Eds.), *Eating disorders and obesity: A comprehensive handbook* (pp. 306–312). New York: Guilford.

Birchall, H. (1999). Interpersonal psychotherapy in the treatment of eating disorders. *European Eating Disorders Review, 7,* 315–320.

Birmingham, C. L., Su, J., Hlynsky, J. A., Goldner, E. M., & Gao, M. (2005). The mortality rate from anorexia nervosa. *International Journal of Eating Disorders, 38,* 143–146.

Booth, D. A. (1988). Culturally corralled into food abuse: The eating disorders as physiologically reinforced excessive appetites. In K. M. Pirke, W. Vandereycken, & D. Ploog (Eds.), *The psychobiology of bulimia nervosa* (pp. 18–32). Berlin: Springer-Verlag.

Bramon-Bosch, E., Troop, N., & Treasure, J. L. (2000). Eating disorders in males: A comparison with female patients. *European Eating Disorders Review, 8,* 321–328.

Braun, D. L., Sunday, S. R., Huang, A., & Halmi, K. A. (1999). More males seek treatment for eating disorders. *International Journal of Eating Disorders, 25,* 415–424.

Bruch, H. (1975). Obesity and anorexia nervosa: Psychosocial aspects. *Australia & New Zealand Journal of Psychiatry, 9,* 159–161.

Bruch, H. (1978). *The golden cage: The enigma of anorexia nervosa.* Cambridge, MA: Harvard University Press.

Cachelin, F. M., & Maher, B. A. (1998). Is amenorrhea a critical criterion for anorexia nervosa? *Journal of Psychosomatic Research, 44*, 435–440.

Cachelin, F. M., Veisel, C., Barzegarnazari, E., & Striegel-Moore, R. H. (2000). Disordered eating, acculturation, and treatment-seeking in a community sample of Hispanic, Asian, Black, and White women. *Psychology of Women Quarterly, 24*, 244–253.

Carter, J. C., Stewart, D. A., Dunn, V. J., & Fairburn, C. G. (1997). Primary prevention of eating disorders: Might it do more harm than good? *International Journal of Eating Disorders, 22*, 167–172.

Carter, W. P., Hudson, J. I., Lalonde, J. K., Pindyck, L., McElroy, S. L., & Pope, H. G. J. (2003). Pharmacologic treatment of binge eating disorder. *International Journal of Eating Disorders, 34*(Suppl.), S74–S88.

Carter, W. P., & Pindyck, L. J. (2003). Pharmacological treatment of binge eating disorder. *Primary Psychiatry, 10* (10), 31–36.

Casper, R. C., & Jabine, L. N. (1996). An eight-year follow-up: outcome from adolescent compared to adult onset anorexia nervosa. *Journal of Youth and Adolescence, 25*, 499–517.

Cockell, S. J., Zaitsoff, S. L., & Geller, J. (2004). Maintaining change following eating disorder treatment. *Professional Psychology: Research and Practice, 35*(5), 527–534.

Collier, D. A., & Treasure, J. L. (2004). The aetiology of eating disorders. *British Journal of Psychiatry, 185*, 363–365.

Corcos, M., Flament, M. F., Giraud, M. J., Paterniti, S., Ledoux, S., Atger, F., & Jeammet, P. (2000). Early psychopathological signs in bulimia nervosa. A retrospective comparison of the period of puberty in bulimic and control girls. *European Child & Adolescent Psychiatry, 9*, 115–121.

Dansky, B. S., Brewerton, T. D., & Kilpatrick, D. G. (2000). Comorbidity of bulimia nervosa and alcohol use disorders: Results from the national women's study. *International Journal of Eating Disorders, 27*, 180–190.

Dare, C., & Eisler, I. (2000). A multi-family group day treatment program for adolescent eating disorder. *European Eating Disorders Review, 81*, 4–18.

Davis, C., & Claridge, G. (1998). The eating disorders as addiction: A psychobiological perspective. *Addictive Behaviors, 23*, 463–475.

Davis, C., & Katzman, M. (1999). Perfectionism as acculturation: Psychological correlates of eating problems in Chinese male and female students living in the United States. *International Journal of Eating Disorders, 25*, 65–70.

Davison, K. K., Earnest, M. B., & Birch, L. L. (2002). Participation in aesthetic sports and girls' weight concerns at ages 5 and 7 years. *International Journal of Eating Disorders, 31*, 312–317.

Devlin, M. J., Goldfein, J. A., Carino, J. S., & Wolk, S. L. (2000). Open treatment of overweight binge eaters with phentermine and fluoxetine as an adjunct to cognitive-behavioral therapy. *International Journal of Eating Disorders, 28*, 325–332.

de Zwaan, M., Mitchell, J. E., Crosby, R. D., Mussell, M. P., Raymond, N. C., Specker, S. M., et al. (2005). Short-term cognitive behavioral treatment does not improve outcome of a comprehensive very-low-calorie diet program in obese women with binge eating disorder. *Behavior Therapy, 36*(1), 89–99.

Dittmar, H. (2005). Vulnerability factors and processes linking sociocultural pressures and body dissatisfaction [Special issue]. *Journal of Social & Clinical Psychology, 24*, 1081–1087.

Drewnowski, A., Kurth, C. L., & Krahn, D. D. (1995). Effects of body image on dieting, exercise, and anabolic steroid use in adolescent males. *International Journal of Eating Disorders, 17*, 381–386.

Eldredge, K. L., & Agras, W. S. (1997). The relationship between perceived evaluation of weight and treatment outcome among individuals with binge-eating disorder. *International Journal of Eating Disorders, 22*, 43–49.

Fairburn, C. G. (1981). A cognitive behavioral approach to the management of bulimia. *Psychological Medicine, 11*, 707–711.

Fairburn, C. G., Cooper, Z., Doll, H. A., Norman, P., & O'Connor, M. (2000). The natural course of bulimia nervosa and binge eating disorder in young women. *Archives of General Psychiatry, 57*, 659–665.

Fairburn, C. G., Cooper, Z., Doll, H. A., & Welch, S. L. (1999). Risk factors for anorexia nervosa: Three integrated case-control comparisons. *Archives of General Psychiatry, 56*, 468–476.

Fairburn, C. G., Cooper, Z., & Shafran, R. (2003). Cognitive behaviour therapy for eating disorders: A "transdiagnostic" theory and treatment. *Behaviour Research and Therapy, 41*, 509–529.

Fairburn, C. G., Norman, P. A., Welch, S. L., O'Connor, M. E., Doll, H. A., & Peveler, R. C. (1995). A prospective study of outcome in bulimia nervosa and the long-term effects of three psychological treatments. *Archives of General Psychiatry, 52*, 304–312.

Fairburn, C. G., Shafran, R., & Cooper, Z. (1998). A cognitive behavioral theory of anorexia nervosa. *Behavior Research and Therapy, 37*, 1–13.

Fairburn, C. G., Welch, S. L., Doll, H. A., Davies, B. A., & O'Connor, M. E. (1997). Risk factors for bulimia nervosa—A community-based case-control study. *Archives of General Psychiatry, 54*, 509–517.

Fennig, S., & Roe, D. (2002). Physical recovery in anorexia nervosa: Is this the sole purpose of a child and adolescent medical-psychiatric unit? *General Hospital Psychiatry, 24*, 87–92.

Feld, R., Woodside, D. B., Kaplan, A. S., Olmsted, M. P., & Carter, J. C. (2001). Pretreatment motivational enhancement therapy for eating disorders: A pilot study. *International Journal of Eating Disorders, 29*(4), 393–400.

Fichter, M. M., Krueger, R., Rief, W., Holland, R., & Doehne, J. (1996). Fluvoxamine in prevention of relapse in bulimia nervosa: Effects on eating-specific psychopathology. *Journal of Clinical Psychopharmacology, 16*, 9–18.

Fichter, M. M., Quadflieg, N., & Gnutzmann, A. (1998). Binge eating disorder: Treatment outcome over a 6-year course. *Journal of Psychosomatic Research, 44*, 385–405.

Fisher, M., Schneider, M., Burns, J., Symons, H., & Mandel, F. S. (2001). Differences between adolescents and young adults at presentation to an eating disorders program. *Journal of Adolescent Health, 28*, 222–227.

Fombonne, E. (1996). Is bulimia nervosa increasing in frequency? *International Journal of Eating Disorders, 19*, 287–296.

Freeman, R. J., Beach, B., Davis, R., & Solyom, L. (1985). The prediction of relapse in bulimia nervosa. *Journal of Psychiatric Research, 19*, 349–353.

Garfinkel, P. E., Lin, E., Goering, P., Spegg, C., Goldbloom, D., Kennedy, S., et al. (1996). Should amenorrhoea be necessary for the diagnosis of anorexia nervosa? Evidence from a Canadian community sample. *British Journal of Psychiatry, 168*, 500–506.

Garner, D. M., & Bemis K. M. (1982). A cognitive behavioral approach to the treatment of anorexia nervosa. *Cognitive Therapy and Research, 6*, 123–150.

Garner, D. M., Olmsted, M. P., & Polivy, J. (1983). Development and validation of a multidimensional eating disorder inventory for anorexia nervosa and bulimia. *International Journal of Eating Disorders, 2*, 15–34.

Garner, D. M., Olmsted, M., Polivy, J., & Garfinkel, P. E. (1984). Comparison between weight preoccupied women and anorexia nervosa. *Psychosomatic Medicine, 46*, 255–266.

Geist, R., Heinmaa, M., Stephens, D., Davis, R., & Katzman, D. K. (2000). Comparison of family therapy and family group psychoeducation in adolescents with anorexia nervosa. *Canadian Journal of Psychiatry—Revue Canadienne de Psychiatrie, 45*, 173–178.

George, L., Thornton, C., Touyz, S. W., Waller, G., & Beumont, P. J. V. (2004). Motivational enhancement and schema-focused cognitive behaviour therapy in the treatment of chronic eating disorders [Special issue]. *Clinical Psychologist, 8*(2), 81–85.

Goldner, E. M., Geller, J., Birmingham, C. L., & Remick, H. A. (2000). Comparison of shoplifting behaviours in patients with eating disorders, psychiatric control subjects, and undergraduate control subjects. *Canadian Journal of Psychiatry—Revue Canadienne de Psychiatrie, 45*, 471–475.

Goldstein, D. J., Wilson, M., Thompson, V. L., Potvin, J., & Rampey, A. H. (1995). Long term fluoxetine treatment of bulimia nervosa. *The British Journal of Psychiatry, 166*, 660–666.

Gonzalez, R. G. (1988). Bulimia and adolescence: Individual psychoanalytic treatment. In H. J. Schwartz (Ed.), *Bulimia: Psychoanalytic treatment and theory* (pp. 339–441). Madison, CT: International Universities Press.

Grant, K., Lyons, A., Landis, D., Cho, M., Scudiero, M., Reynolds, L., et al. (1999). Gender, body image, and depressive symptoms among low-income African American adolescents. *Journal of Social Issues, 55*, 299–315.

Grilo, C. M. (2006). *Eating and weight disorders*. New York: Psychology Press.

Grilo, C. M., Masheb, R., & Salant, S. L. (2005). Cognitive behavioral therapy, guided self-help, and orlistat for the treatment of binge eating disorder: A randomized double-blind placebo-controlled trial. *Biological Psychiatry, 57*, 1193–1201.

Grilo, C. M., Masheb, R., & Wilson, G. T. (2005). Efficacy of cognitive-behavioral therapy and fluoxetine for the treatment of binge eating disorder: A randomized double-blind placebo-controlled trial. *Biological Psychiatry, 57*, 301–309.

Haworth-Hoeppner, S. (2000). The critical shapes of body image: The role of culture and family in the production of eating disorders. *Journal of Marriage and the Family, 62*, 212–227.

Hay, P., & Fairburn, C. (1998). The validity of the DSM-IV scheme for classifying bulimic eating disorders. *International Journal of Eating Disorders, 23*, 7–15.

Heatherton, T. F., & Polivy, J. (1992). Chronic dieting and eating disorders: A spiral model. In J. Crowther, S. E. Hobfall, M. A. P. Stephens, & D. L. Tennenbaum (Eds.), *The etiology of bulimia: The individual and familial context* (pp. 133–155). Washington, D.C.: Hemisphere.

Herpertz-Dahlmann, B., Muller, B., Herpertz, S., Heusen, N., Hebebrand, J., & Remschmidt, H. (2001). Prospective 10-year follow-up in adolescent anorexia nervosa—Course, outcome, psychiatric comorbidity, and psychosocial adaptation. *Journal of Child Psychology and Psychiatry and Allied Disciplines, 42*, 603–612.

Herzog, D. B. (1995). Psychodynamic psychotherapy for anorexia nervosa. In K. D. Brownell & C. G. Fairburn (Eds.), *Eating disorders and obesity: A comprehensive handbook* (pp. 330–335). New York: Guilford.

Herzog, D. B., Dorer, D. J., Keel, P. K., Selwyn, S. E., Ekeblad, E. R., Flores, A. T., et al. (1999). Recovery and relapse in anorexia and bulimia nervosa: A 7.5-year follow-up study. *Journal of the American Academy of Child and Adolescent Psychiatry, 38*, 829–837.

Herzog, D. B., Greenwood, D. N., Dorer, D. J., Flores, A. T., Ekeblad, E. R., Richards, A., et al. (2000). Mortality in eating disorders: A descriptive study. *International Journal of Eating Disorders, 28*, 20–26.

Herzog, D. B., Keller, M., Strober, M., Yeh, C., & Pai, S. (1992). Psychiatric comorbidity in treatment seeking anorexics and bulimics. *Journal of the American Academy of Child and Adolescent Psychiatry, 31*, 810–818.

Hoek, H. W. (2002). Distribution of eating disorders. In C. G. Fairburn & K. D. Brownell (Eds.) *Eating disorders and obesity: A comprehensive handbook* (pp. 233–237). New York: Guilford.

Hoek, H. W., van Harten, P. N., Hermans, K. M., Katzman, M. A., Matroos, G. E., & Susser, E. S. (2005). The incidence of anorexia nervosa on Curacao. *American Journal of Psychiatry, 162*, 7748–7752.

Howard, W. T., Evans, K. K., Quintero-Howard, C. V., Bowers, W. A., & Andersen, A. E. (1999). Predictors of success or failure of transition to day hospital treatment for inpatients with anorexia nervosa. *American Journal of Psychiatry, 156*, 1697–1702.

Hudson, J. I., Carter, W. P., & Pope, H. G. (1996). Antidepressant treatment of binge-eating disorder: Research findings and clinical guidelines. *Journal of Clinical Psychiatry, 57*(Suppl. 8), 73–79.

Hudson, J. I., Pope, H. G., and Jonas, J. M. (1983). Phenomenologic relationship of eating disorders to major affective disorder. *Psychiatry Research, 9*, 345–354.

Jacobi, C., Hawward, C., de Zwaan, M., Kraemer, H. C., & Agras, W. S. (2004). Coming to terms with risk factors for eating disorders: Application of risk terminology and suggestions for a general taxonomy. *Psychological Bulletin, 130*, 19–65.

Johnson, C. (1995). Psychodynamic treatment of bulimia nervosa. In K. D. Brownell & C. G. Fairburn (Eds.), *Eating disorders and obesity: A comprehensive handbook* (pp. 349–353). New York: Guilford.

Johnson, C., & Connors, M. E. (1987). *The etiology and treatment of bulimia nervosa*. New York: Basic Books.

Johnson, W. G., Boutelle, K. N., Torgrud, L., Davig, J. P., & Turner, S. (2000). What is a binge? The influence of amount, duration, and loss of control criteria on judgments of binge eating. *International Journal of Eating Disorders, 27*, 471–479.

Johnson, W. G., Carr-Nangle, R. E., Nangle, D. W., Antony, M. M., & Zayfert, C. (1997). What is binge eating? A comparison of binge eater, peer, and professional judgments of eating episodes. *Addictive Behaviors, 22*, 631–635.

Joiner, T. E., Vohs, K. D., & Heatherton, T. F. (2000). Three studies on the factorial distinctiveness of binge eating and bulimic symptoms among non-clinical men and women. *International Journal of Eating Disorders, 27*, 198–205.

Kahm, A. (1994). Recovery through nutritional counseling. In B. P. Kinoy (Ed.), *Eating disorders: New directions in treatment and recovery* (pp. 15–47). New York: Columbia University Press.

Katzman, M. A., Hermans, K. M., Van Hoeken, D., & Hoek, H. W. (2004). Not your "typical island woman": Anorexia nervosa is reported only in subcultures in Curaçao. *Cultural Medicine and Psychiatry, 28*, 463–492.

Kaye, W. H. (1997). Anorexia nervosa, obsessional behavior, and serotonin. *Psychopharmacological Bulletin, 33*, 335–344.

Kaye, W. H., Gendall, K., & Strober, M. (1998). Serotonin neuronal function and selective serotonin reuptake inhibitor treatment in anorexia and bulimia nervosa. *Biological Psychiatry, 44*, 825–838.

Kaye, W. H., Weltzin, T., & Hsu, L. G. (1993). Relationship between anorexia nervosa and obsessive and compulsive behaviors. *Psychiatric Annals, 23*, 365–373.

Keel, P. K., Mitchell, J. E., Miller, K. B., Davis, T. L., & Crow, S. (1999). Long-term outcome of bulimia nervosa. *Archives of General Psychiatry, 56*, 63–69.

Keller, M. B., Herzog, D. B., Lavori, P. W., Bradburn, I. S., & Mahoney, E. M. (1992). The naturalistic history of bulimia nervosa: Extraordinarily high rates of chronicity, relapse, recurrence, and psychosocial morbidity. *International Journal of Eating Disorders, 12*, 1–9.

Killick, S., & Allen, C. (1997). "Shifting the balance"—Motivational interviewing to help behaviour change in people with bulimia nervosa. *European Eating Disorders Review, 5*(1), 33–41.

Klump, K. L., & Gobrogge, K. L. (2005). A review and primer of molecular genetic studies of anorexia nervosa. *International Journal of Eating Disorders, 37*, S43–S48..

Kruger, S., & Kennedy, S. H. (2000). Psychopharmacotherapy of anorexia nervosa, bulimia nervosa and binge-eating disorder. *Journal of Psychiatry and Neuroscience, 25*, 497–508.

Laliberte, M., Boland, F. J., & Leichner, P. (1999). Family climates: Family factors specific to disturbed eating and bulimia nervosa. *Journal of Clinical Psychology, 55*, 1021–1040.

Lansky, D., & Levitt, J. L. (1992). Multifaceted treatment of patients with severe eating disorders. In C. E. Stout, J. L. Levitt, & D. H. Ruben (Eds.), *Handbook for assessing and treating addictive disorders* (pp. 181–202). New York: Greenwood.

Leon, G., Fulkerson, J. A., Perry, C., & Early-Zald, M. B. (1995). Prospective analysis of personality and behavioral vulnerabilities and gender influences in the later development of disordered eating. *Journal of Abnormal Psychology, 104*, 140–149.

Leung, F., Geller, J., & Katzman, M. (1996). Issues and concerns associated with different risk models for eating disorders. *International Journal of Eating Disorder, 19*, 249–256.

Levine, M. D., Marcus, M. D., & Moulton, P. (1996). Exercise in the treatment of binge eating disorder. *International Journal of Eating Disorders, 19*, 171–177.

Lilenfeld, L. R. R., Stein, D., Bulik, C. M., Strober, M., Plotnicov, K., Pollice, C., et al. (2000). Personality traits among currently eating disordered, recovered and never ill first-degree female relatives of bulimic and control women. *Psychological Medicine, 30*, 1399–1410.

Loeb, K. L., Wilson, G. T., Gilbert, J. S., & Labouvie, E. (2000). Guided and unguided self-help for binge eating. *Behavior Research & Therapy, 38*, 259–272.

Marx, R. D., Kotwal, R., McElroy, S. L., & Malhotra, S. (2003). What treatment data support topiramate in bulimia nervosa and binge eating disorder? What is the drug's safety profile? How is it used in these conditions? *Eating Disorders: The Journal of Treatment & Prevention, 11*(1), 71–75.

Matsunaga, H., Kaye, W. H., McConaa, C., Plotnicov, K., Pollice, C., & Rao, R. (2000). Personality disorders among subjects recovered from eating disorders. *International Journal of Eating Disorders, 27*, 353–357.

Matsunaga, H., Kiriike, N., Iwasaki, Y., Miyata, A., Matsui, T., Nagata, T., Yamagami, S., & Kaye, W. H. (2000). Multi-impulsivity among bulimic patients in Japan. *International Journal of Eating Disorders, 27*, 348–352.

Mayer, L. E. S., & Walsh, B. T. (1998). The use of selective serotonin reuptake inhibitors in eating disorders. *Journal of Clinical Psychiatry, 59*(Suppl. 15), 28–34.

McCabe, E. B., & Marcus, M. D. (2002). Question: Is dialectical behavior therapy useful in the management of anorexia nervosa? *Eating Disorders: The Journal of Treatment & Prevention, 10*(4), 335–337.

McElroy, S. L., Arnold, L. M., Shapira, N. A., Keck, P. E. J., Rosenthal, N. R., & Karim, M. R., et al. (2003). Topiramate in the treatment of binge eating disorder associated with obesity: A randomized, placebo-controlled trial. *American Journal of Psychiatry, 160*(2), 255–261.

McElroy, S. L., Casuto, L. S., Nelson, E. B., Lake, K. A., Soutullo, C. A., Keck, P. E., et al. (2000). Placebo controlled trial of sertraline in the treatment of binge eating disorder. *The American Journal of Psychiatry, 157*, 1004–1006.

McElroy, S. L., Hudson, J. I., Malhotra, S., Welge, J. A., Nelson, E. B., & Keck, P. E. J. (2003). Citalopram in the treatment of binge-eating disorder: A placebo-controlled trial. *Journal of Clinical Psychiatry, 64*(7), 807–813.

McElroy, S. L., Kotwal, R., Hudson, J. I., Nelson, E. B., & Keck, P. E. J. (2004). Zonisamide in the treatment of binge-eating disorder: An open-label, prospective trial. *Journal of Clinical Psychiatry, 65*(1), 50–56.

McElroy, S. L., Shapira, N. A., Arnold, L. M., Keck, P. E. J., Rosenthal, N. R., & Wu, S., et al. (2004). Topiramate in the long-term treatment of binge-eating disorder associated with obesity. *Journal of Clinical Psychiatry, 65*(11), 1463–1469.

McFarlane, T., Polivy, J., & Herman, C. P. (1998). The effects of false feedback about weight on restrained and unrestrained eaters. *Journal of Abnormal Psychology, 107*, 312–318.

Miller, K. B. (2000). The long-term course of bulimia nervosa: Relapse, recovery, and comorbidity over time. *Dissertation Abstracts International, 61*(1-B), 542.

Miller, W. R. & Rollnick, S. (2002) *Motivational interviewing: Preparing people for change* (2nd ed.). New York: Guilford.

Mills, J., Polivy, J., Herman, C. P., & Tiggemann, M. (2002). Effects of media-portrayed idealized body images on restrained and unrestrained eaters. *Personality and Social Psychology Bulletin, 28*, 1687–1699.

Minuchin, S., Rosman, B. L., & Baker, L. (1978). *Psychosomatic families: Anorexia nervosa in context.* Cambridge, MA: Harvard University Press.

Mitchell, J. E., Davis, L., & Goff, G. (1985). The process of relapse in patients with bulimia. *International Journal of Eating Disorders, 4*, 457–463.

Mulholland, A. M., & Mintz, L. B., (2001). Prevalence of eating disorders among African American women. *Journal of Counseling Psychology, 48*, 111–116.

Nasser, M. (1997). *Culture and weight consciousness.* New York: Routledge.

Nevonen, L., & Broberg, A. G. (2000). The emergence of eating disorders: An exploratory study. *European Eating Disorders Review, 8*, 279–292.

Nisbett, R. E., & Wilson, T. D. (1977). Telling more than we can know: Verbal reports on mental processes. *Psychological Review, 84*, 231–259.

Nowak, M. (1998).The weight-conscious adolescent: Body image, food intake, and weight-related behavior. *Journal of Adolescent Health, 23*, 389–398.

Ogden, J., & Elder, C. (1998). The role of family status and ethnic group on body image and eating behavior. *International Journal of Eating Disorders, 23*, 309–315.

Olmsted, M. P., & Kaplan, A. S. (1995). Psychoeducation in the treatment of eating disorders. In K. D. Brownell & C. G. Fairburn (Eds.), *Eating disorders and obesity: A comprehensive handbook* (pp. 299–305). New York: Guilford.

Olmsted, M. P., Kaplan, A. S., & Rockert, W. (1994). Rate and prediction of relapse in bulimia nervosa. *American Journal of Psychiatry, 151*, 738–743.

Palmer, R. L., Birchall, H., Damani, S., Gatward, N., McGrain, L., & Parker, L. (2003). A dialectical behavior therapy program for people with an eating disorder and borderline personality disorder-description and outcome. *International Journal of Eating Disorders, 33*(3), 281–286.

Peterson, C. B., Crow, S. J., Nugent, S., Mitchell, J. E., Engbloom, S., & Mussell, M. P. (2000). Predictors of treatment outcome for binge eating disorder. *International Journal of Eating Disorders, 28*, 131–138.

Pike, K. M. (1998). Long-term course of anorexia nervosa: Response, relapse, remission, and recovery. *Clinical Psychology Review, 18*, 447–475.

Pinhas, L., Toner, B. B., Ali, A., Garfinkel, P. E., & Stuckless, N. (1999). The effects of the ideal of female beauty on mood and body satisfaction. *International Journal of Eating Disorders, 25*, 223–226.

Polivy, J., & Herman, C. P. (1987). Diagnosis and treatment of normal eating. *Journal of Consulting & Clinical Psychology, 55*, 635–644.

Polivy, J., & Herman, C. P. (1993). Etiology of binge eating: Psychological mechanisms. In C. G. Fairburn and G. T. Wilson (Eds.), *Binge eating: Nature, assessment and treatment* (pp. 173–205). New York: Guilford.

Polivy, J., & Herman, C. P. (2002). Causes of eating disorders. *Annual Review of Psychology, 53*, 187–213.

Polivy, J. & Herman, C.P. (2007). Is the body the self? Women and body image. *Collegium Antropologicum.*

Polivy, J., Herman, C. P., Mills, J., & Wheeler, H. B. (2003). Eating disorders in adolescence. In G. Adams & M. Berzonsky (Eds.), *The Blackwell handbook of adolescence* (pp. 523–549). Oxford: Blackwell.

Prochaska, J. O., & DiClemente, C. C. (1992). The transtheoretical approach. In J. C. Norcross & I. L. Goldfield (Eds.), *Handbook of psychotherapy integration* (pp. 300–334). New York: Basic Books.

Pryor, T., Wiederman, M. W., & McGilley, B. (1996). Laxative abuse among women with eating disorders: An indication of psychopathology? *International Journal of Eating Disorders, 20*, 13–18.

Ro, O., Martinsen, E. W., Hoffart, A., & Rosenvinge, J. H. (2004). Short-term follow-up of adults with long-standing anorexia nervosa or non-specified eating disorder after inpatient treatment. *Eating and Weight Disorders, 9* (1), 62–68.

Rooney, B., McClelland, L., Crisp, A. H., & Sedgwick, P. M. (1995). The incidence and prevalence of anorexia nervosa in three suburban health districts in south west London, UK. *International Journal of Eating Disorders, 18*, 299–307.

Russell, G. F. M., Dare, C., Eisler, I., & Le Grange, P. D. F. (1992). Controlled trials of family treatments in anorexia nervosa. In K. A. Halmi (Ed.), *Psychobiology and treatment of anorexia nervosa and bulimia nervosa* (pp. 237–262). Washington, D.C.: American Psychiatric Press.

Safer, D. L., Lively, T. J., Telch, C. F., & Agras, W. S. (2002). Predictors of relapse following successful dialectical behavior therapy for binge eating disorder. *International Journal of Eating Disorders, 32*(2), 155–163.

Safer, D. L., Telch, C. F., & Agras, W. S. (2001). Dialectical behavior therapy adapted for bulimia: A case report. *International Journal of Eating Disorders, 30*(1), 101–106.

Schlundt, D. G., & Johnson, W. G. (1990). *Eating disorders: Assessment and treatment.* Boston: Allyn & Bacon.

Schork, E. J., Eckert, E. D., & Halmi, K. A. (1994). The relationship between psychopathology, eating disorder diagnosis, and clinical outcome at 10-year follow-up in anorexia nervosa. *Comprehensive Psychiatry, 35*, 113–123.

Shapira, N. A., Goldsmith, T. D., & McElroy, S. L. (2000). Treatment of binge eating disorder with topiramate: A clinical case series. *Journal of Clinical Psychiatry, 61*, 368–372.

Shisslak, C. M., Crago, M., & Estes, L. S. (1995). The spectrum of eating disturbances. *International Journal of Eating Disorders, 18*, 209–219.

Smolak, L., & Levine, M. P. (1996). Adolescent transitions and the development of eating problems. In L. Smolak, M. Levine, & R. Striegel-Moore (Eds.), *The developmental psychopathology of eating disorders: Implications for research, prevention, and treatment* (pp. 210–231). Mahwah, NJ: Erlbaum.

Smolak, L., Levine, M. P., & Schermer, F. (1998). A controlled evaluation of an elementary school primary prevention program for eating problems. *Journal of Psychosomatic Research, 44*, 339–353.

Steiger, H., Young, S. N., Kin, N. M. K., Koerner, N., Israel, M., Lageix, P., et al. (2001). Implications of impulsive and affective symptoms for serotonin function in bulimia nervosa. *Psychological Medicine, 31*, 85–95.

Steinhausen, H. C., Seidel, R., & Metzke, C. W. (2000). Evaluation of treatment and intermediate and long-term outcome of adolescent eating disorders. *Psychological Medicine, 30*, 1089–1098.

Stice, E. (2001). A prospective test of the dual-pathway model of bulimic pathology: Mediating effects of dieting and negative affect. *Journal of Abnormal Psychology, 110*, 1–12.

Stice, E., & Shaw, H. (1994). Adverse effects of the media portrayed thin-ideal on women and linkages to bulimic symptomatology. *Journal of Social and Clinical Psychology, 13*, 288–308.

Striegel-Moore, R. H. (1993). Etiology of binge eating: A developmental perspective. In C. G. Fairburn & G. T. Wilson (Eds.), *Binge eating: Nature, assessment and treatment* (pp. 144–172). New York: Guilford.

Striegel-Moore, R. H., Garvin, V., Dohm, F. A., & Rosenheck, R. A. (1999). Eating disorders in a national sample of hospitalized female and male veterans: Detection rates and psychiatric comorbidity. *International Journal of Eating Disorders, 25*, 405–414.

Striegel-Moore, R. H., Schreiber, G. B., Lo, A., Crawford, P., Obarzanek, E., & Rodin, J. (2000). Eating disorder symptoms in a cohort of 11 to 16-year-old black and white girls: The NHLBI growth and health study. *International Journal of Eating Disorders, 27*, 49–66.

Strober, M. (1980). Personality and symptomatological features in young, nonchronic anorexia nervosa patients. *Journal of Psychosomatic Research, 24*, 353–359.

Strober, M., Freeman, R., Lampert, C., Diamond, J., & Kaye, W. (2000). Controlled family study of anorexia nervosa and bulimia nervosa: Evidence of shared liability and transmission of partial syndromes. *American Journal of Psychiatry, 157*, 393–401.

Strober, M., Freeman, R., & Morell, W. (1997). The long-term course of anorexia nervosa in adolescents: Survival analysis of recovery, relapse, and outcome predictors over 10–15 years in a prospective study. *International Journal of Eating Disorders, 22*, 339–360.

Strober, M., & Humphrey, L. L. (1987). Familial contributions to the etiology and course of anorexia nervosa and bulimia. *Journal of Consulting and Clinical Psychology, 55*, 654–659.

Strober, M., & Katz, J. L. (1988). Depression in the eating disorders: A review and analysis of descriptive, family and biological findings. In D. M. Garner & P. E. Garfinkel (Eds.), *Diagnostic issues in anorexia nervosa and bulimia nervosa* (pp. 80–111). New York: Brunner/Mazel.

Sullivan, P. F. (1995). Mortality in anorexia nervosa. *American Journal of Psychiatry, 152*, 1073–1074.

Tantleff-Dunn, S., Gokee-LaRose, J., & Peterson, R. D. (2004). *Interpersonal psychotherapy for the treatment of anorexia nervosa, bulimia nervosa, and binge eating disorder.* Hoboken, NJ: Wiley.

Tasca, G. A., Ritchie, K., Conrad, G., Balfour, L., Gayton, J., & Lybanon, V., et al. (2006). Attachment scales predict outcome in a randomized controlled trial of two group therapies for binge eating disorder: An aptitude by treatment interaction. *Psychotherapy Research, 16*(1), 106–121.

Telch, C. F., Agras, W. S., & Linehan, M. M. (2000). Group dialectical behavior therapy for binge-eating disorder: A preliminary, uncontrolled trial. *Behavior Therapy, 31*(3), 569–582.

Telch, C. F., Agras, W. S., & Linehan, M. M. (2001). Dialectical behavior therapy for binge eating disorder. *Journal of consulting and clinical psychology, 69*(6), 1061–1065.

Theander, S. (1996). Anorexia nervosa with an early onset: Selection, gender, outcome, and results of a long-term follow-up study. *Journal of Youth and Adolescence, 25*, 419–429.

Thode, N. (1990). A family systems perspective on recovery from an eating disorder. In B. P. Kinoy (Ed.), *Eating disorders: New directions in treatment and recovery* (pp. 61–79). New York: Columbia University Press.

Touyz, S. W., Polivy, J., & Hay, P. (2008). *Advances in psychotherapy—evidence-based practice: Eating disorders.* Cambridge, MA: Hogrefe & Huber.

Tozzi, F., & Bulik, C.M. (2003). Candidate genes in eating disorders. *Current Drug Targets—CNS and Neurological Disorders, 2*, 31–39.

Treasure, J., & Ward, A. (1997). A practical guide to the use of motivational interviewing in anorexia nervosa. *European Eating Disorders Review, 5*(2), 102–114

VanderHam, T., Meulman, J. J., VanStrien, D. C., & vanEngeland, H. (1997). Empirically based subgrouping of eating disorders in adolescents: A longitudinal perspective. *British Journal of Psychiatry, 170*, 363–368.

Vanfurth, E. F., Vanstrien, D. C., Martina, L. M. L., Vanson, M. J. M., Hendrickx, J. J. P., et al. (1996). Expressed emotion and the prediction of outcome in adolescent eating disorders. *International Journal of Eating Disorder, 20*, 19–31.

Vitousek, K. B. (1995). Cognitive behavioral therapy for anorexia nervosa. In K. D. Brownell & C. G. Fairburn (Eds.), *Eating disorders and obesity—A comprehensive handbook* (pp. 324–329). New York: Guilford.

Vogeltanz-Holm, N. D., Wonderlich, S. A., Lewis, B. A., Wilsnack, S. C., Harris, T. R., Wilsnack, R. W., et al. (2000). Longitudinal predictors of binge eating, intense dieting, and weight concerns in a national sample of women. *Behavior Therapy, 31*, 221–235.

Wakeling, A. (1996). Epidemiology of anorexia nervosa. *Psychiatry Research, 62*, 3–9.

Ward, A., Tiller, J., Treasure, J., & Russell, G. (2000). Eating disorders: Psyche or soma? *International Journal of Eating Disorders, 27*, 279–287.

Wheeler, H. B., Polivy, J., & Herman, C. P. (2002). *The precarious identities of restrained eaters: Effects of a threat.* Unpublished manuscript.

Wilfley, D. E., Friedman, M. A., Dounchis, J. Z., Stein, R. I., Welch, R. R., & Ball, S. A. (2000). Comorbid psychopathology in binge eating disorder: Relation to eating disorder severity at baseline and following treatment. *Journal of Consulting and Clinical Psychology, 68*, 641–649.

Wilfley, D. E., Welch, R. R., Stein, R. I., Spurrell, E. B., Cohen, L. R., & Saelens, B. E., et al. (2002). A randomized comparison of group cognitive-behavioral therapy and group interpersonal psychotherapy for the treatment of overweight individuals with binge-eating disorder. *Archives of General Psychiatry, 59*(8), 713–721.

Williamson, D. A., Muller, S. L., Reas, D. L., & Thaw, J. M. (1999). Cognitive bias in eating disorders: Implications for theory and treatment. *Behavior Modification, 23,* 556–577.

Wilson, G. T. (1991). The addiction model of eating disorders: A critical analysis. *Advances in Behavior Research and Therapy, 13,* 27–72.

Wilson, G. T. (1996). Treatment of bulimia nervosa: When CBT fails. *Behavior Research and Therapy, 34,* 197–212.

Wilson, G. T. (1999). Cognitive behavior therapy for eating disorders: Progress and problems. *Behavior Research and Therapy, 37,* S79–S95.

Wilson, G. T., & Fairburn, C. G. (2000). The treatment of binge eating disorder. *European Eating Disorders Review, 8,* 351–354.

Wilson, G. T., & Schlam, T. R. (2004). The transtheoretical model and motivational interviewing in the treatment of eating and weight disorders. *Clinical Psychology Review, 24*(3), 361–378.

Wolfe, B. E., Metzger, E. D., & Jimerson, D. C. (1997). Research update on serotonin function in bulimia nervosa and anorexia nervosa. *Psychopharmacology Bulletin, 33,* 345–357.

Wonderlich, S. (1995). Personality and eating disorders. In K. D. Brownell & C. G. Fairburn (Eds.), *Eating disorders and obesity: A comprehensive handbook* (pp. 171–176). New York: Guilford.

Wonderlich, S., & Mitchell, J. E. (2001). The role of personality in the onset of eating disorders and treatment implications. *Psychiatric Clinics of North America, 24,* 249–258.

Woods, S. C., & Brief, D. J. (1988). Physiological factors. In D. M. Donovan & G. A. Marlatt (Eds.), *Assessment of addictive behaviors* (pp. 296–322). New York: Guilford.

Zubieta, J. K., Demitrack, M. A., Fenick, A., & Krahn, D. D. (1995). Obsessionality in eating disorder patients: Relationship to clinical presentation and two year outcome. *Journal of Psychiatric Research, 29,* 333–342.

13
Sexual Dysfunctions and Disorders

Jennifer T. Gosselin

Sexual behavior has a long history of emotionally charged social and cultural expectations, rules, taboos, myths, and misconceptions. "Normal" versus "dysfunctional" or "deviant" sexual behaviors are determined arbitrarily and are tied to the social norms of a particular time and place (Marecek, Crawford, & Popp, 2004). The social construction of appropriate and inappropriate sexual behavior is best reflected by the historical and cultural changes in what has been considered normal and abnormal. In ancient Greece, for example, a male mentor might have sex with his adolescent student as part of their relationship, which was relatively accepted at that time as a way to demonstrate social standing or hierarchy (King, 1996; Plante, 2006). In the Sambian tribe in New Guinea, an important rite involves younger boys performing oral sex on older boys in order to ingest semen, which is believed to provide strength and masculinity; when they get older they transition into heterosexual adults (Stoller, 1985). In contrast, the Victorian Era in England (during most of the 1800s) was a time of sexual conservatism, although like the Sambians, beliefs about sex were rigid and based on misconceptions about semen. The purpose of sex during this era was to produce children, not to experience pleasure. Modesty was important, and women were supposed to cover their bodies, including their ankles. Masturbation was believed to be a cause of mental or physical illness (including blindness) (King, 1996). In some cases, treatment for masturbation included clitoridectomy (removal of the clitoris), male circumcision, or castration (King, 1996; Lips, 2006).

In many nations around the globe, major developments and changes have occurred, such as improved methods of contraception and movements for the rights of women and homosexuals. Homosexuality was included as a disorder in older editions of the *Diagnostic and Statistical Manual of Mental Disorders (DSM)*, but was downgraded to "ego dystonic homosexuality" in 1980 and was removed as a disorder in the *DSM-III-R* due to political pressure. Other issues have emerged, such as the need to protect minors from sexual activity and exploitation, which is an ongoing area of international concern. Many societies—particularly in Europe and the West in general—have become more open about presenting sexual matters in the media. With this acceptance of sex, however, have come new ways to define and treat problems related to sex. Moreover, today's deviance was yesterday's normalcy, and vice versa.

Sex researchers today owe a great deal to the pioneers in this field, such as Alfred Kinsey, William Masters, Virginia Johnson, Katharine Davis, Havelock Ellis, Gilbert Hamilton, and many others (Irvine, 1990; Kimmel & Plante, 2004). These early researchers paved the way for later researchers by challenging social norms to study the taboo topic of sex. Kinsey gathered data through surveys, beginning his work in the late 1930s to learn about typical sexual behavior and experiences. His data normalized many sexual practices that were thought to be very rare or deviant. Masters and Johnson studied sexual behavior in the laboratory, using volunteers who would masturbate or married couples who would have sex. In the 1960s and 1970s, Masters and Johnson's best-sellers *Human Sexual Response* and *Human Sexual Inadequacy* dispelled many myths about sexual function. Their prominent human sexual response cycle has been a widely used model of normal sexual functioning, and would later be used as a framework for the sexual dysfunction categories in the *DSM* (Masters, Johnson, & Kolodny, 1985).

Categories of Sexual Disorders

The current nomenclature identifies two primary categories of sexual disorders: *sexual dysfunction* (such as erectile dysfunction) and *paraphilias* (such as sexual fetishism). Although most people have had occasional experiences that fall into a sexual dysfunction category—such as the inability to reach orgasm when so desired—sexual difficulties that are more frequent and distressing than an incidental occurrence are considered to be sexual dysfunctions, according to the *Diagnostic and Statistical Manual of Mental Disorders* (*DSM-IV-TR*; American Psychiatric Association, 2000). For ease of understanding, the present chapter will use the term *sexual dysfunction* to indicate problems associated with sexual desire, arousal, orgasm, and pain during sex, while *sexual disorders* will refer to the paraphilias, such as exhibitionism, fetishism, frotteurism, pedophilia, sexual masochism, sexual sadism, transvestic fetishism, and voyeurism. The present chapter will also address *gender identity disorder*, although it is concerned with gender identification, rather than a sexual dysfunction or a sexual disorder. Additionally, *compulsive* or *addictive sexuality* will be presented with the paraphilias, despite its omission from the current *DSM*. Diagnostic descriptions, etiological or causal factors, and treatment approaches will be discussed for each dysfunction or disorder presented.

Sexual Dysfunctions

The *DSM-IV-TR* defines sexual dysfunction as "a disturbance in the processes that characterize the sexual response cycle or by pain associated with sexual intercourse" (APA, 2000, p. 535).

Defining and Describing Sexual Dysfunctions

The sexual response cycle indicated in this definition follows Masters and Johnson's model, including Kaplan's (1979) addition of the initial stage of desire, followed by excitement, plateau, orgasm, and resolution (Masters et al., 1985). Sexual desire involves sexual thoughts and fantasies; sexual excitement involves the physiological arousal of the sex organs; plateau involves physiological changes that may lead to orgasm; the next stage is orgasm; and finally, during the resolution phase, the body returns to its unaroused state (Masters et al., 1985).

The types of sexual dysfunction, according to the *DSM-IV-TR*, are as follows:

- Sexual desire disorders: deficiency or absence of sexual fantasies and desire for sexual activity that causes marked distress or interpersonal difficulty. These include hypoactive sexual desire disorder (absence of sexual fantasies and desire for sex) and sexual aversion disorder (extreme avoidance of sex with a partner).
- Sexual arousal disorders: female sexual arousal disorder (persistent or recurrent inability to attain or maintain an adequate lubrication-swelling response of sexual excitement in females) and male erectile disorder (persistent or recurrent inability to attain or to maintain an adequate erection during sexual activity).

- Orgasmic disorders: persistent or recurrent delay in, or absence of, orgasm following a normal sexual excitement phase. These disorders include female orgasmic disorder, male orgasmic disorder, and premature ejaculation (onset of orgasm and ejaculation with minimal stimulation or before the person wishes it).
- Sexual pain disorders: dyspareunia (genital pain that is associated with sexual intercourse in males and females and is not due to lack of lubrication) and vaginismus (recurrent or persistent involuntary contraction of the perineal muscles surrounding the outer third of the vagina when vaginal penetration is attempted by self or others with an item such as a tampon, speculum, penis, or finger).

The *DSM-IV-TR* also includes several subtypes of sexual dysfunction. The clinician is supposed to indicate whether the dysfunction has been acquired after normal functioning or if it is lifelong, whether the dysfunction is limited to particular partners, types of stimulation, or situations or if it generalizes across these factors, and whether the dysfunction is due to psychological or both psychological and medical (combined) factors. Sexual difficulties must be considered "persistent or recurrent" by the clinician to be considered a disorder, and they cannot be due exclusively to a substance, medication, or medical condition, in which case the clinician should use the diagnosis of sexual dysfunction due to a particular medical condition or substance-induced sexual dysfunction. In order to distinguish between sexual impairment that is not considered a disorder and sexual impairment that is diagnosable, significant distress or interpersonal difficulty or impairment is required for diagnosis.

Critcisms of Sexual Dysfunction Diagnostic Categories

Most of the criticisms of the *DSM*'s sexual dysfunction categories stem from its reliance on the human sexual response cycle as a model, which deemphasizes psychological factors in favor of physiological changes. Critics argue that sexual experience is presented in the model as a relationship- and context-independent phenomenon (Tiefer, 2001). They further argue that the human sexual response cycle is a linear model with seemingly discrete stages, which does not necessarily reflect real sexual experience (Basson, 2005; Basson et al., 2004). Researchers also assert that the model is based on male sexual response and that it superimposes the male cycle onto the female response (Basson, 2005; Basson et al., 2004). Further, the research conducted to establish the model was based on carefully selected participants who, for example, could reach orgasm through masturbation and coitus, which is considered a biased sample (Tiefer, 1991).

Researchers following the medical model have generally attempted to create two categories of individuals with respect to sexual functioning: (1) those who are sexually satisfied and have "normal" sexual functioning, and (2) those who are sexually dissatisfied and are sexually "dysfunctional." Both qualitative and quantitative studies, however, do not support this dichotomy. Sexual dysfunctions and consistency of orgasm tend to be poor predictors of sexual satisfaction (Frank, Anderson, & Rubinstein, 1978; Lavie-Ajayi, 2005; McConaghy, 1993). Over half of women in one study who had difficulty reaching orgasm reported that it did not concern them (Lavie-Ajayi, 2005). Some of these inorgasmic women found their lack of orgasm problematic only to the extent that it resulted in their male partners' feelings of inadequacy (Lavie-Ajayi, 2005). Other research suggests that women's distress about their sexual relationship is better predicted by their feelings toward their partner during sex and their subjective state of well-being than by their physical sexual response (Bancroft, Loftus, & Long, 2003).

Dissatisfaction with the sexual dysfunction categories has not led to major revisions to the *DSM* thus far. Alternatively, the *International Classification of Diseases-10 (ICD-10)*, created by the World Health Organization, defines sexual dysfunction as "the various ways in which an individual is unable to participate in a sexual relationship as he or she would wish," and explains that "Sexual response is a psychosomatic process and both psychological and somatic processes are usually involved in the causation of sexual dysfunction" (World Health Organization, October 23, 2006, Section F52). Although both the *ICD-10* and the *DSM-IV-TR* use the human sexual response cycle as their diagnostic structure, the definition used by the *ICD-10* emphasizes the subjective nature of sexual experience, rather than emphasizing genital response.

Epidemiology

Rates of sexual dysfunctions vary from study to study due to different measures used, methodological differences, and the use of different samples (Rosen & Laumann, 2003). Prevalence estimates may be inflated because many studies do not include diagnostic interviews, and they often do not assess significant personal or interpersonal distress associated with the dysfunction, which are criteria for diagnosis. Research generally indicates that 40 to 45% of women and 20 to 31% of men report experiencing one or more sexual dysfunctions (Laumann, Paik, & Rosen, 1999; Lewis et al., 2004). These figures vary with the study and sample, with rates as low as 27% (Kadri, Alami, & Tahiri, 2002) and as high as 55% for female sexual dysfunction (Fisher, Boroditsky, & Morris, 2004). The most common sexual dysfunctions among women tend to be hypoactive sexual desire disorder, female sexual arousal disorder (Utian et al., 2005), and female orgasmic disorder (Fisher et al., 2004; West, Vinikoor, & Zolnoun, 2004). The most common sexual dysfunctions among men are premature ejaculation and erectile dysfunction (Dunn, Croft, & Hackett, 1999; Nicolosi et al., 2004). Rates of premature ejaculation range from 4 to 29%, and rates of erectile dysfunction vary greatly with age, with less than 10% of men under 40 years of age, 49% of men 40 to 88 years old, and 76% of 50 to 75-year-old men in separate studies reporting erectile dysfunction (Feldman, Goldstein, Hatzichristou, Krane, & McKinlay, 1994; Grover et al., 2006; Lewis et al., 2004; Prins, Blanker, Bohnen, Thomas, & Bosch, 2002; Shiri et al., 2003; Simons & Carey, 2001).

Prevalence estimates often vary widely and are a source of ongoing debate. For example, the suggestion that almost half of women and almost one-third of men (depending on their age) have a sexual difficulty is inconsistent with the finding that the majority of people around the world report that they are satisfied with their sexual functioning (including approximately 80% of men and women in Western nations and 42 to 90% of men and women in mostly South American and Eastern countries) (Laumann et al., 2006).

Etiology

Sexual desire, arousal, and behavior can be explained using a *biopsychosocial model*, meaning that internal processes, such as one's physiological systems, thoughts, and feelings, interact with one's behaviors and with external factors, such as environmental and social forces (Althof et al., 2005; Fagan, 2004). This interactionist approach provides a multidimensional explanation for problems that usually do not have a clear, singular causal factor. Sexual difficulties can have multiple etiologies, and these factors tend to be inextricably linked together.

Biological Factors Sex hormones (produced by the ovaries and testes) play a role in sexual interest and functioning in men and women (Berman, Berman, & Goldstein, 1999). Low levels of androgens, particularly testosterone, have been linked in some studies to loss of sexual arousal and orgasm in women (see Shifren, 2004, for a review), although other studies contradict this finding (Davis, Davison, Donath, & Bell, 2005; Nyunt et al., 2005). In men, testosterone has more consistently been associated with sexual desire and activity (Bradford, 2001; Goldstein, 2004; Rowland, 2006). Low levels of estrogens in women also may be related to diminished sexual desire and sexual functioning, although it is likely that sexual functioning in women is the result of a combination of estrogens and androgens (Berman & Bassuk, 2002; Rowland, 2006).

Neurotransmitters, such as dopamine and serotonin, also play a role in sexual functioning, which is supported by animal and human research as well as by the sexual side effects of medications that affect levels of these neurotransmitters in the synapse (Basson, 2005; Kafka, 1997b; Rowland, 2006). Serotonin is synthesized in the gastrointestinal tract and the central nervous system. This neurotransmitter influences a wide range of physiological, behavioral, and mood-related phenomena, including appetite, nausea, sleep, body temperature, anxiety, depression, suicidality, and impulsivity (Carlson, 2001; Pinel, 2003). Increased levels of serotonin (due to medications that block reuptake of serotonin, for example) tend to inhibit sexual activity and delay orgasm in both humans and rats (McMahon, 2004). Dopamine is involved in motivation and the experience of pleasure or reward, leading to the repetition of rewarding experiences, such as eating and having sex. (Dopaminergic pathways are thus also important in addictive behaviors.) The connection between dopamine and sexual behavior has been established, in part, through research on individuals who suffer from conditions involving dopaminergic pathways, such as Parkinson's disease and schizophrenia. For example, on the one hand, patients with Parkinson's disease (which involves a depletion of dopamine) who are treated with medications that facilitate dopamine transmission also report an increase in sexual activity. Individuals with schizophrenia, on the other hand, who are treated with medications that inhibit dopamine often report diminished sexual desire and may experience sexual dysfunction (Dominguez & Hull, 2005; Pinel, 2003). In addition to the monoamines, nitric oxide—which is a neurotransmitter in the form of a soluble gas—plays a role in physiological sexual responses, such as erection, by relaxing smooth muscle tissue and allowing blood flow to the genitals. Medications such as sildenafil (Viagra) increase erectile functioning by influencing the signaling of nitric oxide (Trussell, Anastasiadis, Padma-Nathan, & Shabsigh, 2004).

Sexual dysfunction in men and women is also associated with chronic diseases, particularly hypertension, cardiovascular disease, and diabetes, as well as urinary tract infections, hypogonadism (malfunction of the ovaries or testes), and spinal cord injuries (Archer, Gragasin, Webster, Bochinski, & Michelakis, 2005; Berman et al., 1999; Burchardt et al., 2002; Carbone & Seftel, 2004; Laumann et al., 1999; Lewis et al., 2004; Michael & O'Keane, 2000; Sipski, 2002). Prostate dysfunction, chronic renal failure, and heavy smoking increase men's risk for developing sexual dysfunction (Carbone & Seftel, 2004; Dunn et al., 1999; Laumann et al., 1999; Lewis et al., 2004; Nicolosi, Moreira, Shirai, Bin Mohd Tambi, & Glasser, 2003). In men and women, a proposed cause of limited physiological arousal is insufficient blood flow to the genitalia. This physiological problem, in turn, may have a number of causes, including illnesses that involve vascular (blood vessel) impairment, such as cardiovascular disease. In addition, women who have suffered pelvic trauma, surgical or obstetrical complications, those who have endometriosis or similar health conditions, or those who have undergone female circumcision or female genital mutilation (a cultural practice in some African and Middle-Eastern regions) are more likely to experience dyspareunia (Berman et al., 1999; Committee on Bioethics, 1998; Elgaali, Strevens, & Mardh, 2005).

Age Sexual dysfunction is also often associated with older age in Western and Eastern samples across the globe (Lewis et al., 2004; Nicolosi et al., 2003; Turkistani, 2004). Research findings are mixed, however, with respect to the specific sexual dysfunction and its relationship with age. For example, some researchers have reported that among women, sexual difficulties actually decrease with age (Kadri et al., 2002; Laumann et al., 1999). Older women tend to have the same sexual partner for a longer period of time than do younger women, which may allow for more consistent sexual behavior and orgasm (Laumann et al., 1999). Although some women may experience more pain during sex as they enter menopause, sexual satisfaction does not appear to be related to menopause status (Cain et al., 2003). Sexual interest or desire, however, may decline with age for both men and women (Bancroft et al., 2003; Laumann et al., 1999; Lewis et al., 2004; Nicolosi et al., 2004). Also, among males, the ability to maintain and sustain an erection and to fully ejaculate tends to decrease with age (Blanker et al., 2001; Helgason et al., 1996; Laumann et al., 1999; Nicolosi et al., 2003), and among females, vaginal dryness may increase with age (Laumann et al., 1999; Nicolosi et al., 2004).

Medications A wide range of medications can influence sexual functioning by affecting the release of neurotransmitters or their receptors or by influencing the vascular system. Antidepressant medications, such as selective serotonin reuptake inhibitors (SSRIs), monoamine oxidase inhibitors (MAOIs), and tricyclic antidepressants (TCAs) are associated with sexual dysfunction (Montgomery, Baldwin, & Riley, 2002). A potential confounding variable is that diminished sexual desire or arousal may be a symptom of depression. While research suggests that a substantial portion (about 40 to 50%) of nonmedicated individuals with depression reported decreased sexual desire or sexual difficulties (Kennedy, Dickens, Eisfeld, & Bagby, 1999), research comparing treatment and control groups indicates that antidepressants also contribute to sexual impairment, particularly delayed or absent orgasm (Montgomery et al., 2002). A host of other medications have been associated with diminished sexual functioning, including: anxiolytics (antianxiety medications), such as benzodiazepines; beta-blockers, which lower blood pressure; antipsychotic medications that increase levels of prolactin; oral contraceptives, and chemotherapy and other treatments for cancer (Gruszecki, Forchuk, & Fisher, 2005; Kao et al., 2003; Knegtering, van der Moolen, Castelein, Kluiter, & van den Bosch, 2003; Rowland, 2006; Segraves, 2002). Physicians often treat sexual side effects by either switching medications or by prescribing more medication. For example, physicians may prescribe bupropion (an antidepressant that influences norepinephrine and dopamine levels) instead of antidepressants that have a higher risk of sexual side effects, or a physician may prescribe sildenafil (Viagra) to counteract sexual side effects of other medications that the patient is taking (Segraves, 2002; Zisook, Rush, Haight, Clines, & Rockett, 2006).

Psychological, Interpersonal, and Cultural Factors Previous sexual experiences, beliefs, and knowledge about sex, as well as current levels of stress, depression, anxiety, relationship issues, and many other factors may play a role in the development of sexual difficulties and dysfunction (Araujo, Durante, Feldman, Goldstein, & McKinlay, 1998; Bancroft et al., 2003; Bodenmann, Ledermann, Blattner, & Galluzzo, 2006; Laumann et al., 1999; van Lankveld & Grotjohann, 2000). For example, an individual may learn to associate sex with pain or fear due to past traumatic experiences. In some studies, male and female survivors of childhood sexual abuse and female sexual assault survivors were more likely to experience sexual dysfunction (Laumann et al., 1999; Oberg, Fugl-Meyer, & Fugl-Meyer, 2002), although not all studies demonstrate the same findings (Dennerstein, Guthrie, & Alford, 2004). Research does show, however, that vaginismus in particular is more likely among females who were sexually abused as children (Reissing, Binik, Khalife, Cohen, & Amsel, 2003).

Cultural and religious beliefs, practices, and expectations may also play a role in sexual difficulties, such as views that women should be subordinate to men and that women should not enjoy sex, as well as the discouragement of masturbation and body exploration, and the prearranged marriage of young girls. In some regions of Asia, individuals may complain of a sudden fear that the penis (or vulva and nipples in females) will retreat into the body; this fear is called *koro* (APA, 2000). Beliefs about the origin of sexual difficulties also vary by culture; for example, over 80% of Moroccan women experiencing sexual dysfunction reported that their dysfunction was due to sorcery by someone who wished them harm (Kadri et al., 2002).

From a social-cognitive perspective, individuals have a cognitive framework that reflects their perception of themselves as sexual beings, termed *sexual self-schemas* that guide attention and information-processing in sexual situations (Cyranowski, Aarestad, & Andersen, 1999; Reissing, Laliberte, & Davis, 2005). Individuals also hold sexual self-efficacy beliefs, meaning beliefs about their ability to perform certain sexual behaviors in a given situation (Cyranowski et al., 1999). Negative self-perceptions in terms of sexual schematic representations and low self-efficacy for sexual behaviors interact with particular situations (such as one's partner not reaching orgasm) to result in particular thoughts in the moment (such as "I'm a failure" or "My partner doesn't find me sexually appealing"). These thoughts influence and interact with feelings, behaviors, and even one's physiology, including sexual response. Research has demonstrated that individuals with erectile disorder, as compared to those without this disorder, are more likely to explain negative sexual events—such as loss of an erection—as the result of something that is wrong with them (internal attribution) and as something that is likely to continue (stable attribution) (Scepkowski et al., 2004). Diminished erectile response can also be evoked among sexually functional males by providing them with prior, bogus, negative erectile feedback and an internal, stable attribution of their supposed diminished erectile response (Weisberg, Brown, Wincze, & Barlow, 2001). Physiological sexual processes thus cannot be separated from psychosocial factors, including cognitive processes, beliefs about the self, interpersonal relationship issues, and the context of the sexual behavior.

Treatment

Treatment options for sexual dysfunction include couples therapy, behavioral therapy, cognitive-behavioral therapy, and medical treatment.

Psychotherapy Sexual difficulties may persist without treatment because these difficulties are one of the most challenging problems for people to discuss with a doctor, therapist, or even with their partner. Moreover, without education about sex, individuals' anxiety and misconceptions about their difficulties may exacerbate the problem (Kadri et al., 2002; Turkistani, 2004). Treatment of sexual dysfunctions involves a learning process; clients must learn not only about sexual functioning in general, but also about their own bodies and the connection between their own psychological and physiological processes. They also must learn about their partner's body and preferences.

Rather than adopting a model of focusing treatment on the "disease" (called a "disease-centered" approach), physicians and clinicians may better serve their patients (or clients) by adopting a *patient-centered approach* to treatment (Hatzichristou et al., 2004). This approach involves an empathic understanding of the patient's perspective of the problem, as well as patient education and active inclusion of the patient (and his or her partner, if possible) in exploring treatment options. Treatment providers should obtain a thorough account of past and present psychosocial, sexual, and physical health functioning, as well as a physical examination and relevant laboratory tests when indicated (Basson et al., 2004; Hatzichristou et al., 2004). This process of data gathering may involve collaboration between multiple specialists in different fields. Throughout assessment and treatment, open, reciprocal communication between the patient and treatment provider is paramount for effective treatment of sexual dysfunctions (Hatzichristou et al., 2004).

COUPLES APPROACHES TO THERAPY Sexual dysfunctions are virtually always interpersonal difficulties by definition and should be addressed as such, including facilitation of interpersonal communication and a sense of trust and shared involvement in treatment, including shared consideration of treatment options. Another reason for shared treatment participation is that when one partner in a relationship has a sexual difficulty or dysfunction, the likelihood increases that the other partner has or will develop a sexual difficulty or decreased sexual desire (Fugl-Meyer & Fugl-Meyer, 2002; Greenstein, Abramov, Matzkin, & Chen, 2006; Gruszecki et al., 2005; Lewis et al., 2004). Clinicians should gather information about the couple's relationship, as well as their sexual functioning and sexual scripts. *Sexual scripts* generally refer to social expectations about sexual thoughts, plans, and behaviors, including with whom it is acceptable to have sex, the appropriate reasons for sex, and where and when sexual activity can take place (Gagnon, Rosen, & Leiblum, 1982). Sexual scripts can further refer to a particular couple's (usually unspoken) rules, expectations, and sequences of sexual activity, including the roles each partner takes on during the sexual activity, such as the "initiator," the "resister," or the "passive participant" (Gagnon et al., 1982; Lips, 2006; Matlin, 2000; McCormick, 1987). Through education and communication, modifications to the script can be made to satisfy both partners and allow more flexibility of the couple's sexual roles and sexual activities (Foley, 1994; Gagnon et al., 1982). Clinicians should also determine to what extent one partner has identified the other partner as having the "problem," and when the heart of the issue is a difference in the desired frequency of sex or the nature of the sexual activity. Hence, power differentials in the relationship may also emerge as part of the problem and should be addressed.

BEHAVIORAL THERAPY Sexual problems are also behavioral problems, and research suggests that addressing the specific sexual difficulty is a critical part of therapy, above and beyond enhancing the couple's relationship in general (Baucom, Shoham, Mueser, Daiuto, & Stickle, 1998). Effective behavioral techniques include learning about and practicing masturbation for treatment of orgasmic disorder (LoPiccolo & Lobitz, 1972), as well as progressive dilation using fingers or plastic dilators for vaginismus (Masters & Johnson, 1970). In some cases, vaginal muscle biofeedback for dyspareunia and vaginismus can be helpful (Basson et al., 2004; Lechtenberg & Ohl, 1994).

Sexual difficulties may also be due to distraction (Barlow, 1986; Beck & Barlow, 1986). One can become distracted by one's thoughts about sexual performance, the appearance of one's own body, possible intrusion by others during sex, and many other concerns. The term *spectatoring* or the *spectator role* refers to heightened self-focused attention that interferes with arousal due to concomitant thoughts of performance failure (Masters et al., 1985). Couples techniques, such as sensate focus, have been used to treat arousal difficulties and spectatoring. *Sensate focus* involves removing the psychological pressure involved in sexual performance by instead engaging in relaxed, sensual touch without the goal of intercourse or orgasm (Masters & Johnson, 1970). Another couples technique is the treatment of premature ejaculation through starting and stopping sexual activity to allow the man to better control and delay ejaculation, as well as through use of the *squeeze technique*, which involves repeatedly squeezing the penis for a few seconds either at the frenulum (near the ridge at the top of the penis) or at the base of the penis to deter ejaculation until desired (Masters & Johnson, 1970; Masters et al., 1985).

Individuals who have come to associate sex with trauma or anxiety can unlearn this association through gradual exposure to sexual activity at home with their partner, which is an application of Wolpe's *systematic desensitization* (Janata & Kingsberg, 2005; Wolpe, 1958). The individual learns relaxation techniques and may start with sexual imagery before moving on to in vivo sexual exercises. He or she should have a sense of control over what occurs (unlike past traumatic experiences, if that is the case), and the exposure should begin with less threatening situations, such as nonsexual touching and progress to increasingly more potentially anxiety-provoking stimuli as he or she feels comfortable. Systematic desensitization has generally shown positive results for erectile disorder and sexual anxiety, although women with orgasmic difficulties seem to be better treated by masturbation exercises (Heiman & Meston, 1997). In most cases, however, much of the outcome of therapy rests on the couple's ability to communicate. Couples need to talk to each other about what they find pleasurable; verbal as well as nonverbal techniques may be used to guide one's partner during sexual activity (Lechtenberg & Ohl, 1994). Providing feedback to one's partner is also likely to increase his or her self-efficacy for sexual activity (Reissing et al., 2005).

COGNITIVE-BEHAVIORAL THERAPY Cognitive-behavioral therapy has also received some research support for the treatment of sexual dysfunctions (McCabe, 2001). The cognitive-behavioral approach to sexual dysfunction treatment involves facilitating the couple's communication, practicing sexual skills, and identifying and modifying maladaptive beliefs about sex that may be exacerbating or even causing the difficulty. For example, men who believe that a man must be ready for sex at any moment and that failure to sustain an erection is indicative of personal failure or that impotence is an affront to a man's masculinity will likely experience more debilitating anxiety and self-doubt when faced with loss of an erection, compared to men who do not add special significance to their body's functioning (Nobre & Pinto-Gouveia, 2006). Unrealistic expectations can also impede women's sexual functioning, such as the belief that women should be able to have an orgasm through intercourse during every sexual encounter, as well as beliefs that virtuous women, mothers, and older women should not be sexual (Nobre & Pinto-Gouveia, 2006). Cognitive-behavioral therapists undermine these erroneous beliefs and their negative effects through psychoeducation, cognitive restructuring, and homework assignments involving behavioral techniques, such as sensate focus (McCabe, 2001).

Medical Treatments The use of medication to treat sexual dysfunctions is generally accepted for men, but remains controversial for the treatment of female sexual dysfunctions (Tiefer, 2001). Most researchers recommend addressing relationship concerns for both men and women before considering medication (Basson et al., 2004; Hatzichristou et al., 2004). Since sexual functioning may decline with age, along with reproductive capacity, some researchers advocate an acceptance of these natural changes, rather than an emphasis on artificial maintenance of abilities associated with youth (Potts, Grace, Vares, & Gavey, 2006). The use of medication to treat sexual dysfunction, particularly erectile disorder, however, has become exceedingly popular. This popularity has overshadowed both the acceptance of sexual changes that occur over time and psychological explanations and treatments of sexual dysfunction, as patients readily seek medication as a simple solution to their difficulties (Tiefer, 2006). Research has also moved away from psychotherapeutic approaches to treating sexual dysfunction and instead toward medical approaches (Baucom et al., 1998).

Anatomically, sexual arousal in men and women is a similar process overall, involving the nervous and vascular systems, such as the dilation of blood vessels and flow of blood to the genitals, although this process has been studied more thoroughly in men than in women (Segraves, 2002). Most medical treatments involve maximizing blood flow to the genitals as well as relaxing smooth muscle tissue. Popular treatments for erectile dysfunction include phosphodiesterase-5 inhibitors, such as sildenafil (Viagra), tadalafil (Cialis), and vardenafil (Levitra). Rather than targeting blood flow to the penis, another strategy is to target areas of the brain believed to be involved in sexual functioning. Apomorphine, a medication that is often prescribed for Parkinson's disease, has been shown to be beneficial to men with erectile dysfunction because of its action on dopamine receptors (Wylie & MacInnes, 2005). Other, less commonly used treatments include the use of a vacuum constriction device that increases blood flow to the penis, intracavernosal injections (injections of medications into the penis), urethral suppository (depositing medication into the urethra), and surgically implanted prostheses (Archer et al., 2005; Sadeghi-Nejad & Seftel, 2004). The usually undesirable sexual side effect of delayed orgasm from antidepressants and other medications is the desired effect for men with premature ejaculation, who may be effectively treated with these medications (Heiman & Meston, 1997). Simply becoming healthier, such as exercising, losing extra weight, and quitting smoking can also improve sexual functioning, including erectile function (Archer et al., 2005).

For women, many treatments have targeted hormones that are thought to be etiological factors in female sexual dysfunction, particularly disorders involving desire and arousal. Androgen therapy—such as treatment with testosterone creams and testosterone transdermal (absorbed through the skin) patches—seems to increase sexual desire and arousal among postmenopausal women and women who have had their ovaries and uterus removed (Berman et al., 1999; Braunstein et al., 2005; Shifren, 2004; Shifren et al., 2000; Shifren et al., 2006). Testosterone is not recommended as a long-term treatment at high doses, however, due to masculinizing effects (such as facial hair growth, deepening of one's voice, and acne), and it is not approved by the Food and Drug Administration to treat female sexual dysfunction (Shifren, 2004). Hormone replacement therapy to increase estrogen levels has also been used, although there may be significant health risks associated with these medications, and findings about their associated benefits are mixed (Archer et al., 2005; Basson et al., 2004; Gonzalez, Viafara, Caba, & Molina, 2004). Given their general success with men, vasoactive drugs, such as sildenafil (taken orally) and alprostadil (applied as a topical cream to the genital area) have been tested among women, although findings are either insignificant (Basson, McInnes, Smith, Hodgson, & Koppiker, 2002), mixed, or should be interpreted cautiously due to a large placebo effect (Heiman, 2002; Heiman et al., 2006). Dopaminergic drugs, such as bupropion and apomorphine, have resulted in some success in treating female sexual dysfunction (Caruso et al., 2004; Segraves, Clayton, Croft, Wolf, & Warnock, 2004). Despite successful outcomes with some medications, future researchers should address the substantial placebo effect in many medication studies with female participants (Bancroft, 2002; Enserink, 2005; Shifren et al., 2000). In addition to medication, women may also benefit from the use of various devices, such as the Food and Drug Administration-approved clitoral vacuum device called the EROS Clitoral Therapy Device, which uses a gentle suction to increase blood flow to the clitoris (Billups et al., 2001).

Paraphilias and Compulsive Sexual Behavior

Paraphilia, literally meaning "lover" (*phile*) of that which is "beyond" or "abnormal" (*para*), can include a wide range of sexual activities, objects, and situations (*Merriam-Webster's Collegiate Dictionary*, 2001). According to the *DSM-IV-TR*, the paraphilias are "recurrent, intense sexually arousing fantasies, sexual urges, or behaviors generally involving (1) nonhuman objects, (2) the suffering or humiliation of oneself or one's partner, or (3) children or other nonconsenting persons that occur over a period of at least 6 months" (2000, p. 566). The paraphilias include: fetishism, transvestic fetishism, voyeurism, exhibitionism, frotteurism, pedophilia, sexual masochism, and sexual sadism. Unlike sexual dysfunctions, some of the paraphilias—specifically those involving nonconsenting partners, including pedophilia, voyeurism, exhibitionism, frotteurism, and sexual sadism with a nonconsenting partner—do not require the criterion of significant personal distress or impairment in order to be diagnosed according to the *DSM-IV-TR*. The following descriptions of the paraphilias are based on the *DSM-IV-TR* diagnostic features.

Sexual Fetishism

Sexual fetishism involves sexual focus on a specific object to the extent that it leads to personal distress or impairment, such as relationship difficulties. Examples of fetish objects include underwear, shoes, stockings, belts, and perfume. While many people find certain objects or items of clothing sexy, an individual with a sexual fetish is different in that the object often must be rubbed or smelled during nearly every sexual activity for sexual satisfaction. Partialism (categorized under "paraphilia not otherwise specified" in the *DSM-IV-TR*) is similar to fetishism, although the item that elicits arousal is a part of the body, such as feet, rather than an inanimate object. Although a common fetish is female undergarments, transvestic fetishism involves sexual arousal from wearing attire of the opposite sex, which usually means men wearing women's clothing. The idea of the self as a woman is often the paraphilic focus. The cross-dressing can range from a single item of clothing to a head-to-toe cross-gendered appearance. Typically, the individual is heterosexual, and the cross-dressing is not due to gender dysphoria (discomfort with one's gender).

Voyeurism

Voyeurism involves observing individuals undress or have sex, through a window, for example, without the individuals' knowledge. The voyeur often masturbates while observing.

Exhibitionism

Exhibitionism—unlike the inconspicuous activities of voyeurism—is the exposure of one's genitals to a stranger in an inappropriate place and without the observer's consent. This may be performed to shock the observer or with the intent to elicit arousal in the observer. Although the exhibitionist may masturbate during exposure, he or she usually does not attempt to sexually assault the observer.

Frotteurism

Like exhibitionism, frotteurism often occurs in public places with an unsuspecting victim, but frotteurism involves touching and rubbing against a person without his or her consent. The frotteur usually touches or tries to touch the victim in sexually explicit areas of the body.

Pedophilia

One of the most potentially damaging forms of victimization is pedophilia. This disorder involves sexual fantasies, impulses, or behaviors directed at prepubescent children (usually under 13 years of age) by individuals who are at least 16 years old and who are also at least five years older than the child. The target is often a child to whom the pedophile has convenient access, such as a family member, foster child, or child involved in some form of organization or activity that allows for time apart from others. Female victimization is more commonly reported than is male victimization, although sex offenders who target boys tend to have more victims than those who target girls (see Cohen & Galynker, 2002 ,for a review). Pedophiles can be attracted to boys, girls, or both, and they can be exclusively attracted to prepubescent children, postpubescent adolescents, or a combination of adults and children or adolescents. Fantasizing about sexual activities with children and experiencing concomitant distress, while not acting on these fantasies still fulfills diagnostic criteria for pedophilia (see Fagan, Wise, Schmidt, & Berlin, 2002, for a review).

Sexual Sadism

Another form of sexual activity that may involve victimization is sexual sadism, which is defined as deriving sexual gratification from making another person suffer physically or psychologically, including acts designed to humiliate. The primary components of the sexual gratification are dominance and control, and specific behaviors vary in degrees of severity, from blindfolding and paddling to cutting, burning, beating, and even killing (*DSM-IV-TR*; Alison, Santtila, Sandnabba, & Nordling, 2004). The partner may be a nonconsenting victim or a sexual masochist. Sexual masochism involves deriving sexual pleasure from one's own suffering or humiliation. Masochists may have a partner perform the behavior, such as binding them, or they may perform the behavior alone. For example, *autoerotic asphyxiation* (a type of *hypoxyphilia* or *asphyxiophilia*, meaning pleasure derived from suffocation) involves depriving oneself of oxygen via a noose, plastic bag, or other means, usually while masturbating (*DSM-IV-TR*; Uva, 1995). In addition to the primary categories of paraphilias, the *DSM* also includes a *paraphilia not otherwise specified* category, which encompasses a range of deviant behaviors, including making obscene phone calls (*scatologia*), having sex with animals or corpses, partialism, and the sexual use of urine, feces, and enemas.

Controversy Over Inclusion and Exclusion of Particular Paraphilias in the DSM

The inclusion of particular paraphilias in the *DSM* is an issue of debate. For example, *transvestism* may be viewed as an uncommon deviation of normal sexual activities that is not inherently problematic. Distress caused by transvestism likely involves social or interpersonal pressure to not engage in this behavior. Researchers have also argued for the exclusion of mild forms of consensual sadomasochism (McConaghy, 1993). The inclusion of other paraphilias in the *DSM* has also been questioned, but for different reasons. Some argue that disorders that involve nonconsenting partners, such as pedophilia and sadism with nonconsenting partners, be excluded from the *DSM* because their inclusion implies that the individual has a mental illness that accounts for their behavior. A concern is that labeling these behaviors "disorders" could be akin to excusing these behaviors, which was the argument used against the inclusion in the *DSM* of "paraphilic coercive disorder" or rape (Holden, 1986).

Compulsive Sexual Behavior

Although the *DSM-IV-TR* includes a diagnostic category for individuals who do not want to have sex often enough, wanting to have sex too often is not included in the *DSM-IV-TR* as a specific disorder. Instead, "distress about a pattern of repeated sexual relationships involving a succession of lovers who are experienced by the individual only as things to be used" is provided as an example under the *sexual disorder not otherwise specified* category of the *DSM-IV-TR* (p. 582). *Excessive sexual drive* is included, however, in the *International Classifications of Diseases-10* (*ICD-10*). Many researchers have suggested that *compulsive sexual behavior* be included in the *DSM* (Bradford, 2001). Excessive sexual drive and behavior has been given a variety of names with varied meanings, including *sexual addiction, sexual impulsivity disorder*, and *hypersexual desire disorder*. Although this problem is not clearly defined and encompasses a wide range of behaviors, most definitions include characteristics such as the lack of control over sexual thoughts or activities, the repetitive, time-consuming nature of these thoughts and activities, and the experience of personal distress, impairment, or other negative consequences that do not deter the behavior (Black, Kehrberg, Flumerfelt, & Schlosser, 1997; Kafka, 2003a; Wiederman, 2004). The use of the term *sexual addiction* is controversial in that it may be perceived as being too similar to drug and alcohol abuse, and it may be viewed as absolving the individual of responsibility for his or her behavior (Herring, 2004).

The problematic sexual behavior may be paraphilic in terms of the sexual activities involved, or the behavior may be common sexual practice that is excessive and that causes distress or negative outcomes (Kafka, 1997a). The sexual activity or preoccupations may include excessively high rates of masturbation, excessive use of pornography or phone sex, excessive sex with multiple partners, with prostitutes, with nonconsenting partners, or with one consenting partner that results in relationship difficulties (Kafka, 2003a; Raymond, Coleman, & Miner, 2003). Operational definitions of hypersexuality have included Kinsey's (1948, as cited in Kafka, 1997a) recommendation of at least seven orgasms a week, through any and all means, for several consecutive months, termed *total sexual outlet*. An additional criterion is the average amount of time spent per week devoted to real or imagined sexual activity (Kafka, 1997a). Other researchers suggest that "impersonal sex" be used as a criterion, meaning that the person disregards the other person (if present) in favor of focus on the sex act itself. This criterion is supported by the finding that high rates of impersonal sexual behavior and interests are linked to less satisfaction with life; further, women who previously experienced sexual abuse or assault are more likely to report excessive impersonal sexual activities (Langstrom & Hanson, 2006).

About 5% of the U.S. population engages in compulsive sexual behavior, according to some estimates (Coleman, Raymond, & McBean, 2003), although individuals may be reluctant to report this problem, and few studies have addressed its prevalence. Compulsive sexual behavior is believed to be an anxiety-mitigating strategy, an impulse control difficulty, or both (Raymond et al., 2003). Although there may be an initial reduction in tension after the sexual act, individuals often feel guilty about engaging in the behavior (Black et al., 1997; Wiederman, 2004).

Treatment of compulsive sexual behavior depends on the nature of the behavior (i.e., whether it is compulsive masturbation, exhibitionism, or indiscriminate sex with others). Compulsive sexual behavior can include high-risk sexual behavior, such as repeated sexual behavior with multiple partners, without condom use. This behavior is a serious health risk, and warrants intervention (Coleman, 2002). Regardless of the types of behaviors involved, however, treatment generally includes cognitive and behavioral techniques to increase alternative behaviors and diminish sexual thoughts and activities. In therapy, individuals are encouraged to develop coping strategies to regulate stress and mood (Coleman et al., 2003). Couples therapy may be useful in some cases, as well as a group therapy format modeled after other addictions treatment (such as 12-step programs); however, the goal is usually to reduce the behavior, such as with overeating, and not necessarily to eliminate the sexual behavior, unless it is harmful (Schneider, 1989). Medications used to treat impulse-control disorders and antidepressants with sexual side effects have been indicated as treatments for compulsive sexual behavior (Raymond, Grant, Kim, & Coleman, 2002). More research is needed to better understand and treat the wide range of sexual compulsive behaviors.

Etiology of Paraphilias

Behavioral, psychosocial, and biological factors have been implicated in the development of the paraphilias.

Behavioral Factors Classical or Pavlovian conditioning has been a widely used model to explain the development of the paraphilias (see Akins, 2004, for a review). The development of a sexual fetish, for example, might be traced to a prior sexual experience that involved simultaneous arousal and presence of the object. This experience may occur during adolescence, which is the age at which most paraphilias begin. Once the association is acquired, the individual touches or smells the object in order to experience or enhance arousal, and repeated pairings during masturbation strengthen the association. In addition to the development of sexual fetishes, the pairing of sexual arousal with a particular object, situation, or type of person is likely to be involved in the development of the other paraphilias. Operant conditioning may also reinforce the behavior, as people who expose themselves, make obscene phone calls, or rub up against unsuspecting victims may be rewarded by the strong reaction of the victim or by the satisfaction of the act itself and the evasion of punishment if they are not caught. The types of sexual stimuli that elicit arousal are likely to be learned to some extent through implicit concepts or beliefs within a society. For example, shoes are more likely to be a fetish object than are tables. Important models, such as parents, may teach the deviant behavior through varying degrees of subtle or blatant modeling of the behavior (Stoller, 1985).

Psychosocial Factors and Comorbid Disorders or Difficulties In addition to behavioral conditioning and modeling, many other factors, including one's psychosocial history and comorbid problems and disorders are also likely to play a role in the paraphilias. For example, a history of sexual abuse may be an etiological factor. A substantial minority of individuals who develop pedophilia, for example, report a history of sexual abuse (Cohen & Galynker, 2002). Substance abuse is often a comorbid condition, and being under the influence of a substance may lower sexual inhibitions or impulses (Kafka & Hennen, 2002; Raymond, Coleman, Ohlerking, Christenson, & Miner, 1999). The paraphilias have been associated with a variety of additional difficulties, including mood disorders, social anxiety, attention-deficit/hyperactivity disorder, and impulse-control difficulties (Kafka & Hennen, 2002). For example, sexual offenders' impaired social skills and social anxiety have been implicated in their disorder (Hoyer, Kunst, & Schmidt, 2001), such that they may have difficulty recognizing social cues and may target vulnerable individuals, such as children, perhaps partly due to their difficulty forming relationships with adults (Emmers-Sommer et al., 2004).

Biological Factors The neurotransmitters that are believed to be involved in impulse control, mood, and sexual functioning, namely the monoamines (including norepinephrine, dopamine, and serotonin) are implicated in the paraphilias and compulsive sexual behavior (Bradford, 2001; Kafka, 2003b). Further, multiple sclerosis, temporal lobe epilepsy, as well as brain lesions and brain tumors in various areas have been associated with the paraphilias and compulsive sexual behavior. For example, the frontal lobe (which is involved in impulse control) and the temporal lobe (believed to be involved in sexual arousal) have both been implicated in these sexual disorders (Bradford, 2001; Cohen & Galynker, 2002). In addition, levels of sex hormones, particularly androgens, are likely to play a role in sexual desire and activity (Bradford, 2001).

The paraphilias tend to be much more common among males than among females (Arndt, 1991; Fagan et al., 2002; Langstrom & Zucker, 2005). These gender differences have primarily been explained either in terms of biological differences (such as hormonal differences), or in terms of socially prescribed gender roles. For example, cross-dressing among men is more likely to be noticed and pathologized compared to cross-dressing among women; further, cases of women who derive sexual pleasure from wearing men's clothing may be underreported (Devor, 1996). In addition, sexual scripts in many cultures specify that (in heterosexual relationships) men should be the pursuers, and women should be pursued. Taken a step further, some men may sexually harass women or violate their rights, as in frotteurism, voyeurism, exhibitionism, scatologia, and the like. These behaviors are not simply about sexual gratification, they also involve dominance and control. Paraphilic behaviors among women, however, can have different motivations and outcomes than among men, as females tend to be more sexualized than males. Female exhibitionists, for example, report exposing themselves to men in order to get positive attention and to experience the excitement of the situation (Hugh-Jones, Gough, & Littlewood, 2005).

Psychological Treatments

Individuals with paraphilias are often reluctant to seek treatment, either because (1) they do not believe their behavior is problematic; (2) they are embarrassed about their unusual sexual activities; or (3) their sexual activities are illegal. Accordingly, much of the research on the treatment of paraphilias includes samples of individuals who have been arrested and found guilty of sexual crimes and are mandated to receive therapy, and these individuals are usually highly motivated to report that the treatment has worked, but may not be motivated to change. Individuals with paraphilias that have caused relationship impairment, such as sexual fetishes, may be more motivated to change their behavior in order to preserve their relationship. Most of the research on treatment of the paraphilias, however, involves treatment of sex offenders.

Cognitive-behavioral therapy, with an emphasis on specific behavioral techniques, has been used to treat the paraphilias. This approach may include extinguishing the arousal response that is triggered by the conditioned stimulus, such as a pair of shoes or a picture of a child. Aversion therapy or *aversive conditioning* includes the presentation of an aversive stimulus with imagined or real presentation of the paraphilic stimulus. For example, the individual may become aroused by a pedophilic scenario and is then presented with a noxious odor or receives an electric shock or nausea-inducing substance (Marshall, 1974). *Covert sensitization* involves creating an imagined scene involving the deviant behavior that results in a negative experience or consequence, such as embarrassment or apprehension (Akins, 2004). Reconditioning the individual to become aroused to acceptable sexual stimuli, such as consenting adults, may also be used (Johnston, Hudson, & Marshall, 1992). Clinicians may also facilitate imagery that involves a new sequence of events, such as a scenario involving control of the unwanted impulses (Akins, 2004). Research findings for the effectiveness of these approaches, particularly among sex offenders, are mixed (Hall, 1995; Hanson, Broom, & Stephenson, 2004), and more research is needed with the paraphilias that involve consenting partners. Further, a major research issue regarding treatment approaches is that a commonly used outcome measure of treatment for sexual offenders, penile circumference, tends to be less accurate than penile volume assessment (McConaghy, 1999).

Cognitive strategies are also an important component of cognitive-behavioral therapy for individuals with paraphilias. Psychoeducation is used to help clients better understand their problem, how this problem has developed over time, and how to develop strategies to control their behavior. Clinicians also refute sexual myths that the client may hold, such as the concept that "no means yes" or that children should be taught about sex through experience. Treatment for sexual offenders may include facilitating their self-esteem development, anger management, empathy for others, and in some cases, enhancing communication skills, including helping the client to interpret social cues. Relapse prevention involves assisting the client in identifying patterns of behavior, as well as cues and situations that may increase risk for reoffending (Emmers-Sommer et al., 2004; Saleh & Guidry, 2003). In addition to cognitive and behavioral techniques, group therapy may be used. For disorders involving nonconsenting partners, such as pedophilia, the group format may be confrontational to address clients' defensiveness, denial, and minimization of the harm they have caused others (Cohen & Galynker, 2002; Fagan et al., 2002).

Medical Treatments

Researchers have reported some success in treating the paraphilias with antidepressants that influence serotonergic pathways (see Kafka, 1997b, for a review), as well as medications that reduce the effects of androgens, which are hormones believed to influence sexual desire and activity. Antiandrogens are medications that reduce the effects of androgens by competing with them at the receptor sites. One type of antiandrogen, cyproterone acetate (CPA), blocks androgen receptors and affects hormones that influence the release of testosterone. Medroxyprogesterone acetate (MPA) (Depo Provera) also results in a decrease in testosterone levels, although through a different mechanism of action. These medications have demonstrated success in treating paraphilias, particularly those involving nonconsenting partners, although they can have serious side effects (see Bradford, 2001, for a review; see also Saleh & Guidry, 2003).

Newer medications with fewer side effects have recently been tested, such as the gonadotropin-releasing hormone agonists (GnRH agonists) or luteinizing hormone-releasing hormone agonists (LHRH agonists). These agonists reduce the effect of the hormones that signal the release of androgens by paradoxically stimulating the hypothalamus to release more hormones, until the downregulation of receptors occurs. In many patients, an initial boost in sexual desire is followed by a steady decrease in desire as feedback mechanisms adjust to this overstimulation of the hypothalamus. One type of LHRH agonist, leuprolide acetate, has shown promising results at reducing sexual thoughts and activities among sexual offending paraphiliacs (Saleh & Guidry, 2003). The term *chemical castration* has been used to describe medications that reduce the effects of androgens, particularly the drug MPA; however, these medications do not necessarily cause impotence and their effects are often reversible, depending on the type of medication used. Mandatory treatment with these medications, however, has been an issue of serious debate (Miller, 1998).

Gender Identity Disorder

One's sex refers to anatomical indicators of being male or female. One's gender refers to the *sense* that one is male or female—in other words, the gender with which one identifies (Lips, 2006). Gender identity disorder is the experience of an inconsistency between one's sex and one's gender. Individuals who take steps toward changing their gender or appearing as the opposite sex may be referred to as *transsexuals*, often specified as male-to-female transsexuals and female-to-male transsexuals (Stoller, 1985). The term *transgender* is used as a broader term to include individuals who opt not to have sex reassignment surgery, but who live as the opposite gender, although the terms *transsexual* and *transgender* are often used inconsistently (see Carroll, Gilroy, & Ryan, 2002, for a comprehensive list of terms). According to the *DSM-IV-TR*, gender identity disorder is a strong and persistent cross-gender identification, such that the person with this disorder feels persistent discomfort with his or her sex and has a strong desire to be the opposite sex. The person asserts that he or she is "in the wrong body," and the experience is significantly distressing or results in impairment in functioning.

In children, gender identity disorder typically involves preference for opposite-sex dress, play behaviors, playmates, and urinary position, as well as the persistent assertion that the child belongs to the opposite sex. Although more boys than girls are generally diagnosed with this disorder, this may be due to greater parental disapproval of stereotypically feminine behaviors in boys than for stereotypically masculine behavior in girls (Devor, 1996; Zucker & Bradley, 1995). The majority of children with gender identity disorder do not continue to have this disorder in adolescence or adulthood, although most individuals with gender identity disorder in adulthood recall having the disorder as children. The majority of boys with this disorder identify as bisexual or homosexual as they mature (Zucker & Bradley, 1995). Although there is little research on gender identity disorder among girls, more lesbians than heterosexual women report being tomboys or feeling like they were boys as children, as compared to heterosexual women's reports (see Devor, 1996, for a review). Since gender identity disorder tends not to persist into adulthood, some researchers argue that this disorder should not be diagnosed among children (Lev, 2005). Additionally, dissatisfaction with one's gender role and desiring the freedoms and privileges of males can be common among females (Devor, 1996), but this dissatisfaction is not considered a disorder according to the *DSM-IV-TR*.

Among adolescents and adults with gender identity disorder, behaviors may include cross-dressing, as well as breast-binding in women to reduce the appearance of their breasts. Unlike transvestic fetishism, however, the aim of cross-dressing in gender identity disorder is usually to appear to be the opposite gender, which is consistent with the person's sense of self, rather than cross-dressing for the purpose of sexual arousal, although a person might have both aims (Buhrich & McConaghy, 1978). Sexual orientation (to whom one is attracted) is separate from gender identity (one's subjective sense of being a male or female). Yet, men with gender identity disorder who do not report transvestic fetishism are more likely to have a homosexual orientation (meaning that once they become the opposite sex, they have a heterosexual orientation), and men with transvestic fetishism alone tend to have a heterosexual orientation, according to penile responses to images of men and women (Buhrich & McConaghy, 1978).

Researchers are beginning to discover that individuals with gender identity disorder are a more heterogeneous group than was previously thought. These individuals vary with respect to their sexual orientation, the presence of paraphilias (such as transvestic fetishism), and age of onset of their gender dysphoria. Lev (2005) reviews several categories of experiences that seem to be missing from the transgender nomenclature, including individuals who do not want medical intervention but who do want to appear as the opposite gender, those who desire hormones but not surgery, those who have more than one gender identity and have or would like to have both male and female genitalia, those who want to appear more masculine or feminine with surgery that does not involve sex reassignment, and those who view their gender as nonstatic and do not wish to identify as one gender or the other.

Epidemiology

Gender identity disorder is relatively rare. Research conducted in the Netherlands estimates that transsexualism occurs in 1 in 11,900 males and 1 in 30,400 females (Bakker, van Kesteren, Gooren, & Bezemer, 1993).

Etiology

The etiology of gender identity disorder is complex and not fully understood, and theories about the development of this disorder are areas of serious debate.

Biological Factors Some evidence points to biological factors in the development of gender identity disorder. One theory holds that prenatal exposure to varying levels of sex hormones influences subsequent gender identity development. Although measuring prenatal hormone levels usually is not feasible or practical, comparative finger length on one's hand, particularly between the index and ring fingers is believed to be related to androgen exposure in the womb (Manning, Scutt, Wilson, & Lewis-Jones, 1998). Among male-to-female transsexuals, there is evidence of a difference in the ratio of length of the second to fourth fingers that is more similar to females than it is to nontranssexual males (Schneider, Pickel, & Stalla, 2006). Although digit ratios are now a popular measure, the validity of this measure as an indicator of prenatal androgen exposure is still being confirmed. Handedness has also been studied, with results showing that both types of transsexuals (male-to-female and female-to-male), as well as boys with gender identity disorder are significantly more likely to be left-handed than are people in the general population (Orlebeke, Boomsma, Gooren, Verschoor, & van den Bree, 1992; Zucker, Beaulieu, Bradley, Grimshaw, & Wilcox, 2001).

Other research has examined chromosomal and gonadal or hormonal anomalies that blur the line between the male and female sexes. For example, infants born with congenital adrenal hyperplasia (CAH) may have female chromosomes, but their bodies produce excessive amounts of androgens (masculinizing hormones) due to adrenal gland dysfunction. At birth, these infants may have large clitorises or even appear male. Regardless of whether they are assigned to the female or male gender, most grow up without developing gender identity disorder, although they do have higher rates of gender identity disorder when compared to the very low rates in the general population. Individuals with CAH who are assigned to the male gender and particularly those whose gender is reassigned later in childhood tend to have higher rates of gender identity issues (Dessens, Slijper, & Drop, 2005).

In addition to CAH, a number of other physiological and chromosomal anomalies can occur that result in ambiguous genitalia. One abnormality (5 alpha-Reductase-2 deficiency), which has been studied among individuals in villages in the Dominican Republic, occurred in genetically male children who had ambiguous genitalia, but appeared female, and most were reared as girls (Imperato-McGinley, Guerrero, Gautier, & Peterson, 1974). These children then developed masculine secondary sex characteristics at puberty, their testes descended, and their ambiguous genitalia developed into penises. They were known in the community as "machihembra," meaning "half man, half woman" or "guevedoces," meaning "penis at age 12." Most of these individuals adopted male gender roles as adults, although follow-up research shows that one of them in particular expressed the desire for sex reassignment surgery in adulthood to become a woman (Sobel & Imperato-McGinley, 2004). Finally, in separate research, the famous case of the boy (John/Joan) with the botched circumcision who was unsuccessfully reared as a girl also points to the role that biology plays in gender identity (Diamond & Sigmundson, 1997). Like any other psychological process, however, gender identity development is likely to be influenced by biological and environmental factors, which interact with each other in a bidirectional manner.

Psychosocial Factors The concepts of gender and anatomical sex are socially constructed. For example, in most societies, there are two sex categories: male and female. In some societies, however, such as in India and Thailand, there is a third category for individuals who wear women's clothing, but have male (or sometimes intersex or ambiguous) genitalia and do not try to pass as female (Marecek et al., 2004). Even in societies with two sexes, research suggests that gender identity occurs along a continuum, rather than being dichotomous. In other words, most people have varying degrees of identification with their own gender and with the opposite gender (Dunne, Bailey, Kirk, & Martin, 2000; McConaghy, 1993).

From a social-cognitive perspective, gender identity development involves learning one's gender role through *observational learning* (learning by viewing a model), experiencing others' evaluative reactions to one's behavior, and being directly rewarded and punished for gender-typical or gender-atypical behavior (Bussey & Bandura, 2004). These environmental forces typically exert pressure on children to conform to gender norms. Despite this pressure to conform, individuals with gender identity disorder may persist in their sex-atypical behavior or their assertion that they are the opposite sex. Many explanations have been provided for this unexpected result. In terms of psychosocial factors, researchers have proposed that children with gender identity disorder have identified with and imitated a person of their same gender, or that they have been reinforced for gender-atypical behaviors (Halle, Schmidt, & Meyer, 1980; King, 1996). More psychodynamically oriented theorists posit that male transsexuals had mothers who were either overly emotionally close or extremely distant, although additional research is needed to substantiate this hypothesis (Arndt, 1991). Further, the causal direction of these factors is unclear, as parent–child relationships involve reciprocal interaction, meaning that parents respond to children just as children respond to parents.

Treatment

Unlike treatments for most disorders, which involve helping individuals to change their thoughts, feelings, and behaviors, successful treatment of gender identity disorder often involves helping individuals change their gender. This transition may include hormone treatments, electrolysis for men to remove unwanted hair, and varying degrees of surgery. The primary focus of psychotherapy may be preparing the client for changes in his or her relationships with others and with the broader society. Addressing emotional wounds from prejudice and discrimination may also be a central part of therapy (Carroll et al., 2002).

The treatment of gender dysphoria in children and adolescents has become a controversial issue. Psychotherapeutic approaches may involve teaching the child or adolescent to develop more gender-consistent behaviors. Opponents argue that this treatment is unethical and that it involves imposing narrowly defined social expectations for gender roles onto children and adolescents (Isay, 1999; Lev, 2005). While some clinicians argue that retraining children to act in a more gender-role consistent manner will reduce peer and other interpersonal problems, Lev (2005) notes that "...in other areas where children are routinely bullied, for example racial or ethnic discrimination and physical or mental disabilities, the focus of intervention has been policy directed towards changing the social conditions that maintain abuse, not on changing children to better fit in to oppressive circumstances" (p. 49). Researchers further assert that children with gender-atypical behavior may simply be gay, lesbian, or bisexual, and thus psychotherapy for these children should follow the American Psychological Association's (2000) *Guidelines for Psychotherapy with Lesbian, Gay, & Bisexual Clients,* which involves support and acceptance of feelings and behaviors that vary from socially prescribed gender roles.

Others argue that detection of gender identity disorder in children can be useful in order to assist them to make a transition to the opposite sex during adolescence. This early transition allows the individual to avoid the continued stress of living life as a gender that is inconsistent with the sense of self. Additionally, secondary sex characteristics become evident during adolescence and can be problematic for adolescents with gender identity disorder. In cases involving extreme, unwavering gender dysphoria since childhood and a clear desire for sex reassignment surgery, hormone therapy and surgery for both male-to-female and female-to-male adolescent transsexuals have resulted in a positive outcome. It is noteworthy, however, that most of these adolescents did not undergo full genital surgery because of their waiting for advances in surgical techniques (Cohen-Kettenis & van Goozen, 1997). Not all researchers agree, however, that adolescents are developmentally ready to make such a consequential decision as a transsexual transformation, and the standard practice guidelines for gender identity disorder state that irreversible procedures should not be performed on individuals under the age of 18 *(Standards of Care for Gender Identity Disorders,* 2001).

Since sex reassignment surgery is such a serious, irreversible, and life-changing transformation, surgeons are cautious about accepting patients for this surgery. The current treatment practice for transsexuals is based on the *Standards of Care for Gender Identity Disorders* (2001) guidelines, provided by the World Professional Association for Transgender Health. These guidelines specify that certain conditions must be met before sex reassignment surgery may be performed, including a gender identity disorder diagnosis, recommendation from one or more psychotherapists (depending on the type of surgery requested), and living as the opposite gender for one year while receiving hormone injections. Some researchers have expressed concern that individuals who want sex reassignment surgery have learned to report certain expected case histories, including that they are homosexual, that they have been gender dysphoric since childhood, and that they do not have transvestic fetishism, because they believe it will increase their chances of being accepted for surgery (see Lev, 2005, for a review). Some argue that transsexualism is not a disorder and that the requirements for sex reassignment surgery are expensive, demeaning, and invalid (Denny, 2004). Moreover, research suggests that patients who do not comply with the one-year transgender experience guideline prior to surgery have postoperative outcomes that are no different from the outcomes of patients who do comply (Lawrence, 2003). In most cases, sex reassignment surgery results in positive mental and physical health outcomes (De Cuypere et al., 2005; Smith, Van Goozen, Kuiper, & Cohen-Kettenis, 2005), and negative outcomes often involve dissatisfaction or problems with the surgical procedure, which usually cannot be predicted (Lawrence, 2003). Yet, physicians and surgeons will likely continue to screen their patients for liability reasons.

Summary, Current Issues, and Future Directions

Sexual dysfunctions, the paraphilias, and gender identity disorder reflect a vast array of behaviors, all of which lie along a continuum and have varying degrees of concomitant distress, including no distress to severe distress. Biological, social, and psychological factors play a role in each of these disorders and one cannot separate the influence of these factors on a given individual. The sexual dysfunction literature, which used to emphasize Masters and Johnson's behavioral techniques, is now dominated by medical research that assesses and treats these problems from a biological perspective. Erectile dysfunction has been a predominant area of research (Winton, 2001), and successful treatment with medications has made this problem profitable to drug manufacturers and easily solved by the consumer. Medical interest in female sexual dysfunction, while historically ignored, is now increasing, largely as a result of the potential for a finding a popular drug that could be the female counterpart to drugs such as Viagra (Hartley, 2006). Nevertheless, conceptualizations and treatments of sexual functioning that consider interpersonal, psychological, and social factors are still recommended (Hatzichristou et al., 2004).

The paraphilias include a variety of behaviors, some of which may simply reflect unusual sexual preferences, while other behaviors involve harmful and illegal activities, such as acting on pedophilic impulses. Behavioral explanations of how deviant sexual behavior is learned are prevalent in this area of research. Much of the research emphasis, however, is devoted to pedophiles and sexual offenders and their treatment, which is a much needed line of research, although more research is needed to address the other paraphilias as well. Behavioral techniques involving punishment or changing learned associations may be used to treat these problems, although particularly for sexual offenders, medications to lower sexual desire are likely to be more prevalent in the future (Saleh & Guidry, 2003).

Gender identity disorder involves a conviction that one is or should have been the opposite sex. This problem reflects a wider range of beliefs about one's gender and desired physical changes than was originally thought, including individuals who want to live as the opposite gender with or without hormone therapy and with or without sex reassignment surgery (Lev, 2005). Individuals may also be intersexed or have ambiguous genitalia at birth. A wide variety of biological and psychosocial factors have been proposed to explain gender identity disorder, although the etiology of gender identity disorder is complicated and not clearly understood. For those individuals who opt for sex reassignment surgery, there are commonly used guidelines that must often be met before the surgery can be performed, but most transsexuals make a successful transition postoperatively and are relieved of their gender dysphoria (Smith et al., 2005).

The *DSM* and Future Potential Diagnostic Categories

If the past is a guide to the future, the number of sexual dysfunctions and disorders in the *DSM* is likely to increase. Recommendations from the committee on the Definitions, Classifications and Epidemiology of Sexual Dysfunction include the addition of *persistent sexual arousal disorder* (recurrent, unwanted genital arousal), as well as the addition of *anejaculation*, meaning orgasm in men that occurs without ejaculation (Lewis et al., 2004). Other committees have discussed the possible addition of *sexual satisfaction disorder*, defined as not being sexually satisfied, despite satisfactory reports of desire, arousal, and orgasm (Basson et al., 2000). Another potential disorder is *noncoital sexual pain disorder* (Basson et al., 2000).

Some argue that female sexual arousal dysfunction does not reflect women's subjective experience of sexual arousal, which may or may not correspond to their physical response. Researchers thus propose that female sexual arousal be divided into three disorders: one indicating the lack of genital arousal, the second including lack of the subjective feeling of sexual arousal and pleasure, and the third including both the first and second symptoms (Basson et al., 2004; Lewis et al., 2004). Further, women may experience sexual desire during, rather than prior to sex, and women may not necessarily be sexually motivated by fantasies and sexual thoughts, which suggests that sexual desire disorder should be revised (Basson, 2005).

Another potential revision to the *DSM* is the addition of *compulsive sexual disorder*, which several researchers have recommended (Bradford, 2001). With increasing attention to female paraphilic behaviors, the paraphilias may also be revised to include behaviors that are more common among females. Lastly, research indicates that gender identity disorder may be subcategorized into a variety of components that reflect the wide range of gender variant identification, behaviors, and desires for treatment (Lev, 2005).

Internet Sexuality

While sexual activities were taboo discussion topics in the past, in many cultures, these topics are receiving more attention, including books, magazine articles, television shows and commercials, and other forms of media that promote ideas about what it means to have a fulfilling sex life. With the advent of the Internet, much more information is readily accessible to people than ever before. At the same time, the Internet can also be a place for pedophilia, sexual addictions, and a host of sexually deviant fantasies to flourish. The 24-hour availability, low cost, relative anonymity, and lack of risk for disease may facilitate excessive Internet sexual activity (termed *internet sexual compulsivity*). This problematic behavior can take the form of either viewing sexual material or sexual *computer mediated relating* (CMR) (Cooper, McLoughlin, & Campbell, 2004). This excessive behavior can damage relationships and result in diminished work productivity and job loss. Attempting to control Internet-mediated sexual activity is a major issue for corporations, families, and educational institutions. Yet, online sexual activity can also add excitement to a committed relationship and can provide a "safe" space to discuss sexual fantasies or sexual issues (Cooper et al., 2004).

The Medicalization of Sexual Dysfunction

Researchers who support the view that sexual dysfunction has been socially constructed argue that any sexual experience, activity, or level of desire that does not fit nicely into the restricted definition of "normal sex" becomes medicalized as a disorder (Lavie-Ajayi, 2005). Proponents of the sexual dysfunction categories assert, however, that these categories allow researchers and treatment professionals to more effectively identify, study, and treat these difficulties. Individuals receiving treatment can also be assured that their problem is a valid concern that warrants attention and treatment, particularly if the problem is framed as a medical one.

A major demographic trend is the aging of the Baby Boomer generation. This trend has important implications for the marketing and selling of medications to treat sexual dysfunctions to this large potential market of consumers, particularly since erectile dysfunction tends to increase with age (Prins et al., 2002). The medicalization of sexual difficulties is supported by the current popularity of biological explanations and drug treatments of sexual dysfunction. As Tiefer (2006) explains, "The trend of looking towards biology for the 'most basic' explanations of complex human behavior, sidelined during the socially conscious 1970s and revived by sociobiology in the 1980s, escalated in the 1990s along with the mania for genetics and molecular biology and their magical promises" (p. 282). With the promotion of medication for sexual problems, the media may also be deemphasizing or omitting alternative explanations for sexual problems, including psychosocial factors (Tiefer, 2002). While sexual functioning clearly has a biological component, many argue that the explanation of sexual dysfunction as purely biological in origin oversimplifies the problem and blames the individual (Tiefer, 2001). Moreover, the use of medication in order to encourage people to want to have sex may be viewed as a symptom of a youth-obsessed and sex-obsessed society, rather than a symptom of a medical condition (Potts, Grace, Gavey, & Vares, 2004). Nevertheless, diagnostic categories that determine "appropriate" sexual behavior will likely continue to be used, for better or for worse.

References

Akins, C. K. (2004). The role of Pavlovian conditioning in sexual behavior: A comparative analysis of human and nonhuman animals. *International Journal of Comparative Psychology, 17,* 241–262.

Alison, L., Santtila, P., Sandnabba, N. K., & Nordling, N. (2004). Sadomasochistically oriented behavior. In M. S. Kimmel & R. F. Plante (Eds.), *Sexualities: Identities, behaviors, and society* (pp. 258–265). New York: Oxford University Press.

Althof, S. E., Leiblum, S. R., Chevret-Measson, M., Hartmann, U., Levine, S. B., McCabe, M., et al. (2005). Psychological and interpersonal dimensions of sexual function and dysfunction. *Journal of Sexual Medicine, 2*(6), 793–800.

American Psychiatric Association. (2000). *Diagnostic and statistical manual of mental disorders* (4th ed., text rev.). Washington, D.C.: Author.

American Psychological Association. (2000). *Guidelines for psychotherapy with lesbian, gay, and bisexual clients.* Retrieved October 31, 2006, from http://www.apa.org/pi/lgbc/guidelines.html

Araujo, A. B., Durante, R., Feldman, H. A., Goldstein, I., & McKinlay, J. B. (1998). The relationship between depressive symptoms and male erectile dysfunction: Cross-sectional results from the Massachusetts Male Aging Study. *Psychosomatic Medicine, 60,* 458–465.

Archer, S. L., Gragasin, F. S., Webster, L., Bochinski, D., & Michelakis, E. D. (2005). Aetiology and management of male erectile dysfunction and female sexual dysfunction in patients with cardiovascular disease. *Drugs and Aging, 22*(10), 823–844.

Arndt, W. B., Jr. (1991). *Gender disorders and the paraphilias.* Madison, CT: International Universities Press.

Bakker, A., van Kesteren, P. J., Gooren, L. J., & Bezemer, P. D. (1993). The prevalence of transsexualism in The Netherlands. *Acta Psychiatrica Scandinavica, 87*(4), 237–238.

Bancroft, J. (2002). The medicalization of female sexual dysfunction: The need for caution. *Archives of Sexual Behavior, 31*(5), 451–455.

Bancroft, J., Loftus, J., & Long, J. S. (2003). Distress about sex: A national survey of women in heterosexual relationships. *Archives of Sexual Behavior, 32*(3), 193–208.

Barlow, D. H. (1986). Causes of sexual dysfunction: The role of anxiety and cognitive interference. *Journal of Consulting and Clinical Psychology, 54*(2), 140–148.

Basson, R. (2005). Women's sexual dysfunction: Revised and expanded definitions. *Canadian Medical Association Journal, 172*(10), 1327–1333.

Basson, R., Althof, S., Davis, S., Fugl-Meyer, K., Goldstein, I., Leiblum, S., et al. (2004). Summary of the recommendations on sexual dysfunctions in women. *Journal of Sexual Medicine, 1*(1), 24–34.

Basson, R., Berman, J., Burnett, A., Derogatis, L., Ferguson, D., Fourcroy, J., et al. (2000). Report of the international consensus development conference on female sexual dysfunction: Definitions and classifications. *Journal of Urology, 163*(3), 888–893.

Basson, R., McInnes, R., Smith, M. D., Hodgson, G., & Koppiker, N. (2002). Efficacy and safety of sildenafil citrate in women with sexual dysfunction associated with female sexual arousal disorder. *Journal of Women's Health and Gender-Based Medicine, 11*(4), 367–377.

Baucom, D. H., Shoham, V., Mueser, K. T., Daiuto, A. D., & Stickle, T. R. (1998). Empirically supported couple and family interventions for marital distress and adult mental health problems. *Journal of Consulting and Clinical Psychology, 66*(1), 53–88.

Beck, J. G., & Barlow, D. H. (1986). The effects of anxiety and attentional focus on sexual responding—II. Cognitive and affective patterns in erectile dysfunction. *Behaviour Research and Therapy, 24*(1), 19–26.

Berman, J. R., & Bassuk, J. (2002). Physiology and pathophysiology of female sexual function and dysfunction. *World Journal of Urology, 20*(2), 111–118.

Berman, J. R., Berman, L., & Goldstein, I. (1999). Female sexual dysfunction: Incidence, pathophysiology, evaluation, and treatment options. *Urology, 54*(3), 385–391.

Billups, K. L., Berman, L., Berman, J., Metz, M. E., Glennon, M. E., & Goldstein, I. (2001). A new non-pharmacological vacuum therapy for female sexual dysfunction. *Journal of Sex and Marital Therapy, 27*(5), 435–441.

Black, D. W., Kehrberg, L. L., Flumerfelt, D. L., & Schlosser, S. S. (1997). Characteristics of 36 subjects reporting compulsive sexual behavior. *American Journal of Psychiatry, 154*(2), 243–249.

Blanker, M. H., Bosch, J. L., Groeneveld, F. P., Bohnen, A. M., Prins, A., Thomas, S., et al. (2001). Erectile and ejaculatory dysfunction in a community-based sample of men 50 to 78 years old: Prevalence, concern, and relation to sexual activity. *Urology, 57*(4), 763–768.

Bodenmann, G., Ledermann, T., Blattner, D., & Galluzzo, C. (2006). Associations among everyday stress, critical life events, and sexual problems. *Journal of Nervous and Mental Disease, 194*(7), 494–501.

Bradford, J. M. (2001). The neurobiology, neuropharmacology, and pharmacological treatment of the paraphilias and compulsive sexual behaviour. *Canadian Journal of Psychiatry, 46*(1), 26–34.

Braunstein, G. D., Sundwall, D. A., Katz, M., Shifren, J. L., Buster, J. E., Simon, J. A., et al. (2005). Safety and efficacy of a testosterone patch for the treatment of hypoactive sexual desire disorder in surgically menopausal women: A randomized, placebo-controlled trial. *Archives of Internal Medicine, 165*(14), 1582–1589.

Buhrich, N., & McConaghy, N. (1978). Two clinically discrete syndromes of transsexualism. *British Journal of Psychiatry, 133*, 73–76.

Burchardt, M., Burchardt, T., Anastasiadis, A. G., Kiss, A. J., Baer, L., Pawar, R. V., et al. (2002). Sexual dysfunction is common and overlooked in female patients with hypertension. *Journal of Sex and Marital Therapy, 28*(1), 17–26.

Bussey, K., & Bandura, A. (2004). Social cognitive theory of gender development and functioning. In A. H. Eagly, A. E. Beall & R. J. Sternberg (Eds.), *The psychology of gender* (2nd ed., pp. 92–119). New York: Guilford.

Cain, V. S., Johannes, C. B., Avis, N. E., Mohr, B., Schocken, M., Skurnick, J., et al. (2003). Sexual functioning and practices in a multi-ethnic study of midlife women: Baseline results from SWAN. *Journal of Sex Research, 40*(3), 266–276.

Carbone, D. J., & Seftel, A. D. (2004). Pathophysiology of male erectile dysfunction. In A. D. Seftel, H. Padma-Nathan, C. G. McMahon, F. Giuliano, & S. E. Althof (Eds.), *Male and female sexual dysfunction* (pp. 19–29). New York: Mosby.

Carlson, N. R. (2001). *Physiology of behavior* (7th ed.). Boston: Allyn & Bacon.

Carroll, L., Gilroy, P. J., & Ryan, J. (2002). Counseling transgendered, transsexual, and gender-variant clients. *Journal of Counseling and Development, 80*, 131–139.

Caruso, S., Agnello, C., Intelisano, G., Farina, M., Di Mari, L., & Cianci, A. (2004). Placebo-controlled study on efficacy and safety of daily apomorphine SL intake in premenopausal women affected by hypoactive sexual desire disorder and sexual arousal disorder. *Urology, 63*(5), 955–959.

Cohen, L. J., & Galynker, I. I. (2002). Clinical features of pedophilia and implications for treatment. *Journal of Psychiatric Practice, 8*(5), 276–289.

Cohen-Kettenis, P. T., & van Goozen, S. H. (1997). Sex reassignment of adolescent transsexuals: A follow-up study. *Journal of the American Academy of Child and Adolescent Psychiatry, 36*(2), 263–271.

Coleman, E. (2002). Promoting sexual health and responsible sexual behavior: An introduction. *The Journal of Sex Research, 39*(1), 3–6.

Coleman, E., Raymond, N., & McBean, A. (2003). Assessment and treatment of compulsive sexual behavior. *Minnesota Medicine, 86*(7), 42-47.

Committee on Bioethics. (1998). Female genital mutilation. *Pediatrics, 102*(1), 153–156.

Cooper, A., McLoughlin, I. P., & Campbell, K. M. (2004). Sexuality in cyberspace. In M. S. Kimmel & R. F. Plante (Eds.), *Sexualities: Identities, behaviors, and society* (pp. 285–298). New York: Oxford University Press.

Cyranowski, J. M., Aarestad, S. L., & Andersen, B. L. (1999). The role of sexual self-schema in a diathesis-stress model of sexual dysfunction. *Applied and Preventive Psychology, 8*, 217–228.

Davis, S. R., Davison, S. L., Donath, S., & Bell, R. J. (2005). Circulating androgen levels and self-reported sexual function in women. *Journal of the American Medical Association, 294*(1), 91–96.

De Cuypere, G., T'Sjoen, G., Beerten, R., Selvaggi, G., De Sutter, P., Hoebeke, P., et al. (2005). Sexual and physical health after sex reassignment surgery. *Archives of Sexual Behavior, 34*(6), 679–690.

Dennerstein, L., Guthrie, J. R., & Alford, S. (2004). Childhood abuse and its association with mid-aged women's sexual functioning. *Journal of Sex and Marital Therapy, 30*(4), 225–234.

Denny, D. (2004). Changing models of transsexualism. *Journal of Gay and Lesbian Psychotherapy, 8*(1–2), 25–40.

Dessens, A. B., Slijper, F. M. E., & Drop, S. L. S. (2005). Gender dysphoria and gender change in chromosomal females with congenital adrenal hyperplasia. *Archives of Sexual Behavior, 34*(4), 389–397.

Devor, H. (1996). Female gender dysphoria in context: Social problem or personal problem. *Annual Review of Sex Research, 7*, 44–89.

Diamond, M., & Sigmundson, H. K. (1997). Sex reassignment at birth: Long-term review and clinical implications. *Archives of Pediatrics and Adolescent Medicine, 151*(3), 298–304.

Dominguez, J. M., & Hull, E. M. (2005). Dopamine, the medial preoptic area, and male sexual behavior. *Physiology & Behavior, 86*, 356–368.

Dunn, K. M., Croft, P. R., & Hackett, G. I. (1999). Association of sexual problems with social, psychological, and physical problems in men and women: A cross sectional population survey. *Journal of Epidemiology and Community Health, 53*(3), 144–148.

Dunne, M. P., Bailey, J. M., Kirk, K. M., & Martin, N. G. (2000). The subtlety of sex-atypicality. *Archives of Sexual Behavior, 29*(6), 549–565.

Elgaali, M., Strevens, H., & Mardh, P. A. (2005). Female genital mutilation—An exported medical hazard. *European Journal of Contraception and Reproductive Health Care, 10*(2), 93–97.

Emmers-Sommer, T. M., Allen, M., Bourhis, J., Sahlstein, E., Laskowski, K., Falato, W. L., et al. (2004). A meta-analysis of the relationship between social skills and sexual offenders. *Communication Reports, 17*(1), 1–10.

Enserink, M. (2005). Let's talk about sex—and drugs. *Science, 308*(5728), 1578–1580.

Fagan, P. J. (2004). *Sexual disorders: Perspectives on diagnosis and treatment.* Baltimore: Johns Hopkins University Press.

Fagan, P. J., Wise, T. N., Schmidt, C. W., Jr., & Berlin, F. S. (2002). Pedophilia. *Journal of the American Medical Association, 288*(19), 2458–2465.

Feldman, H. A., Goldstein, I., Hatzichristou, D. G., Krane, R. J., & McKinlay, J. B. (1994). Impotence and its medical and psychosocial correlates: Results of the Massachusetts Male Aging Study. *The Journal of Urology, 151*(1), 54–61.

Fisher, W., Boroditsky, R., & Morris, B. (2004). The 2002 Canadian Contraception Study: Part 2. *Journal of Obstetrics and Gynaecology Canada, 26*(7), 646–656.

Foley, S. M. (1994). Contemporary sex therapy. In R. Lechtenberg & D. A. Ohl (Eds.), *Sexual dysfunction: Neurologic, urologic, and gynecologic aspects* (pp. 259–274). Baltimore: Lea & Febiger.

Frank, E., Anderson, C., & Rubinstein, D. (1978). Frequency of sexual dysfunction in "normal" couples. *New England Journal of Medicine, 299*(3), 111–115.

Fugl-Meyer, K., & Fugl-Meyer, A. R. (2002). Sexual disabilities are not singularities. *International Journal of Impotence Research, 14*(6), 487–493.

Gagnon, J. H., Rosen, R. C., & Leiblum, S. R. (1982). Cognitive and social aspects of sexual dysfunction: Sexual scripts in sex therapy. *Journal of Sex and Marital Therapy, 8*(1), 44–56.

Goldstein, I. (2004). Androgen physiology in sexual medicine. *Sexuality and Disability, 22*(2), 165–169.

Gonzalez, M., Viafara, G., Caba, F., & Molina, E. (2004). Sexual function, menopause and hormone replacement therapy (HRT). *Maturitas, 48*(4), 411–420.

Greenstein, A., Abramov, L., Matzkin, H., & Chen, J. (2006). Sexual dysfunction in women partners of men with erectile dysfunction. *International Journal of Impotence Research, 18*(1), 44–46.

Grover, S. A., Lowensteyn, I., Kaouache, M., Marchand, S., Coupal, L., DeCarolis, E., et al. (2006). The prevalence of erectile dysfunction in the primary care setting: Importance of risk factors for diabetes and vascular disease. *Archives of Internal Medicine, 166*(2), 213–219.

Gruszecki, L., Forchuk, C., & Fisher, W. A. (2005). Factors associated with common sexual concerns in women: New findings from the Canadian contraception study. *The Canadian Journal of Human Sexuality, 14*(1–2), 1–13.

Hall, G. C. (1995). Sexual offender recidivism revisited: A meta-analysis of recent treatment studies. *Journal of Consulting and Clinical Psychology, 63*(5), 802–809.

Halle, E., Schmidt, C. W., Jr., & Meyer, J. K. (1980). The role of grandmothers in transsexualism. *American Journal of Psychiatry, 137*(4), 497–498.

Hanson, R. K., Broom, I., & Stephenson, M. (2004). Evaluating community sex offender treatment programs: A 12-year follow-up of 724 offenders. *Canadian Journal of Behavioural Science, 36*(2), 87–96.

Hartley, H. (2006). The "pinking" of Viagra culture: Drug industry efforts to create and repackage sex drugs for women. *Sexualities, 9*(3), 363–378.

Hatzichristou, D., Rosen, R. C., Broderick, G., Clayton, A., Cuzin, B., Derogatis, L., et al. (2004). Clinical evaluation and management strategy for sexual dysfunction in men and women. *Journal of Sexual Medicine, 1*(1), 49–57.

Heiman, J. R. (2002). Sexual dysfunction: Overview of prevalence, etiological factors, and treatments. *The Journal of Sex Research, 39*(1), 73–78.

Heiman, J. R., Gittelman, M., Costabile, R., Guay, A., Friedman, A., Heard-Davison, A., et al. (2006). Topical alprostadil (PGE1) for the treatment of female sexual arousal disorder: in-clinic evaluation of safety and efficacy. *Journal of Psychosomatic Obstetrics and Gynecology, 27*(1), 31–41.

Heiman, J. R., & Meston, C. M. (1997). Empirically validated treatment for sexual dysfunction. *Annual Review of Sexual Research, 8*, 148–194.

Helgason, A. R., Adolfsson, J., Dickman, P., Arver, S., Fredrikson, M., Gothberg, M., et al. (1996). Sexual desire, erection, orgasm and ejaculatory functions and their importance to elderly Swedish men: A population-based study. *Age and Ageing, 25*(4), 285–291.

Herring, B. (2004). The next 20 years: The developmental challenges facing the field of compulsive sexual behavior. *Sexual Addiction and Compulsivity, 11*, 35–42.

Holden, C. (1986). Proposed new psychiatric diagnoses raise charges of gender bias. *Science, 231*(4736), 327–328.

Hoyer, J., Kunst, H., & Schmidt, A. (2001). Social phobia as a comorbid condition in sex offenders with paraphilia or impulse control disorder. *Journal of Nervous and Mental Disease, 189*(7), 463–470.

Hugh-Jones, S., Gough, B., & Littlewood, A. (2005). Sexual exhibitionism as "sexuality and individuality": A critique of psycho-medical discourse from the perspectives of women who exhibit. *Sexualities, 8*(3), 259–281.

Imperato-McGinley, J., Guerrero, L., Gautier, T., & Peterson, R. E. (1974). Steroid 5alpha-reductase deficiency in man: An inherited form of male pseudohermaphroditism. *Science, 186*(4170), 1213–1215.

Irvine, J. M. (1990). *Disorders of desire: Sex and gender in modern American sexology.* Philadelphia: Temple University Press.

Isay, R. A. (1999). Gender in homosexual boys: Some developmental and clinical considerations. *Psychiatry: Interpersonal and Biological Processes, 62*(2), 187–194.

Janata, J. W., & Kingsberg, S. A. (2005). Sexual aversion disorder. In R. Balon & R. T. Segraves (Eds.), *Handbook of sexual dysfunction* (pp. 111–121). New York: Taylor & Francis.

Johnston, P., Hudson, S. M., & Marshall, W. L. (1992). The effects of masturbatory reconditioning with nonfamilial child molesters. *Behaviour Research and Therapy, 30*(5), 559–561.

Kadri, N., Alami, K. H. M., & Tahiri, S. M. (2002). Sexual dysfunction in women: Population based epidemiological study. *Archives of Women's Mental Health, 5*(2), 59–63.

Kafka, M. P. (1997a). Hypersexual desire in males: An operational definition and clinical implications for males with paraphilias and paraphilia-related disorders. *Archives of Sexual Behavior, 26*(5), 505–526.

Kafka, M. P. (1997b). A monoamine hypothesis for the pathophysiology of paraphilic disorders. *Archives of Sexual Behavior, 26*(4), 343–358.

Kafka, M. P. (2003a). Sex offending and sexual appetite: The clinical and theoretical relevance of hypersexual desire. *International Journal of Offender Therapy and Comparative Criminology, 47*(4), 439–451.

Kafka, M. P. (2003b). The monoamine hypothesis for the pathophysiology of paraphilic disorders: An update. *Annals of the New York Academy of Sciences, 989,* 144–153.

Kafka, M. P., & Hennen, J. (2002). A *DSM-IV* Axis I comorbidity study of males ($n = 120$) with paraphilias and paraphilia-related disorders. *Sexual Abuse: A Journal of Research and Treatment, 14*(4), 349–366.

Kao, J., Mantz, C., Garofalo, M., Milano, M. T., Vijayakumar, S., Jani, A. (2003). Treatment-related sexual dysfunction in male nonprostate pelvic malignancies. *Sexuality and Disability, 21*(1), 3–20.

Kaplan, H. S. (1979). *Disorders of sexual desire.* New York: Brunner/Mazel.

Kennedy, S. H., Dickens, S. E., Eisfeld, B. S., & Bagby, R. M. (1999). Sexual dysfunction before antidepressant therapy in major depression. *Journal of Affective Disorders, 56*(2–3), 201–208.

Kimmel, M. S., & Plante, R. F. (2004). *Sexualities: Identities, behaviors, and society.* New York: Oxford University Press.

King, B. M. (1996). *Human sexuality today* (2nd ed.). Upper Saddle River, NJ: Prentice-Hall.

Knegtering, H., van der Moolen, A. E. G. M., Castelein, S., Kluiter, H., & van den Bosch, R. J. (2003). What are the effects of antipsychotics on sexual dysfunctions and endocrine functioning? *Psychoneuroendocrinology, 28,* 109–123.

Langstrom, N., & Hanson, R. K. (2006). High rates of sexual behavior in the general population: Correlates and predictors. *Archives of Sexual Behavior, 35*(1), 37–52.

Langstrom, N., & Zucker, K. J. (2005). Transvestic fetishism in the general population: Prevalence and correlates. *Journal of Sex and Marital Therapy, 31*(2), 87–95.

Laumann, E. O., Paik, A., Glasser, D. B., Kang, J. H., Wang, T., Levinson, B., et al. (2006). A cross-national study of subjective sexual well-being among older women and men: Findings from the Global Study of Sexual Attitudes and Behaviors. *Archives of Sexual Behavior, 35*(2), 145–161.

Laumann, E. O., Paik, A., & Rosen, R. C. (1999). Sexual dysfunction in the United States: Prevalence and predictors. *Journal of the American Medical Association, 281*(6), 537–544.

Lavie-Ajayi, M. (2005). "Because all real women do": The construction and deconstruction of "female orgasmic disorder". *Sexualities, Evolution, and Gender, 7*(1), 57–72.

Lawrence, A. A. (2003). Factors associated with satisfaction or regret following male-to-female sex reassignment surgery. *Archives of Sexual Behavior, 32*(4), 299–315.

Lechtenberg, R., & Ohl, D. A. (1994). *Sexual dysfunction: Neurologic, urologic, and gynecologic aspects.* Philadelphia: Lea and Febiger.

Lev, A. I. (2005). Disordering gender identity: Gender identity disorder in the *DSM-IV-TR. Journal of Psychology and Human Sexuality, 17*(3/4), 35–69.

Lewis, R. W., Fugl-Meyer, K. S., Bosch, R., Fugl-Meyer, A. R., Laumann, E. O., Lizza, E., et al. (2004). Epidemiology/risk factors of sexual dysfunction. *Journal of Sexual Medicine, 1*(1), 35–39.

Lips, H. M. (2006). *A new psychology of women: Gender, culture, and ethnicity* (3rd ed.). New York: McGraw-Hill.

LoPiccolo, J., & Lobitz, W. C. (1972). The role of masturbation in the treatment of orgasmic dysfunction. *Archives of Sexual Behavior, 2*(2), 163–171.

Manning, J. T., Scutt, D., Wilson, J., & Lewis-Jones, D. I. (1998). The ratio of 2nd to 4th digit length: A predictor of sperm numbers and concentrations of testosterone, luteinizing hormone and oestrogen. *Human Reproduction, 13*(11), 3000–3004.

Marecek, J., Crawford, M., & Popp, D. (2004). On the construction of gender, sex, and sexualities. In A. H. Eagly, A. E. Beall, & R. J. Sternberg (Eds.), *The psychology of gender.* New York: Guilford.

Marshall, W. L. (1974). A combined treatment approach to the reduction of multiple fetish-related behaviors. *Journal of Consulting and Clinical Psychology, 42*(4), 613–616.

Masters, W. H., & Johnson, V. E. (1970). *Human sexual inadequacy.* Boston: Little, Brown.

Masters, W. H., Johnson, V. E., & Kolodny, R. C. (1985). *Masters and Johnson on sex and human loving.* Boston: Little, Brown.

Matlin, M. W. (2000). *The psychology of women* (4th ed.). New York: Harcourt.

McCabe, M. P. (2001). Evaluation of a cognitive behavior therapy program for people with sexual dysfunction. *Journal of Sex and Marital Therapy, 27*(3), 259–271.

McConaghy, N. (1993). *Sexual behavior: Problems and management.* New York: Plenum.

McConaghy, N. (1999). Unresolved issues in scientific sexology. *Archives of Sexual Behavior, 28*(4), 285–318.

McCormick, N. B. (1987). Sexual scripts: Social and therapeutic implications. *Sexual and Marital Therapy, 2*(1), 3–27.

McMahon, C. G. (2004). The ejaculatory response. In A. D. Seftel, H. Padma-Nathan, C. G. McMahon, F. Giuliano, & S. E. Althof (Eds.), *Male and female sexual dysfunction* (pp. 43–57). New York: Mosby.

Merriam-Webster's collegiate dictionary (10th ed.). (2001). Springfield, MA: Merriam-Webster.

Michael, A., & O'Keane, V. (2000). Sexual dysfunction in depression. *Human Psychopharmacology, 15,* 337–345.

Miller, R. D. (1998). Forced administration of sex-drive reducing medications to sex offenders: Treatment or punishment? *Psychology, Public Policy, and Law, 4*(1–2), 175–199.

Montgomery, S. A., Baldwin, D. S., & Riley, A. (2002). Antidepressant medications: A review of the evidence for drug-induced sexual dysfunction. *Journal of Affective Disorders, 69*(1–3), 119–140.

Nicolosi, A., Laumann, E. O., Glasser, D. B., Moreira, E. D., Jr., Paik, A., & Gingell, C. (2004). Sexual behavior and sexual dysfunctions after age 40: The global study of sexual attitudes and behaviors. *Urology, 64(5),* 991–997.

Nicolosi, A., Moreira, E. D., Jr., Shirai, M., Bin Mohd Tambi, M. I., & Glasser, D. B. (2003). Epidemiology of erectile dysfunction in four countries: Cross-national study of the prevalence and correlates of erectile dysfunction. *Urology, 61*(1), 201–206.

Nobre, P. J., & Pinto-Gouveia, J. (2006). Dysfunctional sexual beliefs as vulnerability factors to sexual dysfunction. *The Journal of Sex Research, 43*(1), 68–75.

Nyunt, A., Stephen, G., Gibbin, J., Durgan, L., Fielding, A. M., Wheeler, M., et al. (2005). Androgen status in healthy premenopausal women with loss of libido. *Journal of Sex and Marital Therapy, 31*(1), 73–80.

Oberg, K., Fugl-Meyer, K. S., & Fugl-Meyer, A. R. (2002). On sexual well-being in sexually abused Swedish women: Epidemiological aspects. *Sexual and Relationship Therapy, 17*(4), 329–341.

Orlebeke, J. F., Boomsma, D. I., Gooren, L. J. G., Verschoor, A. M., & van den Bree, M. J. M. (1992). Elevated sinistrality in transsexuals. *Neuropsychology, 6*(4), 351–355.

Pinel, J. P. J. (2003). *Biopsychology* (5th ed.). New York: Allyn & Bacon.

Plante, R. F. (2006). *Sexualities in context: A social perspective.* Boulder, CO: Westview.

Potts, A., Grace, V., Gavey, N., & Vares, T. (2004). "Viagra stories": Challenging "erectile dysfunction." *Social Science and Medicine, 59*(3), 489–499.

Potts, A., Grace, V. M., Vares, T., & Gavey, N. (2006). "Sex for life"? Men's counter-stories on "erectile dysfunction," male sexuality and aging. *Sociolology of Health and Illness, 28*(3), 306–329.

Prins, J., Blanker, M. H., Bohnen, A. M., Thomas, S., & Bosch, J. L. (2002). Prevalence of erectile dysfunction: A systematic review of population-based studies. *International Journal of Impotence Research, 14*(6), 422–432.

Raymond, N. C., Coleman, E., & Miner, M. H. (2003). Psychiatric comorbidity and compulsive/impulsive traits in compulsive sexual behavior. *Comprehensive Psychiatry, 44*(5), 370–380.

Raymond, N. C., Coleman, E., Ohlerking, F., Christenson, G. A., & Miner, M. (1999). Psychiatric comorbidity in pedophilic sex offenders. *American Journal of Psychiatry, 156*(5), 786–788.

Raymond, N. C., Grant, J. E., Kim, S. W., & Coleman, E. (2002). Treatment of compulsive sexual behaviour with naltrexone and serotonin reuptake inhibitors: Two case studies. *International Clinical Psychopharmacology, 17*(4), 201–205.

Reissing, E. D., Binik, Y. M., Khalife, S., Cohen, D., & Amsel, R. (2003). Etiological correlates of vaginismus: Sexual and physical abuse, sexual knowledge, sexual self-schema, and relationship adjustment. *Journal of Sex and Marital Therapy, 29*(1), 47–59.

Reissing, E. D., Laliberte, G. M., & Davis, H. J. (2005). Young women's sexual adjustment: The role of sexual self-schema, sexual self-efficacy, sexual aversion and body attitudes. *The Canadian Journal of Human Sexuality, 14*(3-4), 77–85.

Rosen, R. C., & Laumann, E. O. (2003). The prevalence of sexual problems in women: How valid are comparisons across studies? Commentary on Bancroft, Loftus, and Long's (2003) "Distress about sex: A national survey of women in heterosexual relationships." *Archives of Sexual Behavior, 32*(3), 209–211.

Rowland, D. L. (2006). Neurobiology of sexual response in men and women. *CNS Spectrums, 11*(8, Suppl 9), 6–12.

Sadeghi-Nejad, H., & Seftel, A. D. (2004). Vacuum devices and penile implants. In A. D. Seftel, H. Padma-Nathan, C. G. McMahon, F. Giuliano, & S. E. Althof (Eds.), *Male and Female Sexual Dysfunction* (pp. 129–143). New York: Mosby.

Saleh, F. M., & Guidry, L. L. (2003). Psychosocial and biological treatment considerations for the paraphilic and nonparaphilic sex offender. *The Journal of the American Academy of Psychiatry and the Law, 31*(4), 486–493.

Scepkowski, L. A., Wiegel, M., Bach, A. K., Weisberg, R. B., Brown, T. A., & Barlow, D. H. (2004). Attributions for sexual situations in men with and without erectile disorder: Evidence from a sex-specific attributional style measure. *Archives of Sexual Behavior, 33*(6), 559–569.

Schneider, H. J., Pickel, J., & Stalla, G. K. (2006). Typical female 2nd-4th finger length (2D:4D) ratios in male-to-female transsexuals—Possible implications for prenatal androgen exposure. *Psychoneuroendocrinology, 31*(2), 265–269.

Schneider, J. P. (1989). Rebuilding the marriage during recovery from compulsive sexual behavior. *Family Relations, 38*(3), 288–294.

Segraves, R. T. (2002). Female sexual disorders: Psychiatric aspects. *Canadian Journal of Psychiatry, 47*(5), 419–425.

Segraves, R. T., Clayton, A., Croft, H., Wolf, A., & Warnock, J. (2004). Bupropion sustained release for the treatment of hypoactive sexual desire disorder in premenopausal women. *Journal of Clinical Psychopharmacology, 24*(3), 339–342.

Shifren, J. L. (2004). The role of androgens in female sexual dysfunction. *Mayo Clinic Proceedings, 79*(4 Suppl), S19–S24.

Shifren, J. L., Braunstein, G. D., Simon, J. A., Casson, P. R., Buster, J. E., Redmond, G. P., et al. (2000). Transdermal testosterone treatment in women with impaired sexual function after oophorectomy. *New England Journal of Medicine, 343*(10), 682–688.

Shifren, J. L., Davis, S. R., Moreau, M., Waldbaum, A., Bouchard, C., DeRogatis, L., et al. (2006). Testosterone patch for the treatment of hypoactive sexual desire disorder in naturally menopausal women: Results from the INTIMATE NM1 Study. *Menopause, 13*(5), 770–779.

Shiri, R., Koskimaki, J., Hakama, M., Hakkinen, J., Tammela, T. L., Huhtala, H., et al. (2003). Prevalence and severity of erectile dysfunction in 50 to 75-year-old Finnish men. *Journal of Urology, 170*(6), 2342–2344.

Simons, J. S., & Carey, M. P. (2001). Prevalence of sexual dysfunctions: Results from a decade of research. *Archives of Sexual Behavior, 30*(2), 177–219.

Sipski, M. L. (2002). Central nervous system based neurogenic female sexual dysfunction: Current status and future trends. *Archives of Sexual Behavior, 31*(5), 421–424.

Smith, Y. L., Van Goozen, S. H., Kuiper, A. J., & Cohen-Kettenis, P. T. (2005). Sex reassignment: Outcomes and predictors of treatment for adolescent and adult transsexuals. *Psychological Medicine, 35*(1), 89–99.

Sobel, V., & Imperato-McGinley, J. (2004). Gender identity in XY intersexuality. *Child and Adolescent Psychiatric Clinics of North America, 13*(3), 609–622.

Stoller, R. J. (1985). *Presentations of gender.* New Haven, CT: Yale University Press.

Tiefer, L. (1991). Historical, scientific, clinical and feminist criticisms of "The Human Sexual Response Cycle" model. *Annual Review of Sex Research, 2,* 1–23.

Tiefer, L. (2001). A new view of women's sexual problems: Why new? Why now? *The Journal of Sex Research, 38*(2), 89–96.

Tiefer, L. (2002). Beyond the medical model of women's sexual problems: A campaign to resist the promotion of "female sexual dysfunction." *Sexual and Relationship Therapy, 17*(2), 127–135.

Tiefer, L. (2006). The Viagra phenomenon. *Sexualities, 9*(3), 273–294.

Trussell, J. C., Anastasiadis, A. G., Padma-Nathan, H., & Shabsigh, R. (2004). Oral Type 5 Phosphodiesterase therapy for male and female sexual dysfunction. In A. D. Seftel, H. Padma-Nathan, C. G. McMahon, F. Giuliano, & S. E. Althof (Eds.), *Male and Female Sexual Dysfunction* (pp. 107–119). New York: Mosby.

Turkistani, I. Y. A. (2004). Sexual dysfunction in Saudi depressed male patients. *International Journal of Psychiatry in Clinical Practice, 8,* 101–107.

Utian, W. H., MacLean, D. B., Symonds, T., Symons, J., Somayaji, V., & Sisson, M. (2005). A methodology study to validate a structured diagnostic method used to diagnose female sexual dysfunction and its subtypes in postmenopausal women. *Journal of Sex and Marital Therapy, 31*(4), 271–283.

Uva, J. L. (1995). Review: Autoerotic asphyxiation in the United States. *Journal of Forensic Sciences, 40*(4), 574–581.

van Lankveld, J. J., & Grotjohann, Y. (2000). Psychiatric comorbidity in heterosexual couples with sexual dysfunction assessed with the composite international diagnostic interview. *Archives of Sexual Behavior, 29*(5), 479–498.

Weisberg, R. B., Brown, T. A., Wincze, J. P., & Barlow, D. H. (2001). Causal attributions and male sexual arousal: the impact of attributions for a bogus erectile difficulty on sexual arousal, cognitions, and affect. *Journal of Abnormal Psychology, 110*(2), 324–334.

West, S. L., Vinikoor, L. C., & Zolnoun, D. (2004). A systematic review of the literature on female sexual dysfunction prevalence and predictors. *Annual Review of Sexual Research, 15,* 40–172.

Wiederman, M. W. (2004). Self-control and sexual behavior. In R. F. Baumeister & K. D. Vohs (Eds.), *Handbook of self-regulation: Research, Theory, and Applications* (pp. 525–536). New York: Guilford.

Winton, M. A. (2001). Gender, sexual dysfunctions, and the *Journal of Sex & Marital Therapy. Journal of Sex and Marital Therapy, 27*(4), 333–337.

Wolpe, J. (1958). *Psychotherapy by reciprocal inhibition.* Stanford, CA: Stanford University Press.

World Health Organization. (2006). *International classification of diseases* (10th ed., Section F52). Retrieved October 23, 2006, from http://www.who.int/classifications/apps/icd/icd10online/

World Professional Association for Transgender Health, Inc. (2001). *Standards of care for gender identity disorders (Version 6).* Retrieved November 1, 2006, from http://www.hbigda.org/Documents2/socv6.pdf

Wylie, K., & MacInnes, I. (2005). Erectile dysfunction. In R. Balon & R. T. Segraves (Eds.), *Handbook of sexual dysfunction* (pp. 155–191). New York: Taylor & Francis.

Zisook, S., Rush, A. J., Haight, B. R., Clines, D. C., & Rockett, C. B. (2006). Use of bupropion in combination with serotonin reuptake inhibitors. *Biological Psychiatry, 59*(3), 203–210.

Zucker, K. J., Beaulieu, N., Bradley, S. J., Grimshaw, G. M., & Wilcox, A. (2001). Handedness in boys with gender identity disorder. *Journal of Child Psychology and Psychiatry, 42*(6), 767–776.

Zucker, K. J., & Bradley, S. J. (1995). *Gender identity disorder and psychosexual problems in children and adolescents.* New York: Guilford.

14

Somatoform Disorders

Nature, Psychological Processes, and Treatment Strategies

Georg H. Eifert, Michael J. Zvolensky, and Ashleigh Louis

Individuals exhibiting multiple somatic symptoms often present to medical practitioners believing that they are physically ill, yet upon evaluation, are informed that there is no known physiological source underlying their reports of distress. Although many of these patients will be satisfied with negative medical examination results, a significant subgroup will anxiously continue to worry about the possibility of suffering from a yet undiagnosed physical disease—a phenomenon known as *somatization*, which denotes the presence of physical symptoms (e.g., chest pain) for which no demonstrable disease process or bodily-oriented pathology can be identified as the cause of the symptoms. These individuals are likely to continue to seek help for their physical symptoms, demand more physical examinations and specialist referrals, undergo costly laboratory tests, and in rare cases, even end up on an operating table (Warwick & Salkovskis, 1990). At the extreme, such somatization behavior can interfere with life activities and goals, resulting in clinically significant impairment—a phenomenon typically classified as *somatization disorder*. Yet, somatization processes frequently occur in other "somatic disorders," including hypochondriasis, pain disorder, conversion disorder, and body dysmorphic disorder, as well as many other psychiatric conditions (e.g., panic disorder, major depressive disorder).

Somatization is a relatively common occurrence in the general medical system. For instance, van Hemert, Hengeveld, Bolk, Rooijmans, and Vandenbroucke (1993) found that among 191 new referrals to a general medical outpatient clinic, 52% of patients had symptoms that ultimately remained unexplained. An earlier study reported that of 95 patients visiting a general practitioner and presenting with somatic complaints, 41% had no demonstrable somatic pathology (Pilowsky, Smith, & Katsikitis, 1987). Comparable percentages have been reported in different countries (Eifert, 1992; Harvey, Salih, & Read, 1983; Mayou, Bryant, Forbar, & Clark, 1994), highlighting the cross-cultural relevance of this problem.

Somatization can cause a high degree of personal suffering measured in both financial and human terms. For example, somatization is a common cause of absenteeism and many physicians spend large amounts of time working with individuals who exhibit multiple somatic symptoms (Kellner, 1990). Estimates indicate that the per capita expenditure for the health care service for individuals demonstrating somatization behavior are approximately nine times the average per capita amount for other individuals.

It is important to note from the onset that somatization does not necessarily rule out the possibility of a true physical illness. In fact, many physical healthcare problems, typically quite mild, can be found among individuals with somatization problems (e.g., hypertension). Thus, somatization denotes an excess degree of worry about physical health and overuse of medical services, relative to the severity of *identifiable* illness. Perhaps not surprisingly, these same individuals report a higher degree of physical, social, and occupational impairment compared to individuals who have identifiable medical illnesses (Kellner, 1990). Typically, these impairments are long-standing (occur across most phases of life) and tend to be exacerbated by concurrent stressors in everyday life. Although somatization is indeed a vexing healthcare problem, this domain represents an exciting opportunity for researchers from diverse disciplines to work together in a collaborative manner to better understand the relations between "body and mind" and health and disease.

The main goal of this chapter is to provide a contemporary overview of the process of somatization as it applies to somatoform disorders. To some extent, our discussion is necessarily organized around the categories and classification of somatoform disorders in the *Diagnostic and Statistical Manual of Mental Disorders* (*DSM-IV*; American Psychiatric Association, 1994). However, we attempt to move beyond *DSM* categories toward a more function-based dimensional perspective of somatization problems. We believe such an approach is potentially useful because it targets analyses at fundamental biobehavioral processes and thereby provides information that is likely to be directly useful for the design of clinical interventions.

The first section of the chapter briefly reviews somatoform disorders from a traditional *DSM-IV* perspective highlighting the prevalence, nature, and the diagnostic validity of such diagnoses. We then outline how a *dimensional perspective* that focuses on key biobehavioral processes may be a more useful approach for understanding somatoform disorders than the *DSM*'s categorical approach. We then address some key vulnerability processes for somatoform disorders. Finally, we address how a dimensional perspective and focus on dysfunctional processes related to illness behavior can be translated into treatments for somatoform disorders.

Classification, Prevalence, and Course of Somatoform Disorders

According to *DSM-IV*, the common feature of the somatoform disorders is the presence of physical symptoms that suggest a general medical condition (hence, the term *somatoform*) but are not fully (currently) explained by a general medical condition, the direct effects of substance, or by another mental disorder. The physical symptoms must result in substantial personal, social, and occupational impairment, and are not feigned or voluntarily produced, as in malingering or factitious disorder. Although symptoms are not feigned, the fact that no medical explanation can be found for patient complaints makes it difficult at times to differentiate somatoform disorders from malingering.

Although the exact prevalence of specific somatoform disorders is not exactly known, most estimates place these problems collectively at under 1% of the general population. *DSM-IV* distinguishes between five somatoform disorders: somatization disorder, hypochondriasis, pain disorder, conversion disorder, and body dysmorphic disorder. By way of background, we begin our discussion with a brief overview of these categories.

Somatization disorder is characterized by many physical complaints without clear or known physical causes. The condition may last for many years and, in some cases, extend over the entire adult life span. To meet the *DSM-IV* diagnostic criteria, an individual needs to present with a history of pain related to at least four different sites or functions (e.g., head, back, abdomen, joints), two gastrointestinal symptoms (e.g., diarrhea, food intolerance), one sexual symptom (e.g., irregular menses, indifference to sex), and one pseudoneurological symptom (e.g., poor balance, numbness, paralysis). These symptoms lead to frequent and multiple medical consultations, complex medical history, and to alterations of the person's lifestyle. Physical and laboratory findings cannot detect a plausible medical condition as the cause of the symptoms. Somatization disorder is a relatively rare phenomenon with recent community and epidemiological studies citing prevalence rates between 0.4 and 0.7% (4–7 per 1,000; Bass & Murphy, 1990). Its onset is in early adulthood, course is often chronic, and prognosis is generally regarded as poor.

Hypochondriasis

Perhaps the best known somatoform disorder is hypochondriasis, defined as fears, suspicions, or convictions that one has a serious and often fatal illness such as heart disease, cancer, or AIDS. Patients frequently seek reassurance, check their bodies, and avoid illness-related situations. Merely informing patients of the absence of a disease process, or explaining the benign nature of the symptoms, only results in temporary reassurance that is followed by renewed worry over symptoms and continuing overuse of medical services (Salkovskis & Warwick, 2001). The onset of hypochondriasis is frequently in early adulthood. The course of hypochondriasis is typically chronic and the condition frequently takes on a dominant role in the person's life and relationships.

Pain Disorder

Pain disorder is characterized by acute or chronic pain in one or more body parts that is not easily understood or cannot be fully accounted for by a known medical condition. Pain is considered acute when it exists for less than six months and chronic when it persists beyond six months. Chronic pain, in particular, is often associated with major changes in behavior such as decreased activity and somatic preoccupation (Pilowsky, Chapman, & Bonica, 1977). Pain disorder is relatively common and may occur in adults of all ages. For example, pain is the most common complaint of individuals presenting to a physician. The proliferation of special pain clinics could be seen as another indication of the high number of pain patients seeking professional help. A study of internal medicine private practice patients found that 13% of patients suffered from chronic pain (Margolis, Zimny, & Miller, 1984).

Conversion Disorder

Conversion disorder is characterized by symptoms suggesting a neurological disorder with medical investigations failing to identify a neurological or general medical disorder. At times, the particular symptoms may even be inconsistent with general neurological knowledge. Patients may present with any one or a combination of motor symptoms (e.g., paralysis), seizures or convulsions, and sensory deficits (e.g., blindness, anesthesia, and aphonia). An important requirement for the diagnosis is the temporal relation between conversion symptoms and a psychological stressor such as acute grief, or victimization. Patients are typically unaware of any psychological basis for their symptoms and report being unable to control them. The diagnosis of conversion disorder is rare and difficult to establish with estimates ranging between 0.001% and 0.3% (1–300 per 100,000; *DSM-IV*). One reason for this difficulty is that symptoms indicative of conversion disorder may later be discovered to be linked to a gradually developing, physical (neurological) disease such as a brain tumor or multiple sclerosis (Fishbain & Goldberg, 1991). Although conversion disorder may occur at any age, onset is typically in late childhood or early adulthood. Onset is often sudden and in response to conflicts or stressful situations such as unresolved grief and sexual trauma (Sharma & Chaturvedi, 1995).

Body Dysmorphic Disorder

Body dysmorphic disorder (BDD) is characterized by a preoccupation with an imagined or exaggerated body disfigurement or an excessive concern that there is something wrong with the shape or appearance of body parts. The perceived defect or abnormality is generally not or barely noticeable to others. Objects of concern typically refer to the face (e.g., shape or size of nose), head (e.g., hearing loss), sexual characteristics (size of penis, breasts), or general body appearance (tallness/shortness). Other concerns may involve scars, wrinkles, or body odor. Cognitive features are excessive preoccupation, intrusive thoughts, and sometimes ideas of reference. For instance, an individual may persist in the belief that he or she is physically ill due to blemishes on the skin or somewhat atypical marks on the skin. Behavioral features include avoidance (e.g., of body exposure, direct social contact, talking about the problem, looking in the mirror), camouflaging or concealing imagined deformities (wearing a hat or glasses), excessive grooming and checking, and reassurance seeking.

Reif et al. (2006) estimate the prevalence of BDD at 1 to 2% of the population. Individuals with BDD had higher somatization scores and higher rates of suicidal ideation and they made more suicide attempts than persons not meeting criteria for BDD. Body dysphoric disorder was also found to be associated with higher rates of unemployment, lower financial income, and lower rates of living with a significant other. Rosen (1995) found virtually no gender differences in prevalence rates of BDD. Onset of BDD may be gradual or sudden, and its course is generally continuous and chronic, though fluctuating in intensity. BDD is thought to start in adolescence when preoccupation with physical appearance is very common. Sociocultural factors influencing people's attitudes toward and dissatisfaction with their bodies seem to play a role in determining the extent to which a real or imagined physical abnormality becomes a cause for concern and preoccupation.

A preoccupation with physical appearance and distorted body image can also be found in persons with eating disorders. The difference is that individuals with eating disorders also exhibit abnormal patterns of eating (binging, purging, extreme dieting), whereas such abnormal eating patterns are not typical for persons with BDD.

Diagnostic Validity of DSM-Defined Somatoform Disorders

The diagnostic validity of somatoform disorders in relation to each other as well as to other clinical syndromes is problematic and continues to be the focus of intense debates (Mayou, Kirmayer, Simon, & Sharpe, 2005). Many scholars have observed that these conditions do not necessarily represent distinct conditions and difficulties distinguishing between symptoms of somatoform disorders and physical health problems abound. These disorders are highly influenced by contextual cultural factors.

The distinctiveness of the somatoform disorders has been questioned repeatedly. As a category, somatoform disorders continue to lack conceptual coherence and clearly defined diagnostic criteria. The only common feature to all the somatoform disorders is that they cannot be explained by a general medical condition. Starcevic (2006) criticized the current group of somatoform disorders as simply too heterogeneous. For example, BDD shares very little with the rest of the group other than people's focus on bodily changes. In fact, BDD shares more conceptual and functional features with mood and anxiety disorders—particularly obsessive-compulsive disorder and social anxiety (Castle, Rossell, & Kyrios, 2006).

Also, the diagnostic criteria overlap greatly with other psychiatric disorders that have associated somatic symptoms. Even the authors of the *DSM-IV* concede that the grouping of these disorders in a single section is based on clinical utility rather than on assumptions regarding shared etiology. Murphy (1990) indicated that the disorders are often not qualitatively distinct but rather merge into each other making distinctions between individual somatoform disorders challenging. Mayou et al. (2005) point out that the subcategories have been found to be unreliable and arbitrary. Many of the subcategories have failed to achieve acceptable standards of reliability, which can negatively affect patient's rights to medical-legal and insurance entitlements.

For example, pain may occur in any of the somatoform disorders. Ambiguous criteria such as "the person's concern is grossly in excess of what would be expected," and "slight physical abnormality," further hamper clear differentiation of these problems. The distinction between BDD and normal concerns about appearance is as difficult to make as the distinction between BDD and delusional disorder (somatic subtype). The distinction between somatoform disorders and personality disorders also has been questioned (Bass & Murphy, 1995). Based upon these limitations, Fava (1992) suggested that the term *somatization* should be replaced by the concept of *abnormal illness behavior* because a focus on actual illness-related behavior might help operationalize the problems we are typically referring to when using the term *somatization*.

Cultural influences on somatization processes are well documented (Zvolensky, Feldner, Eifert, Vujanovic, & Solomon, in press). Based on a review of data from cross-cultural studies, Escobar, Allen, Nervi, and Gara (2001) conclude that there is "considerable cultural variation in the expression of somatizing syndromes. The available evidence elaborates the well-accepted tenet that the presentation of personal/social distress in the form of somatic complaints appears to be the norm for most cultures" (p. 226). Thus, the specific symptoms of certain disorders often appear to be more a function of the individual's culture than of some underlying (distinct) biologically based disease process. Even *DSM-IV* suggests that the types and frequency of somatic symptoms differ across cultures and that symptom lists should be adjusted to the culture. For example, people in Africa and Southern Asia report burning hands and feet or the nondelusional experience of worms in the hands or ants in the head, whereas such reports are virtually unheard of amongst persons in Europe and North America. By comparison, people living in Europe and North America tend to be preoccupied with heart disease and cancer.

Mayou et al. (2005) note that the terms *somatoform* or *somatization* are often found to be unacceptable by patients because the terms imply that the patients' symptoms are in their minds and "not real." Patients doubt that clinicians appreciate the reality and authenticity of their symptoms. At a more fundamental level, Mayou and associates (2005) criticized the distinction between somatic and psychological problems as inherently dualistic, which does not translate well into other cultures that have a less dualistic view of mind and body (e.g., Asia and China) than Western culture. The notion that problems can be neatly divided into those that can and cannot be explained by disease is indeed unlikely at best. Several authors also point to potential pathophysiological mechanisms that may underlie unexplained physical symptoms such as chest pain (Sharpe & Bass, 1992). We often just do not understand them very well—and that is what we should tell patients rather than using terms such as *nonorganic* when describing their symptoms. We also need to recognize that there is frequently a reciprocal relation between health anxiety and somatic symptoms. For instance, anxiety and behaviors designed to reduce it (e.g., constant checking of a lump, scratching skin) may actually increase the physical symptoms that are the focus of anxiety (Salkovskis, 1996).

Toward a Dimensional Framework for Understanding Pathogenic Processes

In light of the current diagnostic problems with the somatoform disorder category in *DSM-IV*, Mayou et al. (2005) suggest abolishing this category in *DSM-V* because the concept and category has consistently failed clinicians and patients alike, and there is not much value in keeping it as a diagnostic entity. They suggest the term *somatic symptoms* as a replacement for *somatoform* and that the term *functional* should be used to emphasize those symptoms that lack an association with a general medical condition. They also suggest redistributing the current somatoform disorders to other diagnostic categories. Specifically, BDD should be moved to the category of obsessive-compulsive disorder and hypochondriasis should be placed with the anxiety disorders and renamed *health anxiety disorder* because it is conceptually and functionally closer to the anxiety disorders than to any of the other somatoform disorders. They also suggest adding some multidimensional descriptors to the diagnostic categories to more accurately describe the complaints of the individual patient.

We have previously argued (Eifert, Lejuez, & Bouman, 1998; Eifert, Zvolensky, & Lejuez, 2000) that overlap between related categories is not a problem of "comorbidity" or inaccurate definitions but a result of similar psychological processes involved in these conditions. Accordingly, we suggest adopting a dimensional approach to understanding illness-related concerns that can identify key biobehavioral processes. To illustrate this approach, we discuss focal dimensions of health anxiety, a psychological process that characterizes, in part, many somatoform disorders as well as related conditions (e.g., panic disorder). We view health anxiety as a psychological process where persons present with problems that fall on a continuum along four dimensions:

1. Preoccupation with the body and its functioning. Such bodily preoccupation, especially when coupled with somatic complaints, may produce a state of somatic uncertainty and form the basis for the other three dimensions of the disorder.
2. Disease suspicion or conviction. The person has the suspicion or is convinced of having a serious physical disease; suspicion and conviction are on a continuum of strength, and in rare cases the conviction may reach delusional intensity.
3. Disease fear. The person fears having a serious physical disease.
4. Safety-seeking behavior such as repeated requests for medical examinations and tests, bodily checking, verbal complaints, and seeking reassurance. The function of such behavior is to reduce worry and anxiety over physical illness (Eifert et al., 2000; Salkovskis & Warwick, 2001).

A person could obtain a high score on any one or all four dimensions of health anxiety. For example, disease suspicion/conviction may or may not be accompanied by a strong fear of the suspected disease. Clinically, this feature is most apparent in patient's resistance to medical reassurance. For instance, patients may remain extremely worried about their health even though their fear of suffering from a specific disease may have been eliminated by a medical examination (Fava & Grandi, 1991). Accordingly, a dimensional classification system could help overcome some challenges inherent to a traditional diagnostic perspective of somatoform disorders. Moreover, identifying dimensions that allow a classification of illness behavior based on the function that such behavior serves, rather than just its topography, might lead to a better understanding and improved treatments of persons with somatoform problems (Eifert & Lau, 2001).

General Vulnerabililty Processes for Abnormal Illness Behavior

Given our previous discussion as to prototypical characteristics of health anxiety, the next logical question pertains to the types of processes that increase or decrease the risk for developing abnormal illness behavior. As discussed at the onset of this chapter, just about all people experience distressing physical sensations at some point in their lives. Moreover, a substantial percentage will even experience robust internal physical (interoceptive) reactions in the form of panic attacks, limited symptom panic attacks, gastrointestinal distress, respiratory infections, strained muscles, and so on. In fact, such bodily distress is so common to the human experience that it seems almost inconceivable to imagine a person going through life without experiencing at least some significant somatic disturbance. These normal experiences of physical symptoms become problematic when they begin to interfere with a person's life due to obsessive preoccupation with them and excessive rigid behaviors designed to control, reduce, or escape from them. Such pervasive experiential avoidance behavior seems to be at the core of many anxiety-related clinical problems (Forsyth, Eifert, & Barrios, 2006).

Although systematic knowledge about causes is lacking, factors such as parental modeling, stressful life events, high negative affect, and aspects of the relationship and communication between patients and doctors appear to be related to the development of somatoform disorders (e.g., Bass & Murphy, 1990). In addition, there are a number of biopsychosocial processes that increase vulnerability for the development of somatoform pathology or abnormal illness behavior generally. The processes that we will discuss in this section include (1) an inherited risk for emotional responsivity to physical sensations; (2) deficits in emotion regulatory skills; and (3) language-based and observational learning. Before this discussion, however, we need to briefly define what we mean by the term *abnormal illness behavior*.

Pilowsky (1993) defined abnormal illness behavior as the

persistence of a maladaptive mode of experiencing, perceiving, evaluating, and responding to one's own health status, despite the fact that a doctor has provided a lucid and accurate appraisal of the situation and management to be followed (if any), with opportunities for discussion, negotiation and clarification, based on adequate assessment of all relevant biological, psychological, social and cultural factors. (p. 62)

Thus abnormal illness behavior refers to the disagreement between the doctor and patient about the sick role to which the patient feels entitled. Sharpe, Mayou, and Bass (1995) argued that the concept of abnormal illness behavior is valuable for understanding not only patients with functional somatic symptoms but also the behavioral aspects of all illness.

Inherited Risk for Emotional Responsivity to Physical Sensations

There is convincing evidence that there is an inherited component or substrate for negative emotionality. Researchers have referred to this inherited disposition by a number of different terms, including *negative affectivity*, *trait anxiety*, and *neuroticism* (Barlow, 2001). These synonymous labels are intended to capture a general predisposition to experience negative affect (e.g., anxiety) and perhaps abrupt emotional reactivity (e.g., panic) to challenging or stressful life events.

Although the characteristics of negative affectivity vary across specific negative emotional experiences (e.g., panic versus anger), they all posit that high degrees of negative emotionality are associated with a lower threshold of initial affective response, slower recovery to baseline, and greater reactivation of arousal with repeated exposure to stressful events. High reactivity is generally associated with inhibited temperament, whereas low reactivity is associated with uninhibited temperament (Kagan, 1989). Thus, individual differences in temperament are often related to the experience and regulation of affect because they constrain or facilitate certain types of responding. For example, the temperamental characteristics of behavioral inhibition are believed to relate to tendencies to experience high levels of autonomic arousal in evocative contexts as well as the propensity to react in a defensive manner in response to threat (e.g., avoidance-oriented coping strategies; Kagan, Snidman, & Arcus, 1992).

As behavioral genetic research continues to make important strides in our understanding of emotional functioning, we may eventually have specific models articulating the extent to which a specific gene or combination of genes contributes to a specific anxiety disorder or health disorder. At this stage, however, it appears that a general disposition for negative affectivity is inherited. The contribution of this inherited component is estimated to be at approximately 30% in the development of somatoform-related disorders (Kendler, Walters, Truett, & Heath, 1995). No research has documented the exact proportion of explained variance for the development of a specific disorder, although there is some evidence that there are both shared and specific genetic vulnerabilities across anxiety-related disorders (Kendler et al., 1995). It is likely that a genetic predisposition creates the biological conditions that make people prone to respond with anxiety and panic reactions to certain bodily changes and processes. One research challenge in this domain will be to specify *how* genetic vulnerabilities (once they are identified) might influence the pathogenesis of a specific disorder.

Development of Emotion Self-Regulatory Skills

Research has shown that early in life humans develop a repertoire of regulatory-oriented skills to deal with elevated levels of bodily arousal and concomitant emotional distress. For example, crying as an infant is a signal to caregivers that the infant is in need of something (e.g., food), and ceasing to cry and related behavioral responses (e.g., smiling) reinforce caregiver behavior (Derryberry & Rothbart, 1984). Thus, the effective management of bodily states, particularly negative emotional experiences, is a critical early step in psychological development. As children mature, they learn to approach and avoid salient environmental stimuli, and the members of society increasingly expect them to gain better emotion regulatory skills (e.g., suppression of crying in school). By adulthood, the individual is expected to have sophisticated emotional control skills and the ability to learn new regulatory skills for a variety of changing sociocultural contexts. For example, adults are not supposed to demonstrate signs of emotional distress in social, performance, or work settings. Research indicates that individuals with low levels of emotional regulation skills, or an inability to readily alter regulation strategies, evidence less capacity to function flexibly and successfully in social environments than do those that have such emotion regulation skills (Rothbart, 1989).

The preceding discussion highlights the notion that emotion regulation skills are expected to increase consistently across the lifespan and are an integral component of mental health (Stewart, Zvolensky, & Eifert, 2002). When individuals lack the ability to effectively alter their emotional experiences, they are more susceptible to physical discomfort, negative affect, and anxiety (Rothbart, Ziaie, & O'Boyle, 1992). An important way in which children learn emotional regulation skills is through exercising their capacity to explore their world, both literally and metaphorically. Developmental researchers have referred to these experiences as *mastery learning opportunities* (Rothbart, 1989). Impoverished environments where parents or caregivers (e.g., teachers) respond to children in a noncontingent manner produce more emotional distress than do environments characterized by contingent outcomes. For example, Chorpita, Brown, and Barlow (1998) found that parents who discourage autonomy (through modeling, vicarious learning, rule governed behavior, or instrumental learning) while simultaneously excessively protecting their children from any potential source of threat are more likely to foster in their children a limited sense of personal control. Similar findings have been observed in studies of nonhuman animals raised in environments with little control over important outcomes (e.g., availability of food; Mineka, Gunnar, & Champoux, 1986). Such findings are important to understanding somatoform disorders because greater degrees of perceived uncontrollability are predictive of the tendency to view ambiguous internal stimuli as threatening (Zvolensky, Eifert, Lejuez, & McNeil, 1999).

Coping with emotional distress is, of course, a multidimensional process. Recent work indicates that coping responses are best viewed from a hierarchical model that includes first-order and higher-order dimensions (Compas, Conner-Smith, Saltzman, Thomsen, & Wadsworth, 2001). Indeed, researchers increasingly suggest that coping with emotional distress involves strategic (voluntary) and automatic (involuntary) responses. Additionally, Compas et al. (2001) have categorized these coping responses along the dimensions of engagement and disengagement. *Engagement* responding includes active, primary control-oriented responding aimed at altering the immediate situation in some sort of direct manner (e.g., leaving a situation that one finds uncomfortable because of cardiac-related distress and tension). *Disengagement* responding includes secondary control-oriented responding aimed at adapting to an uncontrollable situation by purposively altering one's cognitive-affective response to that situation (indirect responding). For instance, an individual might adapt to pain or other aversive bodily sensations by altering their cognitive response to such events (e.g., acceptance, distraction, reframing). Overall, it is likely that individuals will develop a variety of emotion regulatory skills across the lifespan, and these skills are likely to be a product of early learning experiences.

Language-Based Learning

Aside from direct forms of learning, individuals also will experience affective responses to body-related events and sensations through the utilization of language. Language serves important symbolic functions by providing humans with emotional experiences without exposure to the actual physical stimuli or events that ordinarily elicit those responses (Staats & Eifert, 1990). For instance, both "knowing what to do" and "knowing what to feel" involve verbal understanding of the relation between them. Thus, the meaning of health-related anxiety in a psychological sense represents a complex act of relating largely arbitrary verbal-symbolic events with other events and psychological functions within a particular context. For instance, words such as *anxiety* and *fear* either implicitly or explicitly establish relations with other events such as "I am anxious or afraid of…something, some event, or someone."

The relational quality of terms denoting emotions, in turn, must be tied to descriptions of behavior and events with a variety of stimulus functions (e.g., eliciting, evoking, reinforcing, and punishing) and meanings (e.g., good, bad, pleasant, unpleasant, or painful). In turn, people often describe their emotional experiences metaphorically in ways that others can understand (e.g., "When I feel anxious it's like a knife going through my chest"). These metaphorical extensions have no real counterpart inside the person. Instead, they function to communicate the meaning of emotional experience (feeling threatened to the point of fearing death) by identifying and relating events with known stimulus functions (a sharp knife can cut into a chest and cause death).

Society determines what kind of stimuli and events are placed in relation to each other and the nature of that relation (Hayes & Wilson, 1994). These arbitrary relations are learned and function in a variety of ways (Sidman, 1994; Staats & Eifert, 1990). Individuals become anxious about particular health-related experiences or "symptoms" because they read and hear about them in the specific cultural context in which they live. This may be one of the main reasons why cultural variations in somatoform disorders are widespread and can be observed with such great regularity (Escobar, Allen, Nervi, & Gara, 2001). For instance, people in Western societies become anxious when they notice a fast or irregular heart beat because they have seen or heard many times that this event may be a sign of a heart attack.

The most important point is that persons with somatoform disorders have likely developed complex repertoires of verbal and other symbolic responses that elicit negative affect and serve as discriminative stimuli for escape or avoidance behavior (Staats & Eifert, 1990). Thus, for otherwise healthy people, the sensations of a beating heart or chest pain may lead to a sequence of verbal and autonomic events that result in the belief that they are having a heart attack (Eifert, 1992). In this instance, a fast or irregular heartbeat is not just a felt beating heart. Instead, it is an acquired and verbally mediated formulation of what it *means* to have a fast or irregular heartbeat or chest pain (e.g., "I have heart disease" or "I am suffering from a heart attack"). Not only may the person respond to such sensations by rushing to an emergency room, but also any other public or private stimulus events associated with this response may now acquire similar negative functions (e.g., physical exercise, smoking, working hard). In this way, a variety of behaviors and events can come to elicit the physiological event that the person then misconstrues as dangerous.

Observational Learning

It is also likely that persons who develop somatoform disorders have been exposed to negative health-related events to a greater degree than persons who do not develop these disorders. For example, some studies indicate that a significant number of persons with cardiophobia, defined as someone who has an irrational fear of heart disease, have observed heart disease and its potentially lethal effects (e.g., death) in relatives and close friends (Eifert & Forsyth, 1996). These persons had been exposed directly to the physical and emotionally painful consequences of heart disease. As a result, they may also have had more exposure to heart-focused perceptions and interpretations of physical symptoms and physiological processes.

Observational learning is strongly involved in learning pain tolerance, pain ratings, and nonverbal expressions of pain (Flor, Birbaumer, & Turk, 1990). Such observational learning may increase the likelihood of expressing and interpreting arousal and pain in later life as a heart problem because socially acquired perceptions and interpretations of symptoms largely determine how people deal with illness. For instance, if one or both parents have heart disease, children might observe their parent's response to a heart problem. If the behavior that is modeled is maladaptive (e.g., excessive illness behavior), these children will not only be more likely to respond to stress with increased cardiovascular activity, but they will have also learned maladaptive labeling and interpretation of such symptoms and have fewer adaptive coping skills.

Taken together, research suggests a variety of general factors that may promote the development of the type of abnormal illness behavior found in somatoform disorders. These processes are likely nonspecific in the sense that they increase the chance of negative emotional responding and poor affect regulatory strategies. Exposure to specific illnesses or to persons who model the potential dangers of certain physical disorders may increase an individual's general vulnerability. Continued research in each of these general domains will improve our ability to predict who will develop a specific type of somatoform disorder.

Treatment of Somatoform Disorders

Cognitive-behavioral theories and research have been helpful in providing a fledgling basis for a better understanding and treatment of persons with somatization problems. Important progress has been made in particular for persons with health anxiety (Eifert & Lau, 2001; Salkovskis & Warwick, 2001) and chronic pain (e.g., Flor, Birbaumer, & Turk, 1990; Schermelleh-Engel, Eifert, Moosbrugger, & Frank, 1997). We now overview these treatment strategies at a general level and how they can be applied to specific types of somatoform disorders.

General Strategies

Psychologically distressed patients who present with unexplained somatic symptoms are high users of medical care and their doctors regard them as frustrating and difficult to treat (Mayou & Sharpe, 1995). There is often a mismatch between the expectations of these patients and their doctors' abilities and communication skills. For instance, terms such as *functional heart problem, nervous heart, atypical chest pain,* and *pseudoangina,* when used to "diagnose" unexplained chest pain, can easily be misinterpreted by a patient who is determined to believe that some significant cardiac disease is being described (Eifert et al., 2000). Health care providers often feel frustrated and emotionally drained because these patients obviously need psychological support but resent being referred to a psychologist or psychiatrist.

Patients often perceive the use of diagnostic labels such as hypochondriasis as an insult because these labels seem to imply that the patients' problems are not real and "just in their head." Accepting and understanding, rather than refuting or arguing with the patient's symptoms, is therefore the more important strategy for engaging the patient in a therapeutic working relationship (cf. Bass & Benjamin, 1993). Lipsitt and Starcevic (2006) state that it is extremely important for health care providers to treat the somatizing patient in a warm, respectful manner, without prejudice based on previous assessments from other clinicians. Health care professionals can help make the patient feel listened to and let them know that they regard their symptoms as "real" and do not view them as "crazy." They can also ease the patient's anxieties and enhance the relationship with the patient by telling the patient that worrying about their symptoms is reasonable and legitimate. A solid and trusting working relationship is essential for optimal help. In the engagement stage of treatment, patients can also be told that there may be alternative explanations for the difficulties they are experiencing (Salkovskis, 1996). The general treatment strategy is to test such alternative or benign medical explanations for symptoms and to conduct therapy in the context of an experiment that provides an opportunity for testing alternative hypotheses (Eifert & Lau, 2001; Salkovskis, 1996).

Rather than merely telling patients there is no "organic" reason for their chest pain, an explanation of symptoms that overcomes the nonorganic-organic dualism provides the patient with a more acceptable rationale and reassurance (Eifert, Hodson, Tracey, Seville, & Gunawardane, 1996). For instance, to provide a patient with a credible explanation of how anxiety and chest wall muscle tension can result in chest pain, patients may be given a chest-focused relaxation with EMG feedback that literally shows them how they can change their chest tension levels. Salkovskis and Warwick (2001) found that reassurance which only informs the patients that there is nothing organically wrong with their bodies will actually increase future reassurance-seeking rather than decrease it. Appropriate reassurance and feedback that provides the patient with new and alternative explanations is the key to successful treatment and may help prevent the development of chronic somatization problems. In a controlled case study, Eifert and Lau (2001) found that behavioral experiments were not only useful in developing alternative symptom explanations but also in teaching the patient to reassure herself rather than seeking therapist reassurance. The treatment strategies and techniques targeting the dimensions of abnormal illness behavior related to heart-focused anxiety are summarized in Table 14.1. Although this example deals with heart-focused anxiety, the process dimensions are adaptable and applicable to other somatization problems.

Medical professionals need to be trained to provide alternative explanations rather than vague pseudo-medical labels and to acknowledge rather than dismiss patients' concerns. At the same time, withholding unnecessary medication and medical examinations (response prevention for safety-seeking behavior) is a crucial part of treatment. For example, Goldberg, Gask, and O'Dowd (1989) developed a training program for primary care physicians that included empathic listening to complaints and symptoms, thus changing the agenda of the actions to be undertaken from a somato-medical focus on bodily symptoms to a psychological perspective focusing on emotional distress. Physicians were also taught how to help patients reattribute bodily symptoms to psychological factors. Two other studies (Rost, Kashner, & Smith, 1995; Smith, Rost, & Kashner, 1995) also focused on changing physician behavior in primary care settings. Physicians were taught to use empathic listening techniques with their patients and to not reinforce patients' abnormal illness behavior by providing expensive diagnostic procedures, surgeries, and hospitalizations. Withholding such procedures also prevents iatrogenic diseases and counteracts patients' disease convictions. The results of these studies suggest

Table 14.1 Key treatment components targeting various dimensions and symptoms of heart-focused anxiety (adopted from Eifert and Lau, 2001)

Dimensions, treatment strategies, and techniques	
Preoccupation with heart	Demonstrate that chest pain/heart sensations are not dangerous • *reduce avoidance/expose to cardiac-related stimuli*
Disease fear	Extinguish fear and exposure to avoided activities • *exposure to interoceptive (particularly cardioceptive) cues* • *reinforce "dangerous" behavior (e.g., strenuous exercise)*
Disease conviction	Test alternative symptom explanations • *explain impact of anxiety & tension on body (chest pain)* • *conduct behavioral experiments to test hypotheses* • *review evidence for/against heart disease* • *review evidence for cardiac vs. tension chest pain*
Safety/reassurance seeking	Extinguish help and reassurance seeking • *review results of previous tests* • *withhold reassurance* • *refuse further tests* • *do physical exercise while preventing pulse checking*
Physical (panic) symptoms	Reduce chronic tension and overbreathing • *chest muscle relaxation* • *teach slow diaphragmatic vs. thoracic breathing*

that this balanced approach to patient care can reduce health care costs and at the same time increase the psychological adjustment of patients.

Finally, it is essential that we move patients from an almost exclusive focus on symptoms, which may or may not be changeable or controllable, to goals and behaviors that are controllable and changeable. For instance, Rief, Hiller, Geissner, and Fichter (1995) suggest that after an initial empathic discussion of symptoms, treatment needs to shift towards more changeable behavioral targets, such as occupational problem solving, social skills training, and quality of life enhancement. Behavioral activation treatment programs (Lejuez, Hopko, & Hopko, 2001) appear to be valuable therapist tools to help move patients in their "valued direction" (Hayes, Strosahl, & Wilson, 1999) and at the same time reduce negative affect.

Acceptance and commitment therapy (ACT), a new acceptance-based behavior therapy, has shown great promise in the treatment of anxiety disorders (Eifert & Forsyth, 2005). In future, this approach could easily be extended to people suffering from health-related anxiety and concerns because it directly targets the experiential avoidance behavior that tends to interfere with people's daily functioning. ACT helps people refocus their efforts on areas in their lives where they can effect change, and where they are in control, rather than wasting their time with fruitless attempts to control or change bodily sensations and their evaluations of them, which are very difficult, if not impossible, to control.

Specific Treatment Recommendations

It may be most useful to think of somatic problems as requiring management rather than treatment (e.g., Bass & Benjamin, 1993). Early diagnosis and the prevention of unnecessary medical and surgical investigation are of primary importance. Most somatization patients have specific expectations regarding treatment goals and procedures and try to persuade their doctors to follow their wishes for further medical investigations and treatments. Bass and Murphy (1990) state that treatment often involves long-term supportive psychotherapy and must be directed toward controlling the demands on medical care as well as the treatment of symptoms and social disability. They recommend the following five steps:

1. Encourage a long-term supportive relationship with only one understanding primary care physician to prevent doctor-shopping and to coordinate all actions;
2. See patients on regular appointments rather than on demand to prevent reinforcement of illness behavior;
3. View patient's physical complaints as a form of communication rather than as evidence of disease; and
4. Minimize the use of psychotropic drugs and/or analgesic medication.

In general, adaptive behavior is encouraged and promoted, whereas sick role behavior is ignored as much as possible. A study by Kashner, Rost, Cohen, Anderson, and Smith (1995) focused on coping with the nature and consequences of the physical symptoms, general problem solving, and helping patients take more control of their lives. These authors found that eight sessions of brief group therapy improved physical and mental health at one year follow-up.

A randomized controlled trial examining a comprehensive cognitive-behavioral approach for dealing with medically unexplained physical symptoms was conducted by Speckens and associates (1996). A cognitive-behavioral intervention group of 39 general medical outpatients was compared with a control group of 40 patients receiving optimized medical care. Treatment included imaginary exposure and distraction techniques to break the vicious circles of cognitive avoidance and preoccupation; activity scheduling, exposure in vivo, and response prevention to decrease avoidance behavior; relaxation training, breathing exercises, and physical exercises; and problem-solving or social skills training to overcome any problems in interpersonal relationships. At both 6- and 12-months follow-up, the intervention group reported lower intensity and frequency of symptoms, reduced illness behavior, less sleep impairment, and fewer limitations in social and leisure activities than did the control group.

Hypochondriasis

Traditionally, individuals with hypochondriasis have been considered difficult to treat and their prognosis has been regarded as poor. For instance, early studies assessing the effectiveness of a variety of psychological interventions available at that time (e.g., Kenyon, 1964) found 40% of patients with primary hypochondriasis to be unchanged or worse following treatment. Although patients with unexplained physical symptoms or health anxiety still pose a considerable challenge for therapists, cognitive-behavioral interventions have yielded encouraging results.

The first comprehensive cognitive-behavioral treatment formulations were provided by Warwick and Salkovskis (1990). Patients are instructed to self-monitor during hypochondriacal episodes, paying careful attention to environmental events, physical symptoms, associated cognitions, and their resulting hypochondriacal behavior. As indicated, their treatment is directed at evaluating alternative, nonthreatening explanations of body-related observations that the patient misinterprets as signs of serious disease. Two possible explanations for the patient's problem are considered together rather than as mutually exclusive alternatives (Salkovskis, 1996). Patients are then asked to engage in a variety of behavioral experiments to test these new explanations and therapy proceeds as an evaluation of the relative merits of the alternative views. Salkovskis (1996) emphasizes that the inappropriate safety-seeking of hypochondriacal individuals prevents them from discovering that their fears are groundless. Hence, the key function of exposure exercises and response prevention is to bring patients into contact with the actual rather than expected consequences of their symptoms (Eifert & Lau, 2001). By allowing patients to repeatedly experience feared bodily sensations without the dreaded consequences, they learn that what they are afraid of does not actually happen. Using a similar approach, Martinez and Botella (2005) found that cognitive-behavioral treatment resulted in significant statistical and clinical improvement in hypochondriacal patients that was maintained at six-month follow-up with 75% of patients reporting noticeable improvement.

A system of differential reinforcement may need to be added for individuals who gain sympathy or interest for their physical complaints but little attention otherwise. In those cases, family members and other individuals the patient has contact with (including the therapist) should reinforce patient initiation of conversation on any topic other than symptoms (healthy conversation). This reinforcement could consist of praise or increased attention. As the patient engages in more healthy conversation, the natural contingencies (e.g., reduced medical bills, more pleasant interactions with others) should begin to maintain behavior and the frequency and magnitude of artificial reinforcement can be slowly reduced.

Salkovskis and Warwick (1986) reported two successfully treated single cases of primary hypochondriasis using cognitive-behavioral methods. In another study, Visser and Bouman (1992) found that four of six hypochondriacal patients improved significantly following in vivo exposure, response suppression, and cognitive therapy. In this study, exposure and response suppression (behavioral components) appeared to have accounted for more of the improvement than the cognitive component (i.e., attempting to change directly the patient's misconceptions about symptoms). The positive results of this series of single case studies were supported in a first controlled trial that showed cognitive-behavioral therapy to be superior to a wait-list control condition (Warwick, Clark, Cobb, & Salkovskis, 1996).

For patients whose main concern is fear of a specific disease, without significant conviction of having the disease, a more focused program of tension reduction (e.g., through relaxation), exposure to the feared stimuli, and prevention of checking and safety-seeking can be sufficient (Eifert, 1992). For instance, Warwick and Marks (1988) employed exposure to feared stimuli, paradox (deliberate attempts to induce a panic attack), and response prevention such as banning reassurance seeking and physician visits. There was a significant decrease in illness fear and an increase in work and social adjustment for the group of 17 patients that were treated. Psychoeducation has also shown some success in reducing hypochondriacal beliefs and fears. Bouman (2002) found that group psychoeducation was an effective intervention with a mean 40% reduction in the frequency of medical service utilization.

Overall, cognitive-behavioral treatments are the most promising interventions for patients with hypochondriasis. Also, the prognosis for patients who are treated with cognitive-behavioral interventions seems more favorable than previously thought. In general, patients with mild, short-lived hypochondriasis that is not associated with any complicating factors have the best prognosis for recovery. More extensive and controlled studies are needed to determine the most crucial treatment components and the mechanisms that explain their success.

Pain Disorder

Earlier approaches for pain management were based on psychodynamic principles and used hypnotic suggestions to help people deal with pain. A review by Turk, Meichenbaum, and Genest (1983) found that these techniques are ineffective when used alone and that treatment effects are due to the unwitting inclusion of behavioral and cognitive treatment components.

Pain behavior is not an expression or side-effect of a pain problem, instead it is *the* problem (Rachlin, 1985). Therefore, the goal of treatment is to extinguish maladaptive pain behavior and teach and reinforce the use of more adaptive pain coping strategies (Nicholas, Wilson, & Goyen, 1991). Treatment begins with a thorough functional analysis of current pain behavior and the environmental contingencies associated with that behavior. Once the consequences that maintain the maladaptive pain behavior are determined, attempts are made to reduce reinforcement for that behavior and increase reinforcement for adaptive pain coping behavior (cf. Fordyce, Roberts, & Sternbach, 1985; Nicholas et al., 1991). In addition to changing a patient's maladaptive pain behavior, cognitive-behavioral therapy also attempts to alter associated thought patterns and the patient's perceived competence in dealing with pain (Schermelleh-Engel et al., 1997). Pain management programs typically require active patient participation and include fostering a patient's real and perceived competence to deal with pain, teaching skills and adaptive responses to problems (including self-attribution for change and success), and planning maintenance.

Based on the assumption that pain is mediated by thoughts and images, cognitive methods involving imagery and distraction have often been added to pain management programs (Turk et al., 1983). Patients are encouraged to create and focus on those thoughts and images that alleviate pain, while ignoring those that exacerbate pain. Particularly for patients who engage in few activities, a *behavioral* activation program is beneficial in more than one way (Lejuez et al., 2001). Such programs encourage and reinforce patients engaging in a host of activities. As patients continue with these activities, they frequently recognize the intrinsically reinforcing value of the activities and their mood enhancing effects.

Although the cognitive-behavioral approach to pain management has been identified as an empirically validated treatment by the Task Force on Promotion and Dissemination of Psychological Procedures (Chambless, 1995), patients are often reluctant to get involved in such programs. Acceptance-based behavior therapy, or Acceptance and Commitment Therapy (ACT), is focused on motivating people to change what they can change and accept what they cannot change. Specifically, ACT teaches people how to bring compassion and acceptance to the pain they cannot control while engaging in life-goal related actions that they can control (Dahl & Lundgren, 2006). This intriguing new approach has been successful in reducing long-term disability resulting from chronic pain (Dahl, Wilson, & Nilsson, 2004).

Conversion Disorder

An important first step in the treatment of conversion symptoms is their early recognition in which a physical examination plays a crucial role. In many cases, a positive diagnosis can be made on the basis of the rather untypical or bizarre symptoms. Since conversion symptoms vary widely across patients, treatment needs to be individualized. Identifying precipitating stressors is crucial so that patients can be taught more adaptive ways of coping with these stressors. Occasionally, manipulation of the patient's social environment is necessary to reduce the influence of secondary gain, such as attention from family and friends. Partners and significant others may have to learn how to reinforce the patients nonsymptomatic behavior.

Behavior therapy has shown some efficacy in the treatment of conversion disorder, particularly for patients that primarily exhibit motor symptoms and gait disturbances (Lipsitt & Starcevic, 2006; Speed, 1996). The program consisted of providing or withholding reinforcement depending on the patient's attempt at normalizing gait and increasing motor movement through specific exercises.

Body Dysmorphic Disorder

Behavioral interventions for BDD aim at changing avoidance behavior, reassurance seeking, checking, and excessive grooming. Exposure in vivo is used to counter avoidance of social situations (meeting people, having a conversation, being in the spotlight) and prevent individuals from attempting to cover their ostensible blemishes (e.g., by wearing camouflaging clothing such as baggy pants, long hair, sun glasses). Patients are encouraged to expose themselves to social situations rather than avoid them and to observe the reactions of other people to their imagined deformity. Rosen (1995) suggests exposure assignments such as wearing trendy clothes, using makeup to accentuate features, standing closer to people, and undressing in front of one's spouse. Response prevention may involve refraining from looking in the mirror for excessive periods of time, the use of makeup, and inspecting skin blemishes.

A few treatment studies for BDD have examined the use of exposure and response prevention (Neziroglu & Yaryura-Tobias, 1993) and social skills training (Braddock, 1982). Schmidt and Harrington (1995) describe a successful cognitive-behavioral therapy in a 24-year-old male who was preoccupied with having small hands. Nine one-hour sessions with behavioral experiments were aimed at challenging beliefs about the size of his hands and other people's attention to his hands. Treatment resulted in a decrease in BDD-related cognitions, distress, and avoidance behavior, and Beck Depression and Beck Anxiety Inventory scores.

The first controlled outcome study of the treatment of BDD (Rosen, Reiter, & Orosan, 1995) compared the effectiveness of cognitive-behavioral therapy with a wait-list control condition in 54 females. Treatment involved eight two-hour small group sessions and was aimed at modifying dysfunctional thoughts about the patients' body image, reducing checking of their appearance, and increasing exposure to avoided situations. Results at posttest and four months follow-up showed improvement in the active treatment condition on several measures of body image, whereas no such changes occurred in the control condition. The results of this study are promising, but more controlled studies are needed to corroborate existing data and to examine the role of the various treatment components.

Conclusions

Unexplained and unexplainable somatic symptoms, complaints, and concerns are very common in the general population. These problems are costly to the individuals concerned in terms of distress and financial expense as well as to society in terms of lost productivity and health care costs. Compared to other common psychological dysfunctions (e.g., anxiety and depression), our present conceptual understanding of somatoform disorders is poor, and comprehensive integrative models are still lacking.

One factor that has impeded a better understanding of the somatoform disorders is the unsatisfactory and somewhat arbitrary nature of their current *DSM* classification. In view of the existing conceptual and diagnostic confusion, vagueness, and imprecision, we question the utility of the current criteria for and distinctions among somatoform disorders and the wisdom of keeping hypochondriasis in particular separate from the anxiety disorders. "Comorbidity" of somatoform disorders with anxiety disorders and depression is not a diagnostic problem but an indication that there are similarities in the underlying psychopathological processes (Aikens, Zvolensky, & Eifert, 2001). We have outlined some commonalities in emotional dysregulation processes particularly in relation to anxiety. A practical consequence for researchers and clinicians is to give up their focus on the individual disorders and increase their efforts at identifying the common functions of symptoms in persons with different somatoform problems (Eifert, 1996).

The complex relationships between the physical and psychological aspects of somatoform disorders have led to much confusion. We caution against an overreliance upon medical diagnostic procedures and medical theory. At the same time, research and service delivery would benefit from a more balanced approach. This approach should focus not just on finding or excluding somatic abnormalities but also on combining current medical knowledge and diagnostic techniques with the psychological assessments of a patient's behavior, cognitive processes, and social relationships (cf. Fink, 1996). In our work with cardiac patients we observed how a simple reliance on one source of information (medical or psychological) was inadequate for many patients. Instead, it was the combination of sophisticated medical tests and psychological information that yielded the type of knowledge that was most useful for recommending and designing the most appropriate treatment for the individual patient.

Hence, one of the most compelling conclusions arising from this chapter is that somatoform disorders cannot be adequately understood, assessed, and treated from a single perspective. Both the classification and research could be improved by adopting a multidisciplinary approach and an integrated biopsychosocial perspective. For example, Mayou, Bass, and Sharpe (1995) propose a multidimensional classification of patients with functional somatic symptoms along five dimensions: (1) number and type of somatic symptoms; (2) mental state (mood and psychiatric disorder); (3) cognitions (e.g., symptom misinterpretations, disease conviction); (4) behavioral and functional impairment (illness behavior, avoidance, use of health services); and (5) pathophysiological disturbance (organic diseases, physiological mechanisms such as hyperventilation). As indicated in the section on health anxiety, individuals may be assigned different positions on all of these dimensions across the various types of somatoform disorders. Rather than attempting to find the "correct diagnosis," we recommend assessment along the crucial dimensions involved in the regulation of maladaptive illness behavior and devising treatment programs based on such assessments. Beyond the number and type of physical complaints, some of these dimensions include the presence and extent of preoccupation with body and health, disease suspicion or conviction, disease fear, and safety-seeking behavior.

A multicausal perspective suggests several potentially fruitful lines for future psychological research into somatoform disorders such as an increased focus on information processing behavior (attribution, attention, and memory) and environmental contingencies for illness behavior (e.g., social, occupational, medical). Psychoneuro-immunological studies may help clarify particular aspects of the nature of the interface between pathophysiological changes and individual responses to such changes as exemplified in some chronic pain research (cf. Flor et al., 1990). Although the past emphasis on the problems of patients with no demonstrable physical pathology was worthwhile and deserves continued attention, the gray area of persons with some organic pathology, bodily symptoms, and psychological distress deserves greater recognition and needs to be investigated more carefully.

Treatment programs and outcomes are likely to be enhanced by an improved conceptual understanding of these problems. The need for better theories and treatments is even more pressing for those somatoform problems that have been particularly neglected in the past such as BDD and conversion problems. The relative success of recent cognitive-behavioral treatment programs for persons with unexplained physical symptoms, health anxiety, or chronic pain is promising. These treatment successes may help change the common perception of health-care providers that people with such problems are just a "pain in the neck" and invariably difficult, or even impossible, to treat.

References

Aikens, J. E., Zvolensky, M. J., & Eifert, G. H. (2001). Fear of cardiopulmonary sensations in emergency room noncardiac chest pain patients. *Journal of Behavioral Medicine. 24*, 155–167.

American Psychiatric Association. (1994). *Diagnostic and statistical manual of mental disorders* (4th ed.). Washington, D.C.: Author.

Barlow, D. H. (2001). *Anxiety and its disorders: The nature and treatment of anxiety and panic* (2nd. ed.). New York: Guilford.

Bass, C. M., & Benjamin, S. (1993). The management of the chronic somatizer. *British Journal of Psychiatry, 162*, 472–480.

Bass, C. M., & Murphy, M. R. (1990). Somatization disorder: Critique of the concept and suggestions for future research. In C. M. Bass (Ed.), *Somatization physical symptoms and psychological illness* (pp. 301–332). Oxford: Blackwell.

Bass, C. M., & Murphy, M. R. (1995). Somatoform and personality disorders: Syndromal comorbidity and overlapping developmental pathways. *Journal of Psychosomatic Research, 39*, 403–427.

Bouman, T. K. (2002). A community-based psychoeducational group approach to hypochondriasis. *Psychotherapy and Psychosomatics, 71*, 326–332.

Castle, D., Rossell, S., & Kyrios, M. (2006). Body dysmorphic disorder. *Psychiatric Clinics of North America, 29*, 521–538.

Chambless, D. L. (1995). Training in and dissemination of empirically validated psychological treatments: Report and recommendations by the Task Force on Psychological Procedures. *The Clinical Psychologist, 48*, 3–23.

Chorpita, B. F., Brown, T. A., & Barlow, D. H. (1998). Perceived control as a mediator of family environment in etiological models of childhood anxiety. *Behavior Therapy, 29*, 457–476.

Compas, B. E., Conner-Smith, J. K., Saltzman, H., Thomsen, A. H., & Wadsworth, M. E. (2001). Coping with stress during childhood and adolescent: Problems, progress, and potential in theory and research. *Psychological Bulletin, 127*, 87–127.

Derryberry, D., & Rothbart, M. K. (1984). Emotion, attention, and temperament. In C. Izard, J. Kagan, & R. Zajonc (Eds.), *Emotion, cognition, and behavior* (pp. 132–166). Cambridge: Cambridge University Press.

Dahl, J., & Lundgren, T. (2006). *Living beyond your pain*. Oakland, CA: New Harbinger.

Dahl, J., Wilson, K. G., & Nilsson, A. (2004). Acceptance and commitment therapy and the treatment of persons at risk for long-term disability resulting from stress and pain symptoms: A preliminary randomized trial. *Behavior Therapy, 35*, 785–802.

Eifert, G. H. (1992). Cardiophobia: A paradigmatic behavioral model of heart-focused anxiety and non-anginal chest pain. *Behaviour Research and Therapy, 30*, 329–345.

Eifert, G. H. (1996). More theory-driven and less diagnosis-based behavior therapy. *Journal of Behavior Therapy and Experimental Psychiatry, 27*, 75–86.

Eifert, G. H., & Forsyth, J. F. (1996). Heart-focused and general illness fears in relation to parental medical history and separation experiences. *Behaviour Research and Therapy, 34*, 735–739.

Eifert, G. H., & Forsyth, J. F. (2005). *Acceptance and commitment therapy for anxiety disorders*. Oakland, CA: New Harbinger.

Eifert, G. H., Hodson, S. E., Tracey, D. R., Seville, J. L., & Gunawardane, K. (1996). Heart-focused anxiety, illness beliefs, and behavioral impairment: Comparing healthy heart-anxious patients with cardiac and surgical inpatients. *Journal of Behavioral Medicine, 19*, 385–399.

Eifert, G. H., & Lau, A. (2001). Using behavioral experiments in the treatment of cardiophobia: A case study. *Cognitive and Behavioral Practice, 8*, 305–317.

Eifert, G. H., Lejuez, C. W., & Bouman, T. K. (1998). Somatoform disorders. In A. S. Bellack & M. Hersen (Series Eds.). *Comprehensive clinical psychology* (Vol. 6, pp. 543–565). Oxford: Pergamon.

Eifert, G. H., Zvolensky, M. J., & Lejuez, C. W. (2000). Heart-focused anxiety and chest pain: A conceptual and clinical review. *Clinical Psychology: Science and Practice, 7*, 403–417.

Escobar, J. I., Allen, L. A., Nervi, C. H., & Gara, M. A. (2001). General and cross-cultural considerations in a medical setting for patients presenting with medically unexplained symptoms. In G. J. G. Asmundson, S. Taylor, & B. Cox (Eds.), *Health anxiety: Clinical research perspectives on hypochondriasis and related disorders* (pp. 220–245). New York: Wiley.

Fava, G. A. (1992). The concept of psychosomatic disorder. *Psychotherapy and Psychosomatics, 58*, 1–12.

Fava, G., & Grandi, S. (1991). Differential diagnosis of hypochondriacal fears and beliefs. *Psychotherapy and Psychosomatics, 55*, 114–119.

Fink, P. (1996). Somatization—Beyond symptom count. *Journal of Psychosomatic Research, 40*, 7–10.

Fishbain, D. A., & Goldberg, M. (1991). The misdiagnosis of conversion disorder in a psychiatric emergency service. *General Hospital Psychiatry, 13*, 177–181.

Flor, F., Birbaumer, N., & Turk, D. C. (1990). The psychobiology of chronic pain. *Advances in Behaviour Research and Therapy, 12*, 47–84.

Fordyce, W. E., Roberts, A. H., & Sternbach, R. A. (1985). The behavioural management of chronic pain: A response to critics. *Pain, 22*, 113–125.

Forsyth, J. P., Eifert, G. H., & Barrios, V. (2006). Fear conditioning research as a clinical analog: What makes fear learning disordered? In M. G. Craske, D. Hermans, & D. Vansteenwegen (Eds.), *Fear and learning: Basic science to clinical application* (pp. 133–153). Washington, D.C.: American Psychological Association.

Goldberg, D., Gask, L., & O'Dowd, T. (1989). The treatment of somatization: Teaching techniques of reattribution. *Journal of Psychosomatic Research, 33,* 689–695.

Harvey, R. F., Salih, W. Y., & Read, A. E. (1983). Organic and functional disorders in 2000 gastroenterology outpatients. *Lancet, i,* 632–634.

Hayes, S. C., Strosahl, K., & Wilson, K. (1999). *Acceptance and commitment therapy: Understanding and treating human suffering.* New York: Guilford.

Hayes, S. C., & Wilson, K. G. (1994). Acceptance and commitment therapy: Altering the verbal support for experiential avoidance. *The Behavior Analyst, 17,* 289–303.

Kagan, J. (1989). Temperamental contributions to social behavior. *American Psychologist, 44,* 668–674.

Kagan, J., Snidman, N., & Arcus, D. M. (1992) Initial reactions to unfamiliarity. *Current Directions in Psychological Science, 1,* 171–174.

Kashner, T. M., Rost, K., Cohen, B., Anderson, M., & Smith. G. R. (1995). Enhancing the health of somatization disorder patients: Effectiveness of short-term group therapy. *Psychosomatics, 36,* 462–470.

Kellner, R. (1990) Somatization: Theories and research. *The Journal of Nervous and Mental Disease 178,* 150–160.

Kendler, K.S., Walters, E. E., Truett, K. R., & Heath, A. C. (1995). A twin-family study of self-report symptoms of panic, phobia, and somatization. *Behavior Genetics, 25,* 499–515.

Kenyon, F. E. (1964). Hypochondriasis: A clinical study. *British Journal of Psychiatry, 110,* 478–488.

Lejuez, C. W., Hopko, D. R., & Hopko, S. D.. (2001). A brief behavioral activation treatment for depression. *Behavior Modification, 25,* 255–286.

Lipsitt, D. R., & Starcevic, V. (2006). Psychotherapy and pharmacotherapy in the treatment of somatoform disorders. *Psychiatric Annals, 36,* 341–350.

Margolis, R. B., Zimny, G. H., & Miller, D. (1984). Internists and the chronic pain patient. *Pain, 20,* 151–156.

Martinez, M. P., & Botella, C. (2005). An exploratory study of the efficacy of a cognitive-behavioral treatment for *hypochondriasis* using different measures of change. *Psychotherapy Research, 15,* 392–408.

Mayou, R., Bass, C. M., & Sharpe, M. (Eds.). (1995). *Treatment of functional somatic symptoms.* Oxford: Oxford University Press.

Mayou, R., Bryant, B., Forbar, C., & Clark, D. (1994). Non-cardiac chest pain and benign palpitations in the cardiac clinic. *British Heart Journal, 72,* 548–553.

Mayou, R., Kirmayer, L., Simon, G., & Sharpe, M. (2005). Somatoform disorders: Time for a new approach in DSM-V. *American Journal of Psychiatry, 162,* 847–855.

Mayou, R., & Sharpe, M. (1995). Patients whom doctors find difficult to help. *Psychosomatics, 36,* 323–325.

Mineka, S., Gunnar, M., & Champoux, M. (1986). Control and early socioemotional development: Infant rhesus monkeys reared in controllable versus uncontrollable environments. *Child Development, 57,* 1241–1256.

Murphy, M. R. (1990). Classification of the somatoform disorders. In C. M. Bass (Ed.) *Somatization. Physical symptoms and psychological illness* (pp. 10–39). Oxford: Blackwell.

Nicholas, M. K., Wilson, P. H., & Goyen, J. (1991). Operant-behavioural and cognitive-behavioural treatment of chronic low back pain. *Behaviour Research and Therapy, 29,* 225–238.

Pilowsky, I. (1993). Aspects of abnormal illness behaviour. *Psychotherapy and Psychosomatics, 60,* 62–74.

Pilowsky, I., Chapman, C. R., & Bonica, J. J. (1977). Pain, depression, and illness behavior in a pain clinic population. *Pain, 4,* 183–192.

Pilowsky, I., Smith, Q. P., Katsikitis, M. (1987). Illness behavior and general practice utilisation: A prospective study. *Psychosomatic Research, 31,* 177–183.

Rachlin, H. C. (1985). Pain and behavior. *Behavioral and Brain Sciences, 8,* 43–83.

Razran, G. (1939). A quantitative study of meaning by conditioned salivary technique (semantic conditioning). *Science, 90,* 89–91.

Rief, W., Buhlmann, U., Wilhelm, S., Borkenhagen, A, & Brahler, E. (2006). The prevalence of *body dysmorphic disorder*: A population-based survey. *Psychological Medicine, 36,* 877–885.

Rief, W., Hiller, W., Geissner, E., & Fichter, M. M. (1995). A two-year follow-up study of patients with somatoform disorders. *Psychosomatics, 36,* 376–386.

Robbins, J. M., & Kirmayer, L. J. (1991). Attributions of common somatic symptoms. *Psychological Medicine, 21,* 1029–1045.

Rosen, J. C. (1995). The nature of body dysmorphic disorder and treatment with cognitive behavior therapy. *Cognitive and Behavioral Practice, 2,* 143–166.

Rost, K., Kashner, T. M., & Smith, G. R. (1995). Effectiveness of psychiatric intervention with somatization disorder patients. *General Hospital Psychiatry, 16,* 381–387.

Rothbart, M. K. (1989). Temperament and development. In G. Kohnstamm, J. Bates, & M. Rothbart, M. K. (Eds.), *Temperament in childhood* (pp. 187–248). Chichester, UK: Wiley.

Rothbart, M. K., Ziaie, H., & O'Boyle, C. G. (1992). Self-regulation and emotion in infancy. In N. Eisenberg & R. A. Fabes (Eds.), *Emotion and its regulation in early development: New Directions For Child Development, 55,* 7–24.

Salkovskis, P. M. (1996). The cognitive approach to anxiety: Threat beliefs, safety seeking behavior, and the special case of health anxiety and obsessions. In P. M. Salkovskis (Ed.) *Frontiers of cognitive therapy* (pp. 49–74). New York: Guilford.

Salkovskis, P. M. & Warwick, H. M. C. (1986). Morbid preoccupations, health anxiety and reassurance: A cognitive-behavioural approach to hypochondriasis. *Behaviour Research and Therapy, 24,* 597–602.

Salkovskis, P. M., & Warwick, H. M. C. (2001). Making sense of hypochondriasis: A cognitive model of health anxiety. In G. J. G. Asmundson, S. Taylor, & B. Cox (Eds.), *Health anxiety: Clinical research perspectives on hypochondriasis and related disorders* (pp. 46–64). New York: Wiley.

Schermelleh-Engel, K., Eifert, G. H., Moosbrugger, H., & Frank, D. (1997). Perceived competence and anxiety as determinants of maladaptive and adaptive coping strategies of chronic pain patients. *Personality and Individual Differences, 22,* 1–10.

Sharma, P., & Chaturvedi, S. K. (1995). Conversion disorder revisited. *Acta Psychiatria Scandinavica, 92*, 301–304.

Sharpe, M., & Bass, C. M. (1992). Pathophysiological mechanisms in somatization. *International Review of Psychiatry, 4*, 81–97.

Sharpe, M., Mayou, R., & Bass, C. M. (1995). Concepts, theories, and terminology. In R. Mayou, C. M. Bass, & M. Sharpe (Eds.), *Treatment of functional somatic symptoms* (pp. 3–16). Oxford: Oxford University Press.

Sidman, M. (1994). *Equivalence relations and behavior: A research story.* Boston, MA: Authors Cooperative.

Smith, G. R., Rost, K., & Kashner, T. M. (1995). A trial of the effect of a standardized psychiatric consultation of health outcomes and cost in somatizing patients. *Archives of General Psychiatry, 52*, 238–243.

Speckens, A. E. M., van Hemert, A. M., Spinhoven, P., Hawton, K. E., Bolk, J. H., & Rooijmans, H. G. M. (1996). Cognitive behavioral therapy for medically unexplained physical symptoms: A randomised controlled trial. *British Medical Journal, 311*, 1328–1332.

Speed, J. (1996). Behavioral management of conversion disorder: Retrospective study. *Archives of Physical and Medical Rehabilitation, 77*, 147–154.

Staats, A. W. & Eifert, G. H. (1990). A paradigmatic behaviorism theory of emotion: Basis for unification. *Clinical Psychology Review, 10*, 539–566.

Stewart, S. H., Zvolensky, M. J., & Eifert, G. H. (2002). The relations of anxiety sensitivity, experiential avoidance, and alexithymic coping to young adults' motivations for drinking. *Behavior Modification, 26*, 274–296.

Turk, D. C., Meichenbaum, D., & Genest, M. (1983). *Pain and behavioral medicine: A cognitive-behavioral perspective.* New York: Guilford.

Van Hemert, A. M., Hengeveld, M. W., Bolk, J. H., Rooijmans, H. G. M., & Vandenbroucke, J. P. (1993). Psychiatric disorders in relation to medical illness among patients of a general outpatient clinic. *Psychological Medicine, 23*, 167–173.

Visser, S., & Bouman, T. (1992). Cognitive-behavioural approaches in the treatment of hypochondriasis: Six single case crossover studies. *Behaviour Research and Therapy, 30*, 301–306.

Warwick, H. M. C., Clark, D. M., Cobb, A. M., & Salkovskis, P. M. (1996). A controlled trial of cognitive-behavioural treatment of hypochondriasis. *British Journal of Psychiatry, 169*, 189–195.

Warwick, H. M. C., & Marks, I. M. (1988). Behavioural treatment of illness phobia. *British Journal of Psychiatry, 152*, 239–241.

Warwick, H. M. C., & Salkovskis, P. M. (1990). Hypochondriasis. *Behaviour Research and Therapy, 28*, 105–117.

Zvolensky, M. J., Feldner, M. T., Eifert, G. H., Vujanovic, A. A., & Solomon, S. E. (in press). Cardiophobia: A critical analysis. *Transcultural Psychiatry.*

Zvolensky, M. J., Lejuez, C. W., & Eifert, G. H. (2000). Prediction and control: Operational definitions for the experimental analysis of anxiety. *Behaviour Research and Therapy, 38*, 653–663.

15
Substance Use Disorders

William Fals-Stewart and Keith Klostermann

Of the major public health concerns of the 20th century, alcoholism and drug addiction certainly are among the most insidious and devastating. However defined, excessive use of alcohol and other drugs is an all-too-common problem, not only in the United States but across the globe. For example, the National Survey on Drug Use and Health reports more than half of the U.S. population, aged 12 and older, uses alcohol. Of these, 30% engage in binge drinking (i.e., drinking five or more drinks on the same occasion at least once in the past month), and more than 10% are heavy drinkers (U.S. Office of Applied Studies, 2003). Although the prevalences of other drug use disorders are much lower than alcohol, they are sizable by nearly any standard. For illicit psychoactive substances, the lifetime prevalence of drug abuse or dependence is roughly 6% in the United States, with lifetime cannabis abuse (i.e., 4.6%) being the most common after alcohol (e.g., Haynes, 2002). The World Health Organization estimates that 28 million people worldwide incur significant health risks by using psychoactive substances other than alcohol (Uchtenhagen, 2004).

Annually, substance use in the United States claims 600,000 lives, including 440,000 attributable to nicotine use, 125,000 from alcohol use, and 10,000 from heroin and cocaine use (exclusive of deaths from HIV; McCrady & Epstein, 1999). Alcoholism is the third major cause of preventable death in the United States (behind coronary heart disease and cancer), with the life span of individuals with alcoholism being about 12 years shorter than their nonalcoholic counterparts (Mokdad, Marks, Stroup, & Gerberding, 2004). In addition to the serious problems individuals with alcohol or drug problems create for themselves, victims of family violence, accidents, and violent crime add to the numbers of those adversely affected. In the home, drug and alcohol use by husbands is associated with a 1- to 15-fold increase in physical violence against their partners (Fals-Stewart, 2003; Fals-Stewart, Golden, & Schumacher, 2003). Parental substance use is associated with a host of emotional, behavioral, and social problems for children who live in the environments these caregivers provide (e.g., Fals-Stewart, Kelley, Cooke, & Golden, 2002), which often evolve into problems with alcohol and drugs as these children enter adolescence and adulthood. Thus, the effects of alcoholism and substance abuse can be accurately described as being part of an intransigent multigenerational vicious cycle.

Aside from the toll in human suffering, estimates of yearly direct and indirect economic social costs arising from substance abuse are substantial. Individuals who abuse alcohol and other drugs consume a disproportionately large share of social resources from a variety of sources, some of which include specialized drug abuse treatment (Institute of Medicine, 1990), treatment of secondary health effects (Langenbucher, 1994), use of social welfare programs (Plotnick, 1994), and criminal justice system use (e.g., arrests, incarceration, parole, and probation; Deschenes, Anglin, & Speckart, 1991; Harwood, Hubbard, Collins, & Rachal, 1988). In the United States, the most recent estimate of the societal cost of drug abuse (focusing on the cost of health care, productivity losses, criminal justice system, and crime victim costs) was $180.9 billion for the year 2002, with an average annual rise in costs of 5.3% per year since 1992 (U.S. Office of National Drug Control Policy, 2004).

The size and scope of substance abuse and dependence in our society has drawn significant and increasing scientific and public attention. Although our understanding of addiction to alcohol and drugs is far from complete, there has been great progress in the understanding of the etiology, course, and treatment of alcoholism and drug abuse. However, progress is not to be confused with consensus. There remains much controversy, not only about the etiology and treatment of substance misuse, but also, on a far more fundamental level, about how to conceptualize and operationalize substance use disorders.

Definition and Description of Substance Use Disorders

For most of U.S. history, chronic and excessive substance use has been viewed either as immoral conduct or as a disease. More recently, with the rising influence of the behavioral sciences in this dialogue, addictive behavior has also been viewed as maladaptive behavior subject to reinforcement contingencies that govern all learned human behavior. In turn, the definition and description of addictive behavior can vary considerably, based on which view (i.e., moral, disease, or behavioral) is emphasized.

Defining Addictive Behavior

The evolution in thinking about what defines addictive behavior is based in large part on the observation that a number of processes are common to excessive behaviors that have been characterized as addictive. Miller (1995) defines addiction as consisting of three primary components: (1) preoccupation, (2) compulsion, and (3) relapse. In the *preoccupation* phase, individuals place a great deal of emphasis on acquiring drugs. As such, social relationships and employment are jeopardized in the continuous search for drugs, and also suffer as a consequence of using drugs. In the *compulsion* phase, the individual continues to use drugs, despite serious negative consequences. During *relapse*, the individual stops using drugs, however, eventually resumes using drugs at an abnormal level. To capture the essence of addiction that spans these behaviors, a broad definition has evolved that can be generally applied to all addictions, including addiction to psychoactive substances. From this vantage point, addiction is viewed as a complex, progressive behavior pattern having biological, psychological, and sociological components. What distinguishes this pattern of behavior from others is the individual's overwhelming pathological involvement in or attachment to it, subjective compulsion to continue it, and reduced ability to exert control over it. The behavior pattern continues despite its negative impact on the physical, psychological, and social functioning of the individual.

Although this depiction provides an overarching description of addictive behavior, it provides little insight into how to discern when use of drugs or alcohol crosses over from normal to problematic use, and from problematic use to disorder. More specifically, because of widely divergent social attitudes toward and prejudices about alcohol and drug use, there have been few generally accepted and agreed-on operational criteria for what level of use constitutes social use, abuse, and dependence. Substance use can follow one of several patterns; addiction "is not an all-or-nothing" phenomenon, but a continuum from recreational use to severe compulsion (Peele, Brodsky, & Arnold, 1991, p. 133).

Labels and Diagnostic Systems

Over the centuries, various value-laden terminologies have been used to describe individuals who use alcohol and other drugs, as well as the problems such use can create (Carroll & Miller, 2006). Labels matter; names used to describe a given phenomenon have great influence in the way one thinks about a problem and how to address it. Individuals who have problems with drinking have been called, at various times, "drunks," "dipsomaniacs," "alcoholics," "alcohol abusers," and so on. Those who use illicit drugs have been called "addicts," "dope fiends," "freaks," and "criminals." Of course, these names have important implications, in terms of who these people are that have these problems and what can be done about it. In a certain sense, more formal diagnostic systems have come to the fore in recognition of the importance of labels and to bring order to any meaningful labeling system.

Although *use, abuse,* and *addiction* are best viewed as a continuum of behavior, much effort has been put forth to delineate boundaries between different critical points on this continuum. There are several different definitional frameworks used to categorize various levels of addictive behavior that are widely referenced in the scientific and lay press. The most widely used framework is the psychiatric diagnostic approach, exemplified in the *Diagnostic and Statistical Manual of Mental Disorders* (*DSM-IV-TR*; American Psychiatric Association, 2000) and the *International Classification of Diseases* (*ICD-10*; World Health Organization, 1992). Using the *DSM-IV* system as an example, the diagnosis of alcohol or psychoactive substance use disorders includes two general subcategories: abuse and dependence. *Substance dependence* is marked by a cluster of cognitive, behavioral, and physiological symptoms indicating that the individual continues to use a given psychoactive substance despite significant substance-related problems. To meet diagnostic criteria for dependence on a psychoactive substance, an individual must display at least three of the following seven symptoms:

1. Physical tolerance.
2. Withdrawal.
3. Unsuccessful attempts to stop or control substance use.
4. Use of larger amounts of the substance than intended.
5. Loss or reduction in important recreational, social, or occupational activities.
6. Continued use of the substance despite knowledge of physical or psychological problems that are likely to have been caused or exacerbated by the substance.
7. Excessive time spent using the substance or recovering from its effects.

In contrast, the essential feature of *substance abuse* is a maladaptive pattern of problem use leading to significant adverse consequences. This includes one or more of the following:

1. Failure to fulfill major social obligations in the context of work, school, or home.
2. Recurrent substance use in situations that create the potential for harm (e.g., drinking and driving).
3. Recurrent substance-related legal problems.
4. Continued substance use despite having persistent social or interpersonal problems caused or exacerbated by the effects of the substance.

However, given the complexity of addictive behavior, it appears that a binary, either–or view implicit in the psychiatric diagnostic approach is too simplistic and provides little understanding of the complexities of the addictive process and how to change it. As noted by Shaffer and Neuhaus (1985), addictive behavior is not easily categorized and, as such, is not easily defined by a set of consensually agreed-on criteria. Indeed, different diagnostic systems often place greater emphases on different aspects of behavioral and physiological functioning in their definitions. In turn, these differences lead to fairly divergent estimates about the prevalence of alcohol and drug use disorders in the general population (for a review of this issue, see Grant & Dawson, 1999).

A Biopsychosocial Perspective

Behavioral scientists have proposed an alternative biopsychosocial approach to defining alcoholism and drug abuse. In this framework, alcohol and drug use disorders are not defined as a unitary disease, nor is it implicitly assumed the observed substance use symptoms are the manifestation of a disease state. Symptoms are viewed as acquired habits that emerge from a combination of genetic, social, pharmacological, and behavioral factors. Addiction is viewed as involving physiological changes in individuals (many of whom may be genetically or psychologically predisposed) and the complex interaction of environmental stressors and individual aspects of the person (including his or her experiential history) that produce and maintain addictive behavior.

A comprehensive understanding of the synergistic relationship among these factors is essential not only to understanding the degree and severity of substance use, but also for understanding treatment when use becomes abuse. Labeling is largely deemphasized, and greater emphasis is placed on understanding the interplay between multiple factors that have led to and maintained the observed behavior.

Cultural and Social Issues

Definitions of substance abuse do not develop in isolation; the point at which substance use moves from recreational to disordered is determined by the social and cultural context in which the behavior occurs (e.g., Thombs, 2006). Thus, societal norms and definitions of substance use and abuse are inextricably intertwined. How we determine what qualifies as an alcohol or drug problem is derived from the boundaries implicitly (e.g., social stigma associated with being labeled an alcoholic or drug addict) or explicitly (e.g., laws prohibiting use of certain substances) drawn by society where the behavior takes place. In many respects, the norms for acceptable drinking and other drug use are delineated and implicitly or explicitly communicated to members of the society by the way the culture defines addiction.

A Sociocultural View of Alcoholism and Drug Abuse

From a sociological perspective, clinical diagnostic criteria for alcoholism and other drug abuse are derived from societal norms and thus vary depending on when and where the diagnosis is made. More specifically, drinking or drug-taking behaviors that are considered disordered are those that deviate from what are considered socially acceptable standards. Perhaps the cultural foundations of alcoholism, which can also be applied to other addictive behaviors, are best captured by Vaillant (1990), who stated: "Normal drinking merges imperceptibly with pathological drinking. Culture and idiosyncratic viewpoints will always determine where the line is drawn" (p. 6).

The sociocultural foundations of substance use diagnoses have certain important implications, even calling into question the veneer of objectivity in our official definitions of substance use disorder. Diagnosing a person as being alcohol dependent may not be very different from offering a personal opinion about his or her alcohol or drug use. The application of the label may be based not so much on scientific evidence as on the values, beliefs, and experiences of the person making the diagnosis. From a sociological perspective, alcoholism and other drug addiction are forms of social deviance, and the deviance is a function of the perceptions and biases of the person observing. Treatment then becomes an effort to force the alcoholic or drug abuser to conform to a socially acceptable standard of conduct.

Moreover, problems with alcoholism and drug abuse have become medicalized, and certain factions appear to have an agenda in viewing these behaviors as symptoms of a disease state and convincing others to view them that way. If addictive behavior is defined as a disease, the label itself gives credibility to physicians' efforts to control, manage, and supervise the care provided to individuals seeking treatment. Thus, the medical community may have a strong, vested interest in defining addictive behavior as a disease. Among its other attributes, treatment of substance abuse is a business; as with all business, economics play a critical role (Carlson, 2006). The label serves to make legitimate such financially lucrative efforts as hospital admissions, insurance billing, expansion of the pool of patients available for hospital admission, consulting fees, and so forth.

However, it would be myopic to assume that societal norms alone shape the parameters for defining alcoholism and drug addiction. In some respects, the process of labeling what constitutes substance abuse or dependence restricts drinking and drug use behavior by members of a given culture. In essence, the definition of alcoholism and substance abuse provides guidelines for drinking and drug use practices for members of a given society. In our culture, obvious drunkenness, drinking early in the morning, drinking while at work, and drinking and driving are considered signs of problem drinking. Such indicators of alcoholism appear in many of our widely used diagnostic instruments, such as the Michigan Alcoholism Screening Test (Selzer, 1971). Clearly, these "symptoms" are culturally derived and are based on a commonly held set of beliefs about acceptable substance use; the nature of the symptoms would likely be different in another culture that had a different set of social norms.

The Disease—Moral Model of Addictive Behavior

The disease model of alcoholism and abuse of other drugs is not the only theoretical conceptualization of these disorders and, in some contexts, not the predominant one. From a social policy perspective, the idea that addictive behavior is deviant and immoral is on at least an equal footing with the disease model. This disease–moral model is summed up by a passage from a turn-of-the-century temperance lecturer, John B. Gough (1881), who wrote that he considered "drunkenness as a sin, but I consider it also a disease. It is a physical as well as moral evil" (p. 443). The disease and moral models of substance abuse are, in many respects, strange bedfellows. These models hold divergent and, at times, inconsistent views about the etiology and maintenance of addictive behavior. In essence, the moral view holds that drinking and drug use are freely chosen acts for which individuals are responsible; the disease model, in many respects, espouses the opposite position. In turn, the conclusions and outcomes of the disease–moral model are, at times, rife with contradiction. For example, it is difficult to reconcile the inherent contradiction in treating the "illness" of psychoactive substance abuse with punishment (e.g., incarceration). How many other illnesses are routinely punished?

At a social policy level, much energy and effort is expended in veering between these two models. Yet, it is the disease–moral model that is the guiding hand that drives alcohol and drug policies today, with neither perspective completely supplanting the other. For instance, judges sentence those convicted of driving while intoxicated (DWI) to attend Alcoholics Anonymous (AA) meetings or face jail. Peele (1996) describes this as the "disease law enforcement model," which perhaps manifests itself most clearly in the debate between those who believe drug abusers should be treated and those who believe they should be incarcerated.

Gender Issues

Although social norms provide a context in which to understand addictive behavior, it is also important to understand that science does not stand above or outside of its social context, but is immersed in and highly influenced by it (Kuhn, 1962). As with all areas of inquiry, social and cultural factors influenced the way scientists study alcoholism and drug abuse. The relationship between addictive behavior and gender is an important case in point. Alcoholism and other addictions have traditionally been considered problems of men; as such, it has been the study of addictive behavior among men that has shaped our understanding of the nature and course of these disorders. Two of the most widely known and influential investigations of alcoholism, Jellinek's (1952) on the phases of alcoholism and Vaillant's (1995) 45-year prospective longitudinal study of alcohol abuse in inner-city and college cohorts, were limited to male participants. Treatment methods and programs were also initially designed to treat male substance abuse; it was not unusual for women who needed treatment for addictive disorders to be placed in psychiatric wards, whereas men were treated in specialized alcoholism or drug abuse treatment programs (Blume, 1998).

Because the majority of research conducted in the area of substance abuse has been based largely on studies with male participants, a significant concern is that conclusions drawn from these studies may not generalize to women with substance use disorders (Straussner & Zelvin, 1997). More recently, women have become the focus of increased attention by the research and treatment communities. Comparisons of substance use by men and women have revealed several important differences in terms of epidemiology, development, and treatment.

Epidemiological and Etiological Comparisons

Data from the 2004 National Survey on Drug Use and Health (U.S. Substance Abuse and Mental Health Services Administration, 2005) reveal males 12 and older were twice as likely as females to be dependent on or abuse alcohol or other illicit drugs during the previous year. Moreover, changes in use patterns over time appear to be different based on gender. For example, since the mid-1970s, the proportion of U.S. men who smoke tobacco products has fallen at a much greater rate (52 to 28%) than the corresponding decrease among women (34 to 22%). Although the National Comorbidity Study (Warner, Kessler, Hughes, Anthony, & Nelson, 1995) revealed the prevalence of substance use disorders in the general population are higher for men than women, other important gender differences did emerge. Women between the ages of 45 and 54 years reported a higher lifetime prevalence of drug dependence (other than alcohol or nicotine) than did men (3.8% compared to 2.1% for men). This finding reflects the higher prevalence of prescription drug dependence in women, whereas men have higher rates of dependence on illicit drugs.

Several important risk factors for the development of problems with alcohol or other drugs have also been identified in women. For example, Winfield, George, Swartz, and Blazer (1990) found the lifetime prevalence of alcohol abuse or dependence was three times higher and that of other drug abuse was four times higher among women who reported a history of sexual assault. It also appears that male significant others who use drugs have a significant influence on women's patterns of substance use. In comparison to women, men are more likely to introduce their female partners to the use of drugs and to supply drugs to them (e.g., Amaro & Hardy-Fosta, 1995).

Another area of difference between men and women are the reasons they give for drinking and drug use. Women misuse psychoactive substances in response to current psychosocial stressors more often than do men; this may be particularly problematic for middle-aged women because several stressful life events often occur during midlife (e.g., children leaving the home, death of parents, divorce; Allan & Cooke, 1985). Female alcoholics and substance abusers have higher rates of comorbid (i.e., co-occurring) psychiatric disorders, especially depressive and anxiety disorders, than do men (Brady & Randall, 1999). Moreover, Annis and Graham (1995) found women were more likely to drink in response to negative emotional states and interpersonal conflict than men. Taken together, these findings suggest that women rely on substance use as a form of self-medication for mood disturbances more than men do.

The Stigma of Addiction for Women

Sociocultural factors also play important roles in the substance use patterns of men and women. In nearly all societies in which alcohol or other drugs are consumed, the cultural norms, attitudes, stereotypes, and legal sanctions often differ for men and women. Most cultures expect that women will drink less alcohol than men. These expectations may serve as a protective factor, reducing the incidence of alcohol use disorders among women (e.g., Kubicka, Csemy, & Kozeny, 1995).

However, the intense stigma associated with drinking and drug use by women can also create serious social problems. Society tolerates some behaviors exhibited by intoxicated men, but views the same behavior as scandalous if exhibited by intoxicated women. As Blume (1991) argues, women who are intoxicated are often the object of unwanted sexual overtures, and men believe that intoxicated women who say "No" to these advances really mean "Yes." In a study of beliefs about rape, participants viewed rapists who were intoxicated as less responsible for their crimes than sober rapists and viewed rape victims who had been drinking as more to blame for the rape than victims who had not been drinking (Richardson & Campbell, 1982). Thus, it is not surprising that alcoholic women are much more likely to be victims of violent crime, including rape, than their nonalcoholic counterparts (e.g., McClelland & Teplin, 2001). Some contend that society at large views women who abuse alcohol or other drugs as partially or fully responsible for sexual advances made by men, thus making these women acceptable targets for physical and sexual aggression (e.g., Stormo, Lang, & Stritzke, 1997).

An important result of the stigma associated with women's alcohol and drug use is denial by the person, the family, and society. These various forms of denial, in turn, are barriers that may prevent women from seeking treatment. As noted by Schober and Annis (1996), women often are reluctant to acknowledge a substance use problem publicly by seeking treatment because of intense fear of being stigmatized as a substance abuser. In comparison to their male counterparts, fears about the stigma associated with the label of *alcoholic* or *substance abuser* may be more powerful disincentives for women to seek treatment than denial of having a problem or accessibility and cost of treatment (Marlatt, Tucker, Donovan, & Vuchinich, 1997).

Along with personal denial, family denial is also a significant barrier to women entering treatment for substance abuse. In fact, the response by family members to women entering treatment appears to be more negative than it is for men. For example, Beckman and Amaro (1986) found that nearly 25% of women in a treatment sample reported opposition from family or friends, compared to only 2% of men. In addition, child-care and child custody issues influence the decision to seek treatment.

Women often fear that entering treatment will lead to the perception that they are unfit as mothers and may be deprived of custody of their children. These fears are not unfounded. Recently, women who use alcohol and other drugs during pregnancy have been prosecuted on charges of prenatal child abuse or delivery of a controlled substance to a minor (via the umbilical cord). Such practices have not prevented substance use during pregnancy, but have discouraged pregnant substance users from seeking prenatal or addiction treatment (Blume, 1997).

In addition to these personal and familial barriers, several factors related to the type and process of treatment have increased women's reluctance to seek help. Less than 14% of all women who need treatment for substance abuse receive it; less than 12% of pregnant women receive help (Center on Addiction and Substance Abuse, 1996). In a recent investigation, Dawson, Grant, Stinson and Chou (2006) supported this notion of gender differences in help-seeking behaviors and found individuals who seek treatment differ in many ways, with men being more likely to seek help than women. These findings, although disturbing, are not surprising; most treatments for addictive behaviors have been developed largely to meet the needs of men and thus may not be as effective for women (e.g., Ramlow, White, Watson, & Luekefeld, 1997). A major reason women do not enter treatment is that most programs do not provide services (e.g., child care, obstetrician services) that make it easier for women to enter treatment (Nelson-Zlupko, Dore, Kauffman, & Kaltenbach, 1996). Some studies do, in fact, suggest that treatment programs designed specifically to meet the treatment needs of substance-abusing women have higher retention and better outcomes than standard outpatient or residential treatment programs (e.g., Dahlgren & Willander, 1989; Roberts & Nishimoto, 1996).

Etiology of Alcohol and Other Drug Use Disorders

Research on the etiology of substance use disorders is a multidimensional, multidisciplinary effort, and findings that have appeared in the literature are truly voluminous. This is a consequence of the multiple theoretical conceptualizations of the development and maintenance of these disorders. For instance, investigators who view alcoholism and drug abuse as diseases are often most interested in examining genetic and biological contributions. Behavior-oriented researchers are more apt to explore antecedent and consequent events that may serve to initiate and reinforce substance use. Sociologists examine macrolevel variables, such as peer and societal influences that contribute to the onset and maintenance of addictive behavior. Development of an addiction to alcohol or other drugs is a complex process involving many factors; however, the exact role of each of these ingredients has not been fully determined and operates differently for each individual. Genetics, biology, environment, sociocultural factors, and the biochemical properties of the psychoactive substances themselves appear to contribute substantially to the process (e.g., Sandbak, Murison, Sarviharju, & Hyytiae, 1998).

Neurobiology of Addiction

Psychoactive substances vary widely in terms of their biochemical properties, how they enter the body, and how they ultimately enter the brain. Central to the neurochemical process underlying addiction is the process by which alcohol or other drugs become reinforcing. Most neurobiological studies of addiction have focused on the dopamine system, which is considered to be the neurotransmitter system through which most drugs of abuse exert their reinforcing effects (Koob & Bloom, 1988). A *reinforcer* is operationally defined as an event that increases the likelihood of a subsequent response; drugs of abuse, which appear to have substantial effects on the dopamine system, are much stronger reinforcers than natural reinforcers, such as food and sex (Wightman & Robinson, 2002).

As described by Volkow, Fowler, and Wang (2003), it is believed that there is a network of four circuits that is largely responsible for drug abuse and addiction: (1) reward, located in the nucleus accumbens and the ventral pallidum; (2) motivation/drive, located in the orbitofrontal cortex and the subcallosal cortex; (3) memory and learning, located in the amygdala and the hippocampus; and (4) control, located in the prefrontal cortex and the anterior cingulate gyrus. These four circuits receive innervations (i.e., are stimulated into action) from dopaminergic neurons, but are also connected to one another through direct and indirect pathways. The circuits work together and can be changed with experience. Thus, during the development and maintenance of addiction to a psychoactive substance, the enhanced value of the substance in the reward, motivation, and memory circuits eventually overcomes any inhibitory control exerted by other parts of the brain (e.g., the prefrontal cortex). This, in turn, creates a positive feedback loop that is initiated by the ingestion of the psychoactive substance and then perpetuated by the activation of the motivation/drive and memory circuits. For an individual addicted to drugs, the value of the drug of abuse is enhanced in the reward and motivation/drive circuits; increases in dopamine induced by drugs are three to five times higher than those of natural reinforcers (Wise, 2002).

Genetic Propensity

Many studies have examined the genetic predisposition to alcohol and drug abuse and addiction, and a substantial literature suggests addiction problems and disorders have a genetic component. The familial nature of alcoholism has long been recognized and is well documented (e.g., Bierut et al., 1998; Merikangas et al., 1998). While alcoholism appears to run in families, it is difficult to separate genetic factors from environmental influences because members of nuclear families typically share both genetic and environmental factors. Adoption studies enable the separation of genetic and environmental factors and usually reveal a strong link between paternal alcoholism and the development of alcoholism, particularly among biological male offspring (e.g., Goodwin et al., 1974). Studies of twins also support the role of genetic factors in the development of alcoholism. The level of twin-pair concordance for a disorder or trait can be compared between identical (monozygotic, or MZ) and fraternal (dizygotic, or DZ) twins. If concordance is higher for MZ than DZ twins, this is an indication of genetic heritability; 100% heritability indicates a disorder is entirely genetic, 50% heritability means there is a substantial contribution from genetic and environmental factors, and 0% indicating genetic factors do not play a role. In general, adult twin studies of alcohol dependence show a heritability of 50 to 60% (Hasin, Hatzenbuehler, & Waxman, 2006). Heritability is much stronger for alcohol dependence than for abuse and has been shown to be stronger for men than for women (National Institute on Alcohol Abuse and Alcoholism, 1993).

Research on the genetic risk factors for abuse of drugs other than alcohol is far less evolved to date; only a few studies have sought to determine a familial influence in the development of substance use disorders other than alcohol. Compton and colleagues (Compton, Thomas, Conway, & Colliver, 2005) estimated that 40 to 60% of variability in the risk of addiction is accounted for by genetic factors (including genetic-environmental interactions). In addition, a preference for specific types of drugs may occur among family members of drug abusers; monozygotic twins appear to display a greater similarity than dizygotic twin pairs in their preference for, and response to, certain types of drugs (Schuckit, 1987).

Examining the genetic link for the abuse of drugs other than alcohol, compared to alcoholism, is often far more difficult because individuals must be exposed to the psychoactive substance for the behavioral manifestation of the genetic propensity toward a certain behavior to appear. Most individuals in the world have extensive exposure to alcohol; this is not the case for many other drugs of abuse (e.g., heroin, cocaine).

Family Environment Influences

Not only do individuals who abuse alcohol and other drugs often develop physiological dependence, they can also develop a strong psychological dependence. Essentially, they become dependent on the drug to help them cope with negative emotional states and stressful social situations. Because substance use so often leads to significant problems for people across multiple domains of functioning, we must ask, "How is psychological dependence on alcohol or other drugs learned?"

As has been argued by many investigators, the family is an extremely important molding influence for children. Although the misuse of alcohol and other psychoactive substances by adults often has serious physical, emotional, behavioral, and economic consequences, the ancillary short-and long-term negative effects on those who live with these adults are often no less destructive. In particular, children who live with parents who abuse alcohol and other drugs may be victimized by the deleterious environments these caregivers frequently create. Findings from several studies suggest that children who live in homes with substance-abusing parents are at an increased risk for developing substance abuse problems and other emotional and behavioral problems in adolescence and early adulthood (e.g., Christensen & Bilenberg, 2000). It appears that alcoholic parents are less likely than nonalcoholic parents to monitor what their children are doing, which can lead to affiliation of their adolescent children with drug-using peers (Chassin, Pillow, Curran, Molina, & Barrera, 1993). Stress and negative affect, which are comparatively high in families with an alcoholic family member, are associated with alcohol use in adolescents (Chassin, Curran, Hussong, & Colder, 1996).

Personality and Psychiatric Factors

Several psychoanalytic explanations for the development and maintenance of alcoholism and drug abuse have been proposed. For example, Wurmser (1984) viewed substance abusers as having overly harsh superegos and proposed these individuals use alcohol and other drugs to escape intense feelings of anger and fear. Khantzian, Halliday, and McAuliffe (1990) theorized inadequacies of the ego underlie substance misuse. In addition, these authors argue that a person's drug of choice has particular self-medicating properties for his or her particular type of ego deficit. Other psychoanalytic formulations also have been put forth (for a review, see Leeds and Morgenstern, 1995); however, because they are difficult to test scientifically, these models have not been widely accepted in the research community.

A related theory that is often used to explain substance abuse (most often in the popular press) is the idea of an *alcoholic personality*—a type of character organization that predisposes a person to use alcohol rather than some other strategy for coping with emotional and social stress. Some investigators have found that persons at high risk for developing alcoholism are significantly more impulsive and aggressive than those at low risk for abusing alcohol (e.g., Morey, Skinner, & Blashfield, 1984). However, results of studies regarding a predisposition to drinking or other drug use have been mixed, and most alcoholism and drug abuse investigators have largely dismissed the traditional notion of the existence of an alcoholic personality. However, there is strong evidence that certain disorders and substance abuse are linked. For example, roughly half of those individuals diagnosed with schizophrenia also are either alcohol or drug dependent (Kosten, 1997). The relationship between antisocial personality and substance use is also strong (Harford & Parker, 1994; Kwapil, 1996), although the direction of the causal link (if there is one at all) is unclear (Carroll, Ball, & Rounsaville, 1993). Some investigators have also suggested that there is a strong relationship between depressive disorders and alcoholism (Kranzler, Del Boca, & Rounsaville, 1997); this relationship may be stronger among women than among men (Moscato et al., 1997).

Although the nature of the relationship between substance abuse and other mental disorders is unclear, this relationship is certainly a very important consideration for treatment. Providing the best possible treatment for substance-abusing clients who have co-occurring psychological disorders requires (1) more cross-disciplinary collaboration; (2) greater integration of substance abuse and mental health treatments; and (3) more comprehensive training to treatment providers in the assessment of and intervention with common co-occurring conditions.

Behavior-Oriented Explanations

Early learning explanations for substance abuse were based on two fundamental assumptions: (1) substance use is a learned behavior, and (2) substance use is reinforced because it reduces anxiety and tension. Perhaps in the most widely known investigation, Masserman, Yum, Nicholson, and Lee (1944) induced an experimental neurosis in cats. After the cats were trained to eat food at a food box, they were given an aversive stimulus (e.g., an air blast to the face or an electric shock) whenever they approached the food. In turn, the cats stopped eating and displayed various symptoms, including anxiety, psychophysiological disturbances, and peculiar behaviors. When the cats were given alcohol, however, their symptoms were alleviated and they were able to eat again. It was concluded the anxiety-reducing properties of the alcohol are reinforcing and are thus responsible for maintaining drinking behavior.

In general, however, the tension reduction model of substance use is difficult to test, and research with alcoholic participants has produced conflicting findings. Paradoxically, in some individuals, prolonged drinking is associated with increased anxiety and depression (e.g., McNamee, Mello, & Mendelson, 1968). In addition, if tension reduction alone explained the development of substance use disorders, anyone who finds drugs or alcohol tension-reducing would be in danger of becoming a substance abuser. We would expect alcoholism and drug abuse to be far more common than it is because psychoactive substances tend to reduce tension for most people who use them.

Recently, several investigators have concluded that expectancies play a central role in the initiation and maintenance of alcohol and drug use disorders (Mendelson & Mello, 1995; Marlatt et al., 1998). Expectancies of the positive effects of substance use develop from repeated pairings of alcohol or other drugs with their reinforcing effects. Thus, expectancies can be conceptualized as conditioned cognitions, which can themselves be associated with positive experiences, or positive subjective responses, to alcohol or other drugs. Positive expectancies can facilitate more frequent use and thus contribute to the development of dependence (Rotgers, 1996). Expectancy theory has been supported by research. For example, expectancies of social benefit can influence adolescents' decisions to start drinking and predict their consumption of alcohol (Christiansen, Smith, Roehling, & Goldman, 1989).

Sociocultural Factors in the Etiology of Substance Abuse

What is ultimately labeled alcoholism or drug addiction varies based on the temporal, geographic, and religious context. In the mid-1800s, the average American consumed roughly three times more alcohol than he or she consumes today. Thus, what would be considered alcoholic drinking then would differ substantially from our present-day definition. During the 1600s and much of the 1700s, alcohol was not even seen as an addictive substance and habitual drunkenness was not, by and large, seen as problematic (Levine, 1978).

Additionally, the effect of cultural attitudes toward drinking is well illustrated by Mormons and Muslims, whose religious values prohibit the use of alcohol. As such, the prevalence of alcoholism using standard diagnostic systems is extremely low in these groups. Any use of alcohol is considered problem use by members of these religious groups. This is not dissimilar from many cultures that consider any use of "hard drugs" (e.g., heroin, cocaine) to be problematic use.

Although alcohol plays a significant role in Jewish family rituals (Lawson & Lawson, 1998), excessive consumption is viewed as inexcusable behavior. Thus, within Jewish culture, norms are for frequent drinking of alcohol, but in small amounts. These cultural norms serve to protect Jewish people from developing problems with alcohol (Glassner & Berg, 1980). In general, among cultures where drinking is integrated into religious rites and social customs and where self-control, sociability, and "knowing how to hold one's liquor" are important, alcoholism is rare (e.g., Blum & Blum, 1969).

In comparison, the prevalence of alcoholism is high in Europe and those countries that have been highly influenced by European culture (i.e., Argentina, Canada, Chile, Japan, the United States, and New Zealand). Although these countries make up less than 20% of the world's population, they consume 80% of the alcohol (Barry, 1982). In particular, the French have the highest rate of alcoholism in the world (i.e., roughly 15% of the population); France is also marked by the highest per capita alcohol consumption and the highest death rate from cirrhosis of the liver (Noble, 1979).

It is also generally accepted that Irish Catholics have a comparatively high rate of alcoholism (Lawson & Lawson, 1998). Vaillant (1983) found Irish subjects in his study on the longitudinal course of alcoholism were more likely to develop alcohol problems than were those from other ethnic groups. Interestingly, Irish subjects were also more likely to abstain as a way of controlling drinking. As noted by Vaillant (1983), "It is consistent with Irish culture to view alcohol in terms of black or white, good or evil, drunkenness or complete abstinence..." (p. 226). Viewing drinking behavior dichotomously, as either good or sinful, may serve to eliminate models of social drinking. In the Irish culture, there appears to be a shared norm that drinking is an acceptable method to deal with personal distress (Bales, 1980).

When comparing cultures that generally engage in moderate drinking and those where a disproportionately large percentage of its members appear to have drinking problems, certain differences consistently emerge (Maloff, Becker, Fonaroff, & Rodin, 1982; Peele & Brodsky, 1996). Cultural groups with comparatively low rates of alcoholism share four characteristics regarding alcohol use. First, drinking alcohol is accepted and is governed by social custom; thus, individuals in these cultures learn constructive norms for drinking. Second, differences between "good" and "bad" patterns of drinking are explicitly taught. Third, skills for drinking responsibly are taught. Fourth, drunkenness and misbehavior under the influence of alcohol are met with disapproval. In cultures where alcohol consumption is more problematic, agreed-on social standards for alcohol use have not been established, so drinkers must rely on an internal standard or their peer group's standards. Drinking is disapproved of by members of the culture and, moreover, abstinence is encouraged; thus, norms of social drinking are not available. Finally, people in these cultures expect that alcohol will overpower the individual's capacity for self-management.

Thus, social customs and cultural norms have an enormous influence on substance use. In addition, the behavior that is displayed while under the influence of psychoactive substances also appears to be affected by cultural factors. For example, Lindman and Lang (1994) studied alcohol-related behavior in eight countries and found participants generally believed aggression frequently would follow many alcoholic drinks. However, the authors found significant national differences in the expectancy that excessive alcohol consumption leads to aggression. These differences were unrelated to self-reported alcoholic beverage preference, frequency of drinking to intoxication, or rates of personal involvement in episodes of alcohol-related aggression. Thus, the expectation that drinking leads to aggression is determined to a significant extent by contextual factors and cultural traditions related to alcohol use. For example, studies using real and mock alcoholic beverages have shown that individuals who believe they have consumed alcohol begin to act more aggressively regardless of the beverage they actually consumed (Bushman, 1997).

Thus, how we learn to drink alcohol and consume other drugs is determined largely by the drinking and drug use we observe and by the people with whom we engage in these behaviors. There is a strong interdependence between the drinking and substance use patterns of those who associate with each other regularly in the same social circle. Indeed, in the broadest sense, each individual is linked, to a greater or lesser extent, to all other members of his or her culture. It is within this social fabric that patterns of belief and behaviors about alcohol and other drug use are modeled through a combination of example, reinforcements, punishments, encouragement, and the many other means that societies use to communicate norms, attitudes, and values (Heath, 1982).

Treatment

The conceptualizations of addiction have varied throughout history and, in turn, different treatment approaches have predominated based largely on the theoretical model holding sway. At present, the range of treatment possibilities is fairly extensive, varying greatly in terms of philosophy and general treatment goals. Thus, those seeking help now have a broad variety of choices in their attempts to resolve substance abuse problems.

Pharmacotherapy

Intuitively, a reasonable solution to drug or alcohol addiction is to identify molecules that oppose the actions of these substances. Much scientific effort has been put forth based on this idea and the results are manifested in the large variety of pharmacotherapies now available to treat addictive behavior. Medications are now used widely as primary or adjunctive interventions to treat alcoholism and other drug abuse. These include medications to reduce cravings to use drugs, to reduce the reinforcing effects of the psychoactive substances, to make taking drugs aversive, and to treat co-occurring mental disorders that may potentially underlie the drinking or drug use (Romach & Sellers, 1998).

Several pharmacotherapies have been developed for the treatment of alcoholism. Disulfiram

(Antabuse) produces a sensitivity to alcohol which results in a highly unpleasant reaction when the patient ingests even small amounts of alcohol. Disulfiram blocks the oxidation of alcohol at the acetaldehyde stage. Accumulation of acetaldehyde in the blood produces a complex of highly unpleasant reactions such as flushing, throbbing in head and neck, throbbing headache, respiratory difficulty, nausea, copious vomiting, sweating, thirst, chest pain, and so forth.

However, the effectiveness of disulfiram has been mixed, particularly if used as the sole intervention. Because it is generally self-administered, the alcoholic client can simply cease taking the disulfiram, wait for the drug to leave his or her system (roughly two weeks), and resume drinking. In fact, controlled clinical trials indicate that, unless its administration is supervised (e.g., by a family member or treatment provider), disulfiram does not significantly improve abstinence rates compared to placebo (e.g., Hughes & Cook, 1997). Conversely, disulfiram has been shown to be effective when another party is enlisted to observe the partner consume the drug (Berglund et al., 2003). In addition, some studies have shown that clients with concurrent alcohol and cocaine problems reduce their intake of both drugs when taking disulfiram (e.g., Carroll et al., 2004; Higgins, Budney, Bickel, Hughes, & Foerg, 1993).

Another medication used to treat alcoholism is naltrexone, which helps to reduce craving for alcohol by blocking the pleasure-producing effects of ethanol. O'Malley and colleagues (1996) have shown that use of naltrexone reduced alcohol intake and lowered the incentive to drink for alcoholics compared to those given a placebo. Volpicelli and colleagues (1992) have shown that, in general, use of naltrexone has a moderate effect in reducing drinking and, in particular, reducing relapse to heavy drinking by alcohol-dependent patients. Although some studies have found naltrexone to be ineffective (Krystal, Cramer, Krol, Kirk, & Rosenheck, 2001), the majority of trials to date support its efficacy and safety (see Bouza, Angeles, Munoz, & Amate, 2004).

Acamprosate has also demonstrated effectiveness in treating alcohol addiction. In a recent metaanalytic review of 17 studies, six-month continuous abstinence rates were significantly higher for those taking acamprosate than a placebo (Mann, Chabac, Lehert, Potgieter, & Henning, 2004). Although acamprosate appears to reduce craving for alcohol, the mechanism underlying acamprosate's action remains unknown, although some evidence suggests that it blocks the glutamate receptor (Harris et al., 2002).

Finally, antidepressant medications have been used to treat alcohol-dependent individuals with co-occurring depression. Mason, Kocsis, Ritvo, and Cutler (1996) reported that tricyclic antidepressants reduced depressive symptoms, and, to a certain extent, drinking behavior. Others have found that selective serotonin reuptake inhibitors, such as Prozac, reduce the frequency of drinking among alcohol-dependent patients with major depression (e.g., Cornelius et al., 1997).

Significant progress also has been made in the pharmacotherapy of opiate addiction. The most effective and commonly used pharmacotherapies for opiate addiction involve the use of agonists (i.e., drugs that occupy and activate the same receptors as opiates). The approach involves administration of drugs with similar action to those of the abuse drug, but with different pharmacotherapeutic effects (e.g., longer acting, less reinforcing, decreased euphoria).

Two widely used agonists, methadone and L-alpha-acetylmethadol (LAAM), have been approved in the United States to treat opiate dependence. Methadone and LAAM reduce the subjective effects of heroin and other opiates through cross-tolerance. Its usefulness in treatment lies in the fact that it satisfies the craving for heroin or other opiate-based illicit drugs, yet it is equally addictive physiologically. Thus, the advantage of methadone and LAAM over heroin is that methadone and LAAM are administered in a controlled environment as part of treatment. Methadone and LAAM are often combined with other psychosocial treatments to be fully effective (e.g., Fals-Stewart, O'Farrell, & Birchler, 2001; McLellan, Arndt, Metzger, Woody, & O'Brien, 1993). LAAM is similar to methadone, but is administered every three days rather than daily. The main difficulty with LAAM is that it takes time to achieve initial stabilization, thus increasing relapse risk (Jaffe, 1995).

Both LAAM and methadone also reduce such concomitant negative behaviors as crime and needle sharing. They also enable those dependent on opiates to function well enough to maintain employment and other social obligations. Many who are involved in LAAM or methadone maintenance programs are also able to function in their communities and their families. The quality and dosing of LAAM and methadone is strictly controlled via well-monitored government standards compared to that of street heroin and other illegal opiate-based substances. However, the practice of weaning drug abusers from heroin only to addict them to a government-controlled substance is considered by many to be morally and ethically questionable. Moreover, LAAM and methadone maintenance treatments are often difficult for participants because they may require secrecy from employers, friends, and family members due to concerns about the stigma associated with being maintained on these drugs. It also is difficult for participants to develop a drug-free social network—a task that many see as a crucial part of successful recovery.

Buprenorphine, an opioid agonist recently approved by the Food and Drug Administration (FDA) for the treatment of opiate addiction, blocks the subjective effects of heroin and other opiates and has been shown to reduce heroin use and increase compliance with psychosocial treatment (Strain et al., 1994). Compared to methadone, an advantage of buprenorphine is that it has less abuse potential and overdose risk. In addition, it can be obtained by prescription from a psychiatrist or primary care physician who has completed approved training rather than through attendance at a specialized methadone clinic (O'Malley & Kosten, 2006).

Naltrexone is another approved treatment for opiate addiction. However, naltrexone is a competitive antagonist; that is, it binds to receptors, but instead of activating these receptors as agonists do, it blocks them. Thus, naltrexone works by preventing receptors from being activated by heroin and other opiates. However, unlike with alcohol treatment, naltrexone has not been very successful in treating opiate dependence, largely because of poor patient compliance (O'Brien & McLellan, 1996). Naltrexone appears to be effective with individuals highly motivated to quit, particularly those in high-level professional positions (attorneys, physicians, etc.; Meandzija & Kosten, 1994), and as part of other psychosocial treatments that include patient monitoring (e.g., Fals-Stewart & O'Farrell, 2003).

Although over 50 different medications have been tried as treatments for cocaine and amphetamine addiction, none is presently FDA approved and none has been demonstrated to be effective (e.g., Mendelson & Mello, 1996). No medications are yet available to treat clients suffering from abuse of other drugs, such as cannabis, phencyclidine, and inhalants (Wilkins & Gorelick, 1994).

Psychosocial Interventions

Although medications are an important part of the treatment armamentarium of clinicians working with clients suffering from psychoactive substance use disorders, most experts agree that the mainstay of treatment for addiction is some form of peer support or psychosocial therapy. Alcoholics Anonymous (AA) and other 12-step peer support groups (e.g., Narcotics Anonymous, Cocaine Anonymous) are the largest and most widely known self-help support groups for treating persons with alcohol and other drug problems. These programs operate primarily as self-help counseling programs in which both person-to-person and group relationships are emphasized. Meetings consist mainly of discussions of participants' problems with alcohol and other drugs, with testimonials from those who have recovered. Participants are encouraged to "work" the 12 steps of AA, which include admitting powerlessness over alcohol, believing a higher power can restore sanity, and making a searching and fearless moral inventory of oneself (Alcoholics Anonymous, 1976). AA promotes total abstinence from alcohol and drugs. Although widely used, evidence for the effectiveness of AA and the related peer support groups is mostly anecdotal rather than based on well-controlled studies, largely because AA does not endorse participation in research. However, Fiorentine (1999) reported affiliation with AA after outpatient treatment was associated with better outcome than non-AA involvement.

A commonly used formal treatment approach derived from AA and the disease model is twelve-step facilitation (TSF). In TSF, substance dependence is viewed not as symptomatic of another illness, but as a primary problem with biological, emotional, and spiritual underpinnings and presenting features. Alcoholism and drug abuse are seen as progressive illnesses, marked largely by denial. The primary goals of treatment are to encourage clients to work through their denial and work the 12 steps of AA. This is typically done in the context of individual and group therapy and involves strong encouragement to attend 12-step self-help groups on a regular basis. Along with individual and group counseling, medical and religious services are also considered important parts of treatment because the disease of alcoholism and other drug use is viewed as affecting the biological and spiritual realms, as well as psychosocial functioning. Although there has been little research on the efficacy of treatments derived from the disease model, it is the most common form of treatment in the United States.

One of the strongest predictors of success of treatment for alcoholism has been motivation to change. A treatment intervention that has grown out of this observation is motivational enhancement therapy (MET), which attempts to get clients to assume responsibility for helping themselves and increasing their desire to change through a technique referred to as motivational interviewing (Gray & Zide, 2006). Motivational interviewing is defined as a directive, client-centered therapy style designed to elicit change by assisting clients with exploring and resolving ambivalence. Exploring ambivalence about change is the central goal of motivational interviewing; therapists are directive in pursuing this objective (Fisher & Harrison, 2000). Several studies have now demonstrated that MET is an effective treatment for alcoholism and other drug abuse (e.g., Vasilaki, Hosier, & Cox, 2006).

Cognitive and behavioral treatments have been among the most widely used and investigated psychosocial treatments for substance dependence. Cognitive-behavioral therapy (CBT) teaches clients coping skills to reduce or eliminate drinking or substance use. Techniques that characterize CBT include identifying high-risk situations for relapse, instruction and rehearsal strategies for coping with those situations, self-monitoring and behavioral analysis of substance use, strategies for recognizing and coping with cravings, coping with lapses, and instruction on problem solving (Carroll & Onken, 2005).

It has long been maintained that treatment for substance use disorders would be more effective if important patient characteristics were taken into account in selecting treatments (e.g., Mattson et al., 1994). This hypothesis was tested in the most comprehensive study of patient–treatment matching for alcoholism, Project MATCH. In this investigation, the efficacy of TSF, MET, and CBT were compared. Overall, the study involved 1,726 participants who were treated in 26 alcohol treatment programs in the United States by 80 different therapists. The investigators evaluated patients on 10 characteristics shown to predict treatment outcome (Project MATCH Group, 1997): diagnosis, cognitive impairment, conceptual ability level, gender, desire to seek meaning in life, motivation, psychiatric severity, severity of alcohol involvement, social support for drinking versus abstinence, and the presence of antisocial personality disorder. The results of the study were somewhat surprising to many in the treatment and research communities—matching the patients to particular treatments did not appear to influence treatment effectiveness. TSF, MET, and CBT were equally effective across multiple domains of functioning. One conclusion drawn from these findings was that clients receiving interventions in competently run programs will do equally well with any of the three treatments (Cooney, Babor, DiClemente, & Del Boca, 2003).

Relapse Prevention

Without question, one of the most vexing problems facing substance abuse treatment providers is relapse. For example, Polich, Armor, and Braiker (1981) found that, over a four-year posttreatment period, only 7% of their total sample (i.e., 922 males) abstained from alcohol during the entire follow-up interval. Abstinence was the goal of treatment, so 7% is a disturbingly low rate of success. Equally disturbing, 54% continued to show alcohol-related problems. Thus, increasing the durability of gains made during any primary intervention has become a major part of overall treatment planning. A cognitive-behavioral approach to preventing relapse that has been widely used is described in the classic work by Marlatt and Gordon (1985), in which relapse is viewed as a key behavior in substance abuse treatment. The behaviors underlying relapse are seen as indulgent behaviors based on an individual's learning history. When a person is abstinent, he or she gains a greater sense of personal control over the indulgent behaviors. The longer the person stays abstinent, the greater his or her sense of self-efficacy. In this model, relapse is a process that begins with a series of small, seemingly irrelevant decisions, even while maintaining abstinence. These decisions make relapse inevitable. For example, an alcoholic who buys beer to keep in his house to be prepared for visits by friends who drink has made a decision that may ultimately lead to relapse.

Another relapse behavior that is also often observed involves the abstinence violation effect, in which any use of drugs or alcohol is viewed by the substance abuser as complete failure. In many respects, this notion is advocated by many treatment programs and grows from an axiom often heard at AA meetings: "One drink, one drunk." Thus, when a substance user who has been abstinent for an extended period drinks or uses drugs, he or she may lose a certain degree of self-efficacy over the ability to control the addictive behavior. Because the goal of complete abstinence has been violated, the individual's self-efficacy for abstinence plummets, and he or she may therefore assume that a return to regular use of the drug is inevitable and then behave in a way that fulfills this prophecy.

As part of the relapse prevention program, clients are taught to recognize the apparently irrelevant decisions that serve as warning signals of the possibility of relapse. High-risk situations are identified and targeted, and the individuals learn to assess their own vulnerability to relapse. To counter the abstinence violation effect, clients are also taught not to become excessively discouraged if they do relapse. Clients are taught that relapse is part of the recovery process and are encouraged to develop plans to address relapse when it does happen.

Controlled Drinking: A Controversial Outcome

Although the goal of the treatments described thus far is abstinence from alcohol and other drugs, other interventions are based on the hypothesis that some individuals need not give up drinking or drug use, but can learn to use moderately (Lang & Kidorf, 1990; Sobell & Sobell, 1995). Several approaches have been used to teach controlled drinking, and some research has suggested that certain alcohol-dependent individuals can control their drinking. For example, self-control training techniques (e.g., behavioral self-control training; BSCT), in which the goal of treatment is to have alcohol-dependent clients reduce their drinking without necessarily abstaining from alcohol, has much appeal for some clients (Harris & Miller, 1990). A computer program is now available that provides instruction on self-control training and has been shown in a well-controlled study to reduce problem drinking (Hester & Delaney, 1997). In general, the best candidates for this type of intervention are young, motivated clients with no biomedical impairment from alcohol abuse (Thombs, 2006). As a result, most proponents of controlled drinking have concluded that controlled drinking may not be a viable intervention for most alcohol-dependent individuals.

In the United States, the vast majority of treatment professionals have rejected the idea that substance abusers can control their drinking or drug use and thus insist on a total abstinence approach. However, controlled drinking interventions are less controversial in other parts of the world (e.g., The Netherlands, Australia), and have been used effectively in other countries (e.g., Dawe & Richmond, 1997). The debate regarding controlled drinking as an acceptable treatment goal has raged for over 25 years. Some investigators have noted that controlled drinking can be efficacious (Heather, 1995; Kahler, 1995), whereas others have argued that alcohol-dependent individuals cannot maintain control over drinking and, as such, controlled drinking is not an acceptable treatment objective (Glatt, 1995).

Conclusion

Substance use disorders are among the most pressing and intransigent mental health problems facing society today. Concerns about abuse of alcohol, tobacco, and other psychoactive substances date as far back as Biblical times: "He shall separate himself from wine and strong drink, and shall drink no vinegar of wine, or vinegar of strong drink, neither shall he drink any liquor of grapes, nor eat moist grapes, or dried" (Num. 6:3). Despite such a long history, scientific scrutiny of these problems is fairly recent. However, an impressive body of knowledge about the epidemiology, etiology, neurobiology, and treatment of addictive behavior has accumulated. These and other aspects of addictive behavior continue to be the focus of extensive clinical and experimental research.

The study of substance use and misuse has been marked by extensive controversy and heated debate. The conflicts have been fueled by a fundamental disagreement among scientists, clinicians, social policy makers, and the public about whether to view addiction as a disease in need of medical treatment, as sin in need of punishment and containment, or as learned behaviors that can be modified by contingencies. The debate is not simply over semantics, but has implications for research, treatment, and social policy. For example, treatments that are shown to be effective in research settings are often ignored in the treatment community because the interventions are viewed as philosophically opposed to a conventional wisdom about what works best. Unfortunately, the conventional wisdom about what constitutes effective treatment is often not supported by the empirical research. Those who view alcoholism and other drug use as diseases are ethically and, in some instances, morally opposed to the use of controlled use treatments, which they view as irresponsible. Drug users fill our criminal justice system, while treatment providers lament the criminalization of these "diseases." Yet, proponents of legalization of drugs, who are in the minority, note that legalization will help contain many of the social ills associated with substance use. Others see such a stance as irresponsible and immoral because it would increase the exposure of those with a genetic propensity for addiction to the substances that would activate the addictive process. In turn, they believe that such policies would contribute to greater social decay. Because the emotional, legal, and economic stakes in the debate are so high, no end to the debate is in sight.

Discussion Questions

1. What are the advantages and limitations of viewing addictive behavior as diseases? As learned behaviors? As immoral and sinful?
2. Should harm reduction approaches to treatment (e.g., controlled drinking, methadone maintenance) be made more widely available in treatment programs?
3. What would be the advantages and disadvantages of legalizing certain illicit substances, such as cannabis?

Acknowledgment

This project was supported, in part, by grants from the National Institute on Drug Abuse (R01DA12189 and R01DA14402) and the Alpha Foundation.

References

Alcoholics Anonymous. (1976). *Living sober: Some methods A.A. members have used for not drinking.* New York: Alcoholics Anonymous World Services.

Allan, C. A., & Cooke, D. J. (1985). Stressful life events and alcohol misuse in women: A critical review. *Journal of Studies on Alcohol, 46,* 147–152.

Amaro, H., & Hardy-Fosta, C. (1995). Gender relations in addiction and recovery. *Journal of Psychoactive Drugs*, *27*, 325–333.

American Psychiatric Association. (2000). *Diagnostic and statistical manual of mental disorders* (4th ed., rev.). Washington, D.C.: Author.

Annis, H. M., & Graham, J. M. (1995). Profile types on the Inventory of Drinking Situations: Implications for relapse prevention counseling. *Psychology of Addictive Behaviors*, *9*, 176–182.

Bales, F. (1980). Cultural differences in roles of alcoholism. In D. Ward (Ed.), *Alcoholism: Introduction to theory and treatment*. Dubuque, IA: Kendall/Hunt.

Barry, H., III. (1982). Cultural variations in alcohol abuse. In I. Al-Issa (Ed.), *Culture and psychopathology* (pp. 309–338). Baltimore: University Park Press.

Beckman, L. J., & Amaro, H. (1986). Personal and social difficulties faced by women and men entering alcoholism treatment. *Journal of Studies on Alcohol*, *47*, 135–145.

Berglund, M., Thelander, S., Salaspuro, M., et al. (2003). Treatment of alcohol abuse: An evidence-based review. *Alcoholism: Clinical & Experimental Research*, *27*, 1645–1656.

Bierut, L. J., Dinwiddie, S. H., Begleiter, H., Crowe, R. R., Hesselbrock, V., Nurnberge, J. I., et al. (1998). Familial transmission of substance dependence: Alcohol, marijuana, cocaine, and habitual smoking. A report from the Collaborative Study on the Genetics of Alcoholism. *Archives of General Psychiatry*, *55*, 982–988.

Blum, R. H., & Blum, E. M. (1969). A cultural case study. In R. H. Blum (Ed.), *Drugs I: Society and drugs* (pp. 226–227). San Francisco: Jossey-Bass.

Blume, S. B. (1991). Sexuality and stigma: The alcoholic woman. *Alcohol Health and Research World*, *15*(2), 139–146.

Blume, S. B. (1997). Women and alcohol: Issues in social policy. In R. Wilsnack & S. Wilsnack (Eds.), *Gender and alcohol: Individual and social perspectives* (pp. 462–489). New Brunswick, NJ: Rutgers Center of Alcohol Studies.

Blume, S. B. (1998). Addictive disorders in women. In R. J. Frances & S. I. Miller (Eds.), *Clinical textbook of addictive disorders* (2nd ed., pp. 413–429). New York: Guilford.

Bouza, C., Angeles, M., Munoz, A., Amate, J. M. (2004). Efficacy and safety of naltrexone and acamprosate in the treatment of alcohol dependence: A systematic review. *Addiction*, *99*, 811–828.

Brady, K. T., & Randall, C. L. (1999). Gender differences in substance use disorders. *Psychiatric Clinics of North America*, *22*, 241–252.

Bushman, B. J. (1997). Effects of alcohol on human aggression: Validity of proposed explanations. In M. Galanter (Ed.), *Recent Developments in Alcoholism* (pp. 227–243). New York: Plenum.

Carlson, R. G. (2006). Ethnography and applied substance misuse research: Anthropologic and cross-cultural factors. In K. M. Carroll & W. R. Miller (Eds.), *Rethinking Substance Abuse: What the Science Shows, and What We Should Do About It* (pp. 201–222). New York: Guilford.

Carroll, K. M., Ball, S. A., & Rounsaville, B. J. (1993). A comparison of alternate systems for diagnosing antisocial personality disorder in cocaine abusers. *Journal of Nervous and Mental Diseases*, *181*, 436–443.

Carroll, K. M., Fenton, L. R., Ball, S. A., Nich, C., Frankforter, T. L., Shi, J., & Rounsaville, B. J. (2004). Efficacy of disulfiram and cognitive behavior therapy in cocaine-dependent outpatients: A randomized placebo-controlled trial. *Archives of General Psychiatry*, *61*, 264–272.

Carroll, K. M., & Miller, W. R. (2006). Defining and addressing the problem. In K. M. Carroll & W. R. Miller (Eds.), *Rethinking Substance Abuse: What the Science Shows, and What We Should Do About It* (pp. 3–7). New York: Guilford.

Carroll, K. M., & Onken, L. S. (2005). Behavioral therapies for drug abuse. *American Journal of Psychiatry*, *162*(8), 1452–1460.

Center on Addiction and Substance Abuse. (1996). *Substance abuse and American women*. New York: Author.

Chassin, L., Curran, P. J., Hussong, A. M., & Colder, C. R. (1996). The relation of parent alcoholism to adolescent substance use: A longitudinal follow-up. *Journal of Abnormal Psychology*, *105*(1), 70–80.

Chassin, L., Pillow, D. R., Curran, P. J., Molina, B. S., & Barrera, M. (1993). Relation of parental alcoholism in early adolescent substance use: A test of three mediating mechanisms. *Journal of Abnormal Psychology*, *102*, 3–19.

Christensen, H. B., & Bilenberg, N. (2000). Behavioural and emotional problems in children of alcoholic mothers and fathers. *European Journal of Child and Adolescent Psychiatry*, *9*, 219–226.

Christiansen, B. A., Smith, G. T., Roehling, P. V., & Goldman, M. S. (1989). Using alcohol expectancies to predict adolescent drinking behavior after one year. *Journal of Consulting and Clinical Psychology*, *57*, 93–99.

Compton, W. M., Thomas, Y. F., Conway, K. P., Colliver, J. D. (2005). Developments in the epidemiology of drug use and drug use disorders. *American Journal of Psychiatry*, *162*, 1494–1502.

Cooney, N. L., Babor, T. F., DiClemente, C. C., & Del Boca, F. K. (2003). Clinical and scientific implications of Project MATCH. In T. F. Babor and F. K. Del Boca (Eds.), *Treatment matching in alcoholism* (pp. 222–237). New York: Cambridge University Press.

Cornelius, J. R., Salloum, I. M., Ehler, J. G., Jarrett, P. J., Cornelius, M. D., Perel, J. M., et al. (1997). Fluoxetine in depressed alcoholics: A double-blind placebo-controlled trial. *Archives of General Psychiatry*, *54*, 700–705.

Dahlgren, L., & Willander, A. (1989). Are special treatment facilities for female alcoholics needed? A controlled 2-year follow-up study from a specialized female unit (EWA) versus a mixed male/female treatment facility. *Alcoholism: Clinical and Experimental Research*, *13*, 499–504.

Dawe, S., & Richmond, R. (1997). Controlled drinking as a treatment goal in Australian alcohol treatment agencies. *Journal of Substance Abuse*, *14*(1), 81–86.

Dawson, D. A., Grant, B. F., Stinson, F. S., & Chou, P. S. (2006). Estimating the effect of help-seeking on achieving recovery from alcohol dependence. *Addiction*, *101*, 824–834.

Deschenes, E. P., Anglin, M. D., & Speckart, G. (1991). Narcotics addiction: Related criminal careers, social and economic costs. *Journal of Drug Issues*, *21*, 383–411.

Fals-Stewart, W. (2003). The occurrence of interpartner violence on days of alcohol consumption: A longitudinal diary study. *Journal of Consulting and Clinical Psychology, 71*, 41–52.

Fals-Stewart, W., Golden, J., & Schumacher, J. A. (2003). Intimate partner violence and substance use: A longitudinal day-to-day examination. *Addictive Behaviors, 28*, 1555–1574.

Fals-Stewart, W., Kelley, M. L., Cooke, C. G., & Golden, J. (2002). Predictors of the psychosocial adjustment of children living in households in which fathers abuse drugs: The effects of postnatal social exposure. *Addictive Behaviors, 27*, 1–19.

Fals-Stewart, W., & O'Farrell, T. J. (2003). Behavioral family counseling and naltrexone for male opioid–dependent patients. *Journal of Consulting and Clinical Psychology, 71*, 432–442.

Fals-Stewart, W., O'Farrell, T. J., & Birchler, G. R. (2001). Behavioral couples therapy for male methadone maintenance patients: Effects on drug-using behavior and relationship adjustment. *Behavior Therapy, 32*, 391–411.

Fiorentine, R. (1999). After drug treatment: Are 12-step programs effective in maintaining abstinence? *American Journal of Drug and Alcohol Abuse, 25*(1), 93–116.

Fisher, G. L., & Harrison, T. C. (2000). *Substance abuse: Information for school counselors, social workers, therapists, and counselors* (2nd ed.). Boston: Allyn & Bacon.

Glassner, B., & Berg, B. (1980). How Jews avoid drinking problems. *American Sociological Review, 45*, 647–664.

Glatt, M. M. (1995). Controlled drinking after a third of a century. *Addiction, 90*, 1157–1160.

Goodwin, D. W., Schulsinger, F., Moller, N., Hermansen, L., Winokur, G., & Guze, S. (1974). Drinking problems in adopted and nonadopted sons of alcoholics. *Archives of General Psychiatry, 31*, 164–169.

Gough, J. B. (1881). *Sunlight and shadow*. Hartford, CT: Worthington.

Grant, B. F., & Dawson, D. A. (1999). Alcohol and drug use, abuse, and dependence: Classification, prevalence, and comorbidity. In B. S. McCrady & E. E. Epstein (Eds.), *Addiction: A comprehensive textbook* (pp. 9–29). New York: Oxford University Press.

Gray, S. W., & Zide, M. R. (2006). *Psychopathology: A competency-based treatment model for social workers*. Belmont, CA: Thomson.

Harford, T. C., & Parker, D. A. (1994). Antisocial behavior, family history, and alcohol dependence symptoms. *Alcoholism, 18*, 265–268.

Harris, K. B., & Miller, W. R. (1990). Behavioral self-control training for problem drinkers: Components of efficacy. *Psychology of Addictive Behaviors, 4*, 82–90.

Harris, B. R., Prendergast, M. A., Gibson, D. A., Rogers, D. T., Blanchard, J. A., Holley, R. C., et al. (2002). Acamprosate inhibits the binding and neurotoxic effects of trans-ACPD, suggesting a novel site of action at metabotropic glutamate receptors. *Alcoholism: Clinical and Experimental Research, 26*, 1779–1793.

Harwood, H. J., Hubbard, R. L., Collins, J. J., & Rachal, J. V. (1988). The costs of crime and the benefits of drug abuse treatment: A cost-benefit analysis using TOPS data. In C. G. Luekefeld & F. M. Tims (Eds.), *Compulsory treatment of drug abuse: Research and clinical practice* (Research Monograph Series 86, pp. 209–235). Rockville, MD: National Institute on Drug Abuse.

Hasin, D., Hatzenbuehler, M., & Waxman, R. (2006). Genetics of substance use disorders. In K. M. Carroll & W. R. Miller (Eds.), *Rethinking Substance Abuse: What the Science Shows, and What We Should Do About It* (pp. 61–80). New York: Guilford.

Haynes, V. D. (2002). Nevada blazes trail for legal marijuana. *Chicago Tribune* (August 9), *1*, 14.

Heath, D. B. (1982). Sociocultural variants in alcoholism. In E. M. Pattison & E. Kaufman (Eds.), *Encyclopedic handbook of alcoholism* (pp. 426–440). New York: Gardner.

Heather, J. (1995). The great controlled drinking consensus. Is it premature? *Addiction, 90*, 1160–1163.

Hester, R. K., & Delaney, H. D. (1997). Behavioral self-control program for Windows: Results of a controlled clinical trial. *Journal of Consulting and Clinical Psychology, 65*, 686–693.

Higgins, S. T., Budney, A. J., Bickel, W. K., Hughes, J. R., & Foerg, F. (1993). Disulfiram therapy in patients abusing cocaine and alcohol. *American Journal of Psychiatry, 150*, 675–676.

Hughes, J. C., & Cook, C. C. (1997). The efficacy of disulfiram: A review of outcome studies. *Addiction, 92*, 381–395.

Institute of Medicine. (1990). *Treating drug problems*. Washington, D.C.: National Academy Press.

Jaffe, J. H. (1995). Pharmacological treatment of opioid dependence: Current techniques and new findings. *Psychiatric Annals, 25*, 369–375.

Jellinek, E. M. (1952). Phases of alcohol addiction. *Quarterly Journal of Studies on Alcohol, 13*, 673–684.

Kahler, C. W. (1995). Current challenges and an old debate. *Addiction, 90*, 1169–1171.

Khantzian, E. J., Halliday, K. S., & McAuliffe, W. E. (1990). *Addiction and the vulnerable self: Modified dynamic group therapy for substance abusers*. New York: Guilford.

Kosten, T. R. (1997). Substance abuse and schizophrenia. *Schizophrenia Bulletin, 23*, 181–186.

Koob, G. F., & Bloom, F. E. (1988). Cellular and molecular mechanisms of drug dependence. *Science, 242*, 715–723.

Kranzler, H. R., Del Boca, F. K., & Rounsaville, B. (1997). Comorbid psychiatric diagnosis predicts three-year outcomes in alcoholics: A posttreatment natural history study. *Journal of Studies on Alcohol, 57*, 619–626.

Krystal, J. H., Cramer, J. A., Krol, W. F., Kirk, G. F., & Rosenheck, R. A. (2001). Naltrexone in the treatment of alcohol dependence. *The New England Journal of Medicine, 345*,1734–1739.

Kubicka, L., Csemy, L., & Kozeny, J. (1995). Prague women's drinking before and after the "velvet revolution" of 1989: A longitudinal study. *Addiction, 90*, 1471–1478.

Kuhn, T. (1962). *The structure of scientific revolutions*. Chicago: University of Chicago Press.

Kwapil, T. R. (1996). A longitudinal study of drug and alcohol use by psychosis-prone and impulsive-non-conforming individuals. *Journal of Abnormal Psychology, 105*(1), 114–123.

Lang, A. R., & Kidorf, M. (1990). Problem drinking: Cognitive behavioral strategies for self control. In M. E. Thase, B. A. Edelstein, & M. Hersen (Eds.), *Handbook of outpatient treatment of adults* (pp. 413–442). New York: Plenum.

Langenbucher, J. (1994). Offsets are not add-ons: The place of addictions treatment in American health care reform. *Journal of Substance Abuse, 6*, 117–122.

Lawson, A., & Lawson, G. (1998). *Alcoholism and the family: A guide to treatment and prevention* (2nd ed.). Gaithersburg, MD: Aspen.

Leeds, J., & Morgenstern, J. (1995). Psychoanalytic theories of substance abuse. In F. Rotgers, D. S. Keller, & J. Morgenstern (Eds.), *Treating substance abuse: Theory and technique* (pp. 68–83). New York: Guilford.

Levine, H. G. (1978). The discovery of addiction: Changing conceptions of habitual drunkenness in America. *Journal of Studies on Alcohol, 39*, 143–174.

Lindman, R. E., & Lang, A. R. (1994). The alcohol-aggression stereotype: A cross-cultural comparison of beliefs. *International Journal of Addictions, 29*, 1–13.

Maloff, D., Becker, H. S., Fonaroff, A., & Rodin, J. (1982). Informal social controls and their influence on substance use. In N. E. Zinberg & W. M. Harding (Eds.), *Control over intoxicant use* (pp. 53–76). New York: Human Sciences Press.

Mann, K., Chabac, S., Lehert, P., Potgieter, A., & Henning, S. (2004, December). *Acamprosate improves treatment outcome in alcoholics: A polled analysis of 11 randomized placebo controlled trials in 3338 patients.* Poster presented at the annual conference of the American College of Neuropsychopharmacology, Puerto Rico.

Marlatt, G. A., Baer, J. S., Kivahan, D. R., Dimeoff, L. A., Larimer, M. E., Quigley, L. A., Somers, J. M., & Williams, E. (1998). Screening and brief intervention for high-risk college student drinkers: Results from a 2-year follow up assessment. *Journal of Consulting and Clinical Psychology, 66*, 604–615.

Marlatt, G. A., & Gordon, J. R. (1985). *Relapse prevention: Maintenance strategies in the treatment of addictive behaviors.* New York: Guilford.

Marlatt, G. A., Tucker, J. A., Donovan, D. M., & Vuchinich, R. E. (1997). Help-seeking by substance abusers: The role of harm reduction and behavioral-economic approaches to facilitate treatment entry and retention. In L. S. Onken, J. D. Blaine, & J. J. Boren (Eds.), *Beyond the therapeutic alliance: Keeping the drug-dependent individual in treatment* (pp. 44–84). Rockville, MD: National Institute on Drug Abuse.

Mason, B. J., Kocsis, J. H., Ritvo, E. C., & Cutler, R. B. (1996). A double-blind placebo-controlled trial of desipramine in primary alcoholics stratified on the presence or absence of major depression. *Journal of the American Medical Association, 275*, 1–7.

Masserman, J., Yum, K., Nicholson, J., & Lee, S. (1944). Neurosis and alcohol: An experimental study. *American Journal of Psychiatry, 101*, 389–395.

Mattson, M. E., Allen, J. P., Longabaugh, R., Nickless, C. J., Connors, G. J., & Kadden, R. M. (1994). A chronological review of empirical studies matching alcoholic clients to treatment. *Journal of Studies on Alcohol, 12*, 16–29.

McClelland, G. M., & Teplin, L. A. (2001). Alcohol intoxication and violent crime: Implications for public health policy. *American Journal for Addictions, 10* (Suppl.), 70–85.

McCrady, B. S., & Epstein, E. E. (1999). Introduction. In B. S. McCrady & E. E. Epstein (Eds.), *Addiction: A comprehensive textbook* (pp. 3–8). New York: Oxford University Press.

McLellan, A. T., Arndt, I. O., Metzger, D. S., Woody, G. E., & O'Brien, C. P. (1993). The effects of psycho-social services in substance abuse treatment. *Journal of the American Medical Association, 260*, 1953–1959.

McNamee, H. B., Mello, N. K., & Mendelson, J. H. (1968). Experimental analysis of drinking patterns of alcoholics: Concurrent psychiatric observations. *American Journal of Psychiatry, 124*, 1063–1069.

Meandzija, B., & Kosten, T. R. (1994). Pharmacologic therapies for opioid addiction. In N. S. Miller (Ed.), *Principles of addiction medicine* (sect. 12, chap. 4, pp. 1–5). Chevy Chase, MD: American Society of Addiction Medicine.

Mendelson, J. H., & Mello, N. K. (1995). Alcohol, sex, and aggression. In J. A. Inciardi & K. McElrath (Eds.), *The American Drug Scene: An Anthology* (pp. 331–346). Los Angeles: Roxbury.

Mendelson, J. H., & Mello, N. K. (1996). Management of cocaine abuse and dependence. *New England Journal of Medicine, 334*, 965–972.

Merikangas, K. R., Stolar, M., Stevens, D. E., Goulet, J., Preisig, M. A., Fenton, B., et al. (1998). Familial transmission of substance use disorders. *Archives of General Psychiatry, 55*, 973–979.

Miller, N. S. (1995). *Addiction psychiatry: Current diagnosis and treatment.* New York: Wiley.

Mokdad, A. H., Marks, J. S., Stroup, D. S., & Gerberding, G. L. (2004). Actual causes of death in the United States, 2000. *Journal of the American Medical Association, 291*, 1238–1245.

Morey, L. C., Skinner, H. A., & Blashfield, R. K. (1984). A typology of alcohol abusers: Correlates and implications. *Journal of Abnormal Psychology, 93*, 403–417.

Moscato, B. S., Russell, M., Zielezny, M., Bromet, E., Egri, G., Mudar, P., & Marshall, J. R. (1997). Gender differences in the relation between depressive symptoms and alcohol problems: A longitudinal perspective. *American Journal of Epidemiology, 146*, 966–974.

National Institute on Alcohol Abuse and Alcoholism. (1993). Genetic and other risk factors for alcoholism. In *Alcohol and Health: Eighth Special Report to the U.S. Congress* (NIH Publication No. 94-3699, pp. 61–83). Washington, D.C.: National Institute of Health.

Nelson-Zlupko, L., Dore, M. M., Kauffman, E., & Kaltenbach, K. (1996). Women in recovery: Their perceptions of treatment effectiveness. *Journal of Substance Abuse Treatment, 13*, 51–59.

Noble, E. P. (1979). *Alcohol and health: Technical support document.* Third special report to the U.S. Congress (DHEW Publication No. ADM 79-832). Washington, D.C.: U.S. Government Printing Office.

O'Brien, C. P., & McLellan, A. T. (1996). Myths about the treatment of addiction. *Lancet, 347*, 237–240.

O'Malley, S. S., Jaffe, A. J., Chang, G., Rode, S., Schottenfeld, R., Meyer, R. E., et al. (1996). Six month follow-up of naltrexone and psychotherapy for alcohol dependence. *Archives of General Psychiatry, 53*, 217–224.

O'Malley, S. S., & Kosten, T. R. (2006). Pharmacotherapy of addictive disorders. In K. M. Carroll & W. R. Miller (Eds.), *Rethinking substance abuse: What the science shows, and what we should do about it* (pp. 240–256). New York: Guilford.

Peele, S. (1996). Assumptions about drugs and the marketing of drug policies. In W. K. Bickel & R. J. DeGrandpre (Eds.), *Drug policy and human nature: Psychological perspectives on the prevention, management, and treatment of illicit drug abuse* (pp. 199–220). New York: Plenum.

Peele, S., & Brodsky, A. (1996). The antidote to alcohol abuse: Sensible drinking messages. In S. Peele (Ed.), *Wine in context: Nutrition, physiology, and policy* (pp. 66–70). Davis, CA: American Society for Enology and Viticulture.

Peele, S., Brodsky, A., & Arnold, M. (1991). *The truth about addiction and recovery.* New York: Simon & Schuster.

Plotnick, R. D. (1994). Applying benefit-cost to substance use prevention programs. *International Journal of the Addictions, 29,* 339–359.

Polich, J. M., Armor, D. J., & Braiker, H. B. (1981). *The course of alcoholism: Four years after treatment.* New York: Wiley Interscience.

Project MATCH Group. (1997). Project MATCH: Rationale and methods for a multisite clinical trial matching patients to alcoholism treatment. *Alcoholism: Clinical and Experimental Research, 17,* 1130–1145.

Ramlow, B. E., White, A. L., Watson, M. A., & Luekefeld, C. G. (1997). The needs of women with substance use problems: An expanded vision for treatment. *Substance Use and Misuse, 32,* 1395–1404.

Richardson, D., & Campbell, J. (1982). The effect of alcohol on attributions of blame for rape. *Personality and Social Psychology Bulletin, 8,* 468–476.

Roberts, A. C., & Nishimoto, R. H. (1996). Predicting treatment retention of women dependent on cocaine. *American Journal of Drug and Alcohol Abuse, 22,* 313–333.

Romach, M. K., & Sellers, E. M. (1998). Alcohol dependency: Women, biology, and pharmacotherapy. In E. F. McCance-Katz & T. R. Kosten (Eds.), *New treatments for chemical addictions* (pp. 35–73). Washington, D.C.: American Psychiatric Press.

Rotgers, F. (1996). Behavioral theory of substance abuse treatment: Bringing science to bear on practice. In F. Rotgers & J. Morgenstern (Eds.), *Treating substance abuse: Theory and technique* (pp. 174–201). New York: Guilford.

Sandbak, T., Murison, R., Sarviharju, M., & Hyytiae, P. (1998). Defensive burying and stress gastric erosions in alcohol-preferring AA and alcohol-avoiding ANA rats. *Alcoholism: Clinical and Experimental Research, 22,* 2050–2054.

Schober, R., & Annis, H. M. (1996). Barriers to help-seeking for change in drinking: A gender-focused review of the literature. *Addictive Behaviors, 21,* 81–92.

Schuckit, M. A. (1987). Biological vulnerability to alcoholism. *Journal of Consulting and Clinical Psychology, 55,* 301–310.

Selzer, M. L. (1971). The Michigan Alcoholism Screening Test: The quest for a new diagnostic instrument. *American Journal of Psychiatry, 127,* 1653–1658.

Shaffer, H. J., & Neuhaus, C., Jr. (1985). Testing hypotheses: An approach for the assessment of addictive behaviors. In H. B. Milkman & H. J. Shaffer (Eds.), *The addictions: Multidisciplinary perspectives and treatments* (pp. 87–103). Lexington, MA: Lexington Books.

Sobell, M. B., & Sobell, L. C. (1995). Controlled drinking after 25 years: How important was the great debate? *Addiction, 90,* 1149–1153.

Stormo, K. J., Lang, A. R., & Stritzke, W. G. (1997). Attributions about acquaintance rape: The role of alcohol and individual differences. *Journal of Applied Social Psychology, 279,* 1559–1816.

Strain, E. C., Stitzer, M. L., Liebson, I. A., & Bigelow, G. E. (1994). Comparison of buprenorphine and methadone in the treatment of opioid dependence. *American Journal of Psychiatry, 151,* 1025–1030.

Straussner, S. L. A., & Zelvin, E. (1997). *Gender and addiction: Men and women in treatment.* Northvale, NJ: Jason Aronson.

Thombs, D. L. (2006). *Introduction to addictive behavior* (3rd ed.). New York: Guilford.

Uchtenhagen, A. (2004). Substance use problems in developing countries. *Bulletin of the World Health Organization, 82,* 641.

U.S. Office of Applied Studies. (2003). *Results from the 2002 national survey of drug use and health: National findings.* Rockville, MD: Substance Abuse Services and Mental Health Services Administration.

U.S. Office of National Drug Control Policy. (2004). *The economic costs of drug abuse in the United States: 1992–2002.* Washington, D.C.: Executive Office of the President.

U.S. Substance Abuse and Mental Health Services Administration. (2005). *Overview of findings from the 2004 national survey on drug use and health* (Office of Applied Studies, NSDUH Series H-27, DHHS Publication No. SMA 05-4061). Rockville, MD.

Vaillant, G. E. (1983). *The natural history of alcoholism.* Cambridge, MA: Harvard University Press.

Vaillant, G. E. (1990). We should retain the disease concept of alcoholism. *Harvard Medical School Mental Health Letter, 6,* 4–6.

Vaillant, G. E. (1995). *The natural history of alcoholism revisited.* Cambridge, MA: Harvard University Press.

Vasilaki, E. I., Hosier, S. G., & Cox, W. M. (2006). The efficacy of motivational interviewing as a brief intervention for excessive drinking: A meta-analytic review. *Alcohol and Alcoholism, 41*(3), 332–335.

Volkow, N. D., Fowler, J. S., & Wang, G. J. (2003). The addicted human brain: Insights from imaging studies. *Journal of Clinical Investigation, 111,* 1444–1451.

Volpicelli, J. R., Alterman, A. I., Hayashida, M., & O'Brien, C. P. (1992). Naltrexone in the treatment of alcohol dependence. *Archives of General Psychiatry, 49,* 876–880.

Warner, L. A., Kessler, R. C., Hughes, M., Anthony, J. C., & Nelson, C. B. (1995). Prevalence and correlates of drug use and dependence in the United States. *Archives of General Psychiatry, 52,* 219–228.

Wightman, R. M., & Robinson, D. L. (2002). Transient changes in mesolimbic dopamine and their association with 'reward.' *Journal of Neurochemistry, 82,* 721–735.

Wilkins, J. N., & Gorelick, D. A. (1994). Pharmacologic therapies for other drugs and multiple drug addiction. In N. S. Miller (Ed.), *Principles of addiction medicine* (sect. 12, chap. 6, pp. 1–6). Chevy Chase, MD: American Society of Addiction Medicine.

Winfield, I., George, L. K., Swartz, M., & Blazer, D. G. (1990). Sexual assault and psychiatric disorders among a community sample of women. *American Journal of Psychiatry, 147,* 335–341.

Wise, R. A. (2002). Brain reward circuitry: Insights from unsensed incentives. *Neuron, 36,* 229–240.

World Health Organization. (1992). *ICD-10 classification of mental and behavioral disorders: Clinical descriptions and diagnostic guidelines.* Geneva: Author.

Wurmser, L. (1984). The role of superego conflicts in substance abuse and their treatment. *International Journal of Psychoanalytic Psychotherapy, 10,* 227–258.

16
Externalizing Disorders of Childhood

Paul J. Frick and Eva R. Kimonis

Introduction

There is clear evidence that a significant number of children and adolescents have severe and impairing emotional or behavioral problems (Frick & Silverthorn, 2001). Further, research has indicated that the form that these problems take can largely be conceptualized along two broad dimensions. One dimension, which is the focus of the current chapter, has been labeled as undercontrolled or externalizing and includes various acting out, disruptive, delinquent, hyperactive, and aggressive behaviors. The second dimension has been labeled as overcontrolled or internalizing and includes such behaviors as social withdrawal, anxiety, and depression (see Ollendick, et al., this volume). This basic distinction between internalizing and externalizing problems has been well supported by a number of factor analytic studies (Achenbach, 1995; Achenbach & Edelbrock, 1978; Quay, 1986).

Within the externalizing dimension, there are two major categories of behavior: (1) problems of attention, impulsivity, and hyperactivity associated with the diagnostic category of attention deficit hyperactivity disorder (ADHD) and (2) conduct problems and aggressive behavior associated with the diagnostic categories of oppositional defiant disorder (ODD) and conduct disorders (CD). Research indicates that these two problem domains can be separated in factor analyses and that they have a number of different correlates (Hinshaw, 1987; Lilienfeld & Waldman, 1990; Waschbusch, 2002). For example, ADHD seems to be more specifically associated with parental problems of attention and impulsivity, poor academic achievement, and problems in executive functioning, whereas conduct problems appear to be more specifically associated with parental criminality/antisocial behavior, socioeconomic disadvantage, and dysfunctional family backgrounds. However, twin research suggests that shared environmental risk factors, such as parent–child conflict, may act as a common vulnerability for the development of both ADHD and conduct problems (Burt, Krueger, McGue, & Iacono, 2003). The importance of these correlates for understanding the two types of externalizing disorders is discussed in later sections of this chapter.

While research supports distinguishing between these two forms of externalizing disorders, it is also important to note that they overlap considerably. For example, between 40 and 60% of children with ADHD have a co-occurring conduct problem diagnosis (Hinshaw, 1987; Waschbusch, 2002) and between 65 and 90% of children with either ODD or CD have a co-occurring ADHD diagnosis (Abikoff & Klein, 1992). This overlap is important in understanding research in this area because many studies have failed to control for this comorbidity when studying external-izing disorders. This failure makes it unclear whether the correlates documented in research are due to one or the other types of externalizing disorders or both (Lilienfeld & Waldman, 1990). Further, this comorbidity predicts a more chronic course for both ADHD and conduct disorders (Barkley, Fischer, Smallish, & Fletcher, 2002; Frick & Loney, 1999) and can influence the type of treatment that may be most effective for children with these disorders (Abikoff & Klein, 1992; Arnold et al., 2004; Frick, 1998; 2001; Jensen, Hinshaw et al., 2001). Therefore, although the following sections provide somewhat separate reviews of the two types of externalizing disorders, it is important to recognize that many children show both patterns of behavior. In addition, understanding this overlap can be important for effectively treating children with disruptive behavior problems.

Attention Deficit Hyperactivity Disorder

In the psychiatric literature, there has been a form of childhood psychopathology recognized since the mid-19th century that has, as its primary feature, extreme and impairing levels of motor activity (Barkley, 1997). However, there has been great debate regarding the primary cause of this condition and the best method for diagnosing it in children. This debate is reflected in numerous changes in its name (e.g., minimal brain dysfunction, hyperactive child syndrome, attention deficit disorder) and in the diagnostic criteria used to classify children with the disorder over the years (see Frick & Lahey, 1991, for a review).

Definition and Description

In the most recent revision of the *Diagnostic and Statistical Manual of Mental Disorders* (*DSM-IV-TR*; American Psychiatric Association, 2000), ADHD has two core symptom dimensions—an inattention-disorganization cluster (e.g. difficulty sustaining attention, does not listen when spoken to directly, easily distracted by extraneous stimuli) and a hyperactivity-impulsivity cluster (e.g. fidgets, runs or climbs excessively, talks excessively, difficulty awaiting turn, interrupts others). Dividing symptoms into these two dimensions was based on a substantial number of factor analyses conducted in both clinic-referred and community samples (Lahey, Carlson, & Frick, 1997).

Diagnosis As with all childhood disorders, some level of the above symptoms is normal in childhood. Therefore, the *DSM-IV-TR* specifies

- the severity (i.e., six or more symptoms),
- the duration (i.e., persists for six months and evident before age 7),
- the pervasiveness (i.e., impairment present in two or more settings), and
- the degree of impairment (i.e., clear evidence of impaired social, academic, or occupational functioning)

that is necessary for a diagnosis of ADHD.

Subtypes An important aspect of most recent definitions of ADHD is the specification of several distinct subtypes of the disorder. The most common subtype is the ADHD-combined type (ADHD-CT) in which children show significant problems in both inattention-disorganization and impulsiv-ity-hyperactivity (American Psychiatric Association, 2000). This subtype accounts for about 55% of all children referred to clinics with ADHD (Lahey, Applegate et al., 1994) and much of the research on ADHD has focused on this group of children (Lahey et al., 1997).

A second group of children with ADHD have the predominantly inattentive type (ADHD-PI;

American Psychiatric Association, 2000). This group of children constitutes approximately 27% of children with ADHD who are referred to clinics for treatment and, as the name implies, this subtype includes children who have problems with inattention-disorganization, but who do not show problems of overactivity (Lahey et al., 1994). In fact, rather than being hyperactive, many of these children are described as being hypoactive, drowsy, and sluggish (Carlson & Mann, 2003; McBurnett, Pfiffner, & Frick, 2001). The designation of this subtype was first made in the third edition of the *Diagnostic and Statistical Manual of Mental Disorders* (1980) under the category of attention deficit disorder without hyperactivity. This diagnostic category has prompted debate for a number of reasons. First, in many past definitions of the disorder, hyperactivity was considered a core and defining feature of the diagnostic category (Stewart, Pitts, Craig, & Dieruf, 1966). Inclusion of this subtype explicitly acknowledges that the presence of increased motor activity is neither necessary nor sufficient for the disorder and supports research on the importance of attentional deficits in defining the disorder (Carlson & Mann, 2000; Frick & Lahey, 1991). Second, in addition to the defining difference in the amount of motor activity, children with ADHD-PI are less likely to show conduct problems and aggression, they are less likely to be rejected by peers, they show higher rates of anxiety and depression, and they tend to respond optimally to lower doses of stimulant medication (Barkley, DuPaul, & McMurray, 1991; Carlson & Mann, 2000; Frick & Lahey, 1991; Lahey et al., 1997). Also, their cognitive and attentional difficulties differ from those of other children with ADHD and appear to be characterized by slower retrieval and information processing (as opposed to fast and impulsive processing of information) and low levels of alertness (Carlson & Mann, 2003; Hartman, Willcutt, Rhee, & Pennington, 2004; McBurnett et al., 2001). These differences have led some authors to suggest that this form of ADHD may be a discrete disorder characterized by a different etiology from other forms of ADHD, rather than a subtype of the same disorder (Barkley, 1997, 2003; Milich, Balentine, & Lynam, 2001). Third, because problems of inattention typically are manifested later in development, when demands for sustained attention increase (Loeber, Green, Lahey, Christ, & Frick, 1992), the appropriateness of the diagnostic criterion that symptoms must cause impairment prior to age 7 has been questioned for this subtype. For example, in a sample of clinic-referred youth ages 4 to 17 who were diagnosed with ADHD, 82% who met symptom severity criteria for the ADHD-CT had an onset of impairment prior to age 7, whereas only 57% with ADHD-PI met this age of onset criterion (Applegate et al., 1997). Importantly, in comparing children with ADHD-PI who did and did not meet the age-of-onset criterion, but who met all other criteria for the disorder, there were no differences in their current level of impairment as documented by teachers, parents, and clinicians.

The third and least common of the ADHD subtypes recognized by the *DSM-IV-TR* is the predominantly hyperactive-impulsive type (ADHD-PHI). Children in this category show problems of hyperactivity-impulsivity without problems of inattention-disorganization. This subgroup accounts for about 18% of children diagnosed with ADHD (Lahey, Applegate et al., 1994). Barkley (1997) has proposed that the predominantly hyperactive subtype of ADHD is best considered a developmental precursor to the ADHD-CT subtype, with children in this category not yet experiencing demands for sustained attention. In support of this hypothesis, a study of 276 children diagnosed with ADHD found that the average age for the ADHD-PHI subgroup was 5.68 years, compared to 8.52 years for the ADHD-CT ($n = 152$) and 9.80 years for the ADHD-PI type ($n = 74$) (Lahey, Applegate, et al., 1994). Problems of inattention may become more evident with the increasing demands of school. As a result, ADHD-PHI youth may shift to the combined type following school entry. In general, there seems to be substantial instability of ADHD subtype membership over time (Lahey, Pelham, Loney, Lee, & Wilcutt, 2005).

Developmental Course By definition, ADHD symptoms emerge early in development (before age 7; American Psychiatric Association, 2000). Many studies have documented symptoms of overactivity emerging as early as ages 3 to 4 years of age (Loeber et al., 1992). Although many preschoolers with these symptoms outgrow their problems as they enter school, about 50% of the most hyperactive and disruptive preschoolers will be diagnosed with ADHD at age 6 (Campbell, Ewing, Breaux, & Szumowski, 1986). Until recently, there was a general view that ADHD was limited to childhood and that children with ADHD "outgrew" the disorder by adolescence or, at least, by adulthood (Lambert, 1988). However, there are now several prospective longitudinal studies that have followed children diagnosed with ADHD into adulthood and have called into question this view of a developmentally limited disorder (Barkley et al., 2002).

Importantly, estimates of the stability of ADHD are somewhat dependent on the method and criteria used to assess ADHD in childhood and the method and criteria used to assess later adult adjustment (Barkley et al., 2002). However, there are several general statements that can be made about the developmental course of the disorder. First, there are variations in the manifestation of ADHD symptoms over the life span that need to be considered in estimating the stability of the disorder. For example, the symptoms of inattention-disorganization seem to be much more stable in adolescence than the hyperactive-impulsive symptoms (Hart et al., 1995). However, this difference in stability may be partly due to the fact that the hyperactive-impulsive symptoms show age variations in their manifestations, such as being manifested in driving problems in adolescents (Barkley, Guevremont, Anastopoulos, DuPaul, & Shelton, 1993) or relationship instability in adults (Barkley et al., 2002). There is also evidence for greater stability of the disorder for those with ADHD-CT (Lahey et al., 2005). Second, when the core symptoms of ADHD are assessed first in childhood and then again in adolescence and young adulthood, between 50 and 70% of children with ADHD have clinically significant levels of symptoms in adolescence and between 30 and 45% have clinically significant levels of symptoms in adulthood (Barkley et al., 2002; Mannuzza, Klein, Bessler, Malloy, & LaPadula, 1998; Rasmussen & Gillberg, 2001; Weiss & Hechtman, 1993). Third, although many children with ADHD do not maintain all of the symptoms of ADHD necessary to meet diagnostic criteria as adults, a large proportion still show significant impairments in their social, occupational, or psychological functioning as adults, even if the core symptoms of the disorder have remitted (Barkley et al., 2002).

Co-Occurring Problems While the diagnosis of ADHD focuses on the two main symptom domains of inattention-disorganization and hyperactivity-impulsivity, research has consistently documented that children with ADHD often have a number of co-occurring problems in adjustment, in addition to the primary symptoms. Importantly, these co-occurring or "co-morbid" conditions can have a great impact on the most appropriate treatment for children with ADHD (Abikoff & Klein, 1992; Arnold et al., 2004; Jensen et al., 2001) and the presence of co-occurring problems may be a strong predictor of later adjustment (Weiss & Hechtman, 1993).

As noted above, it is well-established that many children with ADHD (between 40 and 60%) have a comorbid conduct disorder (Hinshaw, 1987; Lilienfeld & Waldman, 1990; Waschbusch, 2002). Importantly, the presence of significant conduct problems may be one of the strongest predictors of poor adult outcome for children diagnosed with ADHD, especially in terms of risk for delinquency and substance abuse (Weiss & Hechtman, 1993). Additionally, about 30 to 50% of children with ADHD have significant academic problems, such as learning disabilities or early school dropout (Frick, Kamphaus, et al., 1991; Jensen, Martin, & Cantwell, 1997; Spira & Fischel, 2005; Weiss & Hechtman, 1993). A similar percentage of children with ADHD (30 to 50%) have comorbid emotional disorders, such as an anxiety or depressive disorder (Jensen et al., 1997; Kitchens, Rosen, & Braaten, 1999; Schatz & Rostain, 2006). Based on these figures, it is evident that comorbid diagnoses are the rule, rather than the exception, for children diagnosed with ADHD.

The families of ADHD children differ from the families of non-ADHD children in several ways. In a review of studies examining family functioning, Johnston and Mash (2001) found that the presence of an ADHD child in the home is associated with a number of difficulties, including poorer parenting practices, more parental negative and controlling behaviors, more parental stress, and higher levels of parental psychopathology. It is unclear whether these familial factors precede the child's development of ADHD or whether the child's ADHD symptoms lead to a change in the family environment. For example, the stress and difficulty involved in parenting a child with ADHD may make it more likely that parents of children with ADHD will engage in less effective parenting strategies (e.g., more negative and controlling parenting) and will be more susceptible to depression (Barkley & Cunningham, 1979; Fischer, 1990). Further, familial factors may play a greater role in maintaining the disorder (Johnston & Mash, 2001) or in predicting the development of some of the co-occurring conditions often found in children with ADHD (e.g., conduct problems; Frick, 1998) than in causing the primary symptoms of the disorder.

Cultural and Gender Issues

Since the late 1960s, research on ADHD has been dominated by American researchers, leading to the impression that ADHD is largely an American disorder. To test this assumption, Faraone, Sergeant, Gillberg, and Biederman (2003) conducted a review of studies reporting on the prevalence of ADHD across countries and cultures. Using only studies that employed *DSM-III, DSM-III-R,* or *DSM-IV* criteria to establish disorder, they concluded that the range in prevalence rates are roughly equivalent in both U.S. and non-U.S. studies. Also, the highest prevalence rates are reported when using *DSM-IV* criteria (Faraone et al., 2003). Some studies conducted outside of the United States have found divergent prevalence rates (Fergusson, Horwood, & Lynskey, 1993; Gomez-Beneyto, Bonet, Catala, & Puche, 1994; Landgren, Pettersson, Kjellman, & Gillberg, 1996; Verhulst, Van der Ende, Ferdinand, & Kasius, 1997; Wang, Chong, & Chou, 1993) and these rates may reflect differences in (1) the diagnostic criteria used to establish disorder; (2) the informants used to assess symptoms (e.g., parents vs. teachers) that could reflect differences in cultural expectations for children's behavior by adults; or (3) the population surveyed (e.g., proportion of males vs. females, age range), rather than true variations in the level and severity of the child's behavior. Importantly, within the United States, studies have not found consistent differences in the prevalence of ADHD across cultural groups (Barkley, 1996).

One consistent finding across countries and cultures is that ADHD shows some of the strongest and most consistent evidence for male predominance of any form of childhood psychopathology, with male-to-female ratios ranging from 2:1 to 6:1 in community samples to 4:1 to 9:1 in clinic referred samples (Barkley, 1996). An important caveat to this overall male predominance is that there is emerging evidence that the male-to-female ratio may not be similar across all types of ADHD. Although boys tend to be more likely to have all forms of ADHD, the male:female ratio seems to be lower for ADHD-PI subtype (Biederman et al., 2002; Lahey et al., 1994). Despite these differences in prevalence rates, when girls do show ADHD, the types and severity of symptoms and the co-occurring problems in adjustment appear to be quite similar to boys with ADHD (Gaub & Carlson, 1997; Gershon, 2002; Silverthorn, Frick, Kuper, & Ott, 1996). The most consistent differences that emerge are that girls tend to show less severe hyperactivity and fewer conduct problems than do boys with ADHD, but greater intellectual impairments, especially deficits in verbal intelligence (e.g., Rucklidge & Tannock, 2001; Silverthorn et al., 1996). In contrast, boys with ADHD tend to show a stronger family history of ADHD, especially a paternal history of ADHD (Silverthorn et al., 1996).

Etiology

Research on the etiology of ADHD has three main foci. The first is defining the core cognitive deficit that can lead to the primary and secondary characteristics of children with ADHD. The second is investigating the neurological substrate to this core deficit. The third is trying to understand the causes of this neurological substrate. This research has made it increasingly clear that the core symptoms of

ADHD are related to a neurological deficit and that, as noted previously, the child's psychosocial context (e.g., family environment, quality of educational services) largely influences the severity and level of impairment associated with the child's symptoms and the development of co-occurring problems (e.g., conduct problems). However, there are two important considerations in this general conceptualization of ADHD. First, because the diagnostic criteria of ADHD are solely based on behavioral criteria, documentation of a cognitive or neurological deficit is not necessary for the diagnosis. Second, although the child's psychosocial context may not be critical in many etiological theories, intervening in the child's social context (e.g., improving parenting skills, improving the child's educational environment) is nonetheless a critical component of treatment. Limiting the impairment associated with ADHD and preventing the development of secondary problems are both critical to effective intervention for children with ADHD. These goals are often best accomplished through interventions into the child's psychosocial context, a point that is discussed later in this chapter.

Core Deficit Although there have been many theories as to the core cognitive deficit that can lead to ADHD symptoms, the most extensive and best articulated theory is Barkley's (1997). This theory posits that ADHD results from a core deficit in behavioral inhibition, which is defined as the ability to inhibit a prepotent response long enough to consider the consequences of the response; the ability to stop an ongoing response in reaction to environmental feedback; and the ability to suppress stimuli that might interfere with a primary response (i.e., interference control) (see also Nigg, 2006). According to Barkley's (1997) theory, the core deficit in behavioral inhibition leads to secondary impairments in several executive functions (EF). Executive functions are cognitive actions that are self-directed and allow for self-regulation. Four EFs depend on behavioral inhibition for their adequate performance: (1) working memory (e.g., maintaining events in the mind, hindsight, forethought); (2) self-regulation of affect, motivation, and arousal (e.g., self-control of emotions, social perspective taking); (3) internalization of speech (e.g., problem-solving, moral reasoning); and (4) reconstitution (e.g., verbal and behavioral fluency).

Barkley (1997) and Nigg (2006) provide comprehensive reviews of a large number of studies documenting impairments in these four EF's in samples of children with ADHD. Furthermore, these impairments can explain a number of the problems in self-regulation exhibited by children with ADHD. Specifically, the deficit in behavioral inhibition and the resulting impairments in the four domains of EF cause the behavior of ADHD individuals to be controlled by the immediate context rather than internal representations of information (Nigg, 2006). Also, these deficits can explain not only the core symptoms of inattention-disorganization and hyperactivity-impulsivity but also a number of secondary features of the disorder, such as an impaired sense of time and higher levels of emotional reactivity. Furthermore, the importance of the immediate context can explain why the behavior of a person with ADHD can be so strongly influenced by his or her immediate environment, such as the novelty of the task, the intrinsic interest of the child in the activity, the level of fatigue of the child, and the degree of immediate reinforcement present in the task (Barkley, 1996; 1997).

Neurological Substrates Attempting to tie the deficits associated with ADHD to specific neurological abnormalities has a long and controversial history (Frick & Lahey, 1991). Early conceptualizations of ADHD assumed a central nervous system dysfunction because of the similarity in symptomatology between persons with ADHD and persons with known brain injury. These similarities led to the use of the term *minimal brain dysfunction* to refer to this syndrome (Strauss & Lehtinen, 1947). However, early research into potential neurological differences between persons with ADHD and controls failed to document clear neurological abnormalities in most persons with the disorder, leading some to question the utility of assuming a neurological deficit without clear evidence that such a deficit exists (Rutter, 1977).

More recent studies employing a variety of neurobiological techniques have provided more consistent evidence for neurological dysfunction and converge to implicate fronto-striatal network abnormalities in children with ADHD (Bush, Valera, & Seidman, 2005). For example, studies using techniques that examine cerebral blood flow, which provides an index of brain function rather than structure, have documented diminished brain function in persons with ADHD, specifically in the prefrontal regions of the brain and pathways connecting to this region from the caudate and striatal regions (Lou, Henriksen, & Bruhn, 1984; Lou, Henriksen, Bruhn, Borner, & Nielson, 1989; Zametkin et al., 1990). This cortical hypoarousal hypothesis is supported by EEG findings of increased slow-wave activity in the frontal regions in individuals with ADHD, particularly the combined subtype (Loo & Barkley, 2005). Structurally, studies using magnetic resonance imaging (MRI) show reduced size in the corpus callosum, reduced cerebellar volume, and overall reduced total brain volume in ADHD individuals (Giedd et al., 1994; Hynd et al., 1991; Zametkin & Liotta, 1998). These neurobiological studies are informative because the implicated brain areas, the prefrontal and associated regions, have been linked with deficits in inhibition and executive functions and, thus, could explain the core deficits described previously (Barkley, 1997; Nigg, 2006). Further, there is evidence that stimulant medication, which reduces the symptoms of ADHD, increases activity in the prefrontal regions of the brain, thus providing rationale for the method of action of this medication in reducing the symptoms of ADHD (Lou et al., 1989).

Despite these promising findings, this research on the neurological underpinnings of ADHD is limited in several ways. First, as in earlier research, it is still evident that many persons with ADHD do not show clear deficits in brain structure or function. Second, the studies documenting neurological deficits are still few in number and have generally used small samples with limited control groups. Therefore, replications of these results are needed before firm conclusions can be made on their importance. Third, the findings of deficits in persons with ADHD have not always been consistent across studies. For example, some studies have found more diffuse abnormalities in cerebral blood flow that is not limited to prefrontal regions of the brain in adults with ADHD (Zametkin et al., 1990). Other studies have found that diminished blood flow is limited to adolescent girls with ADHD and is not found in adolescent boys with ADHD (Ernst et al., 1994; Zametkin et al, 1993). However, some of these inconsistencies may reflect differences in the sample studied (e.g., variations in which subtypes and comorbid conditions are included). Fourth, these studies do not indicate what causes these neurological deficits.

Causes of the Neurological Abnormalities There are many different pathways through which a neurological deficit can develop in the brain systems involved in inhibition. One way is through an inherited deficit. This possibility is supported by family and adoption studies that have shown evidence for a familial transmission of ADHD symptoms (Faraone & Biederman, 2000; Frick, Lahey, et al., 1991; Sprich, Biederman, Crawford, Mundy, & Faraone, 2000). A review of twin studies estimates that approximately 76% of the variance in measures of ADHD can be attributable to genetic influences, making it one of the most heritable forms of childhood psychopathology (Faraone et al., 2005; Stevenson, 1992). Molecular genetics studies have also identified a number of genes, each of small effect, which may increase the risk for developing ADHD (Faraone et al., 2005).

However, it is also quite likely that environmental factors play a role in the development of ADHD (Pauls, 2005). Some evidence suggests that biological trauma could be involved in the development of ADHD for some children. For example, children with ADHD are more likely to be born prematurely than other children because of higher rates of birth complications during pregnancy (James & Taylor, 1990). In addition, exposure to environmental toxins, such as prenatal exposure to alcohol and tobacco (Bennett, Wolin, & Reiss, 1988) and high lead blood levels (Stein, Schettler, Wallinga, & Valenti, 2002) have been linked to ADHD symptoms. Given these findings, it is quite likely that there are multiple pathways leading to any neurological deficit involved in the development of ADHD (Pauls, 2005).

Empirically Validated Treatments

There have been many treatment approaches attempted for ADHD, most of which have received only limited support for their effectiveness (Barkley, 1996; Hinshaw, 1994). Only two treatments have demonstrated consistent effectiveness in controlled treatment outcomes studies (Pelham, Wheeler, & Chronis, 1998): pharmacological intervention using CNS stimulants (e.g., methylphenidate (Ritalin), d-amphetamine (Dexedrine), d- and 1-AMP combination (Adderall)) and behavioral therapy that focuses on developing very structured contingency management systems for the child with ADHD in his or her home and school environments. To illustrate the effectiveness of these two treatment approaches, the National Institute of Mental Health (NIMH) funded the Collaborative Multimodal Treatment Study of Children with ADHD (MTA; Richters et al., 1995). The MTA was a five-year multi-site treatment study of 579 children ages 7 to 9 years diagnosed with ADHD. The controlled treatment trial compared four treatment groups: (1) psychosocial treatment only; (2) stimulant medication only; (3) combined psychosocial and pharmacological treatment; and (4) standard community treatment (being whatever treatment was typically delivered in that specific community). Each treatment lasted for 14 months (Wells et al., 2000).

The choice of stimulant medication as a key component to treatment was based on over 30 years of research indicating that it leads to significant improvements in ADHD symptoms in 70% to 80% of children with this diagnosis (see Swanson, McBurnett, Christian, & Wigal, 1995, for a review). Furthermore, research has shown that stimulant medication not only reduces the core symptoms of ADHD but also alleviates many secondary problems, such as conduct problems, aggression, poor peer relations, academic problems, and problematic interactions with parents and teachers (Pelham, 1993; Richters et al., 1995; Swanson et al., 1995). In addition, the side effects encountered with appropriate and carefully monitored trials of stimulant medication have been fairly mild, with the most common side effects being appetite suppression and increased irritability. In fact, in some studies, the side effects encountered with an active dose of stimulant medication have been no more than those encountered when the child was on a placebo (Barkley, McMurray, Edelbrock, & Robbins, 1990). It is important to note that much of this research has focused on the use of one particular stimulant medication, Ritalin (MPH; methylphenidate), which was also used in the MTA treatment study. Other stimulant medications have been tested in controlled treatment outcome studies, showing similar response profiles, and which typically vary primarily on how quickly they act and the length of time an active dose shows behavioral effects (Greenhill, Halperin, & Abikoff, 1999). There are a number of nonstimulant medications that have been used to treat ADHD, including noradrenergic reuptake inhibitors (e.g., bupropion, atomexetine), tricyclic antidepressants (e.g., imipramine, desipramine), and antihypertensive agents (e.g., clonidine) (Biederman, Spencer, & Wilens, 2004). The limited research on these nonstimulant medications have suggested that they tend to be superior to placebo in reducing symptoms of ADHD, although it is not clear that they are superior to the more extensively researched stimulant medications in their effectiveness (Biederman et al., 2004).

The initial results of the MTA study support the efficacy of stimulant medication. Children on medication showed substantially greater improvements on most outcome measures than did children in the community treatment control group (some of whom were on medication, as well) and even showed greater improvements in most domains than did the group receiving only the behavioral treatment (MTA Cooperative Group, 1999). The superior performance by stimulant medication over behavioral interventions is consistent with other studies directly comparing these treatments (Abikoff et al., 2004; Pelham, 1993). The MTA study found, however, that this level of improvement required a much more carefully controlled medical regimen than is typically administered in many community settings. For example, the MTA trial involved monthly phone contacts with the child's teacher, through which medication levels were adjusted to determine the optimal dosage for each child (MTA Cooperative Group, 1999).

While the effects of medication found in the MTA study and in other controlled trials have been impressive (Swanson et al., 1995), pharmacological interventions for children with ADHD are limited in several important ways. First, many parents have negative feelings about medication and may not administer it consistently or may even refuse this form of treatment (Richters et al., 1995). For example, about 6% of otherwise eligible participants in the MTA study declined participation because they did not want medication and another 9% refused medication once the trial began (Wells et al., 2000). Of note, 17% of eligible participants also declined participation in the MTA because they did not want to forego medication. This suggests that feelings about medication acceptability can be either strongly positive or strongly negative. Second, despite the impressive efficacy found for stimulant medication, its effectiveness is limited in some respects. For example, it still leaves 10 to 20% of children without significant levels of improvement, and even for those who do demonstrate significant improvement, their behavior is often not brought within what would be considered a normal range (Pelham, 1993; Wells et al., 2000). More importantly, there is little evidence that stimulants change the long-term course of ADHD, with most of the beneficial effects being demonstrated in short-term treatment outcome studies (Pelham et al., 2000). Third, some evidence suggests that medication is more effective when it is used in conjunction with behavioral treatments. Specifically, when medication and behavioral treatments are combined, more children show a clinical response to medication, more children's adjustment is brought within a normative range, and children can often be maintained on lower doses of stimulant medication (and thus reduce the number and severity of side effects) than when medication alone is used (Klein & Abikoff, 1997; Pelham et al., 2000).

As a result of this research, the MTA study included a behavioral intervention that consisted of several psychosocial interventions that have proven effective in treating children with ADHD in past research (Pelham et al., 1998; Wells et al., 2000). The first component consisted of 27 sessions of group parent training provided by therapist-consultants over 14 months. In these sessions, parents were taught (1) intensive behavior management skills (e.g., effective commands, token economies in the home, effective discipline); (2) methods to manage their stress, anger, and negative moods to enhance their parenting abilities; and (3) strategies for working effectively with teachers and advocating for their child with school personnel. There was also a school intervention component that involved 16 consultations with teachers over a 14-month period to establish behavioral management techniques in the classroom (e.g., daily report cards, classroom token economies). In addition, paraprofessionals were trained to be in the child's classroom to help in the implementation of these behavioral management programs. The third component of the MTA behavioral intervention was an eight-week Summer Treatment Program that met daily from 8:00 a.m. to 5:00 p.m. on weekdays during the summer. During this program, children experienced intensive and individualized behavioral management programs (e.g., point system, daily report cards) designed to promote positive behavioral changes. The Summer Treatment Program also included daily social skills training and sports skills training components.

Consistent with past research, the intensive behavioral intervention of the MTA resulted in gains that were superior to those found for the community treatment control group (MTA Cooperative Group, 1999). Although initial findings suggested that there was no clear benefit from adding this intensive behavioral intervention to the medication treatment (9-month, Arnold et al., 2004; 14-month, Pelham, 1999), secondary analysis of this data demonstrated a small but important improvement in the adjustment of children in the combined treatment (Conners et al., 2001; Swanson et al., 2001). The combined treatment was also judged as more acceptable by parents than the medication alone treatment (MTA Cooperative Group, 1999) and was more effective for children who had coexisting anxiety problems (Jensen et al., 2001; March et al., 2000). The combined intervention also appeared to be more effective for ethnic minority youth (Arnold et al., 2003). Surprisingly, there was little improvement in peer relationships resulting from any of the treatments studied in the MTA investigation (Hoza et al., 2005).

Summary of Treatment for ADHD The intervention approach used in the MTA study provides an excellent example of the two methods for treating children with ADHD that have proven effective in past treatment outcome studies (although see Barkley, 2000; Greene & Ablon, 2001, for critiques of the intervention). This large-scale treatment trial supports the effectiveness of both stimulant medication and behavioral interventions, with somewhat stronger effects noted for the stimulant medication across outcome domains. These findings support previous research in suggesting that these types of intervention are currently the state-of-the-art in treating children with ADHD, with some support for combining the interventions to optimize the effects for children. However, there is some evidence for the greater cost-effectiveness of pharmacological treatment over more expensive combined interventions for the routine treatment of children with ADHD, particularly those without comorbid disorders (Jensen et al., 2005). Importantly, much of the treatment research has been conducted with preadolescent children who have ADHD. However, there is growing evidence that stimulant medication is effective for reducing symptoms of ADHD in preschool children (Greenhill et al., 2006) and adults (Dowson, 2006), although the effectiveness rate is somewhat lower in both of these age groups compared to findings in preadolescent children.

Unfortunately, despite this well-documented efficacy for these two treatment modalities, there continues to be a proliferation of unproven therapies with very limited evidence for their effectiveness. These have ranged from biofeedback programs to specialized diets (Barkley, 1996; Hinshaw, 1994). The popularity of these unproven approaches to intervention is likely due to the strong biases against the two empirically supported treatments. Many parents, and even many professionals, have strong negative feelings about the use of medication for controlling children's behavioral problems. Further, most parents report having tried a system of rewards and punishments in an effort to control their children's behavior, albeit not at the level of consistency and intensity needed to bring about meaningful changes in the child's behavior. As a result, they are often reluctant to agree to interventions focusing on behavior management strategies. These biases often lead to the unfortunate outcome that many children with ADHD do not receive the optimal treatment approach for this disorder: a combination of a carefully controlled trial of stimulant medication and an intensive behavior management program.

Oppositional Defiant Disorder and Conduct Disorder

Conduct problems are one of the most common reasons that children and adolescents are referred to mental health clinics (Frick & Silverthorn, 2001) or referred to residential treatment centers (Lyman & Campbell, 1996). Also, severe conduct problems are strongly associated with delinquency and violence (Broidy et al., 2003; Moffitt, 2003). As a result, there has been a great deal of research focused on understanding and treating this form of externalizing psychopathology.

Diagnosis DSM-IV-TR (American Psychiatric Association, 2000) specifies two disorders involving conduct problem behavior. Oppositional Defiant Disorder (ODD) is defined as:

- a recurrent pattern of negativistic, defiant, disobedient and hostile behavior toward authority figures
- that persists for at least 6 months and
- is characterized by the frequent occurrence of at least four of the following behaviors: losing temper, arguing with adults, actively defying or refusing to comply with requests or rules of

adults, deliberately doing things that will annoy other people, blaming others for his or her own mistakes or misbehavior, being touchy or easily annoyed by others, being angry and resentful, or being spiteful or vindictive. (p. 100)

Conduct Disorder (CD) is defined as:

- a repetitive and persistent pattern of behavior which violates the rights of others or major age appropriate societal norms or rules are violated;
- these behaviors fall into four main groupings: aggressive conduct that threatens physical harm to other people or animals, nonaggressive conduct that causes property loss or damage, deceitfulness and theft, and serious violations of rules; and
- three or more characteristic behaviors must have been present during the past 12 months. (pp. 934–994)

There has been great debate as to the best way to conceptualize the relationship between these two disorders that involve conduct problems. Research seems to suggest that the less severe ODD symptoms are linked to the more severe CD symptoms both hierarchically and developmentally. For example, research has found that preadolescent children rarely begin showing the severe conduct problem behaviors associated with CD without first showing the milder ODD behaviors earlier in development. Instead, the typical developmental progression is that children start to show oppositional and argumentative behaviors early in life (e.g., between the ages of 3–8) and then gradually progress into increasingly more severe patterns of conduct problem behavior over the course of childhood (Loeber et al., 1992; Shaw, Gilliom, Ingoldsby, & Nagin, 2003). However, there are two important aspects to this developmental trajectory. First, while most children who show the more severe conduct problems of CD start by showing the less severe ODD symptoms, a large number of children with ODD do not progress to showing the more severe conduct problems (Lahey & Loeber, 1994; Shaw et al., 2003). Second, most children who progress on to CD do not *change* the types of behaviors they display but instead *add* the more severe conduct problem behaviors (Lahey & Loeber, 1994).

Developmental Course In addition to this developmental progression in types of conduct problems, a number of studies have documented the stability of conduct problems across development (e.g., Broidy et al., 2003; Shaw et al., 2003). Frick and Loney (1999) reviewed 12 prospective longitudinal studies of the stability of conduct problems over short periods of time (from 8 months to 5 years) and found that the correlations between initial and follow-up assessments generally fell between .42 and .64. In studies that estimated the degree of stability of diagnoses of conduct disorders, about 50% of the children diagnosed with CD at an initial assessment were rediagnosed with CD at a follow-up assessment. Frick and Loney (1999) also summarized the results of 9 prospective longitudinal studies that investigated the stability of conduct problems over longer periods of time (i.e., > 6 years). The correlation coefficients for the long-term follow-up studies generally fell between .20 and .40. The stability of diagnoses was variable across studies depending on the choice of outcome measure. For example, Kratzer and Hodgins (1997) found that about 64% of boys and 17% of girls (ages 12–16) with a diagnosis of CD had committed a crime during a 16-year follow-up period. In contrast, Robins (1966) reported that 31% of boys and 17% of girls referred to a mental health clinic for CD symptoms were diagnosed with an antisocial disorder as adults and 43% of the boys and 12% of girls were later imprisoned at least once as an adult.

Subtypes of Conduct Disorders Although conduct problems are somewhat stable over time, not all children with severe conduct problems continue to show problems through adolescence and into adulthood. In fact, much of the stability of conduct disorders can be accounted for by a small group of children with very severe and chronic conduct problems (Broidy et al., 2003; Moffitt, 2003). This finding has led to many attempts to uncover characteristics that distinguish between more severe and chronic forms of conduct problems and more benign and transient forms.

One of the more consistent predictors of poor outcome for children with CD is the severity of the initial disorder. Importantly, the frequency and intensity of the behavior exhibited, the variety of different types of symptoms displayed, and the presence of symptoms in more than one setting have all been related to a more severe and persistent form of CD (Loeber, 1982; 1991). Also, children with both conduct problems and ADHD seem to have a worse outcome than those with either type of problem alone (Waschbusch, 2002), as do children with conduct problems that have lower intelligence (Farrington, 1991; Moffitt, 1990). In addition, family dysfunction and socioeconomic adversity have been linked to poorer outcome in children with conduct problems (Frick & Loney, 1999; Moffitt, 1990).

Perhaps one of the most consistent predictors of poor outcome is the age at which the child begins to show serious conduct problems (see Frick & Loney, 1999; Moffitt, 2003, for reviews). For example, in a prospective study of the adult outcomes of a birth cohort in New Zealand, Moffitt, Caspi, Harrington, and Milne (2002) compared two groups of adults who had severe conduct problems as youth. One group who began showing serious problems prior to puberty made up only 10% of the birth cohort but accounted for 43% of violent convictions in the sample, 40% of the drug convictions, and 62% of the convictions for violence against women. The second group whose conduct problems emerged in adolescence (26% of the sample) continued to have some problems in adulthood as well, showing greater antisocial behavior than control adults who did not show conduct problems as a youth. However, they were 50% to 60% less likely to be convicted of an offense than the childhood-onset group and their offenses tended to be less serious (e.g., minor theft, public drunkenness) and less violent (e.g., accounting for 50% of the convictions for property offenses). As a result of findings such as these, *DSM-IV-TR* (2000) included a distinction between childhood-onset and adolescent-onset subtypes of conduct disorder.

More recent research has used the presence of a callous and unemotional interpersonal style (e.g., lacking empathy and guilt; constricted emotions) to designate a distinct group of children with severe and chronic conduct problems (Frick, 2006; Frick & Dickens, 2006; Frick & Marsee, 2006, for reviews). While callous-unemotional (CU) traits seem to be more common in the childhood-onset group (Moffitt et al., 2002), they are characteristic of only about a third of these children (Christian, Frick, Hill, Tyler, & Frazer, 1997). However, this minority of children with childhood onset conduct problems seems to show a more severe, aggressive, and stable pattern of behavioral difficulties. Frick and Dickens (2006) reviewed 22 published studies showing that CU traits either co-occurred with (*n* = 10), or predicted (*n* = 12), more serious antisocial and aggressive behavior. They also reviewed 5 studies showing that CU traits were related to poorer treatment response among youth with conduct problems. For example, clinic-referred children with conduct problems who show CU traits show a greater number and variety of conduct problems, more police contacts, and stronger family histories of antisocial personality disorder than other children with conduct problems (Christian et al., 1997) and they are less responsive to typical parenting interventions designed to reduce conduct problems in young children (Hawes & Dadds, 2005). Further, the utility of CU traits for predicting a more severe pattern of conduct problems has been found in samples of preschool children (Kimonis, Frick, Boris et al., 2006), elementary school-aged children (Frick, Stickle, Dandreaux, Farrell, & Kimonis, 2005), and adolescents (Kruh, Frick, & Clements, 2005). It has also been found for both boys and girls (Marsee, Silverthorn, & Frick, 2005).

Cultural and Gender Issues

There is evidence that aggressive, antisocial, and violent behavior varies in rate across cultures. For example, the United States has one of the highest rates of violence of all industrialized societies, showing

4 to 73 times the rates of violence found in other industrialized nations (Fingerhut & Kleinman, 1990; World Health Organization, 2002). This high rate of violence in the United States has been linked to various factors. One such factor is the high rate of exposure to violence experienced by children, both in their homes and neighborhoods (Osofsky, Wewers, Hann, & Fick, 1993) and through media portrayals (Heath, Bresdin, & Rinaldi, 1989; Huesmann, Moise-Titus, Podolski, & Eron, 2003). In addition, the cultural glorification of violence and the availability of handguns have also been considered as factors related to the high rate of violence in this country (O'Donnell, 1995). Still others have focused on the marginalization of ethnic minorities and the structural inequalities in opportunity afforded to minorities in the United States that can increase the risk of antisocial behavior in those without opportunities for obtaining goods and status through socially sanctioned means (McLoyd, 1990).

This latter possibility would predict higher rates of delinquent and antisocial behavior in ethnic minorities, but these associations have not been consistently found. For example, higher rates of delinquency (Gray-Ray & Ray, 1990) and conduct problems (Fabrega, Ulrich, & Mezzich, 1993; Lahey et al., 1995) have been found for African-American youth in some samples, but not others (McCoy, Frick, Loney, & Ellis, 2000). More importantly, it is unclear whether or not this association, when found, could be explained largely by the fact that ethnic minorities are more likely to experience economic hardships and live in urban neighborhoods with higher concentrations of crime than nonminority individuals (Gorman-Smith, 2003; Peeples & Loeber, 1994).

In contrast to this somewhat mixed picture of the relation between ethnicity and conduct problems, there are clear sex differences in the rate of conduct problems, with most studies showing that boys are more likely to show conduct problems than girls (see Silverthorn & Frick, 1999, for a review). However, these sex differences vary somewhat across development. For example, in preschool children, this sex difference is small and sometimes nonexistent (Keenan & Shaw, 1997), whereas throughout childhood there is a male:female ratio of about 4:1 (Silverthorn & Frick, 1999). This ratio closes to about 2:1 in adolescence, the period in which girls are most likely to be diagnosed with conduct disorder (Silverthorn & Frick, 1999). There is some controversy as to whether these differences in prevalence rates in childhood and adolescence are real differences or an artifact of diagnostic criteria that are not sensitive to sex differences in how conduct problems are expressed. For example, it has been argued that girls are less often diagnosed with severe conduct problems than boys because they manifest more indirect or relational aggression (i.e., spreading rumors, hurting others in the context of a relationship), rather than physical aggression (e.g., Crick & Grotpeter, 1995; Underwood, 2003). Others have argued that girls manifest similar types of behaviors as boys, but that they should be diagnosed using more lenient criteria that compares girls to other girls rather than to mixed samples of girls and boys (e.g., Zoccolillo, 1993). Still others have argued that girls manifest antisocial behaviors that are similar to those of boys but are less likely than boys to experience the necessary pathogenic processes (e.g., high levels of impulsivity; deficits in conscience) that can lead to the development of antisocial behavior (Moffitt & Caspi, 2001; Silverthorn & Frick, 1999).

Research generally suggests that boys and girls with conduct problems show similar risk factors (Fergusson & Horwood, 2002; Lahey et al., 2000). However, less research has focused on whether the subtypes of conduct problems described above are applicable for antisocial and aggressive girls. One consistent finding is that a childhood onset of severe antisocial and aggressive behavior is less common in girls than in boys. For example, in an entire birth cohort of New Zealand children, only a very small group of childhood-onset girls ($N = 6$) could be identified compared to larger groups of adolescent-onset girls ($N = 78$), childhood-onset boys ($N = 47$), and adolescent-onset boys ($N = 122$) (Moffitt & Caspi, 2001). Similarly, in an adjudicated sample of adolescent boys and girls, an almost equal number of boys had a childhood-onset (46%) or adolescent-onset (54%) of severe antisocial behavior, whereas 94% of the girls had an adolescent-onset to their antisocial behavior (Silverthorn, Frick, & Reynolds, 2001).

However, despite the predominance of adolescent onset in antisocial girls, there is evidence that girls with severe conduct problems show poor outcomes in adulthood and show a large number of dispositional and contextual risk factors that are very similar to childhood onset boys. For example, girls with severe conduct problems show high rates of criminality, violence, antisocial personality, and other psychiatric disorders in adulthood (Zoccolillo, 1993). In addition, girls with severe conduct problems show autonomic irregularities (Raine, Venables, & Mednick, 1997), problems with emotional regulation (Caspi, Henry, McGee, Moffitt, & Silva, 1995), and deficits in empathy (Cohen & Strayer, 1996).

To explain these findings, Silverthorn and Frick (1999) proposed a delayed-onset pathway to serious conduct problems in girls. These authors proposed that girls who develop serious conduct problems in adolescence often show many risk factors that may have been present in childhood and predate their behavioral problems. However, the onset of conduct problems may be delayed until adolescence, coinciding with biological (e.g., hormonal changes associated with puberty) and psychosocial (e.g., less parental monitoring and supervision; greater contact with deviant peers) changes that encourage antisocial behavior in girls with predisposing vulnerabilities (e.g., callous-unemotional traits; problems in emotional regulation). In an initial test of this theory, adjudicated adolescent girls who largely showed an adolescent onset to their antisocial behavior also showed high levels of CU traits, problems with impulse control, and a number of other social and temperamental vulnerabilities that were more similar to childhood-onset boys than to adolescent-onset boys (Silverthorn et al., 2001). Other tests of this theory have met with more mixed results. In the birth cohort of New Zealand youngsters described previously, girls with adolescent-onset of their conduct problems showed less parenting dysfunction, fewer temperamental vulnerabilities, and fewer neurocognitive deficits than childhood-onset boys, contrary to the predictions made by the delayed-onset model (Moffit & Caspi, 2001). In another community sample, adolescent-onset girls showed less parental antisocial behavior and were less likely to be diagnosed with ADHD than childhood-onset boys and girls but they did not differ from the childhood onset groups on poor parental monitoring and maltreatment history (McCabe, Rodgers, Yeh, & Hough, 2004).

Etiology: Developmental Pathways to Severe Conduct Problems

A substantial body of research on children and adolescents documents a large number of factors that can place a child at risk for developing conduct problems. These factors range from individual risk factors (e.g., poor impulse control, poor emotional regulation, low intelligence, lack of social skills), to problems in the child's immediate psychosocial context (e.g., poverty, parental psychopathology, inadequate parental discipline, association with a deviant peer group, parental prenatal smoking), to problems in the child's broader psychosocial context (e.g., living in a high crime neighborhood, exposure to violence, lack of educational and vocational opportunities) (see Dodge & Pettit, 2003; Frick, 2006; Moffitt, 2003; Raine, 2002, for reviews). However, it has been difficult to weave this broad array of risk factors into a coherent, yet comprehensive, causal model for conduct problems both because of the sheer number of factors and because they involve so many different types of causal processes. Additionally, these risk factors are typically not independent of each other and probably operate in a transactional (e.g., one risk factor having an influence on another risk factor) or multiplicative fashion (Dodge & Pettit, 2003). For example, an impulsive child may be much more difficult to parent effectively than a child who has better emotional and behavioral regulation, thereby making it more likely that he or she will experience less than adequate parenting (Barkley, 1996; Lytton, 1990). However, the impulsive child probably needs effective parenting even more than the well-regulated child to prevent the development of severe conduct problems (Colder, Lochman, & Wells, 1997). Similarly, Jaffee and colleagues (2005) found that maltreated children were most likely to develop childhood-onset conduct problems if they also showed a genetic vulnerability to problem behavior.

As a result, the development of conduct problems for any child is likely the result of a number of different risk factors that interact to place that child at risk for exhibiting behavior that violates the rights of others or major societal norms (Dodge & Pettit, 2003). Another complicating factor is the possibility that the causal mechanisms that lead to conduct problems may differ across subgroups of youth who exhibit antisocial behavior. For example, the distinction between childhood-onset and adolescent-onset patterns of CD not only has important predictive utility, as mentioned previously, but the two groups of youth with CD also show a number of different correlates that could suggest divergent etiologies. Specifically, children in the childhood-onset group show more aggression, more cognitive and neuropsychological disturbances (e.g., executive functioning deficits, autonomic nervous system irregularities), greater impulsivity, greater social alienation, and more dysfunctional family backgrounds than do children in the adolescent-onset group (see Frick, 2006; Moffitt, 2003, for reviews), although, as noted previously, these findings may not be as consistently found for girls.

These differences in the correlates of the two types of CD suggest that children in the adolescent-onset group show less temperamental and psychosocial adversity, yet they still show a severe and impairing pattern of antisocial behavior (Moffitt, Caspi, Dickson, Silva, & Stanton, 1996; Moffitt et al., 2002). Additionally, they tend to reject traditional status hierarchies and religious rules, and they associate with deviant peers (Moffitt et al., 1996). As a result, adolescents in this group seem to show an exaggeration of the normal developmental process involving separation and individuation that is crucial to identity formation in adolescence. Due to this developmental task, engaging in forbidden behaviors with peers can engender feelings of independence and maturity, albeit in a misguided manner (Moffitt, 2003). Further, although they may continue to have problems in adulthood, their adult adjustment is less impaired than that of children in the childhood-onset group. This is because the impairments in children in the adolescent-onset group are less related to enduring psychosocial vulnerabilities (e.g., neuropsychological impairments, deficits in social skills) and usually is a direct consequence of their antisocial behavior (e.g., poor educational attainment, criminal record, early marriage) (Moffitt et al., 2002).

As mentioned previously, the presence of CU traits appears to designate a more severe group of children within the childhood-onset group. These traits also may be a marker for a group of children who have different causal processes leading to their behavioral problems (see Frick, 2006; Frick & Morris, 2004, for reviews). For example, a large twin study compared the relative importance of environmental and genetic influences on the development of conduct problems in 7-year-old children with and without CU traits (Viding, Blair, Moffitt, & Plomin, 2005). This study reported that the genetic influences on conduct problems for children high on both conduct problems and CU traits were over twice that for children with conduct problems who were low on CU traits. Further, other studies have shown that children with conduct problems who display CU traits tend to be more fearless (Pardini, 2006), more thrill and adventure seeking (Frick et al., 2003; Frick, Lilienfeld, Ellis, Loney, & Silverthorn, 1999), and show lower levels of anxiety (Frick et al, 1999; Frick, Cornell et al., 2003; Lynam et al., 2005) than other children with similar levels of conduct problems. Children with CU traits are also less sensitive to cues of punishment when a reward-oriented response set is primed (Fisher & Blair, 1998; Frick, Cornell et al., 2003; O'Brien & Frick, 1996; Pardini, Lochman, & Frick, 2003) and are less reactive to threatening and emotionally distressing stimuli (Blair, 1999; Frick, Cornell et al., 2003; Kimonis, Frick, Fazekas, & Loney, 2006; Loney, Frick, Clements, Ellis, & Kerlin, 2003) than other children with conduct problems.

Children with CU traits appear to have a temperamental style associated with low fearfulness and low emotional reactivity to aversive stimuli (Blair, 1999). This temperamental style can place a child at risk for missing some of the early precursors to empathic concern, which involve emotional arousal evoked by the misfortune and distress of others. Also, it could lead a child to be relatively insensitive to the prohibitions and sanctions of parents and other socializing agents (Frick & Morris,

2004; Kochanska, 1993). Finally, it could create an interpersonal style in which the child becomes so focused on the potential rewards and gains of aggression or other antisocial means to solve interpersonal conflicts, that he or she ignores the potentially harmful effects of this behavior on him- or herself and others. Thus low fearfulness and low emotional reactivity to aversive stimuli may be fundamental characteristics that lead to the development of CU traits. Some research supports these hypotheses. For example, antisocial and delinquent youth who show CU traits are less distressed by the negative effects of their behavior on others (Blair, Jones, Clark, & Smith, 1997; Frick et al., 1999; Pardini et al., 2003), are more impaired in their moral reasoning and empathic concern towards others (Blair, 1999; Pardini et al., 2003), they expect more instrumental gain (e.g., obtaining goods or social goals) from their aggressive actions (Pardini et al., 2003), and they are more predatory in their violence than antisocial youth without these traits (Caputo, Frick, & Brodsky, 1999; Kruh et al., 2005).

In contrast, children with childhood-onset conduct problems without CU traits are more highly reactive to emotional and threatening stimuli (Kimonis, Frick, Fazekas et al., 2006; Loney et al., 2003), more distressed by the negative effects of their behavior on themselves and others (Frick et al., 2003; Frick et al., 1999; Pardini et al., 2003), and more likely to attribute hostile intent to the actions of peers (Frick et al., 2003). Also, their aggressive and antisocial behavior is more strongly associated with dysfunctional parenting practices (Oxford, Cavell, & Hughes, 2003; Wootton, Frick, Shelton, & Silverthorn, 1997) and with deficits in intelligence (Loney, Frick, Ellis, & McCoy, 1998) than for children with conduct problems who are high on CU traits. These findings suggest that children with conduct problems who do not show high rates of CU traits may have difficulties with behavioral and emotional regulation related to high levels of emotional reactivity. Such poor emotional regulation can result from a number of interacting causal factors, such as inadequate socialization in their rearing environments, deficits in intelligence that make it difficult for them to delay gratification and anticipate consequences, or temperamental problems in response inhibition (Frick & Morris, 2004). The problems in emotional regulation can lead to impulsive and unplanned aggressive acts for which the child may be remorseful afterwards, but for which he or she still has difficulty controlling. They can also lead to a higher susceptibility to anger due to perceived provocations from peers leading to violent and aggressive acts within the context of high emotional arousal (Kruh et al., 2005).

Empirically Validated Treatments

Given the link between conduct problems and later violence and delinquency, it is not surprising that the treatment of antisocial and aggressive behavior in youth has been the focus of a large number of controlled treatment outcome studies (Brestan & Eyberg, 1998; Kazdin, 1995). Unfortunately, one of the main conclusions one can reach from this extensive effort to find effective treatments for conduct problem youth is that the vast majority of treatment approaches are largely ineffective (Kazdin, 1995). Of even greater concern is the evidence that some types of intervention, particularly those that involve extensive antisocial peer group interactions, can actually increase the level and severity of antisocial behavior and increase the risk of negative life outcomes in adulthood (Dishion, McCord, & Poulin, 1999). Therefore, uninformed and ill-conceived treatments can do more harm than good.

Four treatments have proven effective in controlled outcome studies (see Frick, 1998, 2001, 2006, for a more extended discussion). The first intervention is the use of contingency management programs. The basic components of contingency management programs are: (1) establishing clear behavioral goals that gradually shape a child's behavior in those areas of specific concern for the child; (2) monitoring the child's progress toward these goals; (3) reinforcing appropriate steps toward reaching these goals; and (4) providing consequences for inappropriate behavior. These programs can bring about behavioral changes for children with conduct problems in a number of different settings such as at home (Ross, 1981), at school (Abramowitz & O'Leary, 1991), and in residential treatment centers (Lyman & Campbell, 1996).

The second effective treatment is parent management training (PMT). A critical goal of PMT programs is to teach parents how to develop and implement very structured contingency management programs in the home (Kazdin, 2005). However, PMT programs also focus on (1) improving the quality of parent–child interactions (e.g., having parents more involved in their children's activities, improving parent–child communication, increasing parental warmth and responsiveness); (2) changing antecedents to behavior that enhance the likelihood that positive prosocial behaviors will be displayed by children (e.g., how to time and present requests, providing clear and explicit rules and expectations); (3) improving parents' ability to monitor and supervise their children; and (4) using more effective discipline strategies (e.g., being more consistent in discipline, using a variety of approaches to discipline). The effectiveness of this type of intervention has been the most consistently documented of any technique used to treat children with severe conduct problems (Kazdin, 1995; Kazdin & Whitley, 2003).

The third type of intervention that has proven effective in treating children with conduct problems is a cognitive-behavioral approach designed to overcome deficits in social cognition and social problem-solving experienced by many children and adolescents with conduct problems. For example, as mentioned previously, some children with conduct problems tend to attribute hostile intent to ambiguous interactions with peers that make them more likely to act aggressively towards peers. Other aggressive children overestimate the likelihood that their aggressive behavior will lead to positive results (e.g., enhanced status, obtaining a desired toy) and this cognitive bias makes them more likely to select aggressive alternatives to solving peer conflict (Dodge, Lochman, Harnish, Bates, & Pettit, 1997). Most cognitive-behavioral skills-building programs teach the child to inhibit impulsive or angry responding. This inhibition allows the child to go through a series of problem-solving steps (e.g., how to recognize problems, how to consider alternative responses and select the most adaptive one) and overcome deficits in the way they process social information (Larson & Lochman, 2003).

The final intervention that has proven to have some effectiveness in reducing conduct problems in children with ADHD is the use of stimulant medication. As mentioned previously, a large proportion of children with conduct problems also show ADHD and the impulsivity associated with ADHD may directly lead to some of the aggressive and other poorly regulated behaviors of children with severe conduct problems. In addition, the presence of ADHD may indirectly contribute to the development of conduct problems through its effect on (1) children's interactions with peers and significant others (e.g., parents and teachers); (2) parents' ability to use effective socialization strategies; or (3) a child's ability to perform academically. Therefore, for many children and adolescents with conduct problems, reducing ADHD symptoms is an important treatment goal. As mentioned previously, one of the more successful treatments for ADHD is the use of stimulant medication. Most importantly, the effectiveness of stimulants for reducing conduct problems in children with ADHD has been demonstrated in several controlled medication trials (e.g., Hinshaw, 1991; Hinshaw, Heller, & McHale, 1992; Pelham et al., 1993).

Limitations Research indicates that each of these interventions also possess substantial limitations (Brestan & Eyberg, 1998; Kazdin, 1995). First, a significant proportion of children with severe conduct problems do not show a positive response to these interventions and, for those that do respond positively, their behavior problems are often not reduced to a normal level. Second, treatment is most effective with younger children (prior to age 8) with less severe behavioral disturbances. Third, the generalizability of treatment effects across settings tends to be poor. That is, treatments that are effective in changing a child's behavior in one setting (e.g., mental health clinics) often do not bring about changes in the child's behavior in other settings (e.g., schools). Fourth, improvements in behavior are often difficult to maintain over time.

Given these limitations, there has been an increasing focus on trying to improve treatments by integrating our knowledge about the causes of conduct problems with the development of innovative approaches to treatment (Frick, 1998; 2001; 2006). Each of the four treatments described previously targets basic processes that research has shown to be important in the development of conduct problems (e.g., family dysfunction, problems in impulse control). However, these treatments have ignored two additional characteristics of children with severe conduct problems. First, research suggests that severe conduct problems are multidetermined and result from a complex interaction of many different types of causal processes. Second, the causes of severe conduct problems are heterogeneous. As a result, any single intervention, even if it targets multiple causal processes, is not likely to be effective for all children with ODD or CD.

Empirical Supported Principles Based on this research, there is not likely to be any single "best" treatment for severe conduct problems. Instead, interventions must be tailored to the individual needs of children with ODD or CD and these needs will likely differ depending on the specific mechanisms underlying the child's behavioral disturbance. For example, interventions for children in the adolescent-onset pathways will likely be somewhat different from interventions for children in the childhood-onset pathway. Even within the childhood-onset pathway, the focus of intervention may be different depending on the presence or absence of CU traits (see Frick, 1998; 2001; 2006, for examples).

By integrating research on developmental models of conduct problems with empirically supported treatments, several general principles for designing and implementing interventions for children with severe conduct problems appear important. First, one must understand the multiple causal processes that can be involved in the development of conduct problems. For example, by recognizing the developmental progressions that often characterize children and adolescents with severe conduct problems, interventions can be implemented as early as possible in the developmental sequence. In addition, this knowledge can help in determining which processes may be involved in the development of severe conduct problems for a particular child and can guide decisions as to the most important targets of interventions. Second, this flexible approach to treatment requires a clear, comprehensive, and individualized case conceptualization that guides the design of a focused and integrated approach to treatment (Frick & McCoy, 2001). A case conceptualization is a "theory" about the factors most likely involved in the development, exacerbation, and maintenance of conduct problems for an individual child or adolescent. It uses the research on developmental pathways to conduct problems and attempts to apply it to an individual child with a conduct disorder. Third, successful intervention for children and adolescents with severe conduct problems typically involves multiple professionals and multiple community agencies all working together to provide a comprehensive and integrated intervention.

One approach to treatment that incorporates many of the features of a developmental approach to treatment is multi-systemic therapy (MST). MST was originally developed as a general approach to intervention for psychopathological conditions (Henggeler & Borduin, 1990) but has been applied extensively to the treatment of severe antisocial behavior in children and adolescents (Henggeler, Schoenwald, Borduin, Rowland, & Cunningham, 1998). The orientation of MST is an expansion of a systems orientation to family therapy. In systemic family therapy, problems in children's adjustment are viewed as being embedded within the larger family context. MST expands this notion to include other contexts, such as the child's peer, school and neighborhood contexts. Most importantly, MST emphasizes a comprehensive and individualized approach to intervention that is consistent with the treatment principles outlined above.

MST involves an initial comprehensive assessment that seeks to understand the level and severity of the child or adolescent's presenting problems and to understand how these problems may be related to factors in the child's familial, peer, and cultural environment. The information from this assessment is used to outline an individualized treatment plan based on the specific needs of the child and his or her family. Unlike the individual interventions described previously, MST does not emphasize the use of specific techniques. Instead, it emphasizes several principles that follow from its orientation to intervention. These principles include:

- the identified problems in the child are understood within the child's familial, peer, and cultural context,
- therapeutic contacts emphasize positive (strength-oriented) levers for change,
- interventions promote responsible behavior among family members,
- interventions are present focused and action oriented, targeting specific and well-defined problems,
- interventions target sequences of behavior within and between multiple systems,
- interventions must be developmentally appropriate,
- interventions are designed to require daily or weekly effort by family members,
- intervention effectiveness must be evaluated continuously from multiple perspectives, and
- interventions are designed to promote maintenance of therapeutic change by empowering caregivers.

A critical component of MST is a system of intensive supervision for the therapists implementing the treatment to determine how these principles should be implemented to meet the needs of each individual case and to ensure that the principles are followed throughout the intervention (Henggeler et al., 1998).

One of the important contributions of MST to the treatment outcome literature is its demonstration that individualized interventions can be rigorously evaluated through controlled treatment outcome studies. The initial findings from studies on the effectiveness of MST in reducing antisocial and aggressive behavior among even very severely disturbed youth have been quite promising. For example, in a controlled treatment outcome study of MST at a university-based outpatient clinic, 88 adolescent repeat offenders underwent MST. To illustrate the individualized nature of the treatment, the length of treatment with MST ranged from 5 to 54 hours (mean of 23 hours). In addition to this variation in intensity, the way in which these hours were utilized varied depending on the needs of the clients. Eighty-three percent of the MST group participated in family therapy and 60% participated in some form of school intervention, which included facilitation of parent–teacher communication, academic remediation, or help in classroom behavior management. In 57% of the cases, there was some form of peer intervention which included coaching and emotional support for integration into prosocial peer groups (e.g., scouts, athletic teams) or direct intervention with peers. In 28% of the cases there was individual therapy with the adolescent which typically involved some form of cognitive-behavioral skills building intervention. Finally, in 26% of the cases the adolescent's parents became involved in marital therapy.

The outcomes of this group of offenders receiving MST were compared to a control group of 68 offenders who received traditional outpatient services, typically focusing on individual psychotherapy (Borduin et al., 1995). At a four-year follow-up, only 26% of the youth who underwent MST were rearrested compared to 71% of the control adolescents. This efficacy was maintained in a long term follow-up 10 to 16 years after treatment. MST participants had significantly lower rates of criminal recidivism (50 vs. 81%, respectively), fewer arrests, and less time in secure confinement over this extended follow-up period (Schaeffer & Borduin, 2005).

In a second outcome study of MST, master's level therapists provided intervention at a community mental health center (Henggeler, Melton, & Smith, 1992). The sample included adolescents who had been adjudicated as delinquent and had multiple arrests. These adolescents were randomly assigned to either receive MST or standard services provided by the juvenile justice system. The group receiving

MST showed half as many arrests and spent an average of 73 fewer days incarcerated than adolescents who received standard services. These studies and others (Curtis, Ronan, & Borduin, 2004; Henggeler & Lee, 2003) illustrate the promise of MST in treating youth with very serious conduct problems.

Overall Summary

As mentioned previously, externalizing disorders of children constitute one of the most common reasons that children are referred to mental health clinics for treatment (Frick & Silverthorn, 2001). This fact is not surprising given the disruptions that children with these disorders often cause to those around them, especially to parents and teachers who are most likely to refer a child for treatment. Further, given the association between externalizing disorders and many costly and impairing outcomes (e.g., substance abuse, delinquency), understanding and effectively treating children with these disorders is an important endeavor for psychologists and other mental health professionals.

Fortunately, there is a large body of research on children with these disorders. As summarized in this chapter, recent research has led to great advances in our understanding of the causes of these disorders and the development of effective interventions to prevent and treat them in youth. Unfortunately, this research is often not translated well into practice and, as a result, many children with these disorders do not receive state-of-the-art treatment. This gap between research and practice can be the result of a number of factors (Frick, 2000). For example, it can be the result of practitioners not being trained in the most current theories and approaches to treatment or not remaining current on this research. Alternatively, the gap between research and practice can be the result of research not being conducted or presented in a way that is useful to the practicing psychologist. In either case, the quality of services provided to children with disruptive behaviors depends heavily on advances in research and our ability to translate these findings into widely used applications. The focus of this chapter was to summarize research on children with externalizing disorders in a way that promotes such a translation.

References

Abikoff, H., Hechtman, L., Klein, R. G., Weiss, G., Fleiss, K., Cousins, L., et al. (2004). Symptomatic improvement in children with ADHD treated with long-term methylphenidate and multimodal psychosocial treatment. *Journal of the American Academy of Child and Adolescent Psychiatry, 43*(7), 802–811.

Abikoff, H., & Klein, R. G. (1992). Attention-deficit hyperactivity and conduct disorder: Comorbidity and implications for treatment. *Journal of Consulting and Clinical Psychology, 60*, 881–892.

Abramowitz, A.. J., & O'Leary, S. G. (1991). Behavioral interventions for the classroom: Implications for students with ADHD. *School Psychology Review, 20*, 220–234.

Achenbach, T. M. (1995). Diagnosis, assessment, and comorbidity in psychosocial treatment research. *Journal of Abnormal Psychology, 23*, 45–65.

Achenbach, T. M. & Edelbrock, C. S. (1978). The classification of child psychopathology: A review and analysis of empirical efforts. *Psychological Bulletin, 85*, 1275–1301.

American Psychiatric Association. (1980). *Diagnostic and statistical manual of mental disorders* (3rd ed.) Washington, D.C.: Author.

American Psychiatric Association. (2000). *Diagnostic and statistical manual of mental disorders* (4th ed., rev.). Washington, D.C.: Author.

Applegate, B., Lahey, B. B., Hart, E. L., Biederman, J., Hynd, G. W., Barkley, R. A., et al. (1997). Validity of the age-of-onset criterion for ADHD: A report from the *DSM-IV* field trials. *Journal of the American Academy of Child and Adolescent Psychiatry, 36*, 1211–1221.

Arnold, L. E., Chuang, S., Davies, M., Abikoff, H. B., Conner, C. K., Elliott, G. R., et al. (2004). Nine months of multicomponent behavioral treatment for ADHD and effectiveness of MTA fading procedures. *Journal of Abnormal Child Psychology, 32*(1), 39–51.

Arnold, L. E., Elliott, M., Sachs, L., Bird, H., Kraemer, H. C., Wells, K. C., et al. (2003). Effects of ethnicity on treatment attendance, stimulant response/dose, and 14-month outcome in ADHD. *Journal of Consulting and Clinical Psychology, 71*(4), 713–727.

Barkley, R. A. (1996). Attention-deficit/hyperactivity disorder. In E. J. Mash & R. A. Barkley (Eds.), *Child Psychopathology* (pp. 63–112). New York: Guilford.

Barkley, R. A. (1997). Behavioral inhibition, sustained attention, and executive functions: Constructing a unifying theory of ADHD. *Psychological Bulletin, 121*, 65–94.

Barkley, R. A. (2000). Commentary on the Multimodal Treatment Study of children with ADHD. *Journal of Abnormal Child Psychology, 28*, 595–599.

Barkley, R. A. (2003). Issues in the diagnosis of attention-deficit/hyperactivity disorder in children. *Brain and Development, 25*, 77–83.

Barkley, R. A., & Cunningham, C. E. (1979). The effects of Ritalin on the mother-child interactions of hyperactive children. *Archives of General Psychiatry, 36*, 201–208.

Barkley, R. A., DuPaul, G. J., & McMurray, M. B. (1991). Attention deficit disorder with and without hyperactivity: Clinical response to three dose levels of methylphenidate. *Pediatrics, 87*, 519–531.

Barkley, R. A., Fischer, M., Smallish, L., & Fletcher, K. (2002). The persistence of attention-deficit/hyperactivity disorder into young adulthood as a function of reporting source and definition of disorder. *Journal of Abnormal Psychology, 111*, 279–289.

Barkley, R. A., Guevremont, D. G., Anastopoulos, A. D., DuPaul, G. J., & Shelton, T. L. (1993). Driving related risks and outcomes of attention deficit hyperactivity disorder in adolescents and young adults: A 3–5 year follow-up survey. *Pediatrics, 92*, 212–218.

Barkley, R. A., McMurray, M. B., Edelbrock, C. S., & Robbins, K. (1990). Side effects of methylphenidate in children with attention deficit hyperactivity disorder: A systematic, placebo-controlled evaluation. *Pediatrics, 86*, 184–192.

Bennett, L. A., Wolin, S. J., & Reiss, D. (1988). Cognitive, behavioral, and emotional problems among school-age children of alcoholic parents. *American Journal of Psychiatry, 145*, 185–190.

Biederman, J., Mick, E., Faraone, S. V., Braaten, E., Doyle, A., Spencer, T., et al. (2002). Influence of gender on attention deficit hyperactivity disorder in children referred to a psychiatric clinic. *American Journal of Psychiatry, 159*, 36–42.

Biederman, J., Spencer, T., & Wilens, T. (2004). Evidence-based pharmacotherapy for attention-deficit hyperactivity disorder. *International Journal of Neuropsychopharmacology, 7*, 77–97.

Blair, R. J. R. (1999). Responsiveness to distress cues in the child with psychopathic tendencies. *Personality and Individual Differences, 27*, 135–145.

Blair, R. J. R., Jones, L., Clark, F., & Smith, M. (1997). The psychopathic individual: A lack of responsiveness to distress cues? *Psychophysiology, 34*, 192–198.

Borduin, C. M., Mann, B. J., Cone, L. T., Henggeler, S. W., Fucci, B. R., Blaske, D. M., et al. (1995). Multisystemic treatment of serious juvenile offenders: Long term prevention of criminality and violence. *Journal of Consulting and Clinical Psychology, 63*, 569–578.

Brestan, E. V., & Eyberg, S. M. (1998). Effective psychosocial treatments conduct disordered children and adolescents. *Journal of Clinical Child Psychology, 27*, 180–189.

Broidy, L. M., Nagin, D. S., Tremblay, R. E., Bates, J. E., Brame, B., Dodge, K.A., et al. (2003). Developmental trajectories of childhood disruptive behaviors and adolescent delinquency: A six-site, cross-national study. *Developmental Psychology, 39*(2), 222–245.

Burt, S. A., Krueger, R. F., McGue, M., & Iacono, W. (2003). Parent-child conflict and the comorbidity among childhood externalizing disorders. *Archives of General Psychiatry, 60*(5), 505–513.

Bush, G., Valera, E. M., & Seidman, L. J. (2005). Functional neuroimaging of Attention-Deficit/Hyperactivity disorder: A review and suggested future directions. *Biological Psychiatry, 57*, 1273–1284.

Campbell, S. B., Ewing, L. J., Breaux, A. M., & Szumowski, E. K. (1986). Parent-referred problem three-year-olds: Follow-up at school entry. *Journal of Child Psychology and Psychiatry, 27*, 473–488.

Caputo, A. A., Frick, P. J., & Brodsky, S. L. (1999). Family violence and juvenile sex offending: Potential mediating roles of psychopathic traits and negative attitudes toward women. *Criminal Justice and Behavior, 26*, 338–356.

Carlson, C. L., & Mann, M. (2000). Attention-deficit/hyperactivity disorder, predominantly inattentive subtype. *Child and Adolescent Psychiatric Clinics of North American, 9*, 499–510.

Carlson, C. L., & Mann, M. (2003). Sluggish cognitive tempo predicts a different pattern of impairment in the attention deficit hyperactivity disorder type. *Journal of Clinical Child and Adolescent Psychology, 31*, 123–129.

Caspi, A. Henry, B., McGee, R. O., Moffitt, T. E., & Silva, P. A. (1995). Temperamental origins of child and adolescent behavior problems: From age three to fifteen. *Child Development, 66*(1), 55–68.

Christian, R., Frick, P. J., Hill, N., Tyler, L. A., & Frazer, D. (1997). Psychopathy and conduct problems in children: II. Subtyping children with conduct problems based on their interpersonal and affective style. *Journal of the American Academy of Child and Adolescent Psychiatry, 36*, 233–241.

Cohen, D., & Strayer, J. (1996). Empathy in conduct-disordered and comparison youth. *Developmental Psychology, 32*(6), 988–998.

Colder, C. R., Lochman, J. E., & Wells, K. C. (1997). The moderating effects of children's fear and activity level on relations between parenting practices and childhood symptomatology. *Journal of Abnormal Child Psychology, 25*, 251–263.

Conners, C. K., Epstein, J. N., March, J., Angold, A., Wells, K. C., Klaric, J., et al. (2001). Multimodal treatment of ADHD in the MTA: An alternative outcome analysis. *Journal of the American Academy of Child and Adolescent Psychiatry, 40*, 159–167.

Crick, N. R., & Grotpeter, J. K. (1995). Relational aggression, gender, and social-psychological adjustment. *Child Development, 66*, 710–722.

Curtis, N. M., Ronan, K. R., & Borduin, C. M. (2004). Multisystemic treatment: A meta-analysis of outcome studies. *Journal of Family Psychology, 18* (3), 411–419.

Dishion, T. J., McCord, J., & Poulin, F. (1999). When interventions harm: Peer groups and problem behavior. *American Psychologist, 54*, 755–764.

Dodge, K. A., Lochman, J. E., Harnish, J. D., Bates, J. E., & Pettit, G. S. (1997). Reactive and proactive aggression in school children and psychiatrically impaired chronically assaultive youth. *Journal of Abnormal Psychology, 106,* 37–51.

Dodge, K. A., & Pettit, G. S. (2003). A biopsychosocial model of the development of chronic conduct problems in adolescence. *Developmental Psychology, 39,* 349–371.

Dowson, J. H. (2006). Pharmacological treatment for attention-deficit hyperactivity disorder (ADHD) in adults. *Current Psychiatry Reviews, 2,* 317–331.

Ernst, M., Liebenauer, L. L., King, A.C., Fitzgerald, G. A., Cohen, R. M., & Zametkin, A. J. (1994). Reduced brain metabolism in hyperactive girls. *Journal of the American Academy of Child and Adolescent Psychiatry, 33,* 858–868.

Fabrega, J. H., Ulrich, R., & Mezzich, J. E. (1993). Do Caucasian and Black adolescents differ at psychiatric intake? *Journal of the American Academy of Child and Adolescent Psychiatry, 32,* 407–413.

Faraone, S. V., & Biederman, J. (2000). Nature, nurture, and Attention Deficit Hyperactivity disorder. *Developmental Research, 20,* 568–581.

Faraone, S. V., Perlis, R. H., Doyle, A. E., Smoller, J. W., Goralnick, J. J., Holmgren, M. A., et al. (2005). Molecular genetics of attention-deficit/hyperactivity disorder. *Biological Psychiatry, 57,* 1313–1323.

Faraone, S. V., Sergeant, J., Gillberg, C., & Biederman, J. (2003). The worldwide prevalence of ADHD: Is it an American condition? *World Psychiatry, 2,* 104–113.

Farrington, D. P. (1991). Childhood aggression and adult violence: Early precursors and later-life outcomes. In D. Pepler & K. H. Rubin (Eds.), *The development and treatment of childhood aggression* (pp. 5–19). Hillsdale, NJ: Erlbaum.

Fergusson, D. M, & Horwood, L. J. (2002). Male and female offending trajectories. *Development and Psychopathology, 14,* 159–177.

Fergusson, D. M., Horwood, L. J., & Lynskey, M. T. (1993). Prevalence and comorbidity of *DSM-III-R* diagnoses in a birth cohort of 15 year olds. *Journal of the American Academy of Child and Adolescent Psychiatry, 32,* 1127–1134.

Fingerhut, L. A., & Kleinman, J. C. (1990). International and interstate comparisons of homicide among young males. *Journal of the American Medical Association, 263,* 3292–3295.

Fischer, M. (1990). Parenting stress and the child with attention deficit hyperactivity disorder. *Journal of Clinical Child Psychology, 19,* 337–346.

Fisher, L., & Blair, R. J. R. (1998). Cognitive impairment and its relationship to psychopathic tendencies in children with emotional and behavioral difficulties. *Journal of Abnormal Child Psychology, 26,* 511–519.

Frick, P. J. (1998). *Conduct disorders and severe antisocial behavior.* New York: Plenum.

Frick, P. J. (2000). Laboratory and performance-based measures of childhood disorders. *Journal of Clinical Child Psychology, 29,* 475–478.

Frick, P. J. (2001). Effective interventions for children and adolescents with conduct disorder. *The Canadian Journal of Psychiatry, 46,* 26–37.

Frick, P. J. (2006). Developmental pathways to conduct disorder. *Child Psychiatric Clinics of North America, 15,* 311–332.

Frick, P. J., Cornell, A. H., Bodin, S. D., Dane, H. E., Barry, C. T., & Loney, B. R. (2003). Callous-unemotional traits and developmental pathways to severe conduct problems. *Developmental Psychology, 39,* 246–260.

Frick, P. J., & Dickens, C. (2006). Current perspectives on conduct disorder. *Current Psychiatry Reports, 59–72.*

Frick, P. J., Kamphaus, R. W., Lahey, B. B., Loeber, R., Christ, M. A. G., Hart, E. L., et al. (1991). Academic underachievement and the disruptive behavior disorders. *Journal of Consulting and Clinical Psychology, 59,* 289–294.

Frick, P. J. & Lahey, B. B. (1991) The nature and characteristics of attention-deficit hyperactivity disorder. *School Psychology Review, 20,* 163–173.

Frick, P. J., Lahey, B., Christ, M. A. G., Loeber, R., & Green, S. (1991). History of childhood behavior problems in biological parents of boys with attention-deficit hyperactivity disorder and conduct disorder. *Journal of Clinical Child Psychology, 20,* 445–451.

Frick, P. J., Lilienfeld, S. O., Ellis, M. L, Loney, B. R., & Silverthorn, P. (1999). The association between anxiety and psychopathy dimensions in children. *Journal of Abnormal Child Psychology, 27,* 381–390.

Frick, P. J., & Loney, B. R. (1999). Outcomes of children and adolescents with conduct disorder and oppositional defiant disorder. In H. C. Quay & A. Hogan (Eds.), *Handbook of disruptive behavior disorders* (pp. 507–524). New York: Plenum.

Frick, P. J., & Marsee, M. A. (2006). Psychopathic traits and developmental pathways to antisocial behavior in youth. In C. J. Patrick (Eds.), *Handbook of psychopathic traits* (pp. 355–374). New York: Guilford.

Frick, P. J., & McCoy, M. G. (2001). Conduct disorder. In H. Orvaschel, J. Faust, & M. Hersen (Eds.), *Handbook of conceptualization and treatment of child psychopathology* (pp. 57–76). Oxford: Elsevier Science.

Frick, P. J., & Morris, A. S. (2004). Temperament and developmental pathways to conduct problems. *Journal of Clinical Child and Adolescent Psychology, 33(1),* 54–68.

Frick, P. J., & Silverthorn, P. (2001). Psychopathology in children. In P. B. Sutker & H. E. Adams (Eds.), *Comprehensive handbook of psychopathology* (3rd ed., pp. 881–920). New York: Kluwer.

Frick, P. J., Stickle, T. R., Dandreaux, D. M., Farrell, J. M., & Kimonis, E. R. (2005). Callous-unemotional traits in predicting the severity and stability of conduct problems and delinquency. *Journal of Abnormal Child Psychology. 33(4),* 471–487.

Gaub, M., & Carlson, C. L. (1997). Gender differences in ADHD: A meta-analysis and critical review. *Journal of the American Academy of Child and Adolescent Psychiatry, 36,* 1036–1045.

Gershon, J. (2002). A meta-analytic review of gender differences in ADHD. *Journal of Attentional Disorders, 5,* 143–154.

Giedd, J. N., Castellanos, F. X., Casey, B. J., Kozuch, P., King, A. C., Hamburger, S. D., et al. (1994). Quantitative morphology of the corpus callosum in attention deficit hyperactivity disorder. *American Journal of Psychiatry, 151,* 665–669.

Gomez-Beneyto, M., Bonet, A., Catala, N.A., & Puche, E. (1994). Prevalence of mental disorders among children in Calencia, Spain. *Acta Psychiatrica Scandinavica, 89,* 352–357.

Gorman-Smith, D. (2003). The social ecology of community and neighborhood risk for antisocial behavior. In C.A. Essau

(Ed.), *Conduct and oppositional defiant disorders: Epidemiology, risk factors, and treatment* (pp. 117–136). Mahwah, NJ: Erlbaum.

Gray-Ray, P., & Ray, M.C. (1990). Juvenile delinquency in the black community. *Youth & Society, 22,* 67–84.

Greene, R.W., & Ablon, J. S. (2001). What does the MTA study tell us about effective psychosocial treatment for ADHD? *Journal of Clinical Child Psychology, 30,* 114–121.

Greenhill, L. L., Halperin, J. M., & Abikoff, H. (1999). Stimulant medications. *Journal of the American Academy of Child and Adolescent Psychiatry, 38,* 503–512.

Greenhill, L., Kollins, S., McCracken, J., Riddle, M., Swanson, J., Wigal, S., et al. (2006). Efficacy and safety of immediate-release methylphenidate treatment for preschoolers with ADHD. *Journal of the American Academy of Child and Adolescent Psychiatry, 45,* 1284–1293.

Hart, E. L., Lahey, B. B., Loeber, R., Applegate, B., Green, S. M., & Frick, P. J. (1995). Developmental change in attention-deficit hyperactivity disorder in boys: A four-year longitudinal study. *Journal of Abnormal Child Psychology, 23,* 729–749.

Hartman, C. A., Willcutt, E. G., Rhee, S. H., & Pennington, B. F. (2004). The relation between sluggish cognitive tempo and DSM-IV ADHD. *Journal of Abnormal Child Psychology, 32,* 491–503.

Hawes, D. J. & Dadds, M. R. (2005). The treatment of conduct problems in children with callous-unemotional traits. *Journal of Consulting and Clinical Psychology, 73*(4), 737–741.

Heath, L., Bresdin, L. B., & Rinaldi, R. C. (1989). Effects of media violence on children: A review of the literature. *Archives of General Psychiatry, 46,* 376–379.

Henggeler, S. W., & Borduin, C. M. (1990). *Family therapy and beyond: A multisystemic approach to treating the behavior problems of children and adolescents.* Pacific Grove, CA: Brooks/Cole.

Henggeler, S.W., & Lee, T. (2003). Multisystemic treatment of serious clinical problems. In A. E. Kazdin & J. R. Weisz (Eds.), *Evidence-Based Psychotherapies for Children and Adolescents* (pp. 301–322). New York: Guilford.

Henggeler, S. W., Melton, G. B., & Smith, L. A. (1992). Family preservation using multisystemic therapy: An effective alternative to incarcerating juvenile offenders. *Journal of Consulting and Clinical Psychology, 60,* 953–961.

Henggeler, S. W., Schoenwald, S. K., Borduin, C. M., Rowland, M. D., & Cunningham, P. B. (1998). *Multisystemic treatment of antisocial behavior in children and adolescents.* New York: Guilford.

Hinshaw, S. P. (1987). On the distinction between attentional deficits/hyperactivity and conduct problems/aggression in child psychopathology. *Psychological-Bulletin, 101,* 443–463.

Hinshaw, S. P. (1991). Stimulant medication and the treatment of aggression in children with attention deficits. *Journal of Clinical Child Psychology, 20,* 301–312.

Hinshaw, S. P. (1994). *Attention deficits and hyperactivity in children.* Thousand Oaks, CA: Sage.

Hinshaw, S. P., Heller, T., & McHale, J. P. (1992). Covert antisocial behavior in boys with attention-deficit hyperactivity disorder: External validation and effects of methylphenidate. *Journal of Consulting and Clinical Psychology, 60,* 274–281.

Hoza, B., Gerdes, A. C., Mrug, S., Hinshaw, S. P., Bukowski, W. M., Gold, J. A., et al. (2005). Peer-assessed outcomes in the multimodal treatment study of children with Attention Deficit Hyperactivity Disorder. *Journal of Child and Adolescent Psychology, 34,* 74–86.

Huesmann, L. R., Moise-Titus, J., Podolski, C. L., & Eron, L. D. (2003). Longitudinal relations between children's exposure to TV violence and their aggressive and violent behavior in young adulthood: 1977–1992. *Developmental Psychology, 39,* 201–221.

Hynd, G. W., Semrud-Clikeman, M., Lorys, A. R., Novey, E. S., Eliopulos, D., & Lyytinen, H. (1991). Corpus callosum morphology in attention deficit hyperactivity disorder: Morphometric analysis of MRI. *Journal of Learning Disabilities, 24,* 141–146.

Jaffee, S. R., Caspi, A., Moffitt, T. E., Dodge, K. A., Rutter, M., Taylor, A., et al. (2005). Nature×nurture: Genetic vulnerabilities interact with physical maltreatment to promote conduct problems. *Development & Psychopathology, 17,* 67–84.

James, A., & Taylor, E. (1990). Sex differences in the hyperkinetic syndrome of childhood. *Journal of Child Psychology and Psychiatry, 31,* 437–446.

Jensen, P. S., Garcia, J. A., Glied, S., Foster, M., Schlander, M., Hinshaw, S., et al. (2005). Cost-effectiveness of ADHD treatments: Findings from the multimodal treatment study of children with ADHD. *American Journal of Psychiatry, 162*(9), 1628–1636.

Jensen, P. S., Hinshaw, S. P., Kraemer, H. C., Lenora, N., Newcorn, J. H., & Abikoff, H. B. (2001). ADHD comorbidity findings from the MTA study: Comparing comorbid subgroups. *Journal of the American Academy of Child & Adolescent Psychiatry, 40*(2), 147–158.

Jensen, P. S., Martin, D., & Cantwell, D. P. (1997). Comorbidity in ADHD: Implications for research, practice, and *DSM-IV. Journal of the American Academy of Child and Adolescent Psychiatry, 36,* 1065–1079.

Johnston, C., & Mash, E. J. (2001). Families of children with attention-deficit/hyperactivity disorder: Review and recommendations for future research. *Clinical Child and Family Psychology Review, 4,* 183–207.

Kazdin, A. E. (1995) *Conduct disorders in childhood and adolescence* (2nd ed.). Thousand Oaks, CA: Sage.

Kazdin, A. E. (2005). *Parent management training: Treatment for oppositional, aggressive, and antisocial behavior in children and adolescents.* New York: Oxford University Press.

Kazdin, A. E., & Whitley, M. K. (2003). Treatment of parental stress to enhance therapeutic change among children referred for aggressive and antisocial behavior. *Journal of Consulting and Clinical Psychology, 71,* 504–515.

Keenan, K., & Shaw, D. (1997). Development and social influences on young girls' early problem behavior. *Psychological Bulletin, 121,* 95–113.

Kimonis, E. R., Frick, P. J., Boris, N. W., Smyke, A. T., Cornell, A.H., Farrell, J. M., et al. (2006). Callous-unemotional features, behavioral inhibition, and parenting: Independent predictors of aggression in a high-risk preschool sample. *Journal of Child and Family Studies, 15*(4),

Kimonis, E. R., Frick, P. J., Fazekas, H., & Loney, B. R. (2006). Psychopathic traits, aggression, and the processing of emotional stimuli in non-referred children. *Behavioral Sciences and the Law, 24*, 21–37.

Kitchens, S. A., Rosen, L. A., & Braaten, E. B. (1999). Differences in anger, aggression, depression, and anxiety between ADHD and non-ADHD children. *Journal of Attention Disorders, 3*, 77–83.

Klein, R. G., & Abikoff, H. (1997). Behavior therapy and methylphenidate in the treatment of children with ADHD. *Journal of Attention Disorders, 2*, 89–114.

Kochanska, G. (1993). Toward a synthesis of parental socialization and child temperament in early development of conscience. *Child Development, 64*, 325–347.

Kratzer, L., & Hodgins, S. (1997). Adult outcomes of child conduct problems: A cohort study. *Journal of Abnormal Child Psychology, 25*, 65 – 81.

Kruh, I. P., Frick, P. J., & Clements, C. B. (2005). Historical and personality correlates to the violence patterns of juveniles tried as adults. *Criminal Justice and Behavior, 32*, 69–96.

Lahey, B. B., Applegate, B., Barkley, R. A., Garfinkel, B., McBurnett, K., Kerdyck, L., et al. (1994). *DSM-IV* field trials for oppositional defiant disorder and conduct disorder in children and adolescents. *American Journal of Psychiatry, 151*, 1163–1171.

Lahey, B. B., Carlson, C. L., & Frick, P. J. (1997). Attention deficit disorder without hyperactivity. In T. A. Widiger, A. J. Frances, H. A. Pincus, R. Ross, M. B. First, & W. Davis (Eds.), *DSM-IV sourcebook* (Vol. 3, pp. 163–188). Washington, D.C.: American Psychiatric Press.

Lahey, B. B., & Loeber, R. (1994). Framework for a developmental model of oppositional defiant disorder and conduct disorder. In D. K. Routh (Ed.), *Disruptive behavior disorders in childhood* (pp. 139–180). New York: Plenum.

Lahey, B. B., Loeber, R., Hart, E. L., Frick, P. J., Applegate, B., Qhang, Q., et al. (1995). Four year longitudinal study of conduct disorder in boys: Patterns and predictors of persistence. *Journal of Abnormal Psychology, 104*, 83–93.

Lahey, B. B., Pelham, W. E., Loney, J., Lee, S. S., & Wilcutt, E. (2005). Instability of the *DSM-IV* subtypes of ADHD from preschool through elementary school. *Archives of General Psychiatry, 62*, 896–902.

Lahey, B. B., Schwab-Stone, M., Goodman, S. H., Waldman, I. D., Canino, G., Rathouz, P. J., et al. (2000). Age and gender differences in oppositional behavior and conduct problems: A cross-sectional household study of middle childhood and adolescence. *Journal of Abnormal Psychology, 109*, 488–503.

Lambert, N. M. (1988). Adolescent outcomes for hyperactive children. *American Psychologist, 43*, 786–799.

Landgren, M., Pettersson, R., Kjellman, B., & Gillberg, C. (1996). ADHD, DAMP, and other neurodevelopmental/ psychiatric disorders in 6-year-old children epidemiology and co-morbidity. *Developmental Medical Child Neurology, 38*, 891–906.

Larson J., & Lochman J. E . (2003). *Helping schoolchildren cope with anger.* New York: Guilford.

Lilienfeld, S. O., & Waldman, I. D. (1990). The relation between childhood attention-deficit hyperactivity disorder and adult antisocial behavior reexamined: The problem of heterogeneity. *Clinical Psychology Review, 10*, 699–725.

Loeber, R. (1982). The stability of antisocial and delinquent child behavior: A review. *Child Development, 53*, 1431–1446.

Loeber, R. (1991). Antisocial behavior: More enduring than changeable? *Journal of the American Academy of Child and Adolescent Psychiatry, 30*, 393-397.

Loeber, R., Green, S. M., Lahey, B. B., Christ, M. A. G., & Frick, P. J. (1992). Developmental sequences in the age of onset of disruptive child behaviors. *Journal of Child and Family Studies, 1*, 21–41.

Loney, B. R., Frick, P. J., Clements, C. B., Ellis, M. L., & Kerlin, K. (2003). Callous-unemotional traits, impulsivity, and emotional processing in antisocial adolescents. *Journal of Clinical Child and Adolescent Psychology, 32*, 66–80.

Loney, B. R., Frick, P. J., Ellis, M., & McCoy, M. G. (1998). Intelligence, psychopathy, and antisocial behavior. *Journal of Psychopathology and Behavioral Assessment, 20*, 231–247.

Loo, S. K., & Barkley, R. A. (2005). Clinical utility of EEG in Attention Deficit Hyperactivity Disorder. *Applied Neuropsychology, 12*(2), 64–76.

Lou, H. C., Henriksen, L., & Bruhn, P. (1984). Focal cerebral hypoperfusion in children with dysphasia and/or attention deficit disorder. *Archives of Neurology, 41*, 825–829.

Lou, H. C., Henrikson, L., Bruhn, P., Borner, H., & Nielson, J. B. (1989). Striatal dysfunction in attention deficit and hyperkinetic disorder. *Archives of Neurology, 46*, 48–52.

Lyman, R. D., & Campbell, N. R. (1996). *Treating children and adolescents in residential and inpatient settings.* Thousand Oaks, CA: Sage.

Lynam, R. D., Caspi A., Moffitt T. E., Raine A., Loeber R., & Stouthamer-Loeber M. (2005). Adolescent psychopathy and the big five: Results from two samples. *Journal of Abnormal Child Psychology, 33*, 431–443.

Lytton, H. (1990). Child and parent effects in boys' conduct disorder: A reinterpretation. *Developmental Psychology, 26*, 683–697.

Mannuzza, S., Klein, R., Bessler, A., Malloy, P., & LaPadula, M. (1998). Adult psychiatric status of hyperactive boys grown up. *American Journal of Psychiatry, 155*, 493–498.

March, J. S., Swanson, J. M., Arnold, E., Hoza, B., Conners, K., Hinshaw, S. P., et al. (2000). Anxiety as a predictor and outcome variable in the multimodal treatment study of children with ADHD (MTA). *Journal of Abnormal Child Psychology, 28*, 527–541.

Marsee, M. A., Silverthorn, P., Frick, P. J. (2005). The association of psychopathic traits with aggression and delinquency in non-referred boys and girls. *Behavioral Sciences and the Law, 23*, 803–817

McBurnett, K., Pfiffner, L. T., & Frick, P. J. (2001). Symptom properties as a function of ADHD type: An argument for continued study of sluggish cognitive tempo. *Journal of Abnormal Child Psychology, 29*(3), 207–213.

McCabe, K. M., Rodgers, C., Yeh, M., & Hough, R. (2004). Gender differences in childhood onset conduct disorder. *Development & Psychopathology, 16*(1), 179–192.

McCoy, M. G., Frick, P. J., Loney, B. R., & Ellis, M. L. (2000). The potential mediating role of parenting practices in the development of conduct problems in a clinic-referred sample. *Journal of Child and Family Studies, 8,* 477–494.

McLoyd, V. C. (1990). The impact of economic hardship on black families and children: Psychological distress, parenting, and socioemotional development. *Child Development, 61,* 311–346.

Milich, R., Balentine, A. C., & Lynam, D. R. (2001). ADHD combined type and ADHD predominantly inattentive type are distinct and unrelated disorders. *Clinical Psychology: Research and Practice, 8,* 463–488.

Moffitt, T. E. (1990). Juvenile delinquency and attention deficit disorder: Boys' developmental trajectories from age 3 to age 15. *Child Development, 61,* 893–910.

Moffitt, T. E. (2003). Life-course persistent and adolescence-limited antisocial behavior: A 10-year research review and research agenda. In B. B. Lahey, T. E., Moffitt, & A. Caspi (Eds.), *Causes of conduct disorder and juvenile delinquency* (pp. 49–75). New York: Guilford.

Moffitt, T. E., & Caspi, A. (2001). Childhood predictors differentiate life-course persistent and adolescent-limited antisocial pathways among males and females. *Development and Psychopathology, 13,* 355–376.

Moffitt, T. E., Caspi, A., Dickson, N., Silva, P., & Stanton, W. (1996). Childhood-onset versus adolescent-onset antisocial conduct problems in males: Natural history from ages 3 to 18 years. *Development and Psychopathology, 8,* 399–424.

Moffitt, T. E., Caspi, A., Harrington, H., & Milne, B. J. (2002). Males on the life-course persistent and adolescent-limited antisocial pathways: Follow-up at age 26 years. *Development and Psychopathology, 14,* 179–207.

MTA Cooperative Group. (1999). A 14-month randomized clinical trial of treatment strategies for attention deficit hyperactivity disorder. *Archives of General Psychology, 56,* 1073–1086.

Nigg, J. T. (2006). *What causes ADHD? Understanding what goes wrong and why.* New York: Guilford.

O'Brien, B. S., & Frick, P. J. (1996). Reward dominance: Associations with anxiety, conduct problems and psychopathy in children. *Journal of Abnormal Child Psychology, 24,* 223–240.

O'Donnell, C. R. (1995). Firearms deaths among children and youth. *American Psychologist, 50,* 771–776.

Osofsky, J. D., Wewers, S., Hann, D. M., & Fick, A. C. (1993). Chronic community violence: What is happening to our children? *Psychiatry, 56,* 36–45.

Oxford, M., Cavell, T. A., & Hughes, J. N. (2003). Callous-unemotional traits moderate the relation between ineffective parenting and child externalizing problems: A partial replication and extension. *Journal of Clinical Child & Adolescent Psychology, 42,* 364–371.

Pardini, D. A. (2006). The callousness pathway to severe and violent delinquency. *Aggressive Behavior, 32,* 1–9.

Pardini, D. A., Lochman, J. E., & Frick, P. J. (2003). Callous/unemotional traits and social cognitive processes in adjudicated youth. *Journal of the American Academy of Child & Adolescent Psychiatry, 42,* 364–371.

Pauls, D. (2005). The genetics of attention-deficit/hyperactivity disorder. *Biological Psychiatry, 57,* 1310–1312.

Peeples, F., & Loeber, R. (1994). Do individual factors and neighborhood context explain ethnic differences in juvenile delinquency? *Journal of Quantitative Criminology, 10,* 141–157.

Pelham, W. E. (1993). Pharmacotherapy for children with attention-deficit hyperactivity disorder. *School Psychology Review, 22,* 199–227.

Pelham, W. E. (1999). The NIMH multimodal treatment study for attention-deficit hyperactivity disorder: Just say yes to drugs alone? *Canadian Journal of Psychiatry, 44,* 765–775.

Pelham, W. E., Carlson, C., Sams, S. E., Vallan, G., Dixon, M. J., & Hoza, B. (1993). Separate and combined effects of methylphenidate and behavior modification on boys with attention deficit-hyperactivity disorder in the classroom. *Journal of Consulting and Clinical Psychology, 61,* 506–515.

Pelham, W. E., Gnagy, E. M., Greiner, A. R., Hoza, B., Hinshaw, S. P., Swanson, J. M., et al. (2000). Behavioral versus behavioral and pharmacological treatment in ADHD children attending a summer treatment program. *Journal of Abnormal Child Psychology, 28,* 507–526.

Pelham, W. E., Wheeler, T., & Chronis, A. (1998). Empirically supported psychosocial treatments for attention deficit hyperactivity disorder. *Journal of Clinical Child Psychology, 27,* 190–205.

Quay, H. C. (1986). Classification. In H. C. Quay & J. S. Weery (Eds.), *Psychopathological disorders of childhood* (pp. 1–34). New York: Wiley.

Raine, A. (2002). Biosocial studies of antisocial and violent behavior in children and adults: A review. *Journal of Abnormal Child Psychology, 30,* 311–326.

Raine, A., Venables, P. H., & Mednick, S. A. (1997). Low resting heart rate at age 3 years predisposes to aggression at age 11 years: Evidence from the Mauritius Child Health Project. *Journal of the American Academy of Child & Adolescent Psychiatry, 36*(10), 1457–1464.

Rasmussen, P., & Gillberg, C. (2001). Natural outcome of ADHD with developmental coordination disorder at 22 years: A controlled, longitudinal, community-based study. *Journal of the American Academic of Child and Adolescent Psychiatry, 39,* 1424–1431.

Richters, J. E., Arnold, L. E., Jensen, P. S., Abikoff, H., Conners, C.K., Greenhill, L. L., et al. (1995). The National Institute of Mental Health collaborative multisite multimodal treatment study of children with attention deficit hyperactivity disorder (MTA): I. Background and rationale. *Journal of the American Academy of Child and Adolescent Psychiatry, 34,* 987–1000.

Robins, L. N. (1966). *Deviant children grown up.* Baltimore, MD: Williams & Wilkins.

Ross, A. O. (1981). *Child behavior therapy: Principles, procedures, and empirical basis.* New York: Wiley

Rucklidge, J. J., & Tannock, R. (2001). Psychiatric, psychosocial, and cognitive functioning of female adolescents with ADHD. *Journal of the American Academy of Child and Adolescent Psychiatry, 40,* 530–540.

Rutter, M. (1977). Brain damage syndromes in childhood: Concepts and findings. *Journal of Child Psychology and Psychiatry, 18,* 1–21.

Schaeffer, C. M., & Borduin, C. M. (2005). Long-term follow-up to a randomized clinical trial of multisystemic therapy with serious and violent juvenile offenders. *Journal of Consulting and Clinical Psychology, 73 ,* 445–453.

Schatz, D. B. & Rostain, A. L. (2006). ADHD with comorbid anxiety: A review of the current literature. *Journal of Attention Disorders, 10,* 141–149.

Shaw, D. S., Gilliom, M., Ingoldsby, E. M., & Nagin, D. S. (2003). Trajectories leading to school-age conduct problems. *Developmental Psychology, 39,* 201–221.

Silverthorn, P., & Frick, P. J. (1999). Developmental pathways to antisocial behavior: The delayed-onset pathway in girls. *Development and Psychopathology, 11,* 101–126.

Silverthorn, P., Frick, P. J., Kuper, K., & Ott, J. (1996). Attention-deficit hyperactivity disorder and sex: A test of two etiological models to explain the male predominance. *Journal of Clinical Child Psychology, 25,* 52–59.

Silverthorn, P., Frick, P. J., & Reynolds, R. (2001). Timing of onset and correlates of severe conduct problems in adjudicated girls and boys. *Journal of Psychopathology and Behavioral Assessment, 23*(3), 171–181.

Spira, E. G., & Fischel, J. E. (2005). The impact of preschool inattention, hyperactivity, and impulsivity on social and academic development: A review. *Journal of Child Psychology and Psychiatry, 46,* 755–773.

Sprich, S., Biederman, J., Crawford, M. H., Mundy, E., & Faraone, S. V. (2000). Adoptive and biological families of children and adolescents with ADHD. *Journal of the American Academy of Child and Adolescent Psychiatry, 39,* 1432–1437.

Stein, J., Schettler, T., Wallinga, D., & Valenti, M. (2002). In harm's way: Toxic threats to child development. *Journal of Developmental and Behavioral Pediatrics, 23,* 13–22.

Stevenson, J. (1992). Evidence for genetic etiology in hyperactivity in children. *Behavior Genetics, 22,* 337–343.

Stewart, M. A., Pitts, F. N., Craig, A. G., & Dieruf, W. (1966). The hyperactive child syndrome. *American Journal of Orthopsychiatry, 36,* 403–407.

Strauss, A. A., & Lehtinen, L. E. (1947). *Psychopathology and education of the brain-injured child.* New York: Grune & Stratton.

Swanson, J. M., Kraemer, H. C., Hinshaw, S. P., Arnold, L. E., Conners, C. K., Abikoff, H. B., et al. (2001). Clinical relevance of the primary findings of the MTA: Success rates based on severity of ADHD and ODD symptoms at the end of treatment. *Journal of the American Academy of Child and Adolescent Psychiatry, 40,* 168–179.

Swanson, J. M., McBurnett, K., Christian, D. L., & Wigal, T. (1995). Stimulant medication and treatment of children with ADHD. In T. H. Ollendick & R. J. Prinz (Eds.), *Advances in clinical child psychology* (Vol.17, pp. 265–322). New York: Plenum.

Underwood, M. K. (2003). *Social aggression among girls.* New York: Guilford.

Verhulst, F. C., Van der Ende, J., Ferdinand, R. F., & Kasius, M. C. (1997). The prevalence of *DSM-III-R* diagnoses in a national sample of Dutch adolescents. *Archives of General Psychiatry, 54,* 329–336.

Viding E., Blair R. J. R., Moffitt T. E., & Plomin, R. (2005). Evidence for substantial genetic risk for psychopathy in 7-year-olds. *Journal of Child Psychology and Psychiatry, 46,* 592–597.

Wang, Y. C., Chong, M. Y., & Chou, W. J. (1993). Prevalence of ADHD in primary school children in Taiwan. *Journal of the Formosan Medical Association, 92,* 133–138.

Waschbusch, D. A. (2002). A meta-analytic examination of comorbid hyperactive-impulsive-attention problems and conduct problems. *Psychological Bulletin, 128,* 118–150.

Weiss, G., & Hechtman, L. T. (1993). *Hyperactive Children Grown Up: ADHD in Children, Adolescents, and Adults.* New York: Guilford.

Wells, K. C., Pelham, W. E., Kotkin, R. A., Hoza, B., Abikoff, H. B., Abramowitz, A., et al. (2000). Psychosocial treatment strategies in the MTA study: Rationale, methods, and critical issues in design and implementation. *Journal of Abnormal Child Psychology, 28,* 483–505.

Wootton, J. M., Frick, P. J., Shelton, K. K., & Silverthorn, P. (1997). Ineffective parenting and childhood conduct problems: The moderating role of callous-unemotional traits. *Journal of Consulting and Clinical Psychology, 65,* 301–308.

World Health Organization (2002). *World report on violence and health.* Geneva: Author.

Zametkin, A. J., Liebenauer, L. L., Fitzgerald, G. A., King, A. C., Minkunas, D.V., Herscovitch, P., et al. (1993). Brain metabolism in teenagers with attention deficit hyperactivity disorder. *Archives of General Psychiatry, 50,* 333–340.

Zametkin, A. J, & Liotta, W. (1998). The neurobiology of attention deficit hyperactivity disorder. *Journal of Clinical Psychiatry, 59,* 17–23.

Zametkin, A. J., Nordahl, T. E., Gross, M., King, A. C., Semple, W. E., Rumsey, J., et al. (1990). Cerebral glucose metabolism in adults with hyperactivity of childhood onset. *New England Journal of Medicine, 323,* 1361–1366.

Zoccolillo, M. (1993). Gender and the development of conduct disorder. *Development and Psychopathology, 5,* 65–78.

17
Internalizing Disorders in Children and Adolescents

Thomas H. Ollendick, Alison L. Shortt, and Janay B. Sander

Internalizing disorders in childhood and adolescence include the anxiety and affective disorders. As such, they consist of problems related to worry, fear, shyness, low self-esteem, sadness, and depression. These "emotional" problems have frequently been found to be interrelated in clinical settings and to be associated statistically with one another in factor analytic studies. Internalizing problems can be contrasted with externalizing problems—problems frequently associated with inattention, bad conduct, and opposition and defiance (see chapter 16). It is of historic interest to note that these two broad dimensions of childhood and adolescent problems have been recognized for some time. Karen Horney (1945), for example, spoke of children who "move against the world" (i.e., externalizing disorder children) and those who "move away from the world" (i.e., internalizing disorder children).

Although there is little question about the existence of internalizing problems in childhood and adolescence and their detrimental effects on the growing child and adolescent (Ollendick & King, 1994), there is considerable controversy about whether they constitute a single broadband internalizing disorder or whether they constitute multiple, narrow-band disorders. At the heart of this issue is the frequent observation that anxiety disorders and affective disorders frequently co-occur with one another (i.e., are comorbid disorders) and that they are rarely observed in their "pure" forms, at least in childhood and adolescence (Ollendick & March, 2004). For example, in an early study, Last, Strauss, and Francis (1987) found that 73% of separation anxious children and adolescents and 79% of overanxious disorder children and adolescents presented at their outpatient clinic for *anxious* children with one or more additional psychiatric disorders, including major depressive disorders. Similarly, Kovacs, Feinberg, Crouse-Novak, Paulauskas, and Finkelstein (1984) demonstrated early on that a majority of children and adolescents who presented at their outpatient clinic for *depressed* children were diagnosed with concurrent disorders. In fact, 79% of youths with a major depressive disorder and 93% of the cases who presented with dysthymic disorder had a concurrent psychiatric disorder, of which one of the most common was an anxiety disorder. Of importance for the developmental sequence of these disorders, Kovacs et al. reported that anxiety disorders tended to precede the depressive disorders when these two conditions were present in the same child or adolescent. Last, Perrin, Hersen, and Kazdin (1992) have reaffirmed these rates of comorbidity and developmental sequellae, as have Seligman and Ollendick (1998).

Although the major anxiety and affective disorders in childhood and adolescence overlap, we will present them as separate entities in this chapter, consistent with nosological approaches, such as the *Diagnostic and Statistical Manual* (*DSM-IV,* 1994; *DSM-IV-TR,* American Psychiatric Association, 2000) and *International Classification of Diseases* (*ICD-10*; World Health Organization, 1992). In doing so, we will point out areas of overlap and draw distinctions between them. We recognize this decision is not without controversy, but it is consistent with much of clinical practice and research, and it allows us to present information about the disorders in a coherent and organized manner. Prior to examining specific aspects of these disorders, however, we first examine basic tenets of developmental psychopathology inasmuch as this approach informs our perspective on clinical disorders in children and adolescents.

Basic Premises of Developmental Psychopathology

Within the field of developmental psychology, theorists have long debated which developmental model best explains the many changes that occur in individuals throughout their development and across their life span.

Developmental Theory

Early debates were focused upon issues of autonomy and organization and were tied to two major worldviews: the *mechanistic* and *organismic* models of development. According to the mechanistic view (Baer, 1982; Skinner, 1938), organisms were viewed as similar to machines that were acted upon largely by forces from the outside world. That is, with regard to development, organisms were viewed primarily as passive recipients of information and relatively passive respondents to increasingly complex and varied stimulus input (i.e., a tabula rasa). Furthermore, it was believed that changes in behavior over time reflected gradual modifications in antecedent and consequent stimuli with explanations for development derived largely from principles of learning theory (e.g., conditioning, reinforcement). Skinner (1938), for example, suggested "the basic premise of behavioral psychology (was) that all organisms, human and subhuman, *young and old* (italics added), were subject to the same law of effect (principle of reinforcement) and could be studied in the same basic manner" (p. 27). From this perspective, many clinicians and researchers viewed development and developmental processes as possessing relatively little clinical significance (see Gelfand & Peterson, 1985; Ollendick & Cerny, 1981, for extended discussions of this point).

In contrast to the passive qualities of the organism portrayed in the mechanistic view, proponents of the organismic model of development (Erickson, 1968; Freud, 1940/1949; Piaget, 1950) asserted that organisms were not passive; rather, they were viewed as agents who were actively involved in the construction of their own environments. Furthermore, organismic theorists often described development as if it passed through discrete and oftentimes invariant stages (e.g., Piaget's stages of cognitive development, Freud's psychosexual stages, and Erickson's stages of identity development). These various theories maintained that basic structures and functions changed across age and that they reflected emerging, qualitatively different ways of interacting with the environment. In its simplest form, this model proposed that change resulted largely from maturational processes that were determined by intrinsic organismic factors rather than by extrinsic environmental ones.

Decades of debate among proponents of these two models as well as recognition of their limitations led to the advent of a third model of development, namely, the *transactional model*. Also known as *developmental contextualism*, the transactional model moved beyond the mechanismic and organismic points of view (Lerner, Hess, & Nitz, 1991; Sameroff, 1995) and was highly consistent with the tenets of social learning/social cognitive theory (cf, Bandura 1977, 1986; Ollendick & Cerny, 1981). According to this model, developmental changes were proposed to occur as a result of continuous reciprocal interactions (i.e., reciprocal determinism, transactions) between an active organism and its active environmental context. Organisms were said to affect their own development by being both producers and products of their environments (Lerner et al., 1991). Although differences in theory and philosophy remain, most developmental theorists agree that development involves systematic, successive, and adaptive changes within and across life periods in the structure, function, and content of the individual's cognitive, emotional, behavioral, social, and interpersonal characteristics (Lease & Ollendick, 2000; Sameroff, 1995; Silverman & Ollendick, 1999). Inasmuch as developmental changes occur in an orderly and sequential fashion (i.e., they are systematic and successive), changes observed at one point in time will influence subsequent events (although not necessarily in a direct linear fashion, see below). Changes that occur at one point in time (whether due to learning, an unfolding of basic predetermined structures, or some complex, interactive/transactional process) have an impact on subsequent development. Thus, the diversity or variety of changes possible at a later point in time are constrained by, but not solely determined by, those that occur at an earlier point in time.

Developmental Psychopathology

Developmental psychopathology is, of course, firmly grounded in developmental theory (Rutter & Garmezy, 1983). Sroufe and Rutter (1984, p.18) define developmental psychopathology as "the study of the origins and course of individual patterns of behavioral maladaptation, whatever the age of onset, whatever the causes, whatever the transformations in behavioral manifestations, and however complex the course of developmental pattern may be." Implicit in this definition is concern with development and developmental deviations (i.e., clinical psychopathologies) that occur throughout and across the life span and the processes associated with those perturbations. The study of psychopathology, from this perspective, is organized around milestones, transitions, and sequences in physical, cognitive, and social-emotional development. Thus, development is viewed as a series of qualitative reorganizations within and among various systems. The character of these reorganizations is determined by factors at various levels of analysis (e.g., genetic, constitutional, physiological, behavioral, psychological, environmental, and sociological) that are in dynamic transaction with one another (Cicchetti, 1989; Lewis, 1990). Pathological development is understood then as a lack of integration among these systems that contributes synergistically to (mal)adaptation at particular developmental levels (i.e., childhood, adolescence).

Although development at any one point in time is assumed to affect later functioning, direct or isomorphic continuity of behavior is not implied nor expected. Rather, multiple pathways through which developmental outcomes may occur are proposed: both normal and abnormal development results from individually distinct and unique transactions between a changing organism and its ever-changing environmental context. This notion is captured in the developmental principle of *equifinality*—the principle that any one outcome (i.e., a depressive disorder) may result from multiple and diverse pathways. From a developmental perspective, the expectation that a singular pathway to a given disorder exists would be the exception, not the rule (Kazdin & Kagan, 1994; Lease & Ollendick, 2000; Toth & Cicchetti, 1999). In contradistinction to the principle of equifinality, the principle of *multifinality* asserts that varied outcomes can eventuate from the same common starting point. Thus, for example, any one risk factor associated with the development of a disorder (e.g., "behavioral inhibition to the unfamiliar," Kagan, 1994) is likely to result in a variety of outcomes, not just anxiety disorders. It is therefore important to identify and understand intra- and extraindividual characteristics that promote or inhibit early deviations or maintain or disrupt early adaptation and development. Toward this end, the field of developmental psychopathology is primarily concerned with the origins and course of a given disorder, its precursors and sequellae, its variations in manifestation with development, and more broadly, its relations to nondisordered behavior patterns (Rutter, 1985; Toth & Cicchetti, 1999).

As may be evident, the developmental psychopathology perspective does not subscribe to a particular theoretical orientation (i.e., medical model, psychodynamic theory, social learning theory) for the understanding of diverse child psychopathologies, nor does it supplant particular theories; rather, it sharpens our awareness about connections among phenomena that may otherwise seem unrelated or disconnected. Achenbach (1990) refers to it as a macroparadigm that serves to bridge a variety of conceptual models (i.e., microparadigms). The utility of this approach has been demonstrated in the conceptualization of a variety of disorders including depression and anxiety in children and adolescents (Cicchetti & Schneider-Rosen, 1986; Lease & Ollendick, 2000; Ollendick & Hirshfeld-Becker, 2002; Vasey & Dadds, 2000).

Anxiety Disorders in Children and Adolescents

For children and adults alike, anxiety is a normal and common emotional response to a perceived threat to one's physical or emotional well-being. Feeling fearful and fleeing from a genuinely dangerous situation is adaptive. However, if the anxiety response is elicited by a situation or object that is not truly dangerous, then the anxiety and the avoidance associated with it are no longer adaptive.

Phenomenology

A diagnosis of an anxiety disorder may be warranted if the anxiety response is excessive in frequency, intensity, or duration, and if it results in significant impairment in functioning. Excessive anxiety is distressing to children and adolescents, and the associated avoidance interferes with their ability to engage in developmentally appropriate tasks and activities. Alarmingly, anxiety disorders are one of the most common psychological difficulties experienced by children and adolescents, and these disorders tend to persist into late adolescence and adulthood unless effective treatment is received (Ollendick & March, 2004; Ollendick & Seligman, 2006).

Consistent with Lang's (1979) tripartite model, anxiety is viewed as a multidimensional construct involving *physiological* features such as increased heart rate and respiration, *cognitive* ideation including catastrophic and unhelpful thoughts (e.g., "I can't do it"; "What if something terrible happens?"), and *behavioral* responses such as avoidance of the anxiety provoking object or situation. Furthermore, there are developmental differences in the expression of anxiety. For example, young children may avoid objects or situations that scare them; however, they may have difficulty identifying the exact cognitions associated with the feared situation. Young children may also have trouble relating or connecting their physiological symptoms to their anxiety. For example, a child with separation anxiety might insist that the reason she has a headache when she has to go to school is because of the flu, not because she is fearful about being separated from her caregivers.

Developmental Considerations For most, if not all, children and adolescents, fears and worries are a normal part of development. Accordingly, clinicians assessing anxiety in children need to be aware of what constitutes "normal" fear and anxiety at each level of development. For example, young infants and toddlers tend to fear aspects of their immediate environment such as loud noises, unfamiliar people, separation from their caregivers, or heights. Fears of animals, being alone, and of the dark begin to emerge during preschool years. As cognitive abilities continue to develop during the early school years, children's fears begin to include abstract, imaginary, or anticipatory fears such as fear of failure or evaluation, death, bodily injury, and supernatural phenomena. Finally, concerns about death, danger, social comparison, personal conduct, and physical appearance extend from adolescence to adulthood (Gullone, 2000; King, Muris, & Ollendick, 2004; Ollendick, King, & Muris, 2002).

Developmentally normal fears are, by definition, age appropriate and transitory in nature. In contrast, a diagnosis of an anxiety disorder is warranted only when a child experiences anxiety that is not typical of a child his or her age, and when a child experiences anxiety that is severe and causes considerable distress, or which impairs a child's functioning at home, at school, or in peer and family relationships.

Gender Differences

Research examining the prevalence of anxiety disorders in boys and girls has produced mixed results. Studies using community samples have found that girls are more likely to report anxiety than boys (Essau, Conradt, & Petermann, 2000; McGee et al., 1990). In contrast, gender differences are usually not found in clinic samples (Strauss & Last, 1993). There are at least two plausible explanations for this discrepancy. First, societal expectations of gender appropriate behavior for boys and girls may mean that girls are more open to reporting anxiety symptoms than boys in community samples. Alternatively, anxiety symptoms may indeed be more common in girls than boys, and the equal ratio of males to females in clinic samples may indicate that boys experiencing anxiety are more likely to be referred for treatment than girls with similar symptoms.

The direction and size of the gender difference is also dependent on the diagnostic category being considered. Generalized anxiety disorder (GAD) appears to be similarly prevalent in boys and girls during childhood, although in adolescence it is more common among females than males (Cohen et al., 1993; Kendall, Pimentel, Rynn, Algelosante, & Webb, 2004; Werry, 1991). Research concerning gender differences for Separation Anxiety Disorder (SAD) has been mixed. Although some studies find no gender differences for SAD (Cohen et al., 1993; Last, Perrin et al., 1992), most studies find that girls outnumber boys (e.g., Anderson Williams, McGee, & Silva, 1987; Kashani, Orvaschel, Rosenberg, & Reid, 1989; Perwien & Bernstein, 2004). The research on social phobia is less clear, although few gender differences have been noted (Albano & Hayward, 2004; Beidel & Morris, 1995; Ollendick & Ingman, 2001).

Epidemiology

Estimated prevalence rates for the childhood anxiety disorders using *DSM* criteria have been found to vary dramatically but typically range between 7 and 12% (e.g., Anderson et al., 1987; Costello, Egger, & Angold, 2004; Kashani, Beck et al., 1987; Kashani, Orvaschel et al., 1989). For example, Anderson et al. showed that 7.4% of 792 children in the Dunedin, New Zealand longitudinal study met criteria for an anxiety disorder when they were 11 years of age. At 15 years of age, McGee et al. (1990) reported that 10.7% of the adolescents in this same sample met criteria for an anxiety disorder. A 3.3% increase in the anxiety disorders was evident over the four-year period of time. Similar prevalence rates for the anxiety disorders have been found by a host of other researchers, with many indicating that the prevalence of some anxiety disorders increases with age (e.g., GAD, social phobia, panic disorder), whereas the prevalence of other disorders tends to decrease with age (e.g., SAD, specific phobia). Thus, overall prevalence rates vary by gender, age, and the diagnostic category being considered, as we shall illustrate next.

DSM-IV Diagnostic Categories and Associated Prevalence

DSM-IV describes separation anxiety disorder (SAD) as developmentally inappropriate and excessive anxiety associated with separation from home or from those to whom the individual is attached. Often children with SAD worry about danger or harm coming to themselves (e.g., being kidnapped) or their loved one (e.g., becoming ill) when they are separated. Children with SAD exhibit distress when they are separated from their attachment figure and will undertake steps to avoid being apart from them. This may result in children refusing to attend school, attend summer camps, and sleep away from home. The evidence indicates that as children become older, the prevalence of SAD declines: in the

Dunedin study, it was shown that the 12-month prevalence rate for SAD was 3.5% for the 11-year-old children but 2.0% for the 15-year-old adolescents. In adolescence, this disorder seems to become less common compared to other disorders such as GAD, social phobia, and panic disorder (Mattis & Ollendick, 2002).

Generalized anxiety disorder (GAD) is characterized as excessive anxiety and worry, which occurs more days than not for at least six months. These children find it difficult to control their worries about a number of events or activities. They tend to worry about what happened yesterday, what is happening now, and what will happen tomorrow. To meet criteria for GAD, children need to experience at least one associated physiological symptom, although typically these children report multiple physical symptoms. Physical symptoms include stomachaches or nausea, headaches, muscle tension, restlessness, irritability, fatigue, and sleep disturbance. The *DSM-IV* category of GAD in children replaced overanxious disorder (OAD; *DSM-III-R*; American Psychiatric Association, 1980). As noted above, there is some evidence to suggest that the prevalence of OAD/GAD increases with age (Kashani et al., 1989).

Specific phobia (SP) is defined as persistent fear of a specific object or situation that is excessive or unreasonable. Phobias of certain animals or insects, the dark, heights, storms, and medical procedures are among the most common in children. A recent study conducted in Germany reported a prevalence rate of 2.5% in 12- to 17-year-olds (Essau et al., 2000). Studies in the United States have reported prevalence rates ranging from 3.6 to 9% (Costello et al., 1988; Kashani, Beck et al., 1987; Kessler et al., 1994). Taken together, studies suggest a prevalence rate of about 5% for specific phobia in children and adolescents (King et al., 2004; Ollendick, Hagopian, & King, 1997).

Social phobia (SOP), also known as social anxiety disorder, in children as in adults is characterized by a marked or persistent fear of social situations or performance situations. Typically, in these situations, the child is exposed to unfamiliar people or is scrutinized by others. SOP is a disorder with a later age of onset (usually around 11 years of age), being rarely diagnosed in children younger than 10 years old (Davidson, Hughes, George, & Blazer, 1993). Of the changes in diagnostic criteria from the *DSM-III-R* to *DSM-IV*, the difference between the previous category of avoidant disorder and the new category of social phobia has been found to be the most significant (Kendall & Warman, 1996). This disparity has made comparison of prevalence rates across studies using these two systems more difficult. Using the *DSM-III-R*, Anderson et al. (1987) found that less than 1% of children aged 11 years and that none of the 15-year-olds in the Dunedin study were diagnosed with avoidant disorder. A later study using *DSM-IV* criteria reported that 6.3% of adolescents were diagnosed with social phobia. Although these results may suggest an increase in prevalence with age, it is more likely that they reflect changes in diagnostic criteria from *DSM-III-R* to *DSM-IV* (Schniering, Hudson, & Rapee, 2000).

Obsessive-compulsive disorder (OCD) is characterized by obsessions, which are recurrent thoughts, images, or impulses that are intrusive and result in an increase in anxiety. These obsessions are most often, though not always, accompanied by compulsions, which are repetitive behaviors that reduce anxiety (e.g., washing hands, or checking). Epidemiological data on the prevalence of OCD in pre-pubertal children has been reported to be less than 1% (Heyman et al., 2001). The prevalence rates for adolescents, however, range from 1.9 to 3.6% (Cook et al., 2001). The results of the Heyman et al. study suggest that prevalence may increase with age.

Differential Diagnosis and Comorbidity

Although recent research using the *DSM* classification system has facilitated the communication of knowledge between researchers and clinicians, the overlap in diagnostic criteria between some of these nosological categories has generated controversy. Briefly, the major problem, as we have noted earlier, is the co-occurrence of multiple disorders (i.e., comorbidity) in the same child or adolescent.

Several authors (e.g., Caron & Rutter, 1991) have argued that the categorical system of diagnosis does not accurately reflect the true nature of childhood anxiety and suggest that a dimensional approach may be preferred in dealing with the overarching issue of comorbidity (see also Widiger, this volume). Others, however, maintain that the current diagnostic system is sufficiently precise and that we need more refined research to clarify the boundaries among the various anxiety disorders (cf. Curry, March, & Hervey, 2004; Ollendick & March, 2004). Undoubtedly, there are positive aspects to both dimensional and categorical systems, depending upon the intended use of the information obtained from these somewhat disparate approaches.

In clinical populations, the most common comorbidity with any specific anxiety disorder is another type of anxiety disorder (Curry et al., 2004; Kendall, Brady, & Verduin, 2001). Across epidemiological and clinical studies using varied methodologies, disorders have been found to co-occur with one another at rates higher than chance (Caron & Rutter, 1991). Evidence of significant comorbidity is troubling because children with comorbid disorders tend to have a greater severity and persistence of symptoms, more interpersonal problems, and may be more refractory to change and clinically challenging for therapists (Manassis & Monga, 2001).

In addition to comorbidity with other anxiety disorders, anxious children may also exhibit high rates of depression (Brady & Kendall, 1992; Seligman, Goza, & Ollendick, 2004), as noted previously. Using a large cohort of 1,710 adolescents, the Oregon Adolescent Depression project found that 49% of the adolescents with an anxiety disorder also had comorbid depressive disorders using *DSM* criteria (Lewinsohn, Hops, Roberts, Seeley, & Andrews, 1993). Similarly, high rates of comorbidity were found in the Dunedin, New Zealand sample of youths (Anderson et al., 1987; McGee et al., 1990; McGee, Feehan, Williams, & Anderson, 1992). This series of studies also found that the rates of comorbid mood disorders increased as the children became older. Rates of comorbidity of anxiety and depressive disorders were higher among adolescents than among younger children.

Rates of comorbidity between anxiety and externalizing problems such as attention-deficit hyperactivity disorder (ADHD) are also high (Caron & Rutter, 1991). Studies examining this relationship have found that between 13 and 24% of children with an anxiety disorder also have ADHD, oppositional defiant disorder, or conduct disorder (Keller et al., 1992; Last et al., 1987). Consistent with these findings, Kendall et al. (2001) reported that 25% of their clinical sample of anxious children also met *DSM* criteria for one of these three disruptive behavior disorders.

Developmental Course and Prognosis

A common misconception is that children and adolescents will "outgrow" their worries and fears. Although this may be true of developmentally normal fears and everyday concerns, research suggests that anxiety disorders tend to persist unless treated (Ollendick & King, 1994). For example, Pfeffer, Lipkins, Plutchik, and Mizruchi (1988) found that for children aged 6 to 12 years who were diagnosed with OAD, 70.6% still met this diagnosis two years later. Similarly, in the Dunedin study, longitudinal results showed that girls diagnosed with an anxiety or depressive disorder at one age were more likely to continue to meet diagnostic criteria in subsequent years (McGee et al., 1990; McGee et al., 1992).

Anxiety disorders have been shown to persist not only over time but also to be associated with the development of more severe symptomatology (Albano, Chorpita, & Barlow, 1996). Older children tend to report more severe anxiety and comorbid symptomatology than do younger children with the same diagnosis (Strauss, Lease, Last, & Francis, 1988). Similarly, many adults with anxiety disorders report a lifelong history of anxiety symptoms beginning in childhood (Markowitz, Weissman, Ouellette, Lish, & Klerman, 1989; Ollendick, Lease, & Cooper, 1993). For example, a longitudinal study conducted in the United States found that children with an anxiety disorder were at greater risk for future anxiety disorders, and they were at increased risk of developing dysthymic disorders as well (Lewinsohn et al., 1993; Orvaschel, Lewinsohn, & Seeley, 1995).

Etiological Theories of Childhood Anxiety

Anxiety disorders in youth are likely the result of a complex interaction of numerous causal mechanisms, including personal characteristics of the child (e.g., genetic vulnerability, behavioral inhibition), problems in their immediate psychosocial context (attachment to caregivers, learning processes that occur within the family), and problems in the broader psychosocial context (e.g., impoverished environments, unsafe neighborhoods, countries at war). Some of these etiological factors will now be addressed briefly.

Genetics and Temperament Anxiety disorders tend to run in families. The etiology of anxiety disorders is likely to involve both environmental and genetic factors, and the interactions between them. Most twin studies support the conclusion that there is a heritable genetic risk for anxiety disorders, although the specific heritability estimates vary across studies according to the sample characteristics and measures used (e.g., Bolton et al., 2005; Eley et al., 2003; Feigon, Waldman, Levy, & Hay, 2001). It is likely that multiple genes are responsible for anxiety disorders, and the identification of these in coming years may enable early identification and prevention in individuals "at risk." However, a complete understanding of human genetics will be only part of the etiological puzzle, and questions about the processes of transmission from gene to behavior, and how environmental factors bring about changes in characteristics with strong genetic influences still have to be addressed (see also Smith, this volume).

One of the proposed mechanisms by which a predisposition for anxiety is transmitted genetically is via inherited temperamental characteristics such as behavioral inhibition. The category of behavioral inhibition, as described earlier, is suggested by Kagan and his colleagues to describe the 15 to 20% of children who react with withdrawal, avoidance, or distress when confronted with unfamiliar people, situations, or objects (Kagan, Reznick, & Snidman, 1987). Numerous studies have found that behaviorally inhibited children have increased risk for anxiety disorders (e.g., Biederman et al., 2001, Shamir-Essakow, Ungerer, & Rapee, 2005) and the most extremely inhibited children have higher risk (Turner, Beidel, & Wolff, 1996), as do those who remain stably inhibited over time (Hirshfeld et al., 1992). However, not all behaviorally inhibited children develop anxiety disorders. and it is best conceptualized as one possible predisposing factor that may lead to anxiety given the "right" set of other contextual conditions (Ollendick & Hirshfeld-Becker, 2002).

Learning Theories There are at least four major learning pathways to anxiety. First, fear and anxiety can be acquired through the pairing of previously neutral stimuli with aversive or traumatic stimuli or events (Wolpe & Rachman, 1960). Second, fears can be learned vicariously through observational learning or modeling (Bandura, 1977). Accordingly, fears may appear after a child has observed his or her parents, siblings, or peers reacting fearfully to certain objects or situations. Third, children may acquire fears by talking about fearful or frightening things and the verbal transmission of information may be sufficient. A fourth major learning pathway is through operant learning processes. If a child learns to cope with normative anxiety and fear responses through avoidance, then normal anxiety responses may be maintained at high levels and can turn into clinical anxiety (Ollendick, Vasey, & King, 2001). The concept of negative reinforcement is frequently used to explain how avoidant behavior maintains anxiety symptoms over time. Specifically when an anxious child avoids a feared situation, the child is reinforced by the resultant reduction in anxiety symptoms. In addition, avoidance behaviors may be positively reinforced by parents or caregivers. Barrett, Rapee, Dadds, and Ryan (1996) found that parents of clinically anxious children attended more to the anxious and avoidant behaviors of their children than to their brave coping behaviors. Although this study was unable to clarify whether this pattern of parenting behavior existed prior to or after the development of their child's anxiety, it does indicate that positive reinforcement from parents may serve to maintain anxiety symptoms.

Cognitive and Information Processing Biases Cognitive theorists suggest that when processing information, anxious people tend to overestimate the threat of danger and underestimate their abilities to cope with that threat (Beck, 1976, 1991). Attentional biases toward threat-related stimuli have been demonstrated in both clinically anxious (Taghavi, Neshat-Doost, Moradi, Yule, & Dalgleish, 1999) and nonclinically anxious children (Kindt, Brosschot, & Everaerd, 1997). Findings of biased attention in anxious children have been complemented by research examining the process of threat interpretation. A series of studies by Barrett and colleagues (Barrett, Rapee, Dadds, & Ryan, 1996; Dadds & Barrett, 1996; Dadds, Barrett, Rapee, & Ryan, 1996) demonstrated that clinically anxious children tended to interpret ambiguous vignettes of social and physical situations as threatening compared to nonclinical controls.

There is also evidence of a judgment bias characterized by negative or lowered estimates of coping ability in anxious children. Youth with anxiety disorders report significantly lower perceived control about anxiety related events (Weems, Silverman, Rapee, & Pina, 2003). Moreover, clinically anxious youth are more likely to choose avoidance responses when presented with vignettes depicting threatening situations (Bell-Dolan, Foster, & Christopher, 1995).

The Role of the Parent–Child Relationship in Child Anxiety Disorders An increasing number of studies have examined the relations between parenting behavior and anxiety in children. In cross-sectional studies, the parents of clinic-referred anxious children have been found to be more controlling (Dumas, La Freniere, & Sereketich, 1995), more restrictive (Krohne & Hock, 1991), more overinvolved emotionally (Hirshfeld, Biederman, Brody, Faraone, & Rosenbaum, 1997), less accepting, and less granting of psychological autonomy (Siqueland, Kendall, & Steinberg, 1996) than parents of nonreferred children. Studies of the observed behavior of anxious parents in both clinic (Whaley, Pinto, & Sigman, 1999) and community (Woodruff-Borden, Marrow, Bourland, & Cambron, 2002) samples have found that anxious mothers are less warm in interactions with their children and grant their children less autonomy. Parental overcontrol may convey the message to the child that she or he is incapable of handling challenging situations, as well as reducing learning opportunities by restricting exposure. Conversely, children with anxious temperaments may elicit protective responses from their parents. In support of the latter, Moore, Whaley and Sigman (2004) found that mothers in general tended to overprotect anxious children, no matter how anxious the mothers themselves were. More longitudinal studies are needed to draw conclusions about whether relations between parent behavior and anxiety represent cause or effect, or, whether it is reciprocal in nature (Dadds & Roth, 2001).

Assessment

Only a brief overview of assessment practices is provided herein (for a more detailed review of assessment practices with anxious youth, see Ollendick & Ollendick, 1997; Silverman & Ollendick, 2005; Silverman & Treffers, 2001). As discussed above, anxiety is recognized as a multidimensional construct and as such a multi-informant and multimethod approach to the assessment of childhood anxiety is recommended. Diagnostic interviews with the child and the child's parent/s are one of the best methods for distinguishing normal, developmentally appropriate fears and anxieties from problematic anxiety disorders. The most commonly used diagnostic interview to assess youth with anxiety disorders is the Anxiety Disorders Interview Schedule for Children (ADIS-C/P) (Silverman & Albano, 1996). This interview can be used to solicit detailed information about a range of individual anxiety symptoms, interference in daily functioning, school refusal behavior, interpersonal functioning, and avoided situations. In addition to the interviews, the child and her or his parents are usually asked to complete self-report questionnaires, and responses on these questionnaires can be compared to available normative data. Frequently used questionnaires include the Multidimensional Anxiety Scale for Children (MASC; March, Parker, Sullivan, Stallings, & Connor, 1997), the Revised Children's

Manifest Anxiety Scale (Reynolds & Richmond, 1985), the Spence Children's Anxiety Scale (Spence, 1998), and the Fear Survey Schedule for Children-Revised (Ollendick, 1983). Parents and teachers can also complete ratings scales such as the Child Behavior Checklist (CBCL) and Teacher Report Form (TRF, Achenbach, 1991). These scales have the advantage of measuring anxiety/depression symptoms as well as externalizing and other related problems. In addition to these measures, it is recommended that behavioral observation, cognitive assessment, and physiological assessment be considered.

Interventions

Interventions include pharmacological, psychosocial, and psychological.

Pharmacological Interventions There are a limited number of controlled pharmacological treatment trials for anxiety in children and adolescents. As but one example, Labellarte, Ginsburg, Walkup, and Riddle (1999) conducted an extensive review of psychopharmacological treatments for anxiety disorders in children and concluded that selective serotonin reuptake inhibitors (*SSRIs*) represent the first-line medical treatment for childhood anxiety disorders (as well as affective disorders). Serotonergic and tricyclic antidepressants are second-line anxiety agents, and Buspirone may be used as a second- or third-line anxiety treatment. Medication alone is rarely the treatment of choice for children with anxiety disorders, and typically medication is used in combination with psychological treatment (Ollendick & March, 2004).

Psychosocial Interventions Cognitive-behavioral therapy (CBT) for childhood anxiety has the strongest empirical support and randomized controlled trials investigating other therapies are unfortunately lacking (In-Albon & Schneider, in press; Ollendick & King, 1998; Ollendick, King, & Chorpita, 2006). CBT consists of four main strategies. First, *exposure* requires the child to approach the object or situation she or he fears or worries about, either directly (in vivo) or by imaging. Exposure is typically conducted in a graduated and progressive manner. Exposure may also take the form of systematic desensitization in which the child receives relaxation training, and then practices relaxation while facing his or her feared situations in vivo or imaginally. In vivo and imaginal desensitization are both effective treatments for childhood anxiety disorders. A strong, positive therapeutic relationship may be needed to help children perform challenging exposure tasks (Chu et al., 2004)

The second strategy implemented to treat childhood anxiety is *modeling*, which involves a person demonstrating approach behavior in situations that the child finds anxiety provoking. Variants of modeling include filmed modeling where the child watches a videotape; live modeling where the person modeling is in the presence of the anxious child; and participant modeling where a model interacts with the child and guides him or her to approach the feared situation. In their review of nine controlled studies that examined the efficacy of modeling as a treatment for childhood fears and phobias, Ollendick and King (1998) concluded that filmed modeling and live modeling are moderately effective procedures and that participant modeling is a highly effective treatment for childhood fears and phobias.

Progressive exposure and modeling assume that fear must be reduced before approach behavior will occur. In contrast, the third CBT strategy—*contingency management*—based on the principles of operant conditioning, encourages increases in approach behavior by altering the consequences of a child's behavior in the anxiety provoking situations. Contingency management involves modifying the antecedents of anxiety or the consequences of anxious behavior through positive reinforcement, punishment, extinction, and shaping. For example, positive reinforcement for "courageous" or approach behaviors to the feared or dreaded stimulus are frequently used in such programs. These procedures are implemented by the therapist during the therapy session, and are often taught to parents and teachers for use in the home, school, and other community settings. Treatments involving reinforced practice have been shown to be superior to no-treatment or wait list control conditions, and other treatments (verbal coping skills, modeling) in reducing phobic symptoms. As such, reinforced practice is considered to be a well-established treatment for childhood fears and phobias (Ollendick & King, 1998).

The fourth strategy used in cognitive-behavioral therapy is primarily a *cognitive* or *information-processing* one. Cognitive interventions include techniques such as identifying self-talk, cognitive restructuring, and problem solving and they are usually taught in combination with one or more of the behavioral strategies reviewed above. Consequently, most published studies have examined treatments combining cognitive and behavioral interventions, and very few have examined the effectiveness of cognitive strategies in isolation. These integrated CBT programs are the most widely used treatments for children suffering from the most common anxiety disorders.

Kendall and his colleagues, for example, pioneered an integrated cognitive-behavioral treatment program for anxiety in children called "Coping Cat" (Kendall, Kane, Howard, & Siqueland, 1989). The four coping strategies taught to anxious children were summarized in an acronym (FEAR) which helped children remember the steps to take when they felt anxious: **F**eeling frightened, **E**xpect good things to happen, **A**ctions and attitudes to take, and **R**eward yourself. Controlled between-group studies provide strong evidence that individual CBT programs such as Coping Cat and its variants are more effective than a wait-list for reducing anxiety related to SAD, SOP, GAD, and school refusal (Barrett, Dadds, & Rapee, 1996; Heyne et al., 2002; Kendall, 1994; Kendall, Flannery-Schroeder et al. 1997; King et al., 1998). Cognitive-behavioral treatments are also effective when delivered using a group format (Barrett, 1998; Flannery-Schroeder & Kendall, 2000; Mendlowitz et al., 1999; Shortt, Barrett, & Fox, 2001; Silverman et al., 1999). Most recently, the Internet delivery of CBT for childhood anxiety has been trialed and early results suggest that Internet delivery of part of the therapy program is both feasible and effective (Spence, Holmes, March, & Lipp, 2006)

Studies have also examined the impact of incorporating parents in the therapeutic process. Informing parents about strategies their children are learning to manage their anxiety and teaching them strategies to manage their own anxiety may lead to better treatment outcomes than interventions which focus solely on the child. This may be particularly true for younger children (Barrett et al., 1996) and when treating children who also have an anxious parent (Cobham, Dadds, & Spence, 1998). However, the role of parents when treating anxious adolescents needs to be carefully considered, and we should not necessarily conclude that including them will result in more efficacious outcomes (Barmish & Kendall, 2005). Less parental involvement, or separate sessions with the parent/s, may be warranted in the case of anxious adolescents who are seeking autonomy as part of normal development (Kendall & Ollendick, 2004). Taking the role of parents one step further from being "collaborators" or "co-clients" as described above, to parents as therapists, Rapee, Abbott, and Lyneham (2006) examined the efficacy of bibliotherapy for children with anxiety disorders. Parents were asked to work through written materials at home with their own child. Rapee et al. found bibliotherapy to be more effective than no treatment, but less effective than standard CBT group treatment.

Summary

Anxiety is a common problem in childhood and adolescence. Anxiety problems are frequently comorbid with other anxiety disorders, depression, or externalizing behaviors, and have a poor prognosis if left untreated. Several etiological theories have been proposed to explain the development and maintenance of anxiety. Although research indicates a familial risk of anxiety, most anxiety problems can be conceptualized as a transaction between temperament and environmental-contextual factors. Anxiety in children and adolescents can be reliably assessed, and promising cognitive-behavioral and pharmacological treatments are available.

Depressive Disorders

Depressive disorders affect a significant number of children and adolescents, and there are important developmental factors to consider when making a diagnosis and in planning effective treatment for youngsters with these disorders (Duggal, Carlson, Sroufe, & Egeland, 2001).

Phenomenology

A thorough understanding of risk factors, development, family factors, and individual cognitive variables, as well as comorbid disorders, assists in both the assessment and treatment of these youngsters (Stark, Sander, Yancy, Bronik, & Hoke, 2000). Although the existence of depressive disorders in children and adolescents is no longer in question as it was in past years, there remain many unanswered questions about etiology, effective treatments, and dealing with depression when it is comorbid with other disorders.

Developmental Considerations In general, children and adolescents who are depressed do not always report feeling sad or "depressed," and developmentally appropriate language is needed to understand and communicate with them about their experiences. In particular, children tend to express their negative emotions as *anhedonia* (i.e., things that once were fun or reinforcing no longer are), rather than as depressed or sad mood as with adolescents and adults. They tend to have less "fun" than other children rather than being sad, forlorn, or depressed. In addition, both children and adolescents often report greater irritability than sadness, and argumentative behavior may also occur (Hammen & Rudolph, 1996). Although some researchers and clinicians suggest that the observed developmental differences in symptoms warrant different diagnostic categories (not unlike developmental differences between oppositional defiant disorder and conduct disorder), the field appears to have accepted these differences in symptom patterns across development and to embrace them.

Children and adolescents also differ in their perceptions of personal control over their depression. Weisz, Southam-Gerow, and McCarty (2001) have reported on developmental differences in perceived *contingency, control,* and *competence* (CCC) as they relate to depression in children and adolescents. Data were collected in several mental health outpatient centers with both children and adolescents. The CCC model defined perceived control as one's power to influence or engineer a desired outcome. Contingency was determined by how much one perceived that one's efforts caused the outcome, considering other possible contributing factors. Competence was defined as the degree to which one actually carried out the necessary behaviors to produce the desired outcomes. Both children and adolescents appeared negatively affected by low perceived control and low perceived competence, but adolescents were also sensitive to the contingency or "fairness" of the circumstances in a more global sense. Such findings may have important implications for current treatments for depression in children and adolescents.

As in many types of clinical distress and disease, certain factors increase the likelihood that youth will develop the disorder. In a prospective, longitudinal study by Duggal and colleagues (2001), significant differences emerged for factors associated with childhood-onset and adolescent-onset depression. Abuse at an early age, higher maternal stress, and less supportive early care differentiated childhood-onset from adolescent-onset depression. In general, adverse family relationships were associated with childhood-onset depression but not adolescent-onset depression. In the adolescent-onset group, adverse family relationships were less significant; however, greater levels of maternal depression were noted.

Gender Differences Prevalence rates of depressive disorders are different for boys and girls. The differences change systematically with development, adding an additional factor to consider. Prior to adolescence, there is an approximately equal proportion of depressive disorders in boys and girls. However, beginning in adolescence and continuing into adulthood, depressive disorders occur more frequently among females than males (Kessler, Avenevoli, & Merikangas, 2001), with ratios upward of 2:1 (Axelson & Birmaher, 2001). The exact reasons for these gender differences remain unclear. Biological, cultural, and interpersonal factors have been proposed, with no clear causes emerging (Nolen-Hoeksema, 1995). Still, these gender differences have been found to be robust across cultures. For example, in a large study of Mexican youth, Benjet and Hernandez-Guzman (2001) reported that the prevalence of depression was similar for boys and girls prepuberty, and increased for females postmenarche but not for males postpuberty.

One theory espoused by Shaw, Kennedy, and Joffe (1995) was that girls are more sensitive to interpersonal rejection, and more focused on dissatisfying interpersonal relationship qualities than boys. Another theory also proposes that the incidence of depression is greater among women of child-rearing age and that their daughters may learn about depressive symptoms, cognitions, and behaviors from them via modeling processes, thus placing the daughters at higher risk for depressive symptoms (Goodman & Gotlib, 1999). Benjet and Hernandez-Guzman (2001) also explored family factors, self-esteem, parental education, and attitudes about menstruation as potential modifiers in the puberty-depression relationship among young Mexican females but did not find support for modifying effects.

In a review, Beardslee and Gladstone (2001) provided an overview of risk factors for the development of depression in boys and girls. These factors included having a biological relative with a mood disorder, presence of severe stressor, low self-esteem or hopelessness, being female, and low socioeconomic status (poverty). Males and females were characterized, at least partially, by a unique set of risk factors. For boys, but not girls, neonatal and subsequent health problems posed risk for depression; in girls, but not boys, death of a parent by age 9 years, poor academic performance, and family dysfunction were related to risk for depression. In another review, Duggal and colleagues (2001) indicated that early caregiving patterns, such as household stress and quality of early childhood care, predicted depression for adolescent males, but not adolescent females, whereas presence of maternal depression predicted depression in adolescent females, but not adolescent males. The patterns of gender differences in prevalence and risk are reasonably well established. Yet, the mechanisms contributing to gender differences remain elusive and the field is ripe for new ideas and investigations (Seligman et al., 2004).

Epidemiology

Prevalence and incidence rates of depressive disorders vary across studies, and large-scale research is sparse in the area of childhood depression. However, on average, narrowly defined *DSM* major depression is thought to affect 1 to 2% of children (Anderson et al., 1987) and 2 to 4% of adolescents at any given point in time (Lewinsohn, Clarke, Seeley, & Rohde, 1994), or between 1 and 6% for point prevalence in youths in general (Kessler et al., 2001). The lifetime prevalence rate for the spectrum of depressive disorders in adolescents is between 5 and 21% in community samples (Hankin et al., 1998; Jonas, Brody, Roper, & Narrow, 2003; Reinherz, Giaconia, Lefkowitz, Pakiz, & Frost, 1993). Of course, rates increase for subclinical levels of depressive symptoms—depressive symptoms are reported by most children and adolescents at one time or another across their development.

DSM-IV Classification of Depressive Disorders

DSM-IV and *DSM-IV-TR* list major depressive disorder, dysthymia, and depressive disorder not otherwise specified within the depressive disorders category (1994, 2000). Some mental health professionals also consider bipolar disorder in the group of depressive disorders due to the depressive features of that disorder. However, given differences in treatment and prognosis for bipolar disorder spectrum illnesses, we do not view them as part of this category of affective disorders and do not discuss them further in this chapter.

The diagnosis of *major depression* is warranted if the child is experiencing five of the nine criterion symptoms of depression over a two-week period—one of those symptoms must be either depressed mood (can be irritable mood in children) or anhedonia—loss of interest or diminished pleasure in what was once enjoyable to the child (American Psychiatric Association, 1994, 2000). *Dysthymia* is chronic and less severe than major depression, but symptoms must be present for at least one year in children (in contrast to two years in adults). In some cases, a depressed child may appear to have brief moments of enjoyment, such as while playing with friends or winning in a game. When depressed children present for treatment, some clinicians may detect momentary childhood positive moods and mistakenly rule out dysthymia. Children who have clinical symptoms of dysthymia or depression may have such moments, but they fade quickly and their overall experiences remain characterized by chronic depressive symptoms.

Depression is a cyclic, often recurrent, disorder. Emslie and Mayes (2001) reported that 90% of youngsters recovered from a depressive episode within two years. Yet, within six to seven years, 25 to 50% of them reexperienced significant symptoms and distress. In addition, within eight years, 54 to 72% had a recurrent episode of depression.

Differential Diagnosis and Comorbidity

Another important (if not vexing) factor in the diagnosis and treatment of depression is the existence of comorbid disorders: these include an anxiety disorder, conduct disorder, and substance abuse, with anxiety being most common, as noted earlier in this chapter. Lewinsohn and colleagues (Lewinsohn, Zinbarg, Seeley, Lewinsohn, & Sack, 1997) reported that depression co-occurs with the anxiety diagnoses of panic, generalized anxiety, separation anxiety, social phobia, and specific phobia. Although depression may be the first onset with some comorbid disorders (especially with substance abuse disorders and conduct problems), in general, anxiety disorders such as panic disorder and GAD frequently precede its onset (Kessler et al., 2001).

Although anxiety disorders are common comorbid disorders with depression, the two classes of disorders appear to be distinct in children, but related through a common construct of negative affectivity (Axelson & Birmaher, 2001; Seligman & Ollendick, 1998). In depressed youth, up to 75% have a lifetime prevalence of a comorbid anxiety disorder, and between 45 and 50% have a disruptive behavior disorder or substance use disorder (Avenevoli et al., 2001; Wolff & Ollendick, 2006). Point prevalence rates for children and adolescents with depression and a comorbid anxiety disorder range from 25 to 50%; in contrast point prevalence rates for anxious youths with depression range between 15 and 20%. In other words, it is more common for depressed children and adolescents to have a comorbid anxiety disorder than for anxious children and adolescents to have a comorbid depressive disorder. Presence of a comorbid disorder appears to relate to severity of symptoms, such that youngsters with major depression and comorbid anxiety possess more severe depressive symptoms (Axelson & Birmaher, 2001).

Comorbidity is particularly relevant in assessment of suicide risk. Youths with substance abuse as either a primary or secondary diagnosis are at increased risk for suicidal behavior. In addition, antisocial behavior, particularly in females, may increase risk for lethal suicidal behaviors (Wannan & Fombonne, 1998).

Etiological Considerations

Risk of depression in children and adolescents is associated with parental depression, likely due to biological, environmental, and interpersonal reasons.

Biological Factors Weissman and colleagues (1987) indicated that childhood-onset depression was more likely in households where the mother was depressed, particularly if the mother's onset of depression was in early adulthood. This implies a genetic or heritable component, but environmental factors, of course, cannot be ruled out.

In addition to inherited factors, specific neurotransmitters have been implicated in the onset and course of depression in children and adolescents. One prominent theory suggests that select neurotransmitters such as the monoamines, norepinephrine, serotonin, and dopamine are not available at receptor sites in sufficient supply (Wagner & Ambrosini, 2001). In adults, pharmacological treatment traditionally includes antidepressant medications in the class of monoamine oxidase inhibitors or tricyclic antidepressants, and more recently the selective serotonin reuptake inhibitors (SSRIs) or serotonin-norepinephrine reuptake (SNRIs) inhibitors. Use of such medications is based on this neurotransmitter deficiency theory. Other theories, which have not yet been demonstrated with children, implicate poor growth hormone stimulation, as well as hypothalamic-pituitary-adrenal axis regulation difficulties (Axelson & Birmaher, 2001). (See also Ingram, this volume, and Smith, this volume.)

Family and Interpersonal Factors Family risk factors have traditionally focused on maternal factors, such as maternal depression or low maternal warmth and availability. However, more recent models include a more complex conceptualization of family risk factors for youth depression, including the contribution of fathers and mothers, genetic risk, and other environmental risks. Sander and McCarty (2005) conducted a comprehensive review of family factors and interventions addressing family factors in depressed youth. Their conclusions were that many factors, including cognitive style of parents, parental psychopathology, emotional availability of parents, coping styles, and family conflict all contribute in important ways to risk for youth depression. Importantly, both mothers and fathers, along with other factors, are important in conceptualizing risk (Sander & McCarty, 2005). Goodman and Gotlib's (1999) integrative model of risk for transmission of depression from mother to child considers heritability, depressive maternal affect and symptoms, stress within a household with a depressed parent, and neuroregulatory consequences from that environmental circumstance. In addition, these authors propose that the timing, severity, and duration of depressive symptoms interact with the developmental tasks and challenges for children (Goodman & Gotlib, 1999). Furthermore, the Oregon Adolescent Depression Project (Allen, Lewinsohn, & Seeley, 1998) examined prenatal, neonatal, developmental, and family relationship factors in psychopathology. They found several factors increased the risk of adolescent depression, including maternal depression and absence of breastfeeding. Yet, relationship quality with parents may not be the most important consideration across developmental stages. In a study by Williams, Connolly, and Segal (2001), the level of intimacy in romantic relationships predicted risk for depression in older adolescents beyond other parental and friendship relationship factors, but not for children or younger adolescents.

The effect of early relationship quality on later depression in children and adolescents is unclear, as is the contribution made by youngsters with a predisposition for depression to the negative quality of their interpersonal interactions. However, depressed youth do appear to have poorer social competence, perceive less support from peers, and spend less time with peers than do nondepressed youths (Hammen & Rudolph, 1996). Professionals need to acknowledge and integrate interpersonal deficits or struggles, including peer and parental relationships, when conceptualizing and implementing treatment programs for depressed youngsters (Mufson, Weissman, Moreau, & Garfinkel, 1999; Seligman et al., 2004; Stark et al., 2000). In addition, depression and its associated cognitive distortions appear to be related to interpersonal factors and, therefore, can or should be treated within an interpersonal context (Joiner, Coyne, & Blalock, 1999).

Consistent with research on the role of interpersonal and cognitive variables in depression in youth, the *cognitive-interpersonal theory* of depression proposes that cognitive style and interpersonal relationship patterns combine to result in depression (Stark et al., 2000). From this perspective, Bowlby's *attachment theory* (1980) plays an important role. In brief, early or primary interpersonal relationships are proposed to either buffer or increase risk for cognitive style associated with depression. According to this theory, early relationship patterns and the caregiver's responsiveness to the child shape the child's expectations of how they will be treated by others and how responsive others will be to their needs. An unresponsive caregiver, such as a depressed parent, could inadvertently communicate the message that the child's needs are unimportant, thus predisposing the child to adopt a negative self-schema (Duggal et al., 2001; Stark et al., 2000). Others suggest similar cognitive-interpersonal pathways and theoretical integration (Gotlib & Hammen, 1992).

Individual and Cognitive Variables Among individual variables, cognitive style, including *attributional style*, has received the most attention. Attributional style refers to the patterns of causality assigned to events, such as how stable, global, and internal those events are perceived to be (Nolen-Hoeksema, Girgus, & Seligman 1992). In brief, the cognitive model of depression includes the concepts of negative thought patterns, depressive self-schema, and pessimistic attributional style about events (Clark, Beck, & Alford, 1999; Stark, Schmidt, & Joiner, 1996). According to cognitive theory, the self-schema guides information processing and may produce errors in perception that are consistent with a depressive self-schema—typically that the self is unlovable or incompetent (Clark et al., 1999). Depressed children and adolescents, in contrast to nondepressed children and adolescents, may often distort events and make information-processing errors that confirm negatively biased assumptions about the self (Stark et al., 1996) and the internal, stable, and global nature of negative events (Nolen-Hoeksema et al., 1992).

Assessment

The scope of this chapter does not allow for thorough review of the assessment process. However, brief recommendations are put forth (see Kendall, Cantwell, & Kazdin, 1989, for a thorough discussion of this topic). Within the field of depression, a common diagnostic interview used for assessing clinical depression is the Kiddie Schedule for Affective Disorders and Schizophrenia (K-SADS; Orvaschel & Puig-Antich, 1987). Various researchers have adopted versions of the K-SADS, including present episode, epidemiologic version, and combined versions with updates for the *DSM-IV* (Ambrosini, 2000). The K-SADS is a semistructured diagnostic interview designed to be used by clinically trained interviewers, and can be administered to the youth and parent separately. The complete interview is cumbersome and was designed for research. However, the specific prompts and questions can be incorporated into an interview for clinical practice (Stark et al., 2000). Other questionnaires and self-report measures can be administered efficiently and used in community or clinic populations, such as the depression scale of the Behavior Assessment Scale for Children, 2nd edition (BASC-2; Reynolds & Kamphaus, 2004), the Beck Youth Inventory—Depression Scales (BDI-Y; Beck, Beck, & Jolly, 2001), or the Children's Depression Inventory (CDI; Kovacs, 1992), but these are recommended only when used in conjunction with a clinician's interview and other sources of information to determine accurate diagnosis.

Assessment of suicide risk and behavior is important. In adolescents, there may be a precipitating stressor that has compromised developmental tasks such as establishing autonomy, acceptance by a desired peer group, or conflict with important peers or with family members. The clinician must remain attuned to these potential events in relation to increased risk for suicide in youth (Rudd & Joiner, 1998), as well as assess for substance use and antisocial behavior, as discussed previously (Wannan & Fombonne, 1998). Several self-report measures listed above include items and clusters of items that address suicidal risk and should be reviewed with the child and her or his parents immediately following administration.

Interventions

The main interventions are pharmacological or psychosocial.

Pharmacological Interventions As with the anxiety disorders, there have been a limited number of controlled, randomized clinical trials of the treatment of depression in children and adolescents, either pharmacological or psychosocial. Pharmacologically, the most promising results have been obtained with the SSRIs (e.g., fluoxetine—marketed as Prozac) to reduce depressive symptoms. However, rates of improvement have been less than 40% (Wagner & Ambrosini, 2001). Importantly, however, the SSRIs are most likely to reduce depressive symptoms and have fewer and less detrimental side effects than other antidepressants (Emslie & Mayes, 2001). In the most extensive multisite medication and psychosocial intervention study with adolescents to date, which included 439 adolescents from 2000 to 2003, the Treatment of Adolescent Depression Study (TADS team, 2004) reported that fluoxetine plus cognitive-behavioral treatment was the most effective intervention to alleviate depression in adolescents. Fluoxetine was superior to cognitive-behavioral treatment alone (TADS team, 2004). However, the methods and specific cognitive-behavioral interventions incorporated for the TADS group were criticized for being less rigorous than those used in cognitive-behavioral treatment studies, requiring further investigation (Hollon, Garber, & Shelton, 2005).

Psychosocial Interventions In a review of psychosocial interventions for depressed children and adolescents, Asarnow, Jaycox, and Tompson (2001) acknowledged the merits of efficacious interventions across a range of modalities, including cognitive-behavioral therapy (CBT) and interpersonal psychotherapy for adolescents (IPT-A), both of which are relatively short-term interventions. However, the relapse rates (40 to 50%) of clinically depressed youths when these psychosocial treatments are the sole treatment modality are relatively high (Asarnow et al., 2001).

CBT has received the most empirical support of the psychosocial treatments (Curry, 2001; Seligman et al., 2004). Components of CBT include affective education, planning positive activities, proactive problem solving, social skills training, coping strategies, and cognitive restructuring. Family and interpersonal components may also be included. CBT has been implemented with children as young as 8 to 9 years of age and up to 18 years of age. Among 15 CBT studies reviewed by Curry (2001), treatment duration ranged from 5 to 16 weeks. Some therapy protocols involved twice weekly sessions, with an average of 11 sessions total. New treatment investigations include an emphasis on family components when combined with cognitive-behavioral approaches (Asarnow et al., 2001; Curry, 2001). Sander and McCarty (2005) reviewed family factors and treatments for depressed youth that incorporated families across theoretical orientations, and concluded that all approaches need to address family intervention components in a more systematic way, and include multicultural populations and long-term follow-up to better inform treatment strategies for depressed youth.

IPT-A has also received promising empirical support. In IPT-A, the focus is on resolving conflicts in current, important, interpersonal relationships and improving communication and relationship skills (Mufson, Moreau et al., 1993). To date, empirical support for this intervention has been limited to one major clinical trial (Mufson, Weissman et al., 1999).

There are two highly controlled clinical trials that address depression in youth from a cognitive-behavioral perspective: the Coping with Depression for Adolescents group treatment (CWD-A; see Clarke et al. 1999; Lewinsohn, Clarke, Hops, & Andrews, 1990) and the ACTION program (Stark et al., 2006). The CWD-A group treatment is based on cognitive-behavioral principles and has been effective in reducing depressive symptoms in youths with a primary diagnosis of depression (Clarke et al., 1999; Lewinsohn et al., 1990), as well as complex multiple-disorder groups, such as those youth involved in juvenile justice systems (Rohde, Clarke, Mace, Jorgensen, & Seeley, 2004). The CWD-A treatment, however, does not appear to address the comorbid conduct disorder symptoms, but did reduce depressive symptoms in this highly challenging and distressed group of youth (Rohde et al., 2004). The ACTION program, a cognitive-behavioral group treatment for young adolescent girls, is still in the evaluative stages but appears highly promising. Participants have a primary diagnosis of depression, but many have dual diagnoses, most often an anxiety disorder (Sander, 2004). There is a parent component to treatment in the ACTION program, and depression appears to be reduced by participation in the group treatment, with the initial 60 participants showing a 70% improvement rate (Stark et al., 2006).

Managing suicidal risk is a necessary skill when working with depressed youngsters, particularly as outpatients. Managing this risk involves several straightforward strategies (Rudd & Joiner, 1998). The first is to have a proactive stance and a plan for potential hospitalization, to be revised or revisited frequently during suicide risk periods. In addition, treatment progress and goals should be revisited and updated often, particularly noting the changes that co-occur with decreased suicidal ideation. Sessions may need to occur more frequently, and the family's involvement and a phone contact list, as well as availability of emergency 24-hour support, is necessary. Furthermore, medication assessment and monitoring, as well as consultation, is recommended.

In summary, although the available treatments for depressed and suicidal children and adolescents show promise, several important caveats need to be kept in mind. Overall, recovery rates across interventions are generally at or below 50% (Asarnow et al., 2001; Curry, 2001; Seligman et al., 2004). Moreover, relapse rates are high. Also, comorbidity has been rarely addressed in treatment efficacy studies, and it remains an important factor to consider in day-to-day clinical practice as well as in major clinical outcome trials (Curry, 2001; Wolff & Ollendick, 2006). Recent studies that include comorbidity as part of the design, rather than focusing on single-diagnosis participants, appear promising. Psychosocial interventions, particularly the traditional CBT approaches, are moving in new directions to reflect a more integrative treatment, incorporating individual, cognitive, relational, and interpersonal factors.

Summary

The research on child and adolescent depression offers a number of exciting and promising findings. Treatment research is ongoing, including new directions involving biological and interpersonal factors. Although efficacious treatments exist, both pharmacological and psychosocial (primarily CBT and IPT-A), not all youth are being helped by these interventions. Furthermore, the issue of comorbidity has not been adequately addressed nor has the role of culture and ethnicity. The protective factors and risk factors associated with different cultural and ethnic practices have yet to be examined in standard research and clinical practice. These could be pivotal factors in understanding and treating childhood depression in our increasingly diverse society.

Summary and Future Directions

The internalizing disorders of children and adolescents represent a major challenge to practicing clinicians and researchers alike. As we have seen, the anxiety and affective disorders are highly prevalent in childhood and adolescence. Their effects are distressing in the short run and can be long lasting.

Although we have attempted to articulate a developmental psychopathology perspective on these disorders, it is evident that the field has not yet fully embraced this way of thinking about these problems. As a result, many studies continue to look at single causal pathways and direct, linear outcomes. As we have suggested, it may be more productive to posit that several very different pathways can lead to any one outcome such as depression or anxiety (i.e., the developmental principle of equifinality) and that any one pathway can lead to diverse outcomes (i.e., the principle of multifinality). Thus, a risk factor such as child sexual abuse can and frequently does lead to multiple outcomes, whether they are an internalizing disorder or one of the externalizing disorders reviewed in chapter 16. Tracking this developmental process is undoubtedly a complex and challenging undertaking, but a necessary one. This effort will benefit greatly from carefully planned, multisite, longitudinal studies (Ollendick & King, 1994; Ollendick & March, 2004).

Moreover, the effects of these risk factors may not be direct and we need to consider conditions that moderate these relations. Direct effects are oftentimes captured by what are referred to as "main effect" models that imply that a risk factor is directly related to the outcome in a linear fashion. Yet, any one risk factor does not invariably result in any one pathological outcome. For example, it is well known that not all sexually abused children have negative outcomes such as the development of internalizing or externalizing disorders—or at least not the same negative outcomes. Often, a significant minority of abused children do not develop any disorders at all, implying a profound interaction between the experience of abuse and some other internal or external moderating conditions (Kazdin & Kagan, 1994). What does seem most important is the context in which the abuse occurs and the interrelated risk factors that are present. As noted by Kazdin and Kagan, "when one begins with the multiplicity of variables that operate, one might better consider nonlinearity to be the better point of departure in our work" (p. 38).

These same issues have important implications for the treatment and prevention of internalizing disorders. Our treatment and prevention programs must move away from a "one size fits all" mentality. Children and adolescents become depressed or anxious through a variety of pathways, and they express these disorders in a variety of ways. We need to take this complexity into consideration in designing, implementing, and evaluating our interventions. Although current empirically supported or evidence-based interventions work with most (i.e., 50 to 70%) of the children and adolescents and families who come into our practices and research clinics, we must do better. An approach that is individualized and prescriptive, and one that is based in developmental theory and grounded in established principles of behavior change (e.g., exposure, cognitive change, interpersonal relationships), is likely to be most effective, although such remains to be carefully documented.

References

Achenbach, T. M. (1990). What is "developmental" about developmental psychopathology? In J. Rolf, A. Matsen, D. Cicchetti, K. Nuechterlein, & S. Weintraub (Eds.), *Risk and protective factors in the development of psychopathology* (pp. 29–48). New York: Cambridge University Press..

Achenbach, T. M. (1991). *Manual for the child behavior checklist/4–18 and 1991 profile.* Burlington: University of Vermont, Department of Psychiatry.

Albano, A. M., Chorpita, B., & Barlow, D. H. (1996). Anxiety disorders in children and adolescents. In E. J. Mash and R. A. Barkley (Eds.), *Child psychopathology* (pp. 196–241). New York: Guilford.

Albano A. M., & Hayward, C. (2004a). The developmental psychopathology approach to understanding and treating social anxiety disorder. In T. H. Ollendick and J. S. March (Eds), *Phobic and anxiety disorders: A clinician's guide to effective psychosocial and pharmacological interventions* (pp. 198–235). New York: Oxford University Press.

Albano, A. M., & Hayward, C. (2004b). Social anxiety disorder. In T. H. Ollendick & J. S. March (Eds.), *Phobic and anxiety disordes in children and adolescents* (pp. 198–235). New York: Oxford University Press.

Allen, N. B., Lewinsohn, P. M., & Seeley, J. R. (1998). Prenatal and perinatal influences on risk for psychopathology in childhood and adolescence. *Development and Psychopathology, 10,* 513–529.

Ambrosini, P. J. (2000). Historical development and present status of the Schedule for Affective Disorders and Schizophrenia for School-Age Children (K-SADS). *Journal of the American Academy of Child & Adolescent Psychiatry, 39*(1), 4–58.

American Psychiatric Association. (1980). *Diagnostic and statistical manual of mental disorders* (3rd rev. ed.) Washington, D.C.: Author.

American Psychiatric Association. (1994). *Diagnostic and statistical manual of mental disorders* (4th ed.). Washington, D.C.: Author.

American Psychiatric Association. (2000).*Diagnostic and statistical manual of mental disorders* (4th ed., rev.). Washington, D.C.: Author.

Anderson, J. C., Williams, S., McGee, R., & Silva, A. (1987). *DSM-III* disorders in pre-adolescent children: Prevalence in a large sample from the general population. *Archives of General Psychiatry, 44,* 69-76.

Asarnow, R., Jaycox, L. H., & Tompson, M. C. (2001). Depression in youth: Psychosocial interventions. *Journal of Clinical Child Psychology, 30,* 33–47.

Avenevoli, S., Stolar, M., Li, J., Dierker, L., & Merikangas, K. R. (2001). Comorbidity of depression in children and adolescents: Models and evidence from a prospective hi-risk family study. *Biological Psychiatry, 49,* 1071–1081.

Axelson, D. A., & Birmaher, B. (2001). Relation between anxiety and depressive disorders in childhood and adolescence. *Depression and Anxiety, 14,* 67–78.

Baer, D. M. (1982). Behavior analysis and development. *Human Development, 25,* 357–361.

Bandura, A. (1977a). *Social learning theory.* Englewood Cliffs, NJ: Prentice-Hall.

Bandura, A. (1977b). Self-efficacy: Toward a unifying theory of behavioral change. *Psychological Review, 84,* 191–215.

Bandura, A. (1986). *Social foundations of thought and action: A social cognitive theory.* Englewood Cliffs, NJ: Prentice-Hall..

Barmish, A. J., & Kendall, P. C. (2005). Should parents be co-clients in cognitive behavior therapy for anxious youth? *Journal of Clinical Child and Adolescent Psychology, 34,* 569–581.

Barrett, P.M. (1998). Evaluation of cognitive-behavioral group treatments for childhood anxiety disorders. *Journal of Clinical Child Psychology, 27,* 459–468.

Barrett, P.M., Dadds, M.R., & Rapee, R.M. (1996). Family treatment of childhood anxiety: A controlled trial. *Journal of Consulting and Clinical Psychology, 64,* 333–342.

Barrett, P. M., Rapee. R. M., Dadds, M. M., & Ryan, S. M. (1996). Family enhancement of cognitive style in anxious and aggressive children. *Journal of Abnormal Child Psychology, 24,* 187–203.

Beardslee, W. R., & Gladstone, T. R. G. (2001). Prevention of childhood depression: Recent findings and future prospects. *Biological Psychiatry, 49,* 1101–1110.

Beck, A. T. (1976). *Cognitive therapy and the emotional disorders.* New York: International Universities Press.

Beck, A. T. (1991). Cognitive therapy: A 30-year retrospective. *American Psychologist, 46,* 368–375.

Beck, J., Beck, A. T., & Jolly, J. B. (2001). *Beck Youth Inventories.* San Diego, CA: The Psychological Corporation (Harcourt Assessment).

Beidel, D. C., & Morris, T. L. (1995). Social phobia. In E. J. Mash & R. A. Barkley (Eds.), *Child psychopathology* (pp. 181–211). New York: Guilford.

Bell-Dolan, D. J., Foster, S. L., & Christopher, J. S. (1995). Girls' peer relations and internalizing problems: Are socially neglected, rejected, and withdrawn girls at risk? *Journal of Clinical Child Psychology, 24,* 463–473.

Benjet, C., & Hernandez-Guzman, L. (2001). Gender differences in psychological well-being of Mexican early adolescents. *Adolescence, 36,* 47–65.

Biederman, J., Hirshfeld-Becker, D.R., Rosenbaum, J. F., Herot, C., Friedman, D., Snidman, N., et al. (2001). Further evidence of association between behavioral inhibition and social anxiety in children. *American Journal of Psychiatry, 158,* 1673–1679.

Bolton, D., Eley, T. C., O'Connor, T. G., Perrin, S., Rabe-Hesketh, S., Rijsdijk, F., et al. (2005). Prevalence and genetic and environmental influences on anxiety disorders in 6-year-old twins. *Psychological Medicine, 36,* 1–10.

Bowlby, J. (1980). *Attachment and loss: Vol 3. Loss, sadness, and depression.* New York: Basic Books.

Brady, E. U., & Kendall, P. C. (1992). Comorbidity of anxiety and depression in children and adolescents. *Psychological Bulletin, 111,* 244–255.

Caron, C., & Rutter, M. (1991). Comorbidity in child psychopathology: Concepts, issues and research strategies. *Journal of Child Psychology and Psychiatry, 32,* 1063–1080.

Chu, B. C., Choudhury, M. S., Shortt, A. L., Pincus, D. B., Creed, T. A., & Kendall, P. C. (2004). Alliance, technology, and outcome in the treatment of anxious youth. *Cognitive and Behavioral Practice, 11,* 44–55.

Cicchetti D (1989). Developmental psychopathology: Past, present, and future. In D. Cicchetti (Ed.), *The emergence of a discipline: The Rochester symposium on developmental psychopathology* (Vol. 1, pp. 1–12.). Hillsdale, NJ: Erlbaum.

Cicchetti, D., & Schneider-Rosen, K. (1986). An organizational approach to childhood depression. In M. Rutter, C. E. Izard, & P. B. Read (Eds.), *Depression in young people: Developmental and clinical perspectives* (pp. 71–134). New York: Guilford.

Clark, D. A., Beck, A. T., & Alford, B. A. (1999). *Scientific foundations of cognitive theory and therapy of depression.* New York: Wiley.

Clarke, G. N., Rohde, P., Lewinsohn, P. M., Hops, H., & Seeley, J. R. (1999). Cognitive-behavioral treatment of adolescent depression: Efficacy of acute group treatment and booster sessions. *Journal of the American Academy of Child and Adolescent Psychiatry, 38,* 272–279.

Cobham, V. E., Dadds, R., & Spence, S. H. (1998). The role of parental anxiety in the treatment of childhood anxiety. *Journal of Consulting and Clinical Psychology, 66,* 893–905.

Cohen, P., Cohen, J., Kaasen, S., Noemi Velez, C., Hartmark, C., Johnson, J., et al. (1993). An epidemiological study of disorders in late childhood and adolescence—1: Age and gender specific prevalence. *Journal of Child Psychology and Psychiatry, 34,* 851–867.

Cook, E. H., Wagner, K. D., March, J. S., Biederman, J., Landau, P., Wolkow, R., et al. (2001). Long-term sertraline treatment of children and adolescents with obsessive-compulsive disorder. *Journal of the American Academy of Child and Adolescent Psychiatry, 40,* 1175–1189.

Costello, E. J., Costello, A. J., Edelbrock, C., Burns, B. J., Dulcan, M. K., Brent, D., et al. (1988). Psychiatric disorders in pediatric primary care. *Archives of General Psychiatry, 45,* 1107–1116.

Costello, E. J., Egger, H. L., & Angold, A. (2004). In T. H. Ollendick & J. S. March (Eds.), *Phobic and anxiety disorders in children and adolescents* (pp. 61–90). New York: Oxford University Press.

Curry, J. F. (2001). Specific psychotherapies for childhood and adolescent depression. *Biological Psychiatry, 49,* 1091–1100.

Curry, J. F., March, J. S., & Hervey, A. S. (2004). Comorbidity of childhood and adolescent anxiety disorders: Prevalence and implications. In T. H. Ollendick & J. S. March (Eds.), *Phobic and anxiety disorders in children and adolescents* (pp. 116–140). New York: Oxford University Press,.

Dadds, M. R., & Barrett, P. M. (1996). Family processes in child and adolescent anxiety and depression. *Behaviour Change, 13*, 231–239.

Dadds, M. R., Barrett, P. M., Rapee, R. M., & Ryan, S. (1996). Family processes and child psychopathology: An observational analysis of the FEAR effect. *Journal of Abnormal Child Psychology, 24*, 715–735.

Dadds, M. R., & Roth, J. H. (2001). Family processes in the development of anxiety problems. In M. W. Vasey and M. R. Dadds (Eds.), *The developmental psychopathology of anxiety disorders in children* (pp. 278–303). New York: Oxford University Press.

Davey, G. C. L. (1992). Classical conditioning and the acquisition of human fears and phobias: A review and synthesis of the literature. *Advances in Behavior Research and Therapy, 14*, 29–66.

Duggal, S., Carlson, E. A., Sroufe, L. A., & Egeland, B. (2001). Depressive symptomatology in childhood and adolescence. *Development and Psychopathology, 13*, 143–164.

Dumas, J. E., La Freniere, P. J., & Sereketich, W. J. (1995). "Balance of power": A transactional analysis of control in mother-child dyads involving socially competent, aggressive, and anxious children. *Journal of Abnormal Psychology, 104*, 104–113.

Eley, T. C., Bolton, D., O'Connor, T., Perrin, S., Smith, P., & Plomin, R. (2003). A twin study of anxiety-related behaviors in young children. *Journal of Child Psychology and Psychiatry, 44*, 945–960.

Eley, T. C., & Stevenson, J. (1999). Exploring the covariation between anxiety and depression symptoms: A genetic analysis of the effects of age and sex. *Journal of Child Psychology and Psychiatry, 40*, 1273–1282.

Emslie, G. J., & Mayes, T. L. (2001). Mood disorders in children and adolescents: Pharmacological treatment. *Biological Psychiatry, 49*, 1082–1090.

Erickson, E. H. (1968). *Identity, youth, and crisis.* New York: W. W. Norton.

Essau, C. A., Conradt, J., & Petermann, F. (2000). Frequency, comorbidity, and psychosocial impairment of specific phobia in adolescents. *Journal of Clinical Child Psychology, 29*, 221–231.

Feigon, S. A., Waldman, I. D., Levy, F., & Hay, D. A. (2001). Genetic and environmental influences on separation anxiety disorder symptoms and their moderation by age and sex. *Behavior Genetics, 31*, 403–411.

Flannery-Schroeder, E. C., & Kendall, P. C. (2000). Group and individual cognitive-behavioral treatments for youth with anxiety disorders: A randomized clinical trial. *Cognitive Therapy and Research, 24*, 251–278.

Freud, S. (1949). An *outline of psychoanalysis.* New York: W. W. Norton. (Original work published 1940)

Gelfand, D. M., & Peterson, L. (1985). *Child development and psychopathology.* Beverly Hills, CA: Sage.

Goodman, S. H., & Gotlib, I. H. (1999). Risk for psychopathology in the children of depressed mothers: A developmental model for understanding mechanisms of transmission. *Psychological Review, 106*, 458–490.

Gotlib, I. H., & Hammen, C. (1992). *Psychological aspects of depression: Toward a cognitive-interpersonal integration.* Chichester, UK: Wiley.

Gullone, E. (2000). The development of normal fear: A century of research. *Clinical Psychology Review, 20*, 429–458.

Hammen, C., & Rudolph, K. D. (1996). Childhood depression. In E. J. Mash & R. A. Barkley, (Eds.), *Child psychopathology* (pp.153–195). New York: Guilford.

Hankin, B. L., Abramson, L. Y., Silva, P. A., McGee, R., Moffitte, T. E., & Angell, K. E. (1998). Development of depression from preadolescence to young adulthood: Emerging gender differences in a 10-year longitudinal study. *Journal of Abnormal Psychology, 107* (1), 128–140.

Heyman, I., Fombonne, E., Simmons, H., Ford, T., Meltzer, H., & Goodman, R. (2001). Prevalence of obsessive-compulsive disorder in the British nationwide survey of child mental health. *British Journal of Psychiatry, 179*, 324–329.

Heyne, D., King, N. J., Tonge, B. J., Rollings, S., Young, D., Pritchard, M. et al. (2002). Evaluation of child therapy and caregiver training in the treatment of school refusal. *Journal of the American Academy of Child and Adolescent Psychiatry, 41*, 687–695.

Hirshfeld, D. R., Biederman, J., Brody, L., Faraone, S. V., & Rosenbaum, J. F. (1997). Expressed emotion toward children with behavioral inhibition: Associations with maternal anxiety disorder. *Journal of the American Academy of Child and Adolescent Psychiatry, 36*, 910–917.

Hirshfeld, D. R., Rosenbaum, J. F., Biederman, J., Bolduc, E. A., Faraone, S. V., Snidman, N., et al. (1992). Stable behavioral inhibition and its association with anxiety disorder. *Journal of the American Academy of Child and Adolescent Psychiatry, 31*, 103–111.

Hollon, S. D., Garber, J., & Shelton, R. C. (2005). Treatment of depression in adolescents with cognitive behavior therapy and medications: A commentary on the TADS Project. *Cognitive and Behavioral Practice, 12*(2), 149–155.

In-Albon, T., & Schneider, S. (in press). Psychotherapy of childhood anxiety disorders: A meta-analysis. *Psychotherapy and Psychosomatics.*

Joiner, T., Coyne, J. C., & Blalock, J. (1999). On the interpersonal nature of depression: Overview and synthesis. In T. Joiner & J. C. Coyne (Eds.), *The interactional nature of depression: Advances in interpersonal approaches* (pp. 3–20). Washington, D.C.: American Psychological Association,.

Jonas, B. S., Brody, D., Roper, M., & Narrow, W. E. (2003). Prevalence of mood disorders in a national sample of young American adults. *Social Psychiatry and Psychiatric Epidemiology, 38*, 618–624.

Kagan, J. (1994). *Galen's prophecy: Temperament in human nature.* New York: Basic Books.

Kagan, J., Reznick, J. S., & Snidman, N. (1987). The physiology and psychology of behavioral inhibition in children. *Child Development, 58*, 1459–1473.

Kagan, J., Snidman, N., Zentner, M., & Peterson, E. (1999). Infant temperament and anxious symptoms in school age children. *Development and Psychopathology, 11*, 209–224.

Kashani, J. H., Beck, N. C., Hoeper, E. W., Falahi, C., Corcoran, C. M., McAllister, J. A., et al. (1987). Psychiatric disorders in a community sample of adolescents. *American Journal of Psychiatry, 144*, 584–589.

Kashani, J. H., Orvaschel, H., Rosenberg, T. K., & Reid, J. C. (1989). Psychopathology in a community sample of children and adolescents: A developmental perspective. *Journal of the American Academy of Child and Adolescent Psychiatry, 28*, 701–706.

Kazdin, A. E., & Kagan, J. (1994). Models of dysfunction in developmental psychopathology. *Clinical Psychology: Science and Practice, 1*, 35–52.

Keller, M. B., Lavori, P., Wunder, J., Beardslee, W. R., Schwarts, C. E., & Roth, J. (1992). Chronic course of anxiety disorders in children and adolescents. *Journal of the American Academy of Child and Adolescent Psychiatry, 312*, 595–599.

Kendall, P. C. (1994). Treating anxiety disorders in children: Results of a randomized clinical trial. *Journal of Consulting and Clinical Psychology, 62*, 100–110.

Kendall, P. C., Brady, E. U., & Verduin, T. L. (2001). Comorbidity in childhood anxiety disorders and treatment outcome. *Journal of the American Academy of Child & Adolescent Psychiatry, 40*, 787–794.

Kendall, P. C., Cantwell, D. A., Kazdin, A. E. (1989). Depression in children and adolescents: Assessment issues and recommendations. *Cognitive Therapy and Research, 13*, 109–146.

Kendall, P. C., Flannery-Schroeder, E., Panichelli-Mindel, S.M., Southam-Gerow, M., Henin, A., & Warman, M. (1997). Treatment of anxiety disorders in youth: A second randomised clinical trial. *Journal of Consulting and Clinical Psychology, 65*, 366–380.

Kendall, P. C., & Ollendick, T. H. (2004). Setting the research and practice agenda for anxiety in children and adolescence: A topic comes of age. *Cognitive and Behavioral Practice, 11*, 65–74.

Kendall, P. C., Pimentel, S., Rynn, M. A., Algelosante, A., & Webb, A. (2004). Generalized anxiety disorder. In T. H. Ollendick & J. S. March (Eds.), *Phobic and anxiety disorders in children and adolescents* (pp. 334–380). New York: Oxford University Press.

Kendall, P. C., & Warman, M. J. (1996). Anxiety disorders in youth: Diagnostic consistency across *DSM-III-R* and *DSM-IV*. *Journal of Anxiety Disorders, 10*, 453–463.

Kendler, K. S., Karkowski, L. M., & Prescott, C. A. (1999). Fears and phobias: Reliability and heritability. *Psychiatric Medicine, 29*, 539–553.

Kendler, K., Neale, M., Kessler, R., Heath, A., & Eaves, L. (1992). The genetic epidemiology of phobias in women: The interrelationship of agoraphobia, social phobia, situational phobia, and simple phobia. *Archives of General Psychiatry, 49*, 273–281.

Kendler, K. S., Walters, E. E., Neale, M. C., Kessler, R. C., Heath, A. C., & Eaves, L. J. (1995). The structure of genetic and environmental risk factors for six major psychiatric disorders in women: Phobia, generalized anxiety disorder, panic disorder, bulimia, major depression, and alcoholism. *Archives of General Psychiatry, 51*, 8–19.

Kessler, R. C., Avenevoli, S., & Merikangas, K. R. (2001). Mood disorders in children and adolescents: An epidemiologic perspective. *Biological Psychiatry, 49*, 1002–1014.

Kessler, R. C., McGonagle, K. A., Shanyang, Z., Nelson, C. B., Hughes, M., Eshleman, S., et al. (1994). Lifetime and 12-month prevalence of *DSM-III-R* psychiatric disorders in the United States. *Archives of General Psychiatry, 51*, 8–19.

Kindt, M., Brosschot, J. F., & Everaerd, W. (1997). Cognitive processing bias of children in real life stress situation and a neutral situation. *Journal of Experimental Child Psychology, 64*, 79–97.

King, N. J., Muris, P., & Ollendick, T. H. (2004). Specific Phobia. In T. L. Morris & J. S. March (Eds.), *Anxiety disorders in children and adolescents* (2nd ed., pp. 263–279). New York: Guilford..

King, N. J., Tonge, B. J., Heyne, D., Pritchard, M., Rollings, S., Young, D., et al. (1998). Cognitive-behavioral treatment of school-refusing children: A controlled evaluation. *Journal of the American Academy of Child and Adolescent Psychiatry, 37*, 395–403.

Kovacs, M. (1981). Rating scales to assess depression in school aged children. *Acta Paedopsychiatrica, 46*, 305–315.

Kovacs, M. (1992). *Children's Depression Inventory manual.* New York: Multi-Health Systems.

Kovacs, M., Feinberg, T. L., Crouse-Novak, M., Paulauskas, S. L., & Finkelstein, R. (1984). Depressive disorders in childhood: I. A longitudinal prospective study of characteristics and recovery. *Archives of General Psychiatry, 41*, 229–237.

Krohne, H. W., & Hock, M. (1991). Relationships between restrictive mother-child interactions and anxiety of the child. *Anxiety Research, 4*, 109–124.

Labellarte, M. J., Ginsburg, G. S., Walkup, J. T., & Riddle, M. A. (1999). The treatment of anxiety disorders in children and adolescents. *Biological Psychiatry, 46*, 1567–1578.

Lang, P. J. (1979). A bio-informational theory of emotional imagery. *Psychophysiology, 6*, 495–511.

Last, C. G., Perrin, S., Hersen, M., & Kazdin, A. E. (1992). *DSM-III-R* anxiety disorders in children: Sociodemographic and clinical characteristics. *Journal of the American Academy of Child and Adolescent Psychiatry, 31*, 1070–1076.

Last, C. L., Strauss, C. C., & Francis, G. (1987). Comorbidity among childhood anxiety disorders. *Journal of Nervous and Mental Disease, 175*, 726–730.

Lease, C. A., & Ollendick, T. H. (2000). Development and psychopathology. In M. Hersen & A. S. Bellack (Eds), *Psychopathology in adulthood* (2nd ed., pp. 131–149). Boston: Allyn & Bacon.

Lerner, R. M., Hess, L. E., & Nitz, K. (1991). A developmental perspective on psychopathology. In M. Hersen & C. G. Last (Eds), *Handbook of child and adult psychopathology: A longitudinal perspective* (pp. 9–32). Elmsford, NY: Pergamon Press.

Lewinsohn, P. M., Clarke, G. N., Hops, H., & Andrews, J. A. (1990). Cognitive-behavioral treatment for depressed adolescents. *Behavior Therapy, 21*, 385–401.

Lewinsohn, P. M., Clarke, G. N., Seeley, J. R., & Rohde, P. (1994). Major depression in community adolescents: Age at onset, episode duration, and time to recurrence. *Journal of the American Academy of Child and Adolescent Psychiatry, 33*, 809–818.

Lewinsohn, P. M., Hops, H., Roberts, R. E., Seeley, J. R., & Andrews, J. A. (1993). Adolescent psychopathology: I. Prevalence and incidence of depression and other *DSM-III-R* disorders in high school students. *Journal of Abnormal Psychology, 102*, 133–144.

Lewinsohn, P. M., Zinbarg, R., Seeley J. R., Lewinsohn, M., & Sack, W. H. (1997). Lifetime comorbidity among anxiety disorders and between anxiety disorders and other mental disorders in adolescents. *Journal of Anxiety Disorders, 11*, 377–394.

Lewis, M. (1990). Models of developmental psychopathology. In M. Lewis & S. M. Miller (Eds), *Handbook of developmental psychopathology* (pp. 15–27). New York: Plenum Press.

Manassis, K., & Monga, S. (2001). A therapeutic approach to children and adolescents with anxiety disorders and associated comorbid conditions. *Journal of the American Academy of Child & Adolescent Psychiatry, 40*, 115–117.

March, J., Parker, J., Sullivan, K., Stallings, P., & Conners, C. K. (1997). The Multidimensional Anxiety Scale for Children (MASC): Factor structure, reliability, and validity. *Journal of the American Academy of Child and Adolescent Psychiatry, 36*, 554–565.

Mattis, S. G., & Ollendick, T. H. (2002). *Panic disorder and anxiety in adolescence.* Oxford: Blackwell.

McClure, E. B, Brennan, P. A., Hammen, C., & Le Brocque, R. M. (2001). Parental anxiety disorders, child anxiety disorders, and the perceived parent-child relationship in an Australian high-risk sample. *Journal of Abnormal Child Psychology, 9*, 1–10.

McGee, R., Feehan, M., Williams, S., & Anderson, J. (1992). *DSM-III disorders from age 11 to 15 years. Journal of the American Academy of Child and Adolescent Psychiatry, 31*, 50–59.

McGee, R., Feehan, M., Williams, S., Partridge, F., Silvia, P. A., & Kelly, J. (1990). DSM III disorders in a large sample of adolescents. *Journal of the American Academy of Child and Adolescent Psychiatry, 29*, 611–619.

Mendlowitz, S. L., Manassis, K., Bradley, S., Scapillato, D., Miezitis, S., & Shaw, B. F. (1999). Cognitive-behavioral group treatments in childhood anxiety disorders: The role of parental involvement. *Journal of the American Academy of Child and Adolescent Psychiatry, 38*, 1233–1229.

Moore, P. S., Whaley, S. E., & Sigman, M. (2004). Interactions between mothers and children: Impacts of maternal and child anxiety. *Journal of Abnormal Psychology, 113*, 471–476.

Mufson, L., Moreau, D., Weissman, M. M., & Klerman, G. L. (1993). *Interpersonal psychotherapy for depressed adolescents.* New York: Guilford.

Mufson, L., Weissman, M. M., Moreau, D., & Garfinkel, R. (1999). Efficacy of interpersonal psychotherapy for depressed adolescents. *Archives of General Psychiatry, 56*, 573–579.

Nolen-Hoeksema, S. (1995). Epidemiology and theories of gender differences in unipolar depression. In M. V. Seeman (Ed.), *Gender and psychopathology* (pp. 63–87). London: American Psychiatric Press.

Nolen-Hoeksema, S., Girgus, J. S., & Seligman, M. E. (1992). Predictors and consequences of childhood depressive symptoms: A 5-year longitudinal study. *Journal of Abnormal Psychology, 101*, 405–422.

Ollendick, T. H. (1983). Reliability and validity of the Fear Survey Schedule for Children-Revised (FSSC-R). *Behaviour Research and Therapy, 21*, 685–692.

Ollendick, T. H., & Cerny, J. A. (1981). *Clinical behavior therapy with children.* New York: Plenum.

Ollendick, T. H., Hagopian, L. P., & King, N. J. (1997). Specific phobias in children. In G. C. L. Davey (Ed.), *Phobias: A handbook of theory, research and treatment* (pp. 201–224). Chichester, UK: Wiley.

Ollendick, T. H., & Hirshfeld-Becker, D. R. (2002). The developmental psychopathology of social anxiety disorder. *Biological Psychiatry.*

Ollendick, T. H., & Ingman, K. (2001). Social phobia. In H. Orvaschel, J. Faust, & M. Hersen (Eds), *Handbook of conceptualization and treatment of child psychopathology* (pp. 191–210). New York: Pergamon Press.

Ollendick, T. H., & King, N. J. (1994). Assessment and treatment of internalizing problems: The role of longitudinal data. *Journal of Consulting and Clinical Psychology, 62*, 918–927.

Ollendick, T. H., & King, N. J. (1998). Empirically supported treatments for children with phobic and anxiety disorders. *Journal of Clinical Child Psychology, 27*, 156–167.

Ollendick, T. H., King, N. J., & Chorpita, B. (2006). Empirically supported treatments for children and adolescents. In P. C. Kendall (Ed.), *Child and adolescent therapy* (3rd ed., pp. 492–520). New York: Guilford

Ollendick, T. H., King, N. J., & Muris, P. (2002). Fears and phobias in children: Phenomenology, epidemiology, and etiology. *Child Psychology and Psychiatry Review.*

Ollendick, T. H., Lease, C. A., & Cooper, C. (1993). Separation anxiety in young adults: A preliminary examination. *Journal of Anxiety Disorders, 7*, 293–305.

Ollendick, T. H., & March, J. S. (Eds.) (2004). *Phobic and anxiety disorders in children and adolescents: A clinician's guide to effective psychosocial and pharmacological interventions.* New York: Oxford University Press.

Ollendick, T. H., & Ollendick, D. G. (1997). General worry and anxiety in children. *In Session: Psychotherapy in Practice, 3*, 89–102.

Ollendick, T. H., & Seligman, L. D. (2006). Anxiety disorders in children and adolescents. In C. Gillberg, R. Harrington, & H.-C. Steinhausen (Eds.), *Clinician's desk book of child and adolescent psychiatry* (pp. 144–187). Cambridge: Cambridge University Press.

Ollendick, T. H., Vasey, M. W., & King, N. J. (2001). Operant conditioning influences in childhood anxiety. In M. W. Vasey & M. R. Dadds (Eds.), *The developmental psychopathology of anxiety* (pp. 231–252). London: Oxford University Press.

Orvaschel, H., Lewinsohn, P. M., & Seeley, R. J. (1995). Continuity of psychopathology in a community sample of adolescents. *Journal of the American Academy of Child and Adolescent Psychiatry, 34*, 1525–1535.

Orvaschel, H., & Puig-Antich, J. H., (1987). *Schedule for affective disorders and schizophrenia for school-age children* (Epidemiologic version, 4th ed.) Pittsburg, PA: Western Psychiatric Institute and Clinic.

Perwien, A. R., & Bernstein, G. A. (2004). In T. H. Ollendick & J. S. March (Eds.), *Phobic and anxiety disorders in children and adolescents* (pp. 272–305). New York: Oxford University Press.

Pfeffer, C. R., Lipkins, R., Plutchik, R., & Mizruchi, M. (1988). Normal children at risk for suicidal behavior: A two-year follow-up study. *Journal of the American Academy of Child and Adolescent Psychiatry, 27*, 34–41.

Piaget, J. (1950): *The psychology of intelligence*. New York: Harcourt Brace Jovanovich.

Pury, C. L., & Mineka, S. (2001). Differential encoding of affective and nonaffective content information in trait anxiety. *Cognition & Emotion, 15*, 659–693.

Rapee, R. M. (1997). Potential role of childrearing practices in the development of anxiety and depression. *Clinical Psychology Review, 17*, 47–68.

Rapee, R. M., Abbott, M. J., & Lyneham, H. J. (2006). Bibliotherapy for children with anxiety disorders using written materials for parents: A randomized controlled trial. *Journal of Consulting and Clinical Psychology, 74*, 436–444.

Reinherz, H. Z., Giaconia, R. M., Lefkowitz, E. S., Pakiz, B. & Frost (1993). Prevalence of psychiatric disorders in a community population of older adolescents. *Journal of the American Academy of Child and Adolescent Psychiatry, 32*(2), 369–377.

Reiss, S. (1980). Pavlovian conditioning and human fear: An expectancy model. *Behavior Therapy, 11*, 380–396.

Reynolds, C. R., & Kamphaus, R. W. (2004). *The Behavior Assessment Scale for Children* (2nd ed.). Circle Pines, MN: Pearson Assessments.

Reynolds, C. R., & Richmond, B. O. (1985). *Revised Children's Manifest Anxiety Scale: Manual*. Los Angeles, CA: Western Psychological Services.

Robinson, J. L., Kagan, J., Reznick, J. S., & Corley, R. (1992). The heritability of inhibited and uninhibited behavior: A twin study. *Developmental Psychology, 28*, 1030–1037.

Rohde, P., Clarke, G., Mace, D., Jorgensen, J., & Seeley, J. R. (2004). An efficacy/effectiveness study of cognitive-behavioral treatment for adolescents with comorbid major depression and conduct disorder. *Journal of the American Academy of Child and Adolescent Psychiatry, 43*(6), 660–669.

Rudd, D. M., & Joiner, T. E. (1998). An integrative conceptual framework for assessing and treating suicidal behavior in adolescents. *Journal of Adolescence, 21*, 489–498.

Rutter, M. (1985). Resilience in the face of adversity: Protective factors and resistance to psychaitric disorder. *British Journal of Psychiatry, 147*, 498–611.

Rutter, M., & Garmezy, N. (1983). Developmental psychopathology. In E. M. Hetherington (Ed.), *Socialization, personality, and social development: Vol. 4. Mussen's handbook of child psychology* (4th ed.) New York: Wiley.

Sameroff, A. J. (1995). General systems theories and developmental psychopathology. *Developmental Psychology, 1*, 659–695.

Sander, J. B. (2004, November). *CBT for depression in young adolescents: how well does it treat comorbid anxiety symptoms?* Paper presented at the Association for the Advancement of Behavior Therapy Annual Convention, New Orleans, Louisiana.

Sander, J. B., & McCarty, C. A. (2005). Youth depression in the family context: Familial risk factors and models of treatment. *Clinical Child and Family Psychology Review, 8*(3), 203–219.

Schniering, C. A., Hudson, J. L., & Rapee, R. M. (2000). Issues in the diagnosis and assessment of anxiety disorders in children and adolescents. *Clinical Psychology Review, 20*, 453–478.

Seligman, L. D., Goza, A. B., & Ollendick, T. H. (2004). Treatment of depressive disorders in children and adolescents. In P. Barrett & T. H. Ollendick (Eds.) *Handbook of interventions that work with children and adolescents: From prevention to treatment* (pp. 301–328). London: Wiley.

Seligman, L. D., & Ollendick, T. H. (1998). Comorbidity of anxiety and depression in children and adolescents: An integrative review. *Clinical Child and Family Psychology Review, 1*, 125–144.

Shamir-Essakow, G., Ungerer, J. A., & Rapee, R. M. (2005). Attachment, behavioural inhibition, and anxiety in preschool children. *Journal of Abnormal Child Psychology, 33*, 131–143.

Shaw, J., Kennedy, S. H., & Joffe (1995). Gender differences in mood disorders. In M. V. Seeman (Ed.), *Gender and psychopathology*. London: American Psychiatric Press.

Shortt, A. L., Barrett, P. M., & Fox, T. (2001). Evaluating the FRIENDS program: A cognitive behavioral group treatment for anxiety children and their parents. *Journal of Clinical Child Psychology, 30*, 525–535.

Silverman, W. K., & Albano, A. M. (1996). *Anxiety disorders interview schedule for DSM-IV: Child version: Parent interview schedule*. San Antonio: Psychological Corporation.

Silverman, W. K., Cerny, J. A., Nelles, W. B., & Burke, A. E. (1988). Behavior problems in children of parents with anxiety disorders. *Journal of the American Academy of Child and Adolescent Psychiatry, 27*, 779–784.

Silverman, W. K., Kurtines, W. M., Ginsburg, G. S., Weems, C. G., Lumpkin, P. W., & Carmichael, D. H. (1999). Treating anxiety disorders in children with group cognitive behavioural therapy: A randomised clinical trial. *Journal of Consulting and Clinical Psychology, 67*, 995–1003.

Silverman, W. K., & Ollendick, T. H. (Eds.) (1999). *Developmental issues in the clinical treatment of children*. Boston: Allyn & Bacon.

Silverman, W. K., & Ollendick, T. H. (2005). Evidence-based assessment of anxiety and its disorders in children and adolescents. *Journal of Clinical Child and Adolescent Psychology, 34*, 380–411.

Silverman, W. K., & Treffers, P. D. A. (2001). *Anxiety disorders in children and adolescents: Research, assessment and intervention*. New York: Cambridge University Press.

Siqueland, L., Kendall, P. C., & Steinberg, L. (1996). Anxiety in children: Perceived family environment and observed family interaction. *Journal of Clinical Child Psychology, 25*, 225–237.

Skinner, B. F. (1938). *The behavior of organisms*. New York: Appelton-Century-Crofts.

Spence, S. H. (1998) A measure of anxiety symptoms among children. *Behaviour Research and Therapy, 36*, 545–566.

Spence, S. H., Holmes, J. M., March, S., & Lipp, O. V. (2006). The feasibility and outcome of clinic plus internet delivery of cognitive-behaviour therapy for childhood anxiety. *Journal of Consulting and Clinical Psychology, 74*, 614–621.

Sroufe, L. A., & Rutter, M. (1984). The domain of developmental psychopathology. *Child Development, 55*, 17–29.

Stark, K. D., Sander, J. B., Yancy, M., Bronik, M., & Hoke, J. (2000). Treatment of depression in childhood and adolescence: Cognitive-behavioral procedures for the individual and family. In P. C. Kendall (Ed.), *Child and adolescent therapy: Cognitive-behavioral procedures* (2nd ed., pp. 173–234). New York: Guilford.

Stark, K. D., Hargrave, J., Sander, J. B., Schnoebelen, S., Simpson, J., & Glenn, R. (2006). Treatment of depression in childhood and adolescence: Cognitive-behavioral procedures for the individual and family. In P. C. Kendall (Ed.), *Child and adolescent therapy: Cognitive-behavioral procedures* (3rd ed.) New York: Guilford.

Stark, K. D., Schmidt, K. L., & Joiner, T. E., Jr. (1996). Cognitive triad: Relationship to depressive symptoms, parents' cognitive triad, and perceived parental messages. *Journal of Abnormal Child Psychology, 24*, 615–631.

Strauss, C. C., & Last, C. G. (1993). Social and simple phobias in children. *Journal of Anxiety Disorders, 7*, 141–152.

Strauss, C., Lease, C., Last, C., & Francis, G. (1988). Overanxious disorder: An examination of developmental differences. *Journal of Abnormal Child Psychology, 11*, 433–443.

Treatment for Adolescents with Depression Study (TADS) Team (2004). Fluoxetine, cognitive-behavioral therapy, and their combination for adolescents with depression: Treatment for Adolescents with Depression Study (TADS) randomized controlled trial. *Journal of the American Medical Association, 292*(7), 807–820.

Taghavi, M. R., Neshat-Doost, H. T., Moradi, A. R., Yule, W., & Dalgleish, T. (1999). Biases in visual attention in children and adolescents with clinical anxiety and mixed anxiety-depression. *Journal of Abnormal Child Psychology, 27*, 215–223.

Thapar, A., & McGuffin, P. (1995). Are anxiety symptoms in childhood heritable? *Journal of Child Psychology and Psychiatry, 36*, 439–447.

Toth, S. L., & Cicchetti, D. (1999). Developmental psychopathology and child psychotherapy. In S. W. Russ & T. H. Ollendick (Eds.), *Handbook of psychotherapies with children and families* (pp. 15–43). New York: Kluwer Academic/Plenum.

Turner, S. M., Beidel, D., & Wolff, P. L. (1996). Is behavioral inhibition related to anxiety disorders? *Clinical Psychology Review, 16*, 57–172.

Vasey, M. W., & Dadds, M. R. (2000). (Eds.). *The developmental psychopathology of anxiety.* New York: Oxford University Press.

Vasey, M. W., & Ollendick, T. H. (2000). Anxiety. In M. Lewis & A. Sameroff (Eds.), *Handbook of developmental psychopathology* (pp. 511–529). New York: Plenum.

Wagner, K. D., & Ambrosini, P. J. (2001). Childhood depression: Pharmacological therapy/treatment (pharmacology of childhood depression). *Journal of Clinical Child Psychology, 30*, 88–97.

Wannan, G., & Fombonne, E. (1998). Gender differences in rates and correlates of suicidal behavior amongst child psychiatric outpatients. *Journal of Adolescence, 21*, 371–381.

Weems, C. F., Silverman, W. K., Rapee, R., & Pina, A. A. (2003). The role of control in childhood anxiety disorders. *Cognitive Therapy and Research, 27*, 557–568.

Weissman, M. M., Gammon, G. D., J. K., Merikangas, K. R., Warner, V., Prusoff, B. A., & Sholomskas, D. (1987). Children of depressed parents: Increased psychpathology and early onset of major depression. *Archives of General Psychiatry, 44*, 847–853.

Weisz, J. R., Southam-Gerow, M. A., & McCarty, C. A. (2001). Control-related beliefs and depressive symptoms in clinic referred children and adolescents: Developmental differences and model specificity. *Journal of Abnormal Psychology, 110*, 97–109.

Werry, J. S. (1991). Overanxious disorder: A review of its taxonomic properties. *Journal of the American Academy of Child and Adolescent Psychiatry, 30*, 533–544.

Whaley, S. E., Pinto, A., & Sigman, M. (1999). Characterizing interactions between anxious mothers and their children. *Journal of Consulting and Clinical Psychology, 67*, 826–836.

Williams, S., Connolly, J., & Segal, Z. V. (2001). Intimacy in relationships and cognitive vulnerability to depression in adolescent girls. *Cognitive Therapy and Research, 25*(4), 477–496.

Wolff, J. A., & Ollendick, T. H. (2006). The comorbidity of conduct problems and depression in childhood and adolescence. *Clinical Child and Family Psychology Review, 9*, 201–220.

Wolpe, J., & Rachman, S. (1960). Psychoanalytic "evidence": A critique based on Freud's case of little Hans. *Journal of Nervous and Mental Disease, 131*, 135–148.

Wood, J., Mathews, A., & Dalgleish, T. (2001). Anxiety and cognitive inhibition. *Emotion, 1*, 166–181.

Woodruff-Borden, J., Marrow, C., Bourland, S., & Cambron, S. (2002). The behavior of anxious parents: Examining mechanisms of transmission of anxiety from parent to child. *Journal of Clinical Child and Adolescent Psychiatry, 31*, 364–374.

World Health Organization. (1992). *The ICD-10 classification of mental and behavioral disorders: Diagnostic criteria for research.* Geneva: Author.

18

Cognitive Disorders of Childhood

Specific Learning and Intellectual Disabilities

Jack Naglieri, Claudia Salter, and Johannes Rojahn

Learning Disabilities

The term *learning disability* (LD) generally refers to a condition where a child's achievement is substantially lower than expected based on the child's intelligence. Simply stated, it means a person's level of achievement is inconsistent with his or her ability when measured using an achievement and IQ test. According to the U.S. Department of Education, up to 11% of school-aged children qualify as having a disability under the Individuals with Disabilities Education Act (IDEA), and approximately half of these children have a specific type of learning disability (U.S. Department of Education, 2000). Although the concept seems simple (ability versus achievement discrepancy) it has proven to be confusing because of a lack of consensus over how to operationalize it and a variety of definitions proposed by professional organizations and government officials. There is also great variability in the way learning disability has been assessed, including varying tests, methods, state and federal definitions, and in ways of using these definitions in professional practice. This variability of definition and method is also a problem because it makes it difficult for professionals to determine whether or not a child qualifies for special services and receives additional instruction. To better understand the current issues in the field of LD it is first important to understand the history of the diagnosis.

Historical Definitions of Learning Disabilities

In this section we discuss the definitions of learning disabilities from the early 20th century to the present time.

1910–1930s: Early Period During the early 1900s, it was first recognized that some children who were intelligent could not learn to read. At that time it was thought that brain damage caused problems that disrupted learning in a specific domain such as reading or writing. Children thought to have such damage were considered intelligent in all areas except in reading or writing. In 1917, James Hinshelwood, a Scottish ophthalmologist, reported case studies of children who had difficulty acquiring reading skills. He attributed their problem to a condition that he called "congenital word blindness," which he thought resulted from damage to an area of the brain that stored visual memories for words and letters (Torgesen, 1998). In 1937, Samuel Orton, a child neurologist, published his influential work on children with reading disabilities that differed from Hinshelwood. Orton used the term *strephosymbolia* or twisted symbols, to describe the condition because these children often reversed words or letters when reading. He attributed the cause to a lack of hemispheric dominance in the brain, which caused visual images to be confused when transferred from one hemisphere to the other (Torgeson, 1998). Their initial concept that brain dysfunction contributes to a learning disability continues to influence the field of learning disabilities today.

Recent studies have evaluated brain functioning in children and adults with learning disabilities. The view that learning can be disrupted in a single area of the brain and influence a specific type of achievement, such as reading, is the basis for the diagnosis of a reading disorder in some current identification systems (see discussion of *DSM-IV-TR* that follows). In addition, Orton's work continues to have influence in the field of reading intervention since his multisensory educational approach for children with reading disabilities is incorporated into the Orton-Gillingham reading method.

1940s–1950s: Werner and Strauss Heinz Werner and Alfred Strauss at the Wayne County Training School in Michigan described a subset of children, presumed to have brain damage, who had problems working with certain kinds of information and displayed behavioral and cognitive problems similar to those of head-injured soldiers described by Kirk Goldstein. For example, these children had problems inhibiting their responses and they seemed hyperactive. Importantly, these children had difficulties that were distinct from and not as broad as those found for persons with intellectual disabilities (Torgesen, 1998). Werner and Strauss's work also differed from that of Orton and Hinshelwood in that they described problems in general learning areas rather than in specific academic skills. Since these children had difficulties similar to the head-injured soldiers, Werner and Strauss concluded that the children must have had brain damage.

Furthermore, Werner and Strauss concluded that these brain-damaged children needed special educational interventions to overcome their weaknesses. This work by Werner and Strauss suggested that children with learning problems were not all alike in their behavior profiles and that educational programming should be individualized. Since then, millions of dollars have been spent in diagnosing LD and developing special education programs in schools across the United States. The concept of individualized instructional plans (IEPs) was then initiated and remains in many rules and regulations to this day (Hallahan & Keogh, 2001).

1960s: Origins of the Concept of a Learning Disability By the 1960s, evidence had accumulated that children with learning problems often had a history of head injury, infections, or difficulties during pregnancy or labor. The International Study Group in Child Neurology suggested that the term *minimal brain dysfunction* be used to describe these children (1962). The suggested definition was broad and included diverse symptoms and etiology. This was not the only revision in the label that was suggested. In fact, numerous terms were used in the 1960s to describe children who were not achieving at the level expected based on their intelligence, including dyslexic and perceptually handicapped. Support organizations as well as the scientific community began to recognize the growing need for a unified term.

In 1963, Samuel Kirk introduced the term *learning disability* at a conference for parents that explored the problems of children who had specific learning problems and did not have mental retardation (intellectual disabilities). One of the important issues addressed at the meeting was what to call these children. Parents were interested in not only a better label for their children, but also a term that would bring together the many small organizations into a more powerful group (Hallahan & Cruickshank, 1973). Kirk was cautious about the use of labels. In his speech he indicated that he preferred descriptions of the problem rather than technical terms such as *strephosymbolia*. However, he said that he recently started to use the term *learning disabilities* to describe children who have "disorders in development in language, speech, reading, and associated communication skills needed for social interaction" (Kirk, 1963). He excluded from this group children who have sensory handicaps such as deafness or blindness and children who have intellectual disabilities. The response to his suggestion was mostly positive and those at the convention voted the following day to organize under the title Association for Children with Learning Disabilities (Hallahan & Cruickshank, 1973).

Kirk's initiation of the term *learning disabilities* was not as much an endorsement of labeling children, as it was a way of getting help for these individuals. He preferred that a child's behavior be analyzed to determine appropriate remediation and training (Kirk, 1972). He also later developed an approach to identifying specific learning disabilities, which was formalized into a test called the Illinois Test of Psycholinguistic Abilities. Although the value of this test would eventually prove to be very limited, it did much to signify the need for a test that would identify the learning problems of children with learning disabilities.

1960s–1970s: Federal Legislation In 1967, the term *minimal brain dysfunction* was replaced by *learning disability* in U.S. federal legislation. The National Advisory Committee on Handicapped Children (NAHC) proposed a definition for learning disabilities that became the basis for the Education for All Handicapped Children Act (PL 94-142). This is the definition that remains in federal policy at this time.

> "Specific learning disability" means a disorder in one or more of the basic psychological processes involved in understanding or in using language, spoken or written, which may manifest itself in an imperfect ability to listen, think, speak, read, write, spell, or to do mathematical calculations. The term includes such conditions as perceptual handicaps, brain injury, minimal brain dysfunction, dyslexia, and developmental aphasia. The term does not include children who have learning problems, which are primarily the result of visual, hearing, or motor handicaps, of intellectual disabilities, of emotional disturbance, or of environmental, cultural, or economic disadvantage.

The word *specific* was added to the term *learning disabilities* to avoid confusion with the learning problems of children with intellectual disabilities. Children with intellectual disabilities have a general difficulty in learning, whereas children with learning disabilities have difficulty in a more limited area (Kirk, 1972).

The Right to Education for All Handicapped Children's Act of 1975 (PL 94-142) retained the definition and added criteria for identifying children with learning disabilities. The law provided a guarantee that children would receive an appropriate public education in "the least restrictive environment." Each individual was entitled to publicly funded special education and special services and protected from discrimination. These laws have had extraordinary influence on public school practices of assessment, diagnosis, and instruction for children identified as having special educational needs.

1980s: National Joint Committee for Learning Disabilities (NJCLD) In 1981, The National Joint Committee for Learning Disabilities (NJCLD) provided a modified definition of learning disabilities to address areas of confusion with the federal definition. This modified definition included recognizing that learning disabilities are a "heterogeneous group of disorders" and that they often co-occur with other disorders (National Joint Committee on Learning Disabilities, 1991).

Around this time, learning disabilities were also included in the third edition of the *Diagnostic and Statistical Manual of Mental Disorders*, published in 1980 (*DSM-III*; American Psychiatric Association, 1980). Under the category of "Specific Delays in Development," the *DSM-III* listed diagnoses of specific reading retardation, specific arithmetical retardation, and other specific learning difficulties. Specific reading retardation was described as a "serious impairment in the development of reading or spelling skills not explicable in terms of general intellectual retardation or of inadequate schooling" (1980). The revised version, *DSM-III-R* (1987), replaced the language of specific retardation with developmental disorder and listed them under the category of "Academic Skills Disorders": Diagnoses included developmental arithmetic disorder, developmental expressive writing disorder, and developmental reading disorder. These are the three main areas of learning disabilities that remain in *DSM-IV-TR*.

1990s: DSM-IV; Individuals with Disabilities Act 1997 The *DSM-IV* was published in 1994 and a revision, which is the current version in use today, was published in 2000 (*DSM-IV-TR*). The diagnoses in the *DSM-IV-TR* remain the same as in *DSM-IV*. The *DSM-IV-TR* uses the term *learning disorders* rather than *academic skills disorders*. Learning disorders are classified into three main types: reading disorder, mathematics disorder, and disorder of written expression. This classification is similar to that of Hinshelwood and Orton from many years before. The *DSM-IV-TR* diagnoses apply to individuals who have a significant discrepancy between their achievement in one of the above areas and their level of intelligence. Their academic achievement score must be substantially lower than their intellectual ability, which according to *DSM-IV-TR*, is usually a score two standard deviations below their score on a measure of intelligence.

The most current legislation regarding children with disabilities is the Amendments of the Individuals with Disabilities Education Act (IDEA '97), which reauthorized PL 94-142 also known as the Right to Education for All Handicapped Children's Act of 1975. The 1975 act was reauthorized as the Individuals with Disabilities Education Act (IDEA) in 1990. No changes were made to the definition or identification of a specific learning disability throughout these reauthorizations of the law. This law had significant influence on the field of learning disabilities because funding for special educational programs are tied directly to the number of children identified with a disability in each school district.

2000s: Ability Achievement Discrepancy Under Fire In recent years there has been growing concern that the intelligence-achievement discrepancy approach is not effective for identification of learning disabilities and that it does not help professionals devise appropriate interventions. For example, in 2002, Robert Pasternack, the assistant secretary to the Office of Special Education and Rehabilitative Services, spoke about the "Demise of IQ Testing" at the National Association of School Psychologists conference. He concluded that IQ testing is not an appropriate way to diagnose LD and that the discrepancy approach should be eliminated. One of his most significant criticisms was that the intelligence–achievement discrepancy approach emphasizes eligibility issues more than the selection of academic interventions. Although the Assistant Secretary supported the definition of LD as a disorder in one or more of the basic psychological processes required for academic performance, the method of using a discrepancy to find these children was deemed ineffective and expensive.

The Commission on Excellence in Special Education also supports the elimination of the ability achievement discrepancy approach for the purpose of diagnosing learning disorders (2001). In the report, concerns are raised that the vague federal definition of LD and the lack of consistency in diagnostic criteria leads to unreliable methods of diagnosis. Another concern is that children are often inappropriately identified as LD and placed in special education because they have not learned, in some cases because they were not taught, how to read. The Commission recommended early screening of children for LD and placing more focus on assessing the child's response to instruction.

Assessment and Diagnosis

The designation of a clear and objective system for identifying children with learning disabilities has turned out to be as elusive as developing a widely accepted way to identify children with this disorder.

Federal and State definitions provide guidelines, but these guidelines lack the precision necessary for identifying children with learning disorders. The result is that professionals have identified children with learning disorders using many different tests and methods in an attempt to follow the intelligence–achievement discrepancy model which is the most widely used definition. Alternatively, some have attempted to identify children who have a disorder in one or more of the basic psychological processes involved in reading. Some issues surrounding each of these approaches will be more fully examined.

In the IQ-achievement discrepancy approach, a child is typically administered a test of intelligence, and this score is compared to a measure of achievement (e.g., score on a standardized test of achievement or performance in school). The most commonly used measure of intelligence for children is the Wechsler Intelligence Scale for Children (WISC-III; Wechsler, 1991), although there are problems with this test for the purpose of identifying LD (discussed below).

The advantage of the IQ-achievement discrepancy approach is that it helps differentiate between learning disorders and intellectual disabilities (i.e., low achievement and low IQ, respectively) and can be used to identify a specific academic problem (not all achievement is low). There are at least two problems with this approach. First, there are several IQ tests available to psychologists and each one has many scores that could be used. Some state regulations only allow the use of a single total IQ score to determine if there is a discrepancy. Federal and state regulators cannot direct practitioners to use a particular IQ or achievement test, which has resulted in considerable variability in the way the IQ-achievement discrepancy is calculated. In fact, different states and school districts mandate different size of discrepancy (e.g., one or two standard deviation differences between IQ and achievement). State and county criteria also vary in how a discrepancy is operationalized including deviation from grade level, expectancy formulas, regression analyses, and standard score comparisons (Mercer, Jordan, Allsopp, & Mercer, 1996).

The second major problem with the IQ-achievement discrepancy is that in order for a discrepancy to occur, the child has to have time to fall behind in an academic area. This means that a child will likely be in second or third grade before the discrepancy becomes obvious. By that time, however, the child is so far behind in acquiring academic skills that catching up may take many years. Some researchers have argued that not only is the IQ-achievement discrepancy ineffective for identification of children with learning disabilities but also that intelligence tests themselves are irrelevant to the diagnosis of learning disabilities (Siegle, 1989). In fact, after careful review of the research, Kaufman and Lichtenberger (2000) concluded that WISC-III subtest profiles "do not have adequate power on which to base differential diagnosis" (p. 205) for LD. This conclusion is reasonable considering that Wechsler's test was not designed to identify children with LD. Scores on verbal/nonverbal tests of intelligence have not been especially helpful for diagnosis of LD or ADHD (Kavale & Forness, 1984; Kaufman & Lichtenberger, 2000). These problems and others with using the IQ-achievement discrepancy have led many in the field to recognize that an alternative should be considered.

The processing disorder method (cognitive processing disorder model) is an alternative to the IQ-achievement discrepancy model and traditional IQ tests. Recall that a

> Specific learning disability means a disorder in one or more of the basic psychological processes involved in understanding or in using language, spoken or written, which may manifest itself in an imperfect ability to listen, think, speak, read, write, spell, or to do mathematical calculations.

If a processing disorder is detected and the child has academic failure, then eligibility could be made. Historically, identification based on a disorder in one or more of the "basic psychological processes" has been limited because there is no definition of basic psychological processes in state and federal regulations. Practitioners have also been reluctant to utilize this approach to identification because of the limited availability of reliable and valid tests of basic cognitive processes. During the last 15 years, however, two methods have been published that offer psychologists well validated tests to assess cognitive processes: the Kaufman Assessment Battery for Children (Kaufman & Kaufman, 1983) and the Cognitive Assessment System (Naglieri & Das, 1997). Both of these tests are nationally normed instruments with excellent reliability that provide a means to identify a disorder in one or more of the basic psychological, also referred to as cognitive, processes (Naglieri, 1999). Additionally, researchers have found that the cognitive processing approach can provide measures of processes that are relevant to diagnosis and treatment (Naglieri, 1999). The use of these methods, however, has been limited because of the dominance of the IQ-achievement method and the relative recent availability of well standardized tests of cognitive processing.

Epidemiology

The prevalence of learning disabilities depends, of course, on how they are defined and identified, which is why prevalence rates have varied widely from study to study. According to the *DSM-IV-TR*, estimates of the prevalence of learning disorders range from 2 to 10%. In the public schools, 4.5% of students are classified as having a "Specific Learning Disability" (U.S. Department of Education, 2000). Students in this category comprise half of the approximately 6 million students served under IDEA, Part B (U.S. Department of Education, 2000). The next largest groups are students with speech and language impairments (1.7%) and intellectual disabilities (0.95%). Since 1976, following the implementation of PL 94-142, the number of children in the specific learning disability group has grown considerably. Of the children identified, the great majority of children with learning disabilities have difficulties with reading. It is estimated that 4% of school-age children can be classified as having a reading disorder (*DSM-IV-TR*).

Etiology of Learning Disabilities

Professionals in the field of learning disabilities have been more focused on describing the disability and developing interventions than on understanding etiology (Torgeson, 1998). The etiology of learning disabilities is unclear, although most researchers think that they result from neurological impairment. There is a broad range or spectrum of learning disabilities, and there are likely many mechanisms involved, each contributing to particular learning disabilities. Studies have provided evidence that both genetic and environmental factors contribute to the development of some learning disabilities.

Neuroimaging studies have provided evidence for both functional and structural abnormalities associated with learning disabilities, adding further support for a biological basis. Functional abnormalities refer to differences in activation of brain regions (assessed by blood flow, oxygen uptake, or cellular metabolism), while structural abnormalities refer to differences in volume or shape. Filipek recently reviewed neuroimaging findings in children with developmental disorders and found structural and functional differences in some studies of individuals with reading disorders (Filipek, 1999). Results suggested that children with reading disorder have abnormalities in regions associated with receptive language (Hynd et al., 1995; Filipek, 1999).

There is also some evidence that genetic factors contribute to the development of learning disabilities. Family studies have shown a high prevalence rate of LD in first-degree relatives of children with LD. Twin studies have shown greater concordance of LD for monozygotic twins than dizygotic twins. Together, these studies suggest a hereditary component for learning disabilities of approximately 50% (Ingalls & Goldstein, 1999). Work by Bishop has suggested that genetic factors are most substantial for severe literacy problems, which includes children with specific language impairment and specific reading disability (Bishop, 2001). In some families, reading disability has been linked to a region of chromosome 6 (Cardon et al., 1994)

Many factors may negatively affect the developing fetal brain, potentially causing neurological impairment and resulting in learning disabilities. Prenatal and postnatal factors are both important. Prenatal factors include hypoxia, maternal infection, maternal cigarette smoking, and maternal alcohol and drug use. Postnatal factors include infection, injury, and exposure to toxins such as lead. Cognitive impairments ranging from subtle cognitive impairment to LD to intellectual disabilities have been associated with lead toxicity (Ingalls & Goldstein, 1999). Traumatic brain injury has also been shown to cause cognitive deficits and learning problems that may present months to years after injury (Fay et al., 1994; Yeates, 2000).

Conclusions

Like other fields in psychology, the field of learning disabilities is evolving in an erratic and nonlinear manner as the various forces of science, practice, and state and federal legislation all converge to address the needs of children with learning problems. Although much progress has been made, considerably more research will be needed in order to resolve the many longstanding issues in this field.

Intellectual Disabilities

Intellectual disability is typically a lifelong condition that can be caused by a variety of different etiologies.

Definition of Intellectual Disabilities

Intellectual disabilities are defined by three criteria:

1. significant limitations in intellectual functioning,
2. significant limitations in adaptive behavior, and
3. the manifestation of these limitations before the age of 18 years.

All major diagnostic classification systems, such as the *DSM-IV-TR* (American Psychiatric Association, 2000), the *International Classification of Diseases* (ICD-10; World Health Organization, 1992), and the *Definition, Classification and Supports* of the American Association on Mental Retardation (AAMR, 2002)[1] concur on these basic criteria.

Intellectual functioning is operationalized by performance on intelligence tests. A "significant limitation" in intellectual functioning is characterized by scores of approximately two standard deviations below the mean or lower on a standardized, individually administered intelligence test. The construct of adaptive behavior, which is not independent of intelligence, is less well established. The latest rendition of the AAMR/AAIDD definition of adaptive behavior proposes three domains of adaptive skills: conceptual, social, and practical adaptive skills (AAMR, 2002). Deficits in adaptive behavior must be relative to standards of personal independence and social responsibility for the same age group within a culture. Depending upon the person's age, different standards apply in assessing adaptive behavior. For example, during infancy and early childhood, sensory motor skills, communication skills, self-help skills, and socialization are emphasized. During childhood and early adolescence, basic academic skills, appropriate reasoning and judgment, and social skills are stressed, and during late adolescence and adult life, vocational and social responsibilities are most important. The third criterion for an individual to be diagnosed as mentally retarded is that the deficits must be manifested during the developmental period, which has been set between birth and 18 years of age. If the intellectual and adaptive deficits appear after the developmental period, the condition is typically designated as dementia. It is important to note that this three-part definition does not make any assumption about the etiology of the condition and is based solely on the individual's current behavior.

Individuals with intellectual disabilities can be classified by their level of cognitive functioning or by the intensity of supports needed. Levels of intellectual functioning are determined by standard deviations below the mean. For example, using the Wechsler scales with a standard deviation of 15, we speak of mild intellectual disabilities if the IQ falls between 55 and 69 (with a window of tolerance up to 75, depending on adaptive behavior), of moderate mental for IQ scores between 40 and 54, severe intellectual disabilities for IQs between 25 and 39; and profound intellectual disabilities for IQ scores below 25. Classification in terms of intensity of supports needed follows a shift in definition by the AAMR in 1992. The definition placed greater emphasis on environmental interactions that influence an individual's level of functioning. Support intensities can be classified as intermittent (as needed basis), limited (e.g., time-limited employment training), extensive (e.g., long term home living support), and pervasive (e.g., life-sustaining technology). Typical areas of support are human development, teaching and education, home living, employment, health and safety, protection and advocacy, social and behavioral (AAMR, 2002).

A variety of factors can complicate a diagnosis of intellectual disabilities. For example, the presence of a severe sensory impairment, such as blindness or deafness, can complicate the process of obtaining a legitimate estimate of IQ performance. Likewise, severe emotional and behavioral disturbance may confound attempts to obtain a reliable estimate of IQ level. In addition, psychotropic drugs may interfere with cognitive neurological functioning, including anticonvulsant drugs. Such effects may or may not be reversible, and they are particularly problematic in the case of individuals with intellectual disabilities, because the signs and symptoms of drug intoxication (e.g., ataxia, confusion, and slurred speech) may be confused with symptoms of intellectual disabilities commonly encountered in this population.

Prevalence of Intellectual Disabilities

Prevalence estimates of intellectual disabilities vary considerably due to methodological variations in case definitions, case finding methods, sampling frames and procedures, survey methods, etc. (McDermott, Durkin, Schupf, & Stein, 2007). Larsen et al. (2000) analyzed the National Health Interview Survey data (National Center for Health Statistics, 1997, 1998) and state agency statistics (Prouty & Lakin, 1999) and found that the prevalence of intellectual disabilities or developmental disabilities in the U.S. population was approximately 1.6%; the prevalence of intellectual disabilities was 0.78% of the general population. Among children between the ages of 6 and 21 years of age who received special education services under the Individuals with Disabilities Education Act (IDEA), Part B, the prevalence of intellectual disabilities during the 1998–1999 school year was 1.03% (U.S. Department of Education, 2000). However, these data also revealed significant over- and underrepresentations of certain ethnic groups, ranging from low of 0.4% of the Asian and Pacific Islanders population to 2.2% of the population of African Americans (see Table 18.1).

Table 18.1 The percentage of children between the ages of 6 and 21 years of age served under the Individuals with Disabilities Education Act (IDEA) Part B during the 1998–1999 school year

	Prevalence in %
American Indians/Alaskan	1.03
Asians/Pacific Islanders	0.43
Black	2.23
Hispanic	0.60
White	0.79

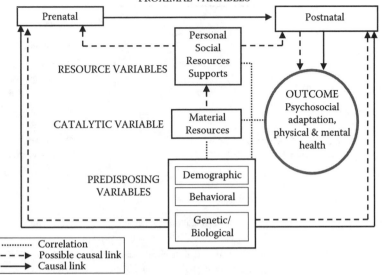

PROXIMAL VARIABLES

Figure 18.1 An interactive model of prenatal and postnatal variables that determine a child's psychosocial, mental, and intellectual outcome (adapted from Baumeister, 1988)..

Etiology of Intellectual Disabilities

The causes of intellectual disabilities are typically complex interactions of biological, behavioral/ psychological, and sociocultural factors. Figure 18.1, which is an adaptation and generalization of a model proposed by Baumeister (1988), delineates the interdependent factors that contribute to a person's psychosocial adaptation. It indicates that genetic endowment, behavioral, and mental health characteristics, and demographic parameters (e.g., level of socioeconomic status) in a family tend to be associated with material resources, which in turn influence access to health services, resources, and supports. These factors also influence the quality of a nurturing and safe environment.

A simplified etiological classification of intellectual disabilities is presented in Table 18.2, organized by known causes and outcomes. There are many inherited conditions due to single gene defects that are associated with intellectual disabilities, including dominant disorders (e.g., tuberous sclerosis and neurofibromatosis), recessive disorders (e.g., phenylketonuria [PKU], microcephaly), and sex-linked disorders (e.g., Fragile X syndrome and Lesch-Nyhan syndrome). Tuberous sclerosis is a multisystem disease that can affect the brain, kidneys, heart, eyes, lungs, and other organs and is characterized by seizures, intellectual disabilities, and skin and eye lesions. Neurofibromatosis (von Recklinghausen's disease) causes nerve sheath tumors and can affect the development of nonnervous tissues such as bones and skin. It can also lead to developmental abnormalities, including a slight increase in frequency of intellectual disabilities. PKU is caused by deficiency of the enzyme phenylalanine hydroxylase, resulting in a marked elevation of phenylalanine and its metabolites. These are toxic to the CNS, and, if the person is not maintained on a low-phenylalanine diet, the toxins can produce brain damage resulting in severe intellectual disabilities, often in combination with seizures and eczema. Lesch-Nyhan syndrome is a rare disorder of purine metabolism. Its most prominent features are intellectual disabilities, often in association with cerebral palsy, and the presence of self-mutilating behavior and other behavior problems. Fragile X syndrome, which is named after an abnormality in the long arm of the X chromosome, usually only affects males. Its most prominent symptoms include long thin faces, prominent jaws, long ears and hands, and large testes after puberty. There are also likely many cases of intellectual disabilities where more than one gene is involved. Understanding of polygenetic

TABLE 18.2   Classification of causes of mental retardation

Causation			Outcome
	Inherited chromosomal conditions	Dominant autosomal	Tuberous sclerosis, Neurofibromatosis
		Recessive autosomal	Phenylketonuria (PKU), Microcephaly, Galactosemia, Tay-Sachs disease
Single gene anomaly		X-Linked	Fragile X, Lesch-Nyhan syndrome
	Noninherited chromo-somal conditions	Autosomal	Down syndrome, Prader-Willi syndrome, Smith-Magenis
		X-Linked	Klinefelter syndrome, Turner syndrome
Polygenetic anomalies			?
Other congenital conditions		Cranial malformations	Anencephaly, Hydrocephaly
		Maternal disease (rubella, AIDS, venereal diseases, and blood group incompatibility, maternal diabetes); substance exposure	Fetal alcohol effects and syndrome
	Prenatal causes	*Biological:* Neurotoxins (alcohol, lead, mercury, exposure to radia-tion, some illicit drugs)	
		Psychosocial: Poverty (maternal malnutrition, lack of prenatal care)	Mental retardation, prematurity
Environmental factors	Perinatal causes	*Biological:* Trauma during birth, oxygen deprivation, brain hemor-rhage, acute maternal herpes	Cerebral palsy, mental retarda-tion, deafness
	Postnatal causes	*Biological:* Infections (encepha-litis, meningitis) head trauma, toxemia, poisons and toxins (lead and carbon monoxide), malnutri-tion, cerebrovascular accidents, degenerative diseases	Mental retardation
		Psychosocial: Secondary effects of poverty, deprivation, neglect, abuse	

determination, which is only in its infancy at this stage, holds great promise for our knowledge about the causation of intellectual disabilities, particularly milder forms of intellectual disabilities.

There are also many chromosomal abnormalities that can cause intellectual disabilities. Down syndrome, the most commonly diagnosed form of intellectual disability (occurring in about one out of every 700 live births) is typically caused by the Trisomy 21 variant, which has an extra chromosome 21. Other forms of Down syndrome are caused by translocation, when a major portion of chromosome 21 is translocated onto another chromosome, usually chromosome 14, and thus three copies of this portion of chromosome 21 are inherited. In Mosaicism, some cells have a normal compliment of 46, whereas others have 47 chromosomes, and such individuals may vary from apparently unaffected to having the typical physical presentation of Down syndrome. Other examples of conditions caused by chromosomal abnormalities are Prader-Willi syndrome and Smith-Magenis syndrome. X-Linked anomalies include Klinefelter syndrome and Turner syndrome.

Congenital malformations are also associated with intellectual disabilities. Such developmental defects include anencephaly, a fatal defect in brain development resulting in small or missing brain hemispheres, and hydrocephaly, an accumulation of cerebrospinal fluid (CSF) in the cranium that causes the ventricles and head to enlarge.

Certain maternal diseases can be transmitted to the fetus either in utero (i.e., prenatally) or during delivery. These include rubella (German measles), cytomegaly virus (the most common viral cause of intellectual disabilities), and mumps. If contracted during the first trimester of pregnancy, the effects of rubella can be devastating to the fetus, with severe intellectual disabilities and a variety of physical disorders ensuing. Other maternal infections that can cause a permanent adverse effect on the offspring include toxoplasmosis, herpes, human immunodeficiency virus (HIV), and syphilis. Maternal diabetes, especially if uncontrolled, can cause excessive or retarded growth, which may be associated with congenital abnormalities. Blood group incompatibility between the mother and fetus can also lead to intellectual disabilities. Finally, toxemia is a metabolic disorder of unknown origin that occurs during pregnancy and is characterized by hypertension, edema, and albuminuria (protein in the urine). It can affect the fetus's brain, heart, kidney, and liver.

Other prenatal causes of intellectual disabilities include exposure to a variety of substances or conditions, including toxins such as lead, mercury, radiation, and some illicit drugs. Mothers who consumed alcohol during pregnancy can pose a threat to the fetus of developing fetal alcohol syndrome. The greatest risk for developing fetal alcohol syndrome appears to be during the first six weeks of pregnancy, when the mother may not even realize she is pregnant.

Perinatal (i.e., at the time of birth) insults can result in neurological injury, which may later be manifested as cerebral palsy, deafness, or intellectual disabilities. The two most common perinatal causes of intellectual disabilities are prematurity and low birth weight. Traditionally, prematurity is defined as birth before 38 weeks of gestation; low birth weight is defined as having a birth weight less than 2,500 grams (5 ½ lb). The major causes of prematurity include maternal health problems, dietary insufficiency, heavy cigarette smoking, and maternal age less than 18 or over 35 years.

Because the premature neonate enters the world with an underdeveloped organ system, it is more susceptible to a variety of problems, such as oxygen deprivation and brain hemorrhage due to structural weakness of the blood vessels (Baroff & Olley, 1999). Low birth weight is also associated with prematurity, but the full-term infant who is born small for gestational age is also at risk for a variety of problems. Physical trauma caused by malpresentation of the fetus or disproportion between the infant's head and the pelvis of the mother can result in physical trauma and intracranial hemorrhage, which in turn can cause motor abnormalities, seizures, and intellectual disabilities. Asphyxia is another perinatal factor sometimes associated with subsequent intellectual disabilities, and it may be due to premature separation of the placenta, prolapse of the umbilical cord, anesthesia, or obstruction of the airways (Baroff, 1999; Kolb & Brodie, 1982). Finally, high birth weight (often associated with maternal diabetes) and herpes transmitted from mother to infant at the time of birth are further complications that can lead to intellectual disabilities.

Of all the postnatal causes of intellectual disabilities, encephalitis (inflammation of the brain) and meningitis (inflammation of the brain's covering membranes) are the most common. Other physical causes include head trauma (from automobile and other accidents), toxemia, poisons and toxins such as lead and carbon monoxide, malnutrition, cerebrovascular accidents or strokes, and degenerative diseases. Another extremely important postnatal cause is psychosocial deprivation. Psychosocial deprivation tends to occur under conditions of poverty, a chaotic living environment, family instability, child abuse and neglect, inadequate care giving, and an emphasis on day-to-day survival rather than on developmentally appropriate intellectual, social, academic, and cultural stimulation.

Assessment of Intellectual Disabilities

To properly establish a diagnosis of intellectual disabilities, the levels of intelligence and adaptive behavior have to be determined. While this seems like a straightforward task, it is complicated by issues such as the definitions of intelligence used by authors of these tests.

Intelligence As with most other clinical populations, tests of intelligence such as the Wechsler Intelligence Scale for Children—Third Edition (WISC-III; Wechsler, 1991) and the Stanford-Binet Intelligence Scales: Fourth Edition (SB:FE; Thorndike, Hagen, & Sattler, 1986) are the typical instruments used to assess intellectual disabilities. These two tests have some similarities that are especially important given the special demands involved with the assessment of persons with intellectual disabilities.

Wechsler's test and the Stanford-Binet are both based on a view of general intelligence that puts emphasis on the total IQ score. Although these tests are comprised of smaller subtests that are organized into three main types: Verbal, Nonverbal (also called Performance), and Quantitative, the tests measure what is called general ability that has a vague definition (Naglieri, 1999). The verbal tests measure general ability using questions that require the subject to define words or describe how two words are alike. Similarly, the nonverbal subtests measure general ability by tests that involve building a geometric design using blocks or combining parts of an object into a whole (like a child's puzzle). Quantitative subtests measure general ability by questions that involve solving arithmetic word problems or working with numbers. These three types of tests of general intelligence have formed the basic ingredients of intelligence tests since the early 1900s (Naglieri, 1999). For persons with intellectual disabilities, however, the achievement-like verbal and quantitative tests pose a particular challenge.

The principal weakness of traditional IQ tests is that they require the examinee to demonstrate knowledge of English and skills at completing math word problems. These skills, also included in many tests of achievement, are particularly difficult for those with a history of school failure and cultural and linguistic differences. The effect that the content of an IQ test has on rates of identification of intellectual disabilities for groups of white and African-American children was illustrated by Naglieri and Rojahn (2000). They found that African-American children who were tested with Wechsler's test (which includes verbal and nonverbal tests) were more likely to earn IQ scores that indicated intellectual disabilities than when assessed using the Cognitive Assessment System, which measures basic psychological or cognitive processes such as planning and attention rather than verbal and arithmetic skills.

The assessment of persons for intellectual disabilities also can be complicated by hearing impairment, visual impairment, motor problems (e.g., cerebral palsy), and speech problems. Additionally, the need to assess children at a very young age may pose problems with the tests discussed so far, particularly with the Wechsler scales. In the case of persons with visual impairments, Sattler (1988), suggests that the Wechsler scales and the Stanford-Binet: Fourth Edition (Thorndike et al., 1986), especially the verbal items, can be used so long as the visual handicap is not too severe. For mentally retarded persons with hearing impairments, verbally based items should be avoided. Suitable nonverbal tests offer well standardized measures of ability that do not involve language tests; for example, the Universal Nonverbal Intelligence Test (UNIT; Bracken & McCallum, 1998) or the Naglieri Nonverbal Ability Test Individual Form (NNAT-I; Naglieri, 2003). Persons with motor problems may be at a particular disadvantage with timed performance tests (Sattler, 1988), making tests like the NNAT-I and UNIT particularly suitable.

Adaptive Behavior Scales The assessment of adaptive behavior plays an important role in both the diagnosis of intellectual disabilities and its ongoing habilitation process. As noted earlier in the chapter, a significant deficit in the ability of a person to behave in such a way as to meet the natural and social demands of his or her environment is one of the defining criteria for the diagnosis of intellectual disabilities. The adaptive behavior assessment also can assist the clinician and other professionals in identifying a person's behavioral strengths and weaknesses, providing for a comparison of the person's behavior across different environments or stimulus conditions (e.g., home vs. school), and providing a relatively uniform and objective method of evaluation for ongoing educational and intervention programs. Sattler (1988) cautions that adaptive behavior scores typically reflect a complex interaction of factors related to the scale itself, the person being rated, the informant who is providing the information for the rating, the examiner who is taking that information, the setting in which the behavior is being observed and reported, and the reasons for the evaluation. Such influences should be kept in mind when interpreting the adaptive behavior scores, and prudent clinical judgment should be applied. Most adaptive behavior scales require an informant such as a parent, teacher, mental health worker, or other direct care staff person (usually relatively naive to the assessment procedures and their standards) to provide detailed information regarding an individual's behavior. Such reports are often subjective and open to potential bias and distortions. For instance, it is relatively common to find that parents rate the overall adaptive behavior of their child higher than the teachers do. The most commonly used instruments for estimating the level of adaptive behavior are the Adaptive Behavior Scales (ABS; Lambert, Nihira, & Leland, 1993; Nihira, Leland, & Lambert, 1993) and the Vineland Adaptive Behavior scales (Sparrow, Balla, & Cicchetti, 2005a, 2005b).

Assessment of Psychopathology and Severe Behavior Problems Individuals with intellectual disabilities often experience mental health and behavior problems, including difficulties with learning, adjustment, integration, and social acceptance. Epidemiological studies have produced variable prevalence rates, but the firm consensus among experts is that people with intellectual disabilities are actually more vulnerable to mental illness than the general population (Nezu, Nezu, & Gill-Weiss, 1992; Rojahn & Tassé, 1996). Unfortunately, providing treatment to persons with a dual diagnosis of mental health problems and intellectual disabilities continues to be hampered by the difficulty of rendering reliable psychiatric diagnoses, particularly in individuals with more severe intellectual disabilities (e.g., Rush & Frances, 2000). Nevertheless, management and treatment of mental health and behavior problems has been a priority for day-to-day care as well as for clinical research, and therefore, assessment and progress monitoring are key issues.

Two kinds of scales can be used for assessment and monitoring of persons with dual diagnosis: generalized and specialized behavior scales. Generalized scales cover a broad band of different conditions, including heterogeneous disorders, such as mood disorders and schizophrenia. Some of these generalized scales were developed deductively to reflect the structure of the *DSM* (e.g., *Reiss Screen for Maladaptive Behavior* [Reiss, 1988], *Diagnostic Assessment for the Severely Handicapped-II* [Matson, 1998]), while others were developed inductively in an empirical fashion (e.g., *Aberrant Behavior Checklist*; Aman, Singh, Stewart, & Field, 1985). Specialized behavior rating scales, on the other hand, such as the *Behavior Problems Inventory* (Rojahn, Matson, Lott, Esbensen, & Smalls, 2001) focus on specific, narrowly defined conditions such as specific behavior problems.

Challenging behaviors such as self-injurious behavior (SIB), aggression, and property destruction are common and pose serious problems in persons with intellectual disabilities. They interfere with learning, threaten self and others, reduce the chances for successful community integration, and diminish the person's quality of life (Repp & Karsh, 1990). The functional-behavioral properties of problem behaviors are an important indicator for behavioral treatment selection. To determine functional properties of an undesirable behavior (e.g., gaining attention from others or avoiding unwanted activities), a variety of assessment methods have been devised, consisting of informal and formal observations to interviews, behavior rating scales and experimental analysis (or functional analysis).

Several functional assessment rating scales have been developed such as the *Motivation Assessment System* (MAS; Durand & Crimmins, 1988) and the *Functional Assessment for Multiple Causality* (FACT; Matson et al., 2003). Functional assessment rating systems have varying psychometric qualities. Typically their greatest shortcoming has been low interrater agreement.

Conclusions

In this chapter we have presented a summary of the history of and important considerations regarding learning disabilities and intellectual disabilities. Although these two areas are quite different in their characteristics, both are associated with controversies over definition and assessment. The very definition of children with learning disabilities is closely tied to how diagnosis is made (intelligence-achievement discrepancy or processing disorder, traditional IQ tests or processing tests, etc.). While the essential definition of intellectual disabilities seems obvious, it has been difficult to operationalize, especially because the type of intelligence test used can influence the results and definitions of adaptive behavior have been varied. Solutions to these complex problems will depend upon the years of research and development to come from future generations of professionals.

Note

1. In 2006 the American Association on Mental Retardation (AAMR) changed its name to the American Association on Intellectual and Developmental Disabilities (AAIDD).

References

Adams, G. L. (1999). *Comprehensive test of adaptive behavior*. Seattle, WA: Educational Achievement Systems.

Aman, M. G., Singh, N. N., Stewart, A., & Field, C. J. (1985). The Aberrant Behavior Checklist: A behavior rating scale for the assessment of treatment effects. *American Journal on Mental Deficiency. 89*, 485–491.

American Association on Mental Retardation. (2002). *Mental retardation: Definition, classification, and systems of supports* (10th ed.). Washington, D.C.: Author.

American Psychiatric Association. (1980). *Diagnostic and statistical manual of mental disorders* (3rd ed.). Washington, D. C.: Author.

American Psychiatric Association. (1987). *Diagnostic and statistical manual of mental disorders* (3rd ed., rev). Washington, D. C.: Author.

American Psychiatric Association. (2000). *Diagnostic and statistical manual of mental disorders* (4th ed., rev.). Washington, D. C.: Author.

Baroff, G. S., & Olley, J. G. (1999) Mental retardation: Nature, cause, and management (3rd ed.). Philadelphia, PA: Brunner/Mazel.

Baumeister, A. A. (1988, August). *The new morbidity and the prevention of mental retardation. Research progress*. John F. Kennedy Center for Research on Education and Human Development, George Peabody College, Vanderbilt University.

Bishop, D. V. M. (2001). Genetic influences on language impairment and literacy problems in children: Same or different? *Journal of Child Psychology and Psychiatry, 42*, 189–198.

Bracken, B. A., & McCallum, R. S. (1998). *Universal nonverbal intelligence test*. Itasca, IL: Riverside.

Bruininks, R. H., Hill, B. K., Weatherman, R. F., & Woodcock, R. W. (1986). *ACAP: Inventory for client and agency planning*. Chicago: Riverside.

Cardon, L. R., Smith, S. D., Fulker, D. W., Kimberling, W. J., Pennington, B. F., & DeFries, J. C. (1994). Quantitative trait locus for reading disability on chromosome 6, *Science, 266*, 276–279.

Fay, G. C., Jaffe, K. M., Polissar, N. L., Liao, S., Rivara, J. B., Martin, K. M. (1994). Outcome of pediatric traumatic brain injury at three years: a cohort study. *Archives of Physical Medicine Rehabilitation, 75*, 733–741.

Filipek, P. A. (1999). Neuroimaging in the developmental disorders: The state of the science. *Journal of Child Psychology and Psychiatry, 40*, 113–128.

Hallahan, D. P., & Cruickshank, W. M. (1973). *Psychoeducational foundations of learning disabilities*. Englewood Cliffs, NJ: Prentice-Hall.

Hallahan, D. P., & Keogh, B. K. (2001). *Research and global perspectives in learning disabilities*. Mahwah, NJ: Erlbaum.

Harrison, P. L., & Oakland, T. (2000). *ABAS: Adaptive behavior assessment system*. San Antonio, TX: Psychological Corporation.

Hynd, G. W., Hall, J., Novey, E., Eliopolus, D., Black, K., Gonzales, J. et al. (1995). Dylexia and corpus callosum morphology. *Archives of Neurology, 52*, 32–38.

Ingalls, S., & Goldstein, S. (1999). Learning disabilities. In S. Goldstein & C. R. Reynolds (Eds.), *Handbook of neurodevelopmental and genetic disorders in children* (pp. 101–153). New York: Guilford.

Jacobson, J. W., & Mulick, J. A. (Eds.). (1996), *Manual on mental retardation and professional practice* (pp. 147–156). Washington, D.C.: American Psychological Association.

Kaufman, A. S., & Kaufman, N. L. (1983). *Kaufman Assessment Battery for Children*. Circle Pines, MN: American Guidance Service.

Kaufman, A. S., Lichtenberger, E. O. (2000) *Essentials of WISC-III and WPPSI-R Assessment*. New York: Wiley.

Kirk, S. A. (1963). Behavioral diagnosis and remediation of learning disabilities. In *Proceedings of the first annual meeting of the ACLD conference on exploration into the problems of the perceptually handicapped child* (pp. 1–7). Chicago, IL:.

Kirk, S. A. (1972). *Educating exceptional children* (2nd ed.). Boston: Houghton Mifflin.

Kolb, L. C., & Brodie, H. K. H. (1982). Mental retardation. In L. C. Kolb & H. K. H. Brodie (Eds.), *Modern clinical psychiatry* (10th ed.; pp. 715–744). Philadelphia: W.B. Saunders.

Lambert, N., Nihira, K., & Leland, H. (1993). *AAMR adaptive behavior scale—School and community*. Austin, TX: Pro-Ed.

Larsen, S., Lakin, C., Andersen, L., Kwak, N., Lee, J. H., & Andersen, D. (2000, April). *MR/DD Data Brief, 2*, No 1. The College of Education and Human Development, University of Minnesota.

Matson, J. L. (1998). *Diagnostic assessment for the severely handicapped II—Manual*. Baton Rouge, LA: Scientific Publishers.

Matson, J. L., Kuhn, D. E., Dixon, D. R., Mayville, S. B., Laud, R. B., Cooper, C. L., et al. (2003). The development and factor structure of the Functional Assessment for Multiple Causality (FACT). *Research in Developmental Disabilities, 24*, 485–495.

McDermott, S., Durkin, M. S., Schupf, N., & Stein, Z. A. (2007). Epidemiology, and etiology of mental retardation. In J. W. Jacobson, J A. Mulick, & J. Rojahn (Eds), *Intellectual and developmental disabilities* (pp. 3–40). New York: Springer.

Mercer, C. D., Jordan, L., Allsopp, D. H., & Mercer, A. R. (1996). Learning disabilities definitions and criteria used by state education departments. *Learning Disability Quarterly, 19*, 217–232.

Naglieri, J. A. (1999). *Essentials of CAS assessment*. New York: Wiley.

Naglieri, J. A. (2003). *Naglieri nonverbal ability test—Individual form*. San Antonio, TX: Psychological Corporation.

Naglieri, J. A., & Das, J. P. (1997). *Cognitive assessment system*. Itasca, IL: Riverside.

National Joint Committee on Learning Disabilities. (1991). Learning disabilities: Issues on definition. *Asha, 33*, 18–20.

Nezu, M. N., Nezu, A. M., & Gill-Weiss, M. J. (1992). *Psychopathology in persons with mental retardation*. Champaign, IL: Research Press.

Nihira, N., Leland, H., & Lambert, N. (1993). *AAMR adaptive behavior scale—Residential and community* (2nd ed.). Austin, TX: Pro-Ed.

O'Neill, R. E., Horner, R. H., Albin, R. W., Sprague, J. R. Storey, K., & Newton, J. S. (1997). *Functional assessment and program development for problem behavior: A practical handbook*. Pacific Grove, CA: Brooks/Cole.

Pasternack, R. H. (2002, March). *The demise of IQ testing for children with learning disabilities*. Paper presented at the meeting of the National Association of School Psychologists, Chicago, Illinois.

Public Law 94-142, Education for All Handicapped Children Act of 1975 (1977, August). 10. U.S. C. 1401 et seq. Federal Register, 42 (163), 42, 474–518.

Prouty, R. W., & Lakin, C. (1999). *Residential services for persons with developmental disabilities: Status and trends through 1998*. Minneapolis: University of Minnesota, Research and Training Center on Community Living, Institute on Community Integration.

Reiss, S. (1988). *Test manual for the Reiss screen for maladaptive behavior*. Orland Park, IL: International Diagnostic Systems.

Repp, A. C., & Karsh, K.G. (1990). A taxonomic approach to the nonaversive treatment of maladaptive behavior of persons with developmental disabilities. In A. C. Repp & N. N. Singh (Eds), *Perspectives on the use of nonaversive and aversive interventions for persons with developmental disabilities* (pp. 331–347). Sycamore, IL: Sycamore.

Rojahn, J., Matson, J. L., Lott, D., Esbensen, A. J., & Smalls, Y. (2001). *The Behavior Problems Inventory*: An instrument for the assessment of self-injury, stereotyped behavior and aggression/destruction in individuals with developmental disabilities. *Journal of Autism and Developmental Disorders, 31*, 577–588.

Rojahn, J., & Tassé, M. J. (1996). Psychopathology in mental retardation. In J. W. Jacobson & J. A. Mulick (Eds.), *Manual on mental retardation and professional practice* (pp. 147–156). Washington, D.C.: American Psychological Association.

Rush, A. J., & Frances, A. (Eds.). (2000). Treatment of psychiatric and behavioral problems in mental retardation [Special issue]. *American Journal on Mental Retardation, 105*(3), 159–228.

Sattler, J. M. (1988). *Assessment of children* (3rd ed.). San Diego: Jerome M. Sattler.

Shepherd, M. J. (2001). History lessons. In A. S. Kaufman & N. L. Kaufman (Eds.), *Specific learning disabilities and difficulties in children and adolescents* (pp. 3–28). Cambridge: Cambridge University Press.

Sparrow, S. S., Cicchetti, D. V., & Balla, D. A. (2005a). *Vineland II—Vineland Adaptive Behavior scales: Survey forms manual*. (2nd ed.). Circle Pines, MN: AGS.

Sparrow, S. S., Cicchetti, D. V., & Balla, D. A. (2005b). *Vineland II—Vineland Adaptive Behavior Scales: Teacher rating form manual* (2nd ed.). Circle Pines, MN: AGS.

Thorndike, R. L., Hagen, E. P., & Sattler, J. M. (1986). *Stanford-Binet intelligence scale* (4th ed.). Chicago: Riverside.

Torgesen, J. K. (1998). Learning disabilities: An historical and conceptual overview. In B. Y. L. Wong (Ed.), *Learning about learning disabilities* (pp. 3–28). San Diego, CA: Academic Press.

U.S. Department of Education. (2000). *Twenty-first annual report to Congress on the implementation of the Individuals with Disabilities Education Act*. Washington, D.C.: U.S. Government Printing Office.

U.S. Department of Education Office of Special Education and Rehabilitative Services. (2002). *A new era: Revitalizing special education for children and their families*. Washington, D.C.: Author.

Wechsler, D. (1991). *Wechsler intelligence scale for children* (3rd ed.; WISC-III). San Antonio, TX: The Psychological Corporation.

World Health Organization. (1993). *International statistical classification of diseases and related health problems* (10th ed.). Geneva: Author.

Yeates, K. O. (2000). Closed-head injury. In K. O. Yeates, M. D. Ris, & H. G. Taylor (Eds.), *Pediatric neuropsychology: Research, theory, and practice* (pp. 92–116). New York: Guilford.

19

Mental Health and Aging

Current Trends and Future Directions

Lisa M. Kinoshita, Kristen H. Sorocco, and Dolores Gallagher-Thompson

Who Are Older Adults?

The population of older adults is growing at a rapid rate. In 2003, the older adult population (65 years and older) reached 35.9 million (U.S. Administration on Aging [AOA], 2004), 21 million of whom were older adults. That is, one out of every eight Americans is an older person, representing 12.4% of the U.S. population. By 2030, the older adult population is projected to double, totaling 71.5 million older persons (AOA, 2004). The growth of ethnic minority older adult populations will contribute substantially to this increase. By the year 2030, the number of older Hispanics is expected to increase by 342%; Asian and Pacific Islanders by 302%; Indians, Eskimos, and Aleuts by 207%; African Americans by 164%; followed by European Americans by 77% (AOA, 2004). This rapid increase in the population of ethnic minority older adults has instigated a mental health initiative to examine the impact of culture on mental disorders (U.S. Department of Health and Human Services, 2001).

According to a 2003 study of the lifestyles of older adults, the majority (71%) of older men were married compared to women (41%; AOA, 2004). However, this ratio is expected to change, due to the increasing rate of divorce. Furthermore, most older adults lived with their spouses (53.9%), 30.8% lived alone, and only a small proportion lived in a nursing home (4.5%). Geographically, about half of the older adult population lived in one of nine states (California, Florida, New York, Texas, Pennsylvania, Ohio, Illinois, Michigan, and New Jersey). Regarding physical health status, only 37.4% of noninstitutionalized older adults assessed their health as excellent or very good (AOA, 2000). There were minimal differences between the sexes in self-reported health, but African American older adults (57.7%) and Hispanic older adults (60.1%) were less likely to rate their health as excellent or very good than were European Americans (76.9%; AOA, 2000).

Given the rapid growth of the older adult population, the physical and mental health needs of older adults will demand future attention. The purpose of this chapter is threefold: (1) to discuss the risks and prevalence rates of several common mental health disorders among older adults; (2) to inform readers of effective and culturally appropriate assessment and treatment interventions for older adults; and (3) to discuss how to meet the future needs of this growing population. The chapter will focus on the following disorders: anxiety, depression, dementia, and alcohol abuse. Other disorders, such as late-life schizophrenia, personality disorders, bereavement and adjustment disorders, and more general substance abuse issues, are not included. Interested readers are referred to the suggested readings at the end of the chapter. Before we examine specific mental health issues, we will first examine the process of normal aging.

Normal Aging

There are a number of myths concerning aging in our society. Dychtwald and Flower (1990) discussed six myths: (1) people over 65 are old; (2) most older people are in poor health; (3) older minds are not as bright as young minds;(4) older people are unproductive; (5) older people are unattractive and sexless; and (6) all older people are the same. As a result of these myths, many individuals spend an enormous amount of time and money fighting the aging process. For example, women and men buy antiaging products and undergo painful, expensive surgical procedures to look younger. Older adult role models or positive images of the aging process are seldom portrayed. This lack is not surprising, given that our society equates beauty with youth. However, as the population of older adults grows, there will be a need to reexamine these negative stereotypes and determine how they influence the mental well-being of older adults.

Clinicians working with older adults need to be aware of these aging myths and also of normal age-related changes. All individuals experience physical, cognitive, and psychosocial changes as they age. When working with older adults, it is important for therapists to normalize age-related changes. Physically, as individuals age, their risk for disease increases. First, body organs lose strength, and as a result, they do not function as efficiently. For example, changes in the immune system put older adults at increased risk of illness. Once ill, they often take longer to heal than younger adults. Second, modest increases in blood pressure, blood sugar, and body weight occur with normal aging, thus placing an older adult at risk for cardiovascular disease, stroke, and diabetes.

Cognitive changes include slowed reaction time and decrease in working memory function. Salthouse (1996) proposed a general slowing hypothesis, positing that the increases in reaction time are due to a general decline of information-processing speed within the aging nervous system (Whitbourne, 2000). Working memory is also affected. It does not function as efficiently with age because of reduced processing speed. Processing speed is slowed by the cognitive difficulty older adults experience when they are required to hold information in storage while simultaneously processing new information. These normal cognitive changes do not mean that older adults are incapable of learning new information, but they have to use different strategies to learn effectively as they age (Zeiss & Steffen, 1996).

Physical and cognitive decline can directly impact the psychosocial functioning of older adults. For example, physical illness can prevent older adults from engaging in enjoyable social activities. Older adults are often forced to examine their mortality as they experience the deaths of loved ones. Those who are caregivers often experience anticipatory grief before the death of their care recipient, due to the strains of caregiving and the role loss they are witnessing (Lindgren, Connelly, & Gaspar, 1999). At any age these are life experiences that might serve as a risk factor for the development of a mental health disorder, but many older adults adapt to these life challenges and experience them successfully.

Whether we are discussing physiological changes associated with aging or psychosocial issues, it is important not to overgeneralize commonalities among "normal" older adults. In fact, variability among individuals tends to increase with age (Knight, 1986). This variability is due to a wide range of cohort differences among the older adult population in addition to other diversity factors, such as ethnicity. In order to better understand the heterogeneity of the older adult population, Knight (1986) proposed that the older adult population be divided into subgroups based on age cohorts: young-old (65 to 74 years), old (75 to 84 years), and old-old (85 years and older). As we discuss mental health issues among older adults, it is important to remember that although some risk factors for mental health problems increase with age, the majority of older adults are able to cope with late life stressors without developing significant mental health problems.

Theories of Adjustment in Aging

Henry and Cumming (1959) proposed the *disengagement theory* of aging which states that there is a gradual withdrawal from life's activities in preparation for death. A contrasting view is *activity theory* (Havighurst, 1961) which proposes that normal aging involves the maintenance of activities and attitudes engaged in during middle age. Activity theory advocates that, to age successfully, people must make adaptations in activities to accommodate any physical, sensory, or cognitive deficits as they age. A primary criticism of both of these theories is that they are too simplistic, leading later theorists to study human development theorists, such as Sigmund Freud and Erik Erikson, who believed that later life adjustment could be understood only by examining earlier life development. Together, these aging theories illustrate the great debate concerning whether human development is continuous (gradual, cumulative from conception to death) or discontinuous (involving distinct changes in the life span) (Halonen & Santrock, 1996). The continuity–discontinuity debate also attempts to answer whether or not our behaviors are stable as we age or if individuals can accommodate and make appropriate changes in their behavior depending on life circumstances (Lerner, 1986).

Recently, aging theorists and health professionals have examined the concept of successful aging to understand optimal adjustment in later life. Successful aging is a key factor involved in the prevention of physical and mental health disorders in older adults. Successful aging, as defined by the MacArthur Foundation study (Rowe & Kahn, 1998), is the ability of an individual to maintain the following three behaviors: (1) low risk of disease and disease-related disability; (2) high mental and physical function; and (3) active engagement in life. Each of these behaviors to some extent is independent from the others, but they are not mutually exclusive. In fact, Rowe and Kahn (1998) suggest that there is a hierarchical organization to these three behaviors. Specifically, the absence of disease and disability makes it easier to maintain high mental and physical function, which are the characteristics that enable us to engage in life as we age. Unfortunately, health care continues to focus on providing medical interventions only when necessary and places less emphasis on prevention. In our opinion, prevention is a key to successful aging. Theories of aging highlight the point that although there are some similarities among all older adults, there are also significant individual differences to consider. Environmental, biological, and psychological factors all affect how an older adult will adjust to normative life events and changes.

Stress and Coping Model

Coping refers to "engaging in behavioral and cognitive efforts to deal with environmental and internal demands and with conflicts between the two" (Rice, 1999, p. 80). Life events may be stressful when individuals perceive them as threatening (either physically or psychologically) and when individuals perceive the demands of the event as exceeding his or her coping resources and skills (Lazarus & Launier, 1978). As individuals evolve and experience the world, they learn ways of coping with stressful events that help get them through such events with little or no problem. They have the resources and skills needed to cope. As individuals age, however, multiple stressors begin to emerge (e.g., death of spouse, relatives, friends; changes in family roles due to illness; increased demands of caregiving), such that old ways of coping that typically worked in the past are no longer effective in coping with these new situations. This situation in turn may lead to increased psychological distress and mental illness in later life.

Common Mental Health Problems of Later Life

The majority of older adults are satisfied with their mental health; however, nearly 20% of those 55 and older experience mental disorders that are not a part of normal aging. Common mental health problems in later life include anxiety disorders and depression.

Anxiety Disorders in Older Adults

Given the number of psychosocial losses that an older adult is likely to experience, one might assume that depression is the most common psychological disorder among older adults; however, research has shown that anxiety disorders are actually more prevalent (Stanley & Beck, 1998). The Epidemiological Catchment Area (ECA) study found that anxiety disorders were the most prevalent problem among older adults (Regier et al., 1988). Anxiety symptoms occur in 10 to 20% of the older adult population (Banazak, 1997; Beekman et al., 1998). However, in comparison to other diagnoses (e.g., depression) less is known about the etiology, including clinical characteristics, course, treatment, and prognosis of anxiety disorders in late life (Lauderdale & Sheikh, 2003; see also Williams, this volume.)

Assessment of Anxiety Disorders Because anxiety disorders are difficult to diagnose in older adults, they are often undiagnosed (Scogin, Floyd, & Forde, 2000). The assessment of anxiety disorders among older adults is difficult because of a number of challenges. The first challenge is the association between anxiety symptoms and other psychiatric disorders, particularly depression, because symptoms of anxiety and depression frequently occur simultaneously (Blazer, 2002). Second, anxiety disorders also co-occur with a number of medical diagnoses (Raj and Sheehan, 1988), including cardiovascular/respiratory disorders (e.g., asthma, hypertension, chronic obstructive pulmonary disease), endocrine disorders (e.g., hyperthyroidism, hypothyroidism, menopause), neurological disorders (e.g., multiple sclerosis, dementia, Huntington's disease), or substance-related disorders (e.g., drug intoxication and withdrawal symptoms). A third challenge is selecting an assessment measure that is reliable and valid for older adult clients.

Due to these challenges, a combined assessment approach, including clinical assessment, age appropriate self-reports, and laboratory findings is suggested (Lauderdale & Sheikh, 2003). A clinical assessment involves an interview with the older adult to determine presenting symptoms, mental health history, medical history, medication usage (including over-the-counter medications and herbal supplements), and family history of anxiety disorders (Lauderdale & Sheikh, 2003). Self-report measures that have been identified as reliable and valid for older adults include the Hamilton Anxiety Rating Scale (HARS; Hamilton, 1959) and Beck Anxiety Inventory (BAI; Beck, Epstein, Brown, & Steer, 1988). Both self-report instruments have been shown to differentiate anxious older adults from older controls (Wetherell & Arean, 1997; Stanley, Beck, & Zebb, 1996). Given the co-occurrence of anxiety disorders with certain medical disorders, laboratory tests can be used to differentiate anxiety disorders from medical diagnoses.

Generalized Anxiety Disorder Generalized anxiety disorder (GAD) is one of the most common anxiety disorders among older adults. Blazer, George, and Hughes (1991) found that 39% of older adults who were surveyed had experienced GAD onset before late adulthood; however, 50% of those diagnosed with GAD had experienced their symptoms for five years or less. More recently, among a sample of 67 older adults enrolled in a psychotherapy study for GAD, 57% reported early onset GAD, with early onset being characteristic of psychiatric comorbidity, medication use, and more severe worry (Le Roux, Gatz, & Wetherell, 2005). Late onset GAD was more characteristic of increased functional limitations as a result of physical problems (Le Roux, Gatz, & Wetherell, 2005).

According to *DSM–IV–TR* (American Psychiatric Association, 2000), the primary symptom of

GAD is unrealistic or excessive worry about two or more life circumstances for a period of at least six months. In addition, individuals need to experience at least three of the following symptoms: restlessness, feeling keyed up or on edge, feeling easily fatigued, difficulty concentrating or mind going blank, irritability, muscle tension, or sleep disturbance. The final criterion for this diagnosis is that the symptoms cause the older adult significant distress or impairment. A diagnosis of GAD in an older adult is an example of a mental health disorder that must take into account age-related factors. Given the number of physiological symptoms associated with GAD there is the possibility for misdiagnosis if physical health factors are not adequately evaluated.

Another threat to proper diagnosis of GAD is the high co-ocurrence of depression and GAD. Among older adults, GAD has been found to either progress to depression or to have an etiology of mixed anxiety depressive disorder suggesting the need for a dimensional rather than categorical classification of anxiety and depression (Schoevers, Deeg, van Tilburg, & Beekman, 2005). However, GAD and depression appear to have different onsets with GAD often preceding depression (Lenze et al., 2005). Properly identifying a mixed anxiety-depressive disorder is necessary due to poorer treatment outcomes and increased vulnerability for older adults with mixed etiologies (Schoevers, Deeg, van Tilburg, & Beekman, 2005; Steffens & McQuoid, 2005).

BEHAVIORAL INTERVENTIONS Limited research has been conducted examining the effectiveness of treatment interventions for older adults suffering from anxiety disorders. Furthermore, most of the research has been conducted with older adults who suffer from general symptoms of anxiety rather than specific disorders such as GAD (Wetherell, 2002). These studies have found that behavioral interventions (e.g., relaxation, exposure therapy, imaginal exposure) are effective with older adults with symptoms of anxiety (Deberry, Davis, & Reinhard, 1989; Scogin, Rickard, Keith, Wilson, & McElreath, 1992). Imaginal relaxation techniques (visualizing peaceful nature scenes) are more appropriate than progressive muscle relaxation with older adults. Progressive muscle relaxation, which involves tensing and relaxing muscles, might be ineffective and even painful to older adults with particular medical problems, such as arthritis.

Even though relatively few studies have examined the effectiveness of cognitive-behavioral therapy (CBT) for GAD among older adults, CBT appears to be a useful intervention, although modifications need to be made for older adult clients (Beck & Stanley, 1997; Wetherell, 1998). CBT teaches clients to identify and modify unhealthy patterns in their thoughts, emotions, and behavioral responses. Stanley, Beck, and Glassco (1996) found that CBT or a supportive therapy group were effective interventions for older adults with GAD and that gains were maintained at six-month follow-up. A more recent study found that both CBT and a discussion group around worry-provoking topics helped to reduce anxiety symptoms among older adults with GAD compared to a wait-list group (Wetherell, Gatz, & Craske, 2003). A large effect was demonstrated for CBT and a medium effect was seen for the discussion group indicating the usefulness of treating late life anxiety. CBT also has been found to reduce psychological symptoms in older adult patients as they begin to reduce their use of anxiolytic medication (Gorenstein et al., 2005). Suggested modifications when using CBT with older adults clients suffering with GAD include using a group format to increase social support networks, teaching at a slower pace, providing multiple examples when teaching the intervention, using handouts, and repeating information (Wetherell, 2002).

PHARMACOLOGICAL INTERVENTIONS Antianxiety medications are frequently used by older adults (Graham & Vidal-Zeballos, 1998). Selective serotonin reuptake inhibitors and serotonin norepinephrine reuptake inhibitors have been identified as the most efficacious and yield fewest side-effects when used with older adults (Lauderdale & Sheikh, 2003). However, a number of cautions need to be taken into consideration when using pharmacological interventions with older adults. First, normal age-related physiological changes that are common in older adulthood (e.g., slower metabolism) impact drug absorption, distribution, metabolism, and sensitivity to side effects (Scogin et al., 2000). Generally, older adults are more susceptible to side effects of medications and are at greater risk of drug interactions than younger adults. Second, older adults often take several medications, therefore they are at greater risk for drug interactions. For some older adults medication is necessary for successful treatment, however, many older adults benefit from nonpharmacological interventions (e.g., psychotherapy).

POSTTRAUMATIC STRESS DISORDER In recent years, posttraumatic stress disorder (PTSD) in older adults has received attention in the literature. Much of the available research in the area primarily focuses on veterans, Holocaust survivors, and to some extent on victims of assault in later life. In a recent study, researchers found that the six-month prevalence of PTSD and of subthreshold PTSD was 0.9 and 13.1%, respectively, suggesting that PTSD in older adults is not a rare disorder (Van Zelst, De Beurs, Beekman, Deeg, & Van Dyck, 2003). However, older adults with PTSD are often not recognized or they are misdiagnosed.

According to the *DSM-IV-TR*, PTSD is characterized by the following: (1) presence of a recognizable stressor that evokes significant symptoms of distress in most individuals; (2) reexperiencing of the trauma;(3) hyperarousal symptoms; and (4) avoidance of stimuli that remind the individual of the traumatic event. Researchers have examined whether PTSD in older adults is the same psychological phenomenon as PTSD in younger adults. Research suggests that the PTSD symptom profile in older adults is similar to those seen in younger individuals; however, the course of the disorder, intensity of PTSD symptoms, and comorbid diagnoses differ in older adults (Averill & Beck, 2000; Hyer, 1999). Furthermore, older veterans are more likely to manifest their PTSD symptomatology as somatic complaints rather than as psychological distress compared to younger veterans.

First, the course of the disorder in some older adult veterans differs from that seen in younger veterans (McLeod, 1994). For example, McLeod found that World War II veterans initially coped well in the immediate years following their wartime period. They later experienced an exacerbation of symptoms that lasted for approximately five years, followed by a time in middle age when their symptoms were masked as they excelled in their careers and family life. As these veterans grew older, their PTSD symptoms again were exacerbated. Thus, another complicating issue related to the investigation of PTSD in later life is the time of the psychiatric assessment. Furthermore, late-onset PTSD also has been documented in older combat veterans (Spiro, Schnurr, & Aldwin, 1994).

In other studies of World War II veterans, it was found that intrusive symptoms decreased over time, whereas avoidance symptoms and isolation from others increased as the veterans grew older (McFarlane, 1990). World War II veterans who were treated in an outpatient mental health clinic commonly complained of insomnia, nightmares, irritability, social isolation, and flashbacks (Kaup, Ruskin, & Nyman, 1994). A 45-year retrospective study of surviving Pearl Harbor veterans found that roughly two thirds of them experience intrusive memories, approximately one half report survivor guilt, and one third report avoidance and hyperarousal symptoms and emotional numbing (Wilson, Harel, & Kahana, 1989). Thus, these PTSD symptoms remained with the veterans even decades after their initial traumatic experience. Overall, however, most studies have found that veterans report a decrease in PTSD symptoms over time, with the most reduction experienced in intrusive thoughts and survivor guilt.

ASSESSMENT OF PTSD Accurate assessment of PTSD in older adults is difficult because few PTSD assessment measures and semistructured interviews have been validated with this population. First, the combat and civilian forms of the Mississippi PTSD Scales (MISS) (Watson, 1990) are 35-item self-report measures. Both forms were found to be highly correlated with other diagnostic measures of PTSD (McFall, Smith, Mackay, & Tarver, 1990). Moreover, the combat form of the MISS was found to be the most accurate measure of PTSD severity in older adults who were former prisoners of war (Neal, Hill, Hughes, Middleton, & Busuttil, 1995). The Clinician Administered PTSD Scale (CAPS; Blake et al., 1990) is a semistructured clinical interview used to assess core and associated symptoms of PTSD based on *DSM-IV* diagnostic criteria. The CAPS has been used with older adults who experienced trauma during wartime events. It was found to have good discriminatory power, with a 93% accuracy rate (Hyer, Summers, Boyd, & Litaker, 1996).

Other validation studies done on PTSD measures have shown inconsistent results. Investigations of the Impact of Events Scale (IES) (Horowitz, Wilner, & Alvarez, 1979), a 15-item, self-report questionnaire used to assess intrusion and avoidance symptoms, suggest equivocal data for its use with older adults. Such inconsistent results suggest that the type of traumatic event is important when assessing PTSD in older adults (Neal et al., 1995). Thus, future research is needed to validate existing and newly created PTSD measures for older adults.

TREATMENT FOR PTSD There is evidence to suggest that psychotherapy, specifically CBT (Gillespie, Duffy, Hackmann, & Clark, 2002) and eye movement desensitization and reprocessing (EMDR; Hyer, 1999), as well as psychopharmacological interventions, such as paroxetine/Paxil (Tucker et al., 2001; Wagstaff, Cheer, Matheson, Ormrod, & Goa, 2002), fluvoxamine/Luvox (Martenyi, Brown, Zhang, Prakah, & Koke, 2002), and gabapentin/Neurontin (Hammer, Brodrick, & Labbbate, 2001) are effective in treating PTSD in young adults. However, treatment paradigms of PTSD in older adults have not been well formulated nor well studied. Furthermore, well-controlled clinical trials with older adults are lacking in the literature which makes the treatment of PTSD in this population challenging.

Initial reports of common psychotherapeutic treatments, such as CBT, for older adults who have PTSD are promising. Hyer et al. (1990) evaluated a 12-session CBT protocol with older patients who had chronic PTSD or acute stress reactions related to loss. The CBT protocol included exploration of irrational beliefs as well as anxiety management training (AMT) that included relaxation. Although objective measures showed no difference between the CBT group and control group, participants reported that they benefited from the cognitive therapy, AMT, and relaxation training (Hyer et al., 1990).

Similarly, preliminary results related to the efficacy of eye movement desensitization and reprocessing (EMDR) treatment for PTSD in older adults are available (Hyer, 1995). EMDR is a type of psychotherapy that integrates successful elements from other therapeutic approaches and combines them with eye movements or other forms of rhythmical stimulation in ways that stimulate the brain's information processing system. Furthermore, EMDR involves limited exposure to specific information related to the trauma (Boudewyns & Hyer, 1997). This type of treatment uses emotions, sensations, cognitions, and images to uncover the traumatic event(s) at a pace set by the client. EMDR is different from CBT treatment in that it is more active and guides the client to uncover the trauma when this information is not readily available and allows for positive patient change (Hyer & Brandsma, 1997). In recent years, however, EMDR has received divergent reactions from researchers and clinicians alike. The confusion in the EMDR literature is based on the following five issues: (1) the lack of an empirically validated model to explain the effects of EMDR; (2) inaccurate and selective reporting of research; (3) poorly designed empirical studies; (4) outcome research with flawed treatment fidelity; and (5) a number of biased or inaccurate literature reviews (Perkins & Rouanzoin, 2002). Thus, sound outcome studies that investigate the efficacy of EMDR with older adults are needed in the future.

The utility of supportive group therapy with older adult veterans has been demonstrated, as a sole treatment (Boehlein & Sparr, 1993; Bonwick, 1997; Molinari & Williams, 1995) and in conjunction with antidepressant or antianxiety medications (Lipton & Schaffer, 1988). Psychiatric symptoms remain stable over a one-year period and social functioning improves (Boehnlein & Sparr, 1993), with reports of both improved quality of life and coping skills (Bonwick, 1997). Individuals in supportive group therapy report lower levels of subjective distress. However, controlled studies on supportive therapy conducted with older adults are not available; therefore, the overall impact of this form of therapy is not clear.

More recently, Maercker (2002) explored a life-review technique as a treatment for PTSD in older adults. The treatment incorporates a discussion of the older adult's chronological life stages while focusing on the individual's memories of the positive and negative aspects of life events, including traumatic ones. The therapist reinforces the individual's positive coping skills during treatment. The utility of the life-review technique was demonstrated in three case studies (Maecker, 2002). Overall, treatment efficacy for PTSD in older adults appears promising; however, additional well-controlled studies are needed.

Depression in Later Life

Clinically significant depression is one of the most common psychiatric disorders reported by older adults with a prevalence of 4.4%, second only to anxiety disorders in prevalence (11.4%) (U.S. Department of Health and Human Services, 1999). Although research suggests that the prevalence of major depressive disorder is relatively rare in community-dwelling older adults (Judd & Kunovac, 1998; Weissman, Bruce, Leaf, Florio, Holzer, 1991), epidemiological studies suggest that 10 to 25% of community-dwelling older adults over the age of 65 years report depressive symptoms that do not meet criteria for major depressive disorder (MDD) (Blazer, 2002; see also Ingram & Smith, this volume).

According to the *DSM–IV–TR*, the diagnostic criteria for MDD includes the following: depressed mood or diminished interest or pleasure in daily activities, weight loss or weight gain, sleep difficulty, psychomotor agitation or retardation, loss of energy, feelings of worthlessness or excessive guilt, decreased ability to concentrate or difficulty making decisions, recurrent thoughts of suicide or death. Bereavement, adjustment disorder, or dysthymia constitute the other portion of the depressive spectrum. However, the initial diagnosis of dysthymia in later life appears to be rare (Blazer, 1986), suggesting that individuals who suffer from chronic depression developed symptoms earlier in life.

Four older adult populations have higher levels of depression than community-dwelling individuals: nursing home patients (Parmelee, Katz, & Lawton, 1989); recently bereaved individuals (Gallagher, Breckenridge, Thompson, & Peterson, 1983; Thompson, Tang, Kaye, & Gallagher-Thompson, 2004); family caregivers (Gallagher, Rose, Rivera, Lovett, & Thompson, 1989); and individuals who are cognitively impaired (Teri & Gallagher-Thompson, 1991; Teri & Logsdon, 1991). In physically impaired, cognitively intact nursing home patients, the prevalence of late-life depression increases, ranging from 20% of new admissions to 42% of nursing home residents (Parmelee, Katz, & Lawton, 1989). This high number likely reflects the many losses (e.g., loss related to physical decline, loss of control and independence) that older adults experience when they are institutionalized in long-term care settings. Similarly, in recently bereaved individuals and cognitively impaired patients, 20 to 30% report significant depression. However, close to 50% of family caregivers are at least mildly depressed, with approximately 25% meeting criteria for MDD.

Assessment of Late Life Depression Accurate, early diagnosis, and treatment of depression in older adults is important because it can improve quality of life and functional status, and may prevent premature death. However, problems with diagnostic systems, assessment measures, and assessment procedures complicate the assessment process. In particular, most commonly used depression inventories for younger adults—for example, the Beck Depression Inventory–II (BDI–II; Beck, Steer, & Brown, 1996) and the Center for Epidemiologic Studies Depression Scale (CES–D; Radloff, 1977)—include items that assess somatic symptoms that are typically more prevalent in older adults. Therefore, these somatically related items may artificially increase the depression score for older adults

TABLE 19.1   Adaptations in treatment with older adults

- Discuss age difference between therapist and client
- Foster independence
- Use slower pace
- Make modifications for sensory or cognitive deficits
- Address common later life themes

---

on these measures. Yesavage et al. (1983) created a 30-item (and 15-item; Sheikh & Yesavage, 1986) depression measure, the Geriatric Depression Scale (GDS) designed specifically to assess depression in older adults (see Table 19.2 on page 430 for additional information). The GDS assesses psychological aspects of depression (e.g., pessimism about the future) with less emphasis on the physical symptoms related to depression, leading to a more accurate assessment for older adults.

Additional older adult issues that cloud the clinical picture are comorbid physical problems and cognitive impairment. Because of the likely presence of concurrent physical health problems, clinicians should consult with medical professionals to rule out a medical basis for the individual's depression. In addition, cognitive impairment can confound the diagnostic picture: depressive symptoms such as decreased ability to concentrate and make decisions are also common among people with cognitive impairment (e.g., Alzheimer's disease, vascular dementia). Therefore, it is important to consider the older adult's level of cognitive impairment when using depression screening instruments. In a study by McGivney and colleagues (1994), the validity of the GDS in a nursing home population was significantly decreased in patients with a Mini-Mental State Examination (MMSE) score of 15 or less, a score that indicates cognitive impairment. For a detailed review of the issues involved in assessing depression among older adults, see Lichtenberg (1996), Mui, Burnette, and Chen (2001), and Powers, Thompson, and Gallagher-Thompson (2002).

One primary question of interest for researchers and clinicians alike is the following: Is depression experienced differently by older adults compared to younger adults? Preliminary research in the area suggests that both the type and severity of depression may be different. Two qualitatively different syndromes, the depressive syndrome and the depletion syndrome, were found through factor analysis (Newmann, Engel, & Jensen, 1991a; Newmann, Engel, & Jenson, 1991b) and help illustrate these differences. The *depressive syndrome* is characterized by the emotional and cognitive features of depression; the *depletion syndrome*, however, is characterized by decreased appetite, lack of interest, feelings of hopelessness, and thoughts of death. Younger adults more readily report features related to the former whereas older adults are more likely to report aspects of the latter (Newmann et al., 1991a, 1991b). However, in actual practice, most older adults who seek treatment for depression do so because of losses that have overwhelmed their capacity to cope. These common losses are typically related to social support network, health problems, and control and independence. Working successfully with older adults requires mental health professionals to receive geropsychology training so that they can accurately assess the most common subtypes of geriatric depressive symptoms (Powers et al., 2002).

Treatment of Depression in Late Life   Many clinicians believe that psychotherapy is essential in the treatment of depression in older adults. Still others posit that psychotherapy in conjunction with psychopharmacologic interventions is beneficial to older adults who are acutely suffering from severe depression or who have recovered from a depressive episode and are now in the maintenance phase of treatment (National Institutes of Health Consensus Development Conference Consensus Statement, 1991). Empirical evidence suggests that both cognitive-behavioral therapy (Fry, 1984; Gallagher-Thompson & Steffen, 1994; Gatz et al., 1998; Thompson, 1996; Thompson, Coon, Gallagher-Thompson, Sommer, & Koin, 2001; Thompson, Gallagher, & Breckenridge, 1987) as well as interpersonal psychotherapy (Klerman, Weissman, Rounsaville, & Chevron, 1984) are effective in decreasing depressive symptoms in older adults. Moreover, advances in psychopharmacologic treatments have made additional effective interventions available to older adults diagnosed with depression.

COGNITIVE-BEHAVIORAL PSYCHOTHERAPY Considerable evidence demonstrates that CBT is effective in the treatment of depression in older adults (see review article by Gatz et al., 1998), including depression treatment in dementia patients (Teri & Gallagher-Thompson, 1991; Teri & Logsdon, 1991). Moreover, cognitive therapy for older adults with severe depressive symptoms was found to be more accepted and preferred by clients than was cognitive bibliotherapy or antidepressant medication (Landreville, Laundry, Baillargeon, Guerette, & Matteau, 2001). CBT has also been shown to be effective in conjunction with other interventions. In a recent study, depressed low-income older adults benefited from increased access to social services either alone or combined with group CBT (Arean et al., 2005).

Manualized CBT treatments have been used to provide individual treatment for late-life depression in outpatients (Laidlaw, Thompson, & Gallagher-Thompson, 2004; Thompson et al., 2001; Thompson et al., 1987; Thompson, Gallagher-Thompson, & Dick, 1996); in family caregivers (Gallagher-Thompson & DeVries, 1994; Gallagher-Thompson & Steffen, 1994), and in Latina family caregivers (Gallagher-Thompson, Ossinalde, Menendez et al., 1996). Similarly, studies suggest that manualized group CBT therapy is effective with Latina and Caucasian caregivers (Gallagher-Thompson, Arean, Rivera, & Thompson, 2001; Gallagher-Thompson, Lovett et al., 2000; Gallagher-Thompson, Haley et al, 2003). These caregiver studies included about 400 participants overall. Compared to telephone support or typical caregiver support groups, CBT was found to be more effective in reducing depressive symptoms and increasing use of adaptive coping strategies. Other studies have found similar positive results, suggesting that CBT is an effective treatment for many common problems in later life.

INTERPERSONAL PSYCHOTHERAPY Interpersonal psychotherapy (IPT) is a type of therapy that was designed to treat depressed patients. IPT is a focused, time-limited therapy that focuses on the patient's current interpersonal relationships. Throughout treatment, the role of genetic, biochemical, developmental, and personality factors are also examined, as they are believed to relate to the patient's vulnerability to depression (Klerman et al., 1984). IPT focuses on past and current interpersonally relevant issues that are related to the current depression. IPT is well established as a successful treatment for depression in younger adult populations (Klerman et al., 1984; see also Ingram & Smith, this volume.) Moreover, evidence suggests that interpersonal psychotherapy is effective in reducing depressive symptoms in older adults (Hinrichsen, 1999). Older adults commonly experience interpersonal changes such as loss of close friends or family members, transitions in social roles, conflicts with others, and the need to acquire new skills to adapt to changes in life that often makes IPT ideal for older adults (Hinrichsen, 1999). Moreover, the combination of nortriptyline, a tricyclic antidepressant, and weekly sessions of ITP in the initial and continuation phases of treatment for depression in late life was shown to benefit older adults (Reynolds et al., 1992).

MEDICATION AND MEDICAL INTERVENTIONS More than 20 years of research suggests that psychopharmacological treatments can be beneficial for depressed older adults (Bell, 1999; Powers et al., 2002). Moreover, there is evidence to suggest that antidepressants are equally effective in older adult patients as they are in younger adults (Katona, 2000; see also Ingram & Smith, this volume.) However, both the safety and efficacy of psychopharmacological treatment for older adults are complicated by pharmacokinetic changes associated with aging, the increased potential for adverse drug interactions and polypharmacy issues, the effect of psychotropic medications on certain concomitant illnesses, and difficulties in the management of common side effects.

In the past, tricyclic antidepressant (TCA) medications were commonly prescribed for depression in older adults. However, adverse side effects related to the anticholinergic effects of the TCAs (e.g., exacerbation of glaucoma, blurry vision, increased confusion, increased risk of urinary tract infection) were found to be intolerable by many older adult patients (Katona, 2000). TCAs are also associated with postural hypotension and dizziness, so older adults are at higher risk of falling when taking TCAs to treat their depression. Moreover, TCAs are potentially fatal at high dosages. Thus, there is increased concern when an older adult is depressed that he or she may attempt suicide via overdose using TCAs (Kasper, Lepine, Mendlewicz, Montgomery, & Rush, 1995).

In recent years, a class of antidepressants called selective serotonin reuptake inhibitors (SSRIs) have been found to be effective in treating depression in older adults and have a safer side-effect profile compared to TCAs (Montgomery, 1998). For instance, SSRIs do not have the same anticholinergic effects of TCAs, and SSRIs have a lower potential for adverse drug interaction compared to TCAs (Katona, 2000). Moreover, in a meta-analysis of studies in which older adult patients took either SSRIs or TCAs to treat their depression, more individuals receiving an SSRI remained in the studies, and they reported fewer adverse events related to the medication (Montgomery & Kasper, 1995). SSRIs were found to be as effective as TCAs in the treatment of late-life depression with better tolerability (Altamura et al., 1989). Thus, SSRIs rather than TCAs are often the current treatment of choice when treating an older adult suffering from depression (see also Ingram & Smith, this volume; Smith, this volume).

More recently, rapid transcranial magnetic stimulation (rTMS) has been shown to produce antidepressant effects in treatment-refractory elderly populations (Mosimann et al., 2004). First introduced in 1985, rTMS involves placement of a small coil over the scalp to induce alternating currents that produce magnetic fields that pass through the brain. Overall, research suggests that psychotherapeutic, medication, and medical interventions have been successful in treating late-life depression.

Suicide in Older Adults Depression in older adulthood is correlated with suicide; therefore, early detection and proper treatment of depression in later life is important. Given the multiple losses that older adults experience (e.g., physical deterioration, bereavement, and grief), suicide in later life has come to the forefront of attention in recent years (Gallagher-Thompson & Osgood, 1997; McIntoch, Santos, Hubbard, & Overholser, 1994; Osgood, 1985; Richman, 1999). Older adults commit suicide at a higher rate than any other age group. Specifically, a high rate of suicide (24.9 cases per 100, 000 of the population) was found in the 75- to 84-year-old age range (Kochanek, & Murphy, 1999, p. 85, Table 26). However, white males who were 85 and older constituted the highest suicide rates (59 cases per 100,000) which is five times the national rate. Furthermore, data suggest that older adults made up 13% of the U.S. population but committed 19% of all suicides (Kochanek & Murphy, 1999). In comparison, younger adults composed 14% of the U.S. population and committed 14% of all suicides. According to Zarit and Zarit (1998), the increase seen in suicide rates in older adults is due to high rates among older men. The ratio of suicide rates of men versus women was 4.2 to 1 in 1990 (Moscicki, 1995). Research shows that suicide rates in men dramatically increase at age 60 and peak in men over the age of 85. Moreover, older men compared to younger men tend to make suicide attempts with more lethal means (e.g., firearms, hanging) and with the serious intent to end their lives compared to women. Differences in suicide rates are related not only to gender but also to ethnicity. Specifically, suicide rates tend to increase over time for Caucasian-, Japanese-, Chinese-, and Filipino-American males, whereas in African-American and Native-American individuals, the suicide rate tends to peak at age 35 and then steadily declines in older age (Zarit & Zarit, 1998).

Researchers have explored numerous risk factors related to suicide in older adults. The two most important risk factors are depression and physical illness, especially when the physical illness involves pain, discomfort, and poor prognosis (Gallagher-Thompson & Osgood, 1997; Zarit & Zarit, 1998). In some cases, the physical illness is not life threatening but causes a decrease in quality of life for the older adult. Furthermore, widows, widowers, and divorced men are more likely to commit suicide than married individuals, particularly if they also have poor social support overall. Additional risk factors include alcoholism, recent losses, and history of prior suicide attempts. Furthermore, although it is not common, some suicides occur in institutional settings, such as nursing homes. Individuals who commit suicide in nursing homes tend to have intact cognitive functioning and no diagnosis of dementia. Similarly, increases in suicide risk in older adults are higher in those individuals who are anticipating nursing home placement.

Dementing Disorders

As the population of older adults exponentially increases in the United States, age-related diseases will inevitably increase. For example, dementia impacts the patient, the family, and the health care system in general. According to Fields (1998), *dementia* is defined as "a deterioration in mental capacities that goes beyond the changes expected to occur with the normal aging process" (p. 211). According to the *DSM–IV*, dementia syndromes are characterized by the "development of multiple cognitive deficits (including memory impairment) that are due to the direct physiological effects of a general medical condition, to the persisting effects of a substance, or to multiple etiologies" (p. 133). Moreover, *dementia* is an all-encompassing term used to refer to cognitive decline and impairment, especially in memory function and learning.

Prevalence of Common Dementing Disorders Over the past several years, research has revealed the complexity and heterogeneity of dementia. Thus, research provides evidence for several variants of the disease (e.g., Alzheimer's disease, vascular dementia, Lewy body dementia, frontotemporal dementia), all with different prevalences and etiologies. Postmortem studies of Alzheimer's disease (AD) patients suggest that AD is the most common form of dementia, accounting for 80% of cases (Luis, Mittenberg, Gass, & Duara, 1999). The second most prevalent subtype is vascular dementia, which accounts for 7 to 18% of all cases (Luis et al., 1999; for discussions of other types of dementia, see Grossman, 2002; Lezak, 1995; Simard, van Reekum, and Cohen, 2000).

Alzheimer's Disease (AD) AD is a progressive neurodegenerative disease in which neurons are lost and abnormalities develop in the neocortical areas of the brain (Kolb & Whishaw, 1996). It has specific neuropathological characteristics, including global neuronal loss, beta-amyloid deposits in cerebral blood vessels, and the development of neuritic plaques and neurofibrillary tangles (U.S. Department of Health and Human Services, 2000). These structural changes in the brain affect the association areas of the cerebral cortex, the hippocampus, and the middle and temporal lobes. Another significant neurological change that occurs in AD is a decrease in the concentration of the neurotransmitter acetylcholine that is related to the severity of the disease (O'Hara, Mumenthaler, & Yesavage, 2000; U.S. Department of Health and Human Services, 2000).

According to the *DSM–IV–TR* (2000), a diagnosis of dementia is given when the following cognitive deficits are present: (1) memory impairment and (2) one or more of the following cognitive impairments: aphasia (language disturbance); apraxia (impaired ability to perform motor tasks given intact motor function); agnosia (inability to recognize or identify objects given intact sensory function); or disturbance of executive function (i.e., planning, organizing, sequencing, abstraction skills).

The first signs of AD include subtle decline in memory functions when the individual is in a clear state of consciousness. This condition leads to impairment in daily functioning (e.g., increased problems handling finances, difficulty participating in conversations; Braak et al., 1999; O'Hara et al., 2000). As the disease progresses, additional cognitive changes occur (e.g., deterioration in language function, impairment in the ability to care for oneself) and quality of life of both the patient and caregiver often deteriorates. Personality changes and behavioral disturbances (e.g., agitation, physical aggression, hallucinations, delusions, sleep disturbance, wandering) may also occur as the disease progresses (O'Hara et al., 2000). In the final stages, the motor system deteriorates, motor reaction to stimuli decreases (often related to muscle spasms), and the individual becomes fully dependent on others for self-care. The individual may require nursing home placement at this point, when the burdens of care overwhelm the caregiver's capacity to respond. On average, an individual lives with AD for approximately 8 to 10 years after the initial diagnosis (U.S. Department of Health and Human Services, 2000).

Vascular Dementia (VaD) VaD is defined by *DSM–IV–TR* as described previously for AD, but also includes the presence of focal neurologic signs and symptoms or laboratory evidence that indicates cerebrovascular disease (CVD; U.S. Department of Veterans Affairs, 1997). CVD is defined by the presence of focal signs on neurological examination, such as hemiparesis (weakness on one side of the body) and evidence of relevant CVD on brain imaging (e.g., multiple large vessel strokes, or a single major stroke placed in an area where multiple cognitive areas are disrupted). In brief, VaD occurs after an individual has experienced either a large stroke that in turn affects multiple cognitive functions or a series of small strokes. When an individual is diagnosed with VaD, it is difficult to know what cognitive deficits to expect because they vary, depending on the location of the stroke in the brain. Moreover, a definitive diagnosis of VaD is complicated because an individual may have a mixed vascular degenerative dementia in which the symptoms of a progressive dementia, like AD is accompanied or complicated by a cerebrovascular accident.

Risk Factors for AD and VaD Researchers have identified a number of risk factors related to AD including the following: genetic predisposition, advanced age, ethnicity, a history of head trauma, and Down syndrome (O'Hara et al., 2000; Petronis, 1999; Teng et al., 1998). Researchers have linked a specific gene to Alzheimer's disease, called apolipoprotein E4 (ApoE4), which can be inherited from one or both parents. Thus, individuals who test positive for one or both of these ApoE4 alleles are at greater risk for eventually developing AD later in life than those who do not have ApoE4 alleles. Individuals who inherited one ApoE4 allele have twice the risk, and individuals with two ApoE4s are 10 times more likely to develop AD (O'Hara et al. 2000). Furthermore, the prevalence and incidence of AD increases as one advances in age. Estimates suggest that the incidence of AD doubles every 5 years after age 60 (Cummings, Vinters, Cole, & Khachaturian, 1998). Ethnicity is another possible risk factor, although research on ethnicity has been inconsistent (Fillenbaum, Heyman, et al., 1998). African Americans and Latino/a Americans may have a higher risk of AD than white Americans (Teng et al., 1998).

Risk factors for VaD include health problems related to CVD and heart disease, such as hypertension, high cholesterol, diabetes, heart rhythm problems, and abnormally high fatty content of the blood (Lezak, 1995). Cigarette smoking, being overweight, and having a family history of heart disease may also increase the risk of a stroke which is associated with VaD. Transient ischemic attacks (TIA) are ministrokes which may warn of an imminent larger stroke, leading to VaD. Medications, surgery, and adopting a healthy lifestyle may decrease an individual's risk for VaD.

Assessment of Dementia The goals of the assessment process are fourfold: (1) to provide an accurate diagnosis; (2) to provide the patient and family with the prognosis; (3) to review treatment options with the patient and family; and (4) to assist the patient and family in planning for the management of the disease (Riley & Carr, 1989). A diagnosis of AD is typically made within the context of an interdisciplinary team that includes physicians, psychologists, nurses, and other health care professionals who have specialty training in geriatrics or geropsychology. In an attempt to make an accurate diagnosis, the diagnostic team gathers a combination of data such as neuroimaging results from computed to-mography (CT) or magnetic resonance imaging (MRI) scans, neuropsychological test results, patient's medical records, and caregiver/informant observations (U.S. Department of Veterans Affairs, 1997). Several assessment measures are commonly administered. The Mini-Mental State Examination (MMSE; Folstein, Folstein, & McHugh, 1975) is typically given to assess global cognitive functioning (see Table 19.2). The Alzheimer's Disease Assessment Scale (ADAS; Rosen, Mohs, & Davis, 1984) assesses both cognitive and noncognitive symptoms related to AD (e.g., memory, language, constructions, ideational praxis, mood and behavioral disturbances; see Table 19.2). The Clinical Dementia Rating Scale (CDR) (Hughes, Berg, Danziger, Cohen, & Martin, 1982) is administered to quantify a large number of func-tional impairments in dementia. The Dementia Rating Scale (DRS; Mattis, 1976) is used to identify dementia and to differentiate among the subtypes of dementia (e.g., AD, VaD).

Treatment of Dementia Currently, there is no known cure for AD. Researchers continue to make advances in understanding the etiology and neuropathology of AD. Thus, the available treatments only slow the progression of the disease and improve the quality of life for AD patients, their caregiv-ers and family.

BEHAVIORAL TREATMENT WITH DEMENTIA PATIENTS Dementia patients often suffer from concurrent depressive symptoms. Roughly 30% of patients with AD also have symptoms of depression that meet diagnostic criteria for major depressive disorder (Teri & Reifler, 1987; Teri & Wagner, 1992). These depressed dementia patients are prone to higher rates of behavioral and functional problems (e.g., increased irritability, agitation, and aggressive behavior), and their caregivers report higher levels of distress (Pearson, Teri, Wagner, Truax, & Logsdon, 1993). In recent years, research has focused on cognitive and behavioral treatments for depressed dementia patients and their family

TABLE 19.2   Summary of geriatric measures

Name of scale	Key citations
Back Anxiety Inventory (BAI)	Beck, Epstein, Brown, & Steer (1988)
Beck Depression Inventory (BDI)	Gallagher, Nies, & Thompson (1982)
Center of Epidemiologic Studies Depression Scale (CES-D)	Radloff (1977)
Geriatric Depression Scale (GDS)	Yesavage, Brink, Rose, Lum, Huang, Adey, & Leirer (1983)
Geriatric Depression Scale-short form	Sheikh & Yesavage (1986)
Mini-Mental State Examination (MMSE)	Folstein et al. (1975)
Alzheimer's Disease Assessment Scale (ADAS)	Rosen, Mohs, & Davis (1984)
The Clinical Dementia Rating Scale (CDR)	Hughes, Berg, Danziger, Cohen, & Martin (1982)
Dementia Rating Scale (DRS)	Mattis (1976)
Mississippi PTSD Scales	Neal et al. (1995)
Clinician Administered PTSD Schedule (CAPS)	Hyer, Summers, Boyd, & Litaker (1996)
Michigan Alcohol Screening Test-Geriatric Version (MAST-G)	Blow et al. (1992)
CAGE Alcohol Screen	Ewing (1984)
Alcohol-Related Problems Survey (ARPS) and Short ARPS (SHARPS)	Moore et al., (2002)
Alcohol Use Disorders Inventory Test (AUDIT)	Babor, de la Fuente, Saunders, & Grant (1989)

caregivers (Teri & Gallagher-Thompson, 1991) as well as on training of health care staff in long-term care settings to treat depressed dementia patients (Teri & McCurry, 1994). Teri (1994) developed a nine-week treatment for both the dementia patient and caregiver in which they were provided with (1) education about AD and behavioral interventions; (2) methods of behavior change; (3) strategies for identifying and increasing patient pleasant events; (4) methods to maximize the patient's cognitive and functional abilities; (5) problem solving related to patient care, including depression behavior; (6) aid for caregiving responsibilities; and (7) plans for maintaining treatment gains. Investigations have shown somewhat promising results of this behavioral treatment (Teri, Logsdon, Peskind et al., 2000; Teri, Logsdon, Uomoto, & McCurry, 1997). Furthermore, behavioral treatment combined with other interventions appears to be effective. In one study, AD patients showed improved physical health and less depressive symptoms when the patient and caregiver received exercise training and the caregiver learned behavioral management techniques for problematic behaviors (Teri, Gibbons et al., 2003).

TREATMENT FOR DISTRESS IN FAMILY CAREGIVERS Caregivers of individuals with dementia experience extensive caregiver stress and often feel progressively overwhelmed as their loved one continues to deteriorate (Coon, Thompson, & Gallagher-Thompson, 2002; Martin-Cook, Trimmer, Svetlik, & Weiner, 2000). Furthermore, the stress of caregiving often has negative effects on the psychological and physical health of the caregiver (Bauer et al., 2000; Schulz, O'Brien, Bookwala, Fleissner; 1995; Vedhara, Shanks, Anderson, & Lightman, 2000). A variety of caregiver interventions have been developed and empirically validated (Coon et al., 2002; Gallagher-Thompson, Coon, Rivera, Powers, & Zeiss, 1998; Gallagher-Thompson, McKibbin et al., 2000). A review of evidence-based psychological treatments (EBT) for reducing distress and improving well-being of family caregivers indicate that psychoeducational programs, psychotherapy, and multicomponent interventions (e.g., family meetings plus individual therapy and support group attendance) received ample empirical support (Gallagher-Thompson & Coon, in press). Furthermore, Gallagher-Thompson, Lovett et al. (2000) found that, in white participants, a cognitive-behavioral psychoeducational "Coping With Caregiving" group reduced caregiver affective distress and increased coping behavior more than a problem-solving psychoeducational class or a wait-list control condition.

Similar results were found with white and Latina samples of dementia caregivers in the Resources for Enhancing Alzheimer's Caregiver Health (REACH I) project, a multisite study that sought to examine culturally sensitive interventions for dementia caregivers. Specifically, participants in the "Coping With Caregiving" class reported a significant reduction in depressive symptoms, increased use of adaptive coping strategies, and a trend toward decreased use of negative coping strategies when compared with those in an Enhanced Support Group condition (guided discussion and empathic listening to develop reciprocal support within the group) (Gallagher-Thompson, Haley et al., 2003). Guidelines for culturally competent services for ethnically diverse dementia caregivers (African American, Cuban American, Mexican American) were developed following the REACH I and II projects (see Gallagher-Thompson, Haley et al., 2003; REACH II investigators, 2006, for review). The results of REACH II (in which the same treatments were administered across five sites to over 600 ethnically diverse caregivers) are now available. They are generally supportive of prior research indicating the positive effects of skill training to improve the quality of life of family caregivers. Training families to cope with the burdens of caregiving has become necessary and increases the family caregiver's effectiveness (Teri, 1999). Thus, the individual living with dementia receives better care from caregivers. Furthermore, providing both the individual with dementia and his or her caregivers with information about local community resources and social services can reduce caregiver stress (Thompson & Thompson, 1999).

MEDICATION INTERVENTIONS In recent years, there have been important developments in medication treatment for dementia, such as the introduction of cholinesterase inhibitors that help slow the progression of brain atrophy. These medications act by inhibiting the enzyme acetylcholinesterase, which slows down the metabolic breakdown of acetylcholine. Unfortunately, the medications do not alter the underlying course of the disease (U.S. Department of Health and Human Services, 2000).

In 1993, tacrine (Cognex) was the first medication approved by the Food and Drug Administration in the United States for treatment of dementia. Efficacy studies of tacrine found only modest improvement in cognitive function (Sirvio, 1999). Furthermore, tacrine had serious side effects including liver toxicity (Nordberg & Swensson, 1998). Thus, the costs of taking tacrine often outweighed the benefits.

With the advent of acetylcholinesterase inhibitors with few serious side effects, tacrine is prescribed less frequently. The newer medications, donepezil (Aricept), rivastigmine (Exelon), and galantamine (Razadyne, formerly named Reminyl), are now more widely used. Clinical trials have found these second-generation cholinesterase inhibitors to be efficacious. Specifically, 5 or 10 mg of donepezil daily was associated with some improvement in cognitive function after 12 or 24 weeks of treatment. Moreover, significant improvements were found in global function and activities of daily living after 24 weeks of treatment (compared with placebo) in patients with mild to moderate AD (Wilkinson, 1999).

The newest medication designed to treat Alzheimer's disease, is memantine (Namenda), a N-methyl-d-aspartate receptor antagonist. Memantine has shown positive results when used to treat mild to moderate AD patients (Peskind et al., 2006) and moderately to severely impaired patients (Reisberg et al., 2003; Tariot et al., 2004; Winblad & Poritis, 1999). Peskind and colleagues (2006) found that cognition, global mental status, and behavioral functioning were significantly better in those individuals taking memantine compared to those taking placebo after 24 weeks. In three pivotal clinical trials involving moderately to severely impaired AD patients, memantine was shown to be effective in slowing the progression of cognitive, behavioral, and functional impairments seen in AD patients (Reisberg et al., 2003; Tariot et al., 2004; Winblad & Poritis, 1999).

Alcohol Use Disorders in Older Adults

The Substance Abuse and Mental Health Services Administration (SAMHSA) has identified alcohol abuse among older adults as one of the fastest growing health problems facing the United States (Arndt, Gunter, & Acion, 2005; SAMHSA, 1998). According to the annual national survey on drug use and health sponsored by SAMHSA (2004), community-dwelling older adults drink alcohol on a regular basis. Among individuals surveyed, between the ages of 60 and 64 years, 49.9% used alcohol in the past month, and 35.3% of individuals aged 65 or older used alcohol in the past month. In terms of binge drinking and heavy drinking, 6.9% of adults aged 65 or older reported binge drinking and 1.8% reported heavy drinking. Binge drinking is defined as five or more drinks on the same occasion on at least one day in the past month, and heavy drinking is defined as five or more drinks on the same occasion on each of five or more days in the past 30 days. Other estimates of problem alcohol use among community-dwelling, noninstitutionalized older adults range from 2 to 15% (Adams, Barry, & Fleming, 1996; Gomberg, 1992). The estimates of alcohol use problems among this age group increases significantly for medical patients. Among older primary care patients, 10 to 15% were found to meet the criteria for problem drinking, defined as drinking habits that led to medical, social, or psychological problems (Callahan & Tierney, 1995; Oslin, 2004). Despite the high prevalence of alcohol use among older adults, they are less likely than younger adults to receive treatment for substance use disorders (Moos, Mertens, & Nrennan, 1993; see also Fals-Stewart & Klosterman, this volume.)

Assessment of Alcohol Abuse and Dependence

There are a number of barriers to early detection of alcohol use among older adults. In fact, alcohol problems among older adults have been called the "*Invisible Epidemic*" (SAMHSA, 1998). First, compared to younger adults, older adults are less likely to seek out and use mental health or substance abuse services. When alcohol abuse is identified, it is often found as a secondary condition within primary care settings. A second barrier is that elders are not routinely screened for alcohol abuse by medical and mental health providers, leading to problems with early detection and treatment of the disorder. Third, older adult drinkers tend to have fewer social indicators of alcohol abuse (e.g., family complaints, DUIs, work impairment). Lastly, symptoms of alcohol problems mimic those of other psychological disorders (e.g., depression) that are common among older adults. As a result, these diagnoses are assessed first without further screening for alcohol use.

The need to increase early detection and treatment of alcohol abuse and dependence among older adults is warranted due to the negative physiological consequences of alcoholism in this age group. In terms of the health consequences, smaller amounts of alcohol have a stronger net effect in older adults because of physiological changes that occur as the body ages. Second, there is significant risk for malnutrition in that excess amounts of alcohol decrease the ability of the stomach to absorb food and thus increase the risk for malnutrition. Third, there is a risk of negative interaction between alcohol and other regularly prescribed medications which is of particular concern because of the high prevalence of substance use problems among older adults with health problems. Finally, substance use has a negative impact on the cognitive functioning of older adults, affecting memory performance on tasks involving frontal lobe activity (e.g., flexibility of thinking) and perceptual-motor deficits (e.g. poor performance on speed-dependent and visual spatial tasks).

Health conditions are often useful indicators of substance abuse among older adults and may suggest a screen for alcohol use (Egbert, 1993). One indicator is encountered when a therapy for a normally treatable medical illness (e.g., hypertension) is not working for an older patient. Second, there are certain physical problems associated with alcohol use in older adults including insomnia, diarrhea, urinary incontinence, weight loss, and malnutrition. Third, older adults who complain of anxiety, experience unexplained postoperative agitation, or those who frequently ask for prescriptions of anxiolytics, sedatives, or hypnotics might be suffering from a substance use disorder and suggests a screening for such a disorder.

Although health conditions can be helpful indicators of a substance use problem in older adult patients, very few admissions to treatment are referred by healthcare providers (Arndt et al., 2005). All adults age 60 or older should be screened for alcohol use problems on a regular basis, preferably at their annual physical exam (SAMHSA, 1998). If patients are younger than 60 years of age, they should be screened if they are undergoing major life changes or exhibiting physical symptoms suggestive of an alcohol use disorder. Table 19.2 includes assessment measures for alcohol use found to be reliable and valid with older adults.

Treatment of Alcohol Abuse and Dependence

Although older adults are less likely than younger adults to receive substance abuse treatment, brief interventions, motivational counseling, and cognitive behavioral therapies have been shown to be effective treatment options for older adults. Practice recommendations suggest that the least intensive treatment options should be explored first with older adults who have been diagnosed with an alcohol problem (SAMHSA, 1998). In terms of brief interventions, 10 to 30% of older problem drinkers, who did not meet criteria for a *DMS–IV* diagnosis of substance dependence, reduced their drinking to moderate levels following a brief intervention (SAMHSA, 1998). The brief intervention consisted of one or more counseling sessions that included: motivations for change strategies, patient education, assessment and direct feedback, contracting and goal setting, behavioral modification techniques, and the use of written material. One approach that facilitates effective brief interventions with older adults is a motivation-to-change strategy developed by Miller and Rollnick (1991, 2002)—feedback, responsibility, advice, menu, empathetic, self-efficacy (FRAMES; SAMHSA, 1998). The FRAMES approach emphasizes providing feedback on personal risk or impairment, personal responsibility for change, clear advice to change, a menu of ways to change, an empathetic counseling style, and enhancing a client's self-efficacy (SAMHSA, 1998). An advantage to brief interventions is they can be used in a variety of settings, including primary care settings where alcohol problems among older adults can be easily identified. Brief interventions in primary care settings for older adults with alcohol problems have been shown to significantly reduce weekly alcohol consumption, episodes of binge drinking, and frequency of excessive drinking (Fleming, Barry, Manwell, Johnson, & London, 1997; Gordon et al., 2003).

Cognitive-behavioral approaches to substance abuse and dependence were found to be successful with older adult clients. These approaches are often structured, short-term psychotherapies in which the client learns new skills (e.g., initiating adaptive behaviors, challenging unhelpful thoughts) to cope with and overcome an addiction to alcohol. The effectiveness of a cognitive-behavioral approach to treat older adults with alcohol problems was demonstrated in the Gerontology Alcohol Project (GAP, 1979–1981; Dupree, Broskowski, & Schonfeld, 1984). GAP used a treatment that included a cognitive-behavioral based analysis of drinking behavior (ABCs of drinking) and self-management groups. Of those who completed the program, 75% maintained abstinence or limited drinking at 1-year follow-up and reported increased social support networks at discharge and at 1-year follow-up. Cognitive-behavioral therapy with an emphasis on developing coping skills for dealing with personal problems has been found to be more effective for adults ages 50 and over who were receiving treatment for substance use in comparison to relationship enhancement and vocational enhancement therapies (Rice, Longabaugh, Beattie, & Noel, 1993).

SAMHSA has developed practice guidelines for treating older adults with substance abuse problems (SAMHSA TIPS no. 26, 1998; Schonfeld & Dupree, 1998). When working with older adults receiving treatment for alcohol use the following is suggested:

- Emphasize age-specific group treatment that is supportive rather than confrontational.
- Treatment facilities should employ staff experienced in working with elders.
- The overall treatment approach should be broad and holistic, recognizing the age-specific psychological, social, and health factors related to substance use.
- The pace of treatment should be slow and the content should attend to negative emotions (e.g., depression, loneliness, overcoming losses).
- Treatment should also teach skills to rebuild social support networks.
- Substance abuse treatment centers for older adults should be linked with aging services to address other needs that could potentially put elders at an increased chance of relapse.

Studies suggest that for older adults, age-specific treatments yield higher attendance rates and treatment completion rates in comparison to treatments for mixed-age groups (Kashner, Rodell, Ogden, Guggenheim, & Karson, 1992; Kofoed et al., 1987). However, Oslin and colleagues (Oslin, Pettinati, & Volpicelli, 2005) demonstrated that mixed-age treatment settings were effective in treating older adults with alcohol dependence as long as other age-appropriate treatment components, such as a nonconfrontational style and individualized techniques, were used.

Psychologcal Assessment of Older Adults

Selecting an assessment instrument for an older individual is a challenge because there are few assessment measures designed specifically for older adults. As discussed in previous sections, some diagnostic criteria for particular disorders are not always applicable to older adults and could result in an inaccurate diagnosis. Once an appropriate assessment measure is selected, modifications in the assessment procedure must be made, beginning with slowing the pace of testing (Zarit & Haynie, 2000). Older adults tire more easily, so assessment procedures need to be accommodating. Test sessions might need to be spread across several days and frequent breaks taken to ensure more accurate results. Instructions and testing materials also should be presented at a slower pace and in multiple modalities if possible. Second, mental health professionals need to be aware of the sensory deficits of their older adult clients. Moreover, it is important to ensure that the testing environment is quiet with minimal distractions, and that older adult clients use sensory aids they require (e.g., glasses, hearing aids). Third, it is important for clinicians working with older adults to collaborate with other health professionals. Ideally, physicians should be involved in the assessment process to rule out any physical health problem that might be associated with the presenting mental health problem, thus leading to more accurate treatment recommendations.

Treatment Issues with Older Adults

Treatment interventions used with older adults who are suffering from mental health problems are not significantly different from those used with younger or middle-aged adults. What differs is the process and content of therapy. The process of therapy differs in three main ways: (1) there is often a need to directly address the age difference between therapist and client; (2) it is necessary to conduct therapy in such a manner as to foster independence in older clients; and (3) it is usually necessary to use a slower pace of treatment and to make appropriate modifications due to cognitive or sensory deficits (Zeiss & Steffen, 1996). Specifically, there is a high likelihood that the mental health provider will be considerably younger than the older adult client. Therefore, it is necessary to openly address any concerns older adult clients have related to the age differential at the onset of therapy. This can be achieved by treating clients with respect and explaining how specific training in geropsychology helps therapists to understand age-related problems and needs (Zarit & Zarit, 1998). The second component, the need to foster independence, can be done primarily through a collaborative relationship, which encourages the older adults' involvement in therapy decisions, such as frequency and time of visits and between-session interventions for the client to do independently. Regarding the third point, the pace of therapy is usually slower with older adult clients, who generally benefit from repetition of information. Reviewing and summarizing what has been discussed in a session helps older clients to learn and remember new information. It is important for mental health providers to be patient with the pace of treatment and not to get discouraged. Change in older adults is possible, but usually occurs in smaller increments (Zeiss & Steffen, 1996).

Another factor influencing the pace of therapy is the need to accommodate sensory deficits. Older adults are able to hear better when they are spoken to in a voice that is loud, slow, and at a low pitch (Zarit & Zarit, 1998). Presenting information in multiple modalities, such as in verbal and written formats, also assists older adults' ability to maintain information. All written material should be presented in a large, easy-to-read font. Daily log books are also useful to help older adults record observations related to treatment between sessions and to take notes during therapy sessions. Some clients also find it helpful to audiotape or videotape sessions for future review.

Zeiss and Steffen (1996) have summarized the basic adaptations needed when treating older adults into five components using the mnemonic MICKS (multimodal, interdisciplinary awareness, clear knowledge of aging challenges and strengths, and slow down). Using the strengths of older clients is a concept that fits well with the notion of successful aging. Zeiss and Steffen (1996) suggest that during the process of therapy, clinicians can foster older adults' strengths by demonstrating respect for the role of the elder, having the older adult identify their personal strengths and how they can be used to alleviate the presenting problem, discussing past experiences in which they handled similar problems, and considering the clients' wisdom.

The content of therapy differs from therapy with younger adults because of the particular life experiences of older adults, including chronic illness and disability, concerns with death and dying, and interpretation of the aging process (Thompson, 1996). Knight (1986) also suggests that the content of therapy should include themes such as empowerment in later life, how to cope with losses and maintain independence, the importance of everyday pleasant activities, and life review.

Meeting the Future Needs of Older Adults

Although there is not a direct causal relationship between growing old and developing psychological disorders, a significant number of older adults do suffer from mental health disorders in later life. Appropriate assessment and treatment of mental health disorders among older adults are going to be a growing concern as the population of older adults continues to grow. Given the projected future increase in the older adult population, a major mental health need of older adults is access and use of mental health services. Relatively few older adults seek treatment for mental health problems (Scogin et al., 2000). Service use is even lower among ethnic minority older adults (U.S. Department of Health and Human Services, 2001). Furthermore, when an older adult receives treatment for a mental health problem, services are often obtained via a primary care physician (Robinson, 1998) rather than a trained mental health professional.

In order to meet the future needs of older adults, mental health professionals need to be able to provide evidenced-based practices in psychology (EBPP) to older adults dealing with mental health disorders (for a review see Gallagher-Thompson & Coon, 2007; Levkoff, Chen, Fisher, & McIntyre, 2006). According to the American Psychological Association Presidential Task Force on Evidenced-Based Practice (2006), "EBPP provides effective psychological practice and enhances public health by applying empirically supported principles of psychological assessment, case formulation, therapeutic relationship, and intervention" (p. 271). In terms of future research directions the Task Force has identified determining the efficacy and effectiveness of psychological treatments with older adults as a priority for future research.

Addressing the future mental health needs of older adults also can be achieved through interdisciplinary collaboration and through promoting health care that uses an interdisciplinary treatment team model. Given the physiological changes associated with normal aging and the related possible psychosocial stressors, both the mental and physical health needs of older adults would be better met with an interdisciplinary treatment team approach. As the population of older adults continues to grow, health professionals are going to be asked how to foster well-being and enhance the quality of life of older adults. We have some answers, but many more need to be discovered.

Discussion Questions

1. To get a better understanding of your stereotypes of aging, create a list of positive and negative images of aging in our society.
2. What do we know about other cultures' views of aging and how can these values be applied to the development of treatment interventions in the United States? How do these views change the way we conceptualize or define mental health problems?

3. Create an outreach program designed to reduce mental health problems among older adults. Address the following issues: prevalent mental health issues, ethnic minority older adults, interdisciplinary health teams, and successful aging.
4. Discuss ways to create a paradigm shift in the current health care system for older adults (e.g., government policies, community programs).

ACKNOWLEDGMENT

This work is supported by grants AG18784, AG17824, AG022252 from the National Institute on Aging, grant AA07222 from the NIAAA, grant IIRG–01–3157 from the National Office of the Alzheimer's Association, and by the Department of Veterans Affairs Sierra-Pacific Mental Illness Research, Education, and Clinical Center (MIRECC).

Suggested Readings

Birren, J. E., & Schaie, K. W. (Eds.). (2006). *Handbook of the psychology of aging* (6th ed.). Boston: Elsevier Academic Press.
Duffy, M. (Ed.). (1999). *Handbook of counseling and psychotherapy with older adults.* New York: Wiley.
Gallagher-Thompson, D., Steffen, A., & Thompson, L.W. (Eds.). (In preparation). *Handbook of behavior and cognitive therapies with older adults.* Oakland, CA: New Harbinger.
Levkoff, S. E., Chen, H., Fisher, J. E., & McIntyre, J. S. (Eds.). (2006). *Evidence-based behavioral health practices for older adults: A guide to implementation.* New York: Springer.
Whitbourne, S. K. (Ed.). (2000). *Psychopathology in later adulthood.* New York: Wiley.
Yeo, G., & Gallagher-Thompson, D. (Eds.). (2006). *Ethnicity and the dementias* (2nd ed.). New York: Taylor & Francis.
Zarit, S. H., & Zarit, J. M. (1998). *Mental disorders in older adults.* New York: Guilford.

References

Adams, W. L., Barry, K. L., & Fleming, M. F. (1996). Screening for problem drinking in older primary care patients. *Journal of the American Medical Association, 276*(24), 1964–1967.
Adams, A. Ockene, J. K., Wheller, E. V., & Hurley, T. G. (1998). Alcohol counseling: Physicians will do it. *Journal of General Internal Medicine, 13,* 692–698.
Altamura, A. C., De Novellis, F., Guercetti, G., Invernizzi, G., Percudano, M., & Montgomery, S. A. (1989). Fluoxetine compared with amitriptyline in elderly depression: A controlled clinical trial. *International Journal of Clinical Pharmacological Research, 9,* 391–396.
American Psychiatric Association. (1980). *Diagnostic and statistical manual of mental disorders* (3rd ed.). Washington, D.C.: Author.
American Psychiatric Association. (1994). *Diagnostic and statistical manual of mental disorders* (4th ed.). Washington, D.C.: Author.
American Psychiatric Association. (2000). *Diagnostic and statistical manual of mental disorders* (4th ed., rev.). Washington, D.C.: Author.
American Psychological Association, Presidential Task Force on Evidence-Based Practice (2006). Evidence-based practice in psychology. *American Psychologist, 61*(4), 271–285.
Arean, P.A., Gum, A., McCulloch, C. E., Bostrom, A., Gallagher-Thompson, D., & Thompson, L. (2005). Treatment of depression in low-income older adults. *Psychology and Aging, 20,* 601–609.
Arndt, S., Gunter, T. D., & Acion, L. (2005). Older admissions to substance use treatment in 2001. *American Journal Geriatric Psychiatry, 13,* 385–392.
Averill, P. M., & Beck, J. G. (2000). Posttraumatic stress disorder in older adults: A conceptual review. *Journal of Anxiety Disorders, 14*(2), 133–156.
Babor, T. F., de la Fuente, J. R., Saunders, J., & Grant, M. (1989). AUDIT The Alcohol Use Disorders Identification Test: Guidelines for use in primary health care. WHO/MNH/DAT 89 (4), World Health Organization, Geneva.
Banazak, D. A. (1997). Anxiety disorders in elderly patients. *Journal of the American Board of Family Practice, 10,* 280–289.
Bauer, M. E., Vedhara, K., Perks, P., Wilcock, G. K., Lightman, S. L., & Shanks, N. (2000). Chronic stress in caregivers of dementia patients is associated with reduced lymphocyte sensitivity to glucocorticoids. *Journal of Neuroimmunology, 103*(1), 84–92.
Beck, A., Epstein, N., Brown, G., & Steer, R. (1988). An inventory for measuring clinical anxiety: Psychometric properties. *Journal of Consulting and Clinical Psychology, 56,* 893–897.
Beck, J. G., & Stanley, M. A. (1997). Anxiety disorders in the elderly: The emerging role of behavior therapy. *Behavior Therapy, 28,* 83–100.
Beck, A. T., Steer, R. A., & Brown, G. K. (1996). *BDI-II manual.* San Antonio, TX: The Psychological Corporation.

Beekman, A. T. F., Bremmer, M. A., Deeg, D. J. H., Van Balkom, A. J. L. M., Smit, J. H., De Beurs, E., et al. (1998). Anxiety disorders in later life: A report from the longitudinal aging study, Amsterdam. *International Journal of Geriatric Psychiatry*, 13, 717–726.

Bell, I. (1999). A guide to current psychopharmacological treatments for affective disorders in older adults: Anxiety, agitation, and depression. In M. Duffy (Ed.), *Handbook of counseling and psychotherapy with older adults* (pp. 561–576). New York: Wiley.

Blake, D. D., Weathers, F. W., Nagy, L. M., Kaloupek, D. G., Klauminzer, G., Charney, D. S., et al.(1990). A clinician rating scale for assessing current and lifetime PTSD: The CAPS–1. *Behavioral Therapist*, 13, 187– 188.

Blazer, D. (1986). Depression. *Generations*, 10, 21–23.

Blazer, D. (2002). *Depression in late life*. New York: Springer.

Blazer, D., George, L. K., & Hughes, D. (1991). The epidemiology of anxiety disorders: An age comparison. In C. Salzman & B. Lebowitz (Eds.), *Anxiety in the elderly* (pp. 17–30). New York: Springer.

Blow, F. C., Brower, K. J., Schulenberg, J. E., Demo-Dananberg, L. M., Young, J. P., & Beresford, T. P. (1992). The Michigan Alcoholism Screening Test—Geriatric Version (MAST-G): A new elderly-specific screening instrument. *Alcoholism: Clinical and Experimental Research*, 16, 372.

Boehlein, J. K., & Sparr, L. F. (1993). Group therapy with WWII ex-POWs: Long-term posttraumatic adjustment in a geriatric population. *American Journal of Psychotherapy*, 47, 273–282.

Bonwick, R. (1997). A group treatment programme for elderly war veterans with post traumatic stress disorder. *Australian and New Zealand Journal of Psychiatry*, 31, A24.

Boudewyns, P., & Hyer, L. (1997). Changes in psychophysiological response to war memories among Vietnam veteran PTSD patients treated with directed therapeutic exposure. *Behavior Therapy*, 21, 63–87.

Braak, E., Griffing, K., Arai, K., Bohl, J., Bratzke, H., & Braak, H. (1999). Neuropathology of Alzheimer's disease: What is new since A. Alzheimer? *European Archives of Psychiatry and Clinical Neuroscience*, 249(Suppl. 3), 14–22.

Callahan, C. M., & Tierney, W. M. (1995). Health services use and mortality among older primary care patients with alcoholism. *Journal of American Geriatrics Society*, 43(12), 1378–1383.

Coon, D., Thompson, L. W., & Gallagher-Thompson, D. G. (Eds.). (2002). *Innovative interventions to reduce dementia caregivers' distress: A sourcebook and clinical guide*. New York: Springer.

Cummings, J. L., Vinters, H. V., Cole, G. M., & Khachaturian, Z. S. (1998). Alzheimer's disease: Etiologies, pathophysiology, cognitive reserve, and treatment opportunities. *Neurology*, 51(Suppl. 1), S2–S17.

Deberry, S., Davis, S., & Reinhard, K. E. (1989). A comparison of meditation-relaxation and cognitive-behavioral techniques for reducing anxiety and depression in a geriatric population. *Journal of Geriatric Psychiatry*, 22, 231–247.

Dupree, L. W., Broskowski, H., & Schonfeld, L. (1984). The gerontology alcohol project: A behavioral treatment program for elderly alcohol abusers. *Gerontologist*, 24, 510–516.

Dychtwald, K., & Flower, J. (1990). *Age wave: How the most important trend of our time will change your future*. New York: Bantam Books.

Egbert, A. M. (1993). The older alcoholic: Recognizing the subtle clinical clues. *Geriatrics*, 48(7), 63–66, 69.

Ewing, J. A. (1984). Detecting alcoholism: CAGE Questionnaire. *Journal of the American Medical Association*, 252, 1905–1907.

Fields, R. B. (1998). The dementias. In P. J. Snyder & P. D. Nussbaum (Eds.), *Clinical neuropsychology: A pocket handbook for assessment* (pp. 211–239). Washington, D.C.: American Psychological Association.

Fillenbaum, G. G., Heyman, A., Huber, M. S., Woodbury, M. A., Leiss, J., Schmader, K. E., et al. (1998). The prevalence and 3-year incidence of dementia in older black and white community residents. *Journal of Clinical Epidemiology*, 51(7), 587–595.

Fleming, M. F., Barry, K. L., Manwell, L. B., Johnson, K., & London, R. (1997). Brief physician advice for problem alcohol drinkers: A randomized controlled trial in community-based primary care practices. *Journal of the American Medical Association*, 277, 1039–1045.

Folstein, M. F., Folstein, S. E., & McHugh, P. R. (1975). "Mini-mental state." A practical method for grading the cognitive state of patients for the clinician. *Journal of Psychiatric Research*, 12, 189–198.

Fry, P. S. (1984). Cognitive training and cognitive-behavioral variables in the treatment of depression in the elderly. *Clinical Gerontologist*, 3, 25–45.

Gallagher, D., Breckenridge, J., Thompson, L. W., & Peterson, J. (1983). Effects of bereavement on indicators of mental health in elderly widows and widowers. *Journal of Gerontology*, 38, 565–571.

Gallagher, D., Nies, G., & Thompson, L. W. (1982). Reliability of the Beck Depression Inventory with older adults. *Journal of Consulting and Clinical Psychology*, 50, 152–153.

Gallagher, D., Rose, J., Rivera, P., Lovett, S., & Thompson, L. W. (1989). Prevalence of depression in family caregivers. *The Gerontologist*, 29, 449–456.

Gallagher-Thompson, D., Arean, P., Rivera, P., Thompson, L. W. (2001). A psychoeducational intervention to reduce distress in Hispanic family caregivers: Results of a pilot study. *Clinical Gerontologist*, 23, 17–32.

Gallagher-Thompson, D., Coon, D.W. (2007). Evidence-based psychological treatments for distress in family caregivers of older adults. *Psychology and Aging*, 22, 37–51.

Gallagher-Thompson, D., Coon, D., Rivera, P., Powers, D., & Zeiss, A. (1998). Family caregiving: Stress, coping, and intervention. In M. Hersen & V. B. Van Hasselt (Eds.), *Handbook of clinical geropsychology* (pp. 469–494). New York: Plenum.

Gallagher-Thompson, D., Coon, D. W., Solano, N., Ambler, C., Rabinowitz, Y., & Thompson, L.W. (2003). Change in indices of distress among Latina and Anglo female caregivers of elderly relatives with dementia: Site specific results from the REACH national collaborative study. *The Gerontologist*, 43(4), 580–591.

Gallagher-Thompson, D. & DeVries, H. (1994). "Coping with Frustration" classes: Development and preliminary outcomes with women who care for relatives with dementia. *The Gerontologist*, 34, 548–552.

Gallagher-Thompson, D., Haley, W., Guy, D., Rupert, M., Arguelles, T., Zeiss, L., et al. (2003). Tailoring psychological interventions for ethnically diverse caregivers. *Clinical Psychology: Science and Practice, 10,* 423–438.

Gallagher-Thompson, D., Lovett, S., Rose, J., McKibbin, C., Coon, D., Futterman, A., et al. (2000). Impact of psychoeducational interventions on distressed family caregivers. *Journal of Clinical Geropsychology, 6*(2), 91–110.

Gallagher-Thompson, D., McKibbin, C., Koonce-Volwiler, D., Menendez, A., Stewart, D., & Thompson, L. W. (2000). Psychotherapy with older adults. In C. R. Snyder & R. Ingram (Eds.), *Handbook of psychological change: Psychotherapy processes and practices for the 21st century* (pp. 614–637). New York: Wiley.

Gallagher-Thompson, D., & Osgood, N. (1997). Suicide in later life. *Behavior Therapy, 28,* 23–41.

Gallagher-Thompson, D., Ossinalde, C., Menendez, A., Fernandez, E., Romero, J., Valverde, I., et al. (1996). *Como mantener su bienestar. Una clase para cuidadores.* Palo Alto, CA: VA Palo Alto Health Care System.

Gallagher-Thompson, D., Ossinalde, C., & Thompson, L. W. (1996). *Coping with caregiving: A class for family caregivers.* Palo Alto, CA: VA Palo Alto Health Care System.

Gallagher-Thompson, D., & Steffen, A. M. (1994). Comparative effects of cognitive behavioral and brief psychodynamic psychotherapies for depressed family caregivers. *Journal of Consulting and Clinical Psychology, 62,* 543–549.

Gatz, M., Fiske, A., Fox, L. S., Kaskie, B., Kasl-Godley, J. E., McCallum, T. J., et al. (1998). Empirically validated psychological treatments for older adults. *Journal of Mental Health and Aging, 4*(1), 9–46.

Gillespie, K., Duffy, M., Hackmann, A., & Clark, D. M. (2002). Community based cognitive therapy in the treatment of post-traumatic stress disorder following the Omagh bomb. *Behavior Research and Therapy, 40,* 345–357.

Gomberg, E. S. (1980). *Drinking and problem drinking among the elderly.* Ann Arbor, MI: Institute of Gerontology, University of Michigan.

Gomberg, E. S. L. (1992). Medication problems and drug abuse. In F. J. Turner (Ed.), *Mental Health and the Elderly* (pp. 355–374). New York: Free Press.

Gordon, A. J., Conigliaro, J., Maisto, S. A., McNeil, M., Kraemer, K. L., & Kelley, M. E. (2003). Comparison of consumption effects of brief interventions for hazardous drinking elderly. *Substance Use and Misuse, 38*(8), 1017–1035.

Gorenstein, E. E., Kleber, M. S., Mohlman, J., DeJesus, M., Gorman, J. M., & Papp, L. A. (2005). Cogntive-behavioral therapy for management of anxiety and medication taper in older adults. *American Journal of Geriatric Psychiatry, 13,* 901–909.

Graham, K., & Vidal-Zeballos, D. (1998). Analysis of the use of tranquilizers and sleeping pills across five surveys of the same population (1985–1991): The relationship with gender, age, and use of other substances. *Social Science and Medicine, 46,* 381–395.

Grossman, M. (2002). Frontotemporal dementia: A review. *Journal of the International Neuropsychological Society, 8,* 566–583.

Halonen, J. S., & Santrock, J. W. (1996). *Psychology: Contexts of behavior.* Chicago: Brown & Benchmark.

Hamilton, M. (1959). The assessment of anxiety states by rating. *British Journal of Medical Psychology, 32,* 50–55.

Hammer, M. B., Brodrick, P. S., & Labbbate, L. A. (2001). Gabapentin in PTSD: A retrospective, clinical series of adjunctive therapy. *Annals of Clinical Psychiatry, 13*(3), 141–146.

Havighurst, R. J. (1961). Successful aging. *Gerontologist, 1,* 8–13.

Henry, W. E., & Cumming, E. (1959). Personality development in adulthood and old age. *Journal of Projective Techniques and Personality Assessment, 34,* 384–390.

Hinrichsen, G. A. (1999). Interpersonal psychotherapy for late-life depression. In M. Duffy (Ed.), *Handbook of counseling and psychotherapy with older adults* (pp. 470–486). New York: Wiley.

Horowitz, M. J., Wilner, N., & Alvarez, W. (1979). Impact of Event Scale: A measure of subjective stress. *Psychosomatic Medicine, 41*(3), 209–218.

Hoyert, D. L., Kochanek, K. D., & Murphy, S. L. (1999). *Deaths: Final data for 1997.* National vital statistics report, 47(19). Hyattsville, MD: National Center for Health Statistics. DHHS Publication No. PHS 99–1120.

Hughes, C. P., Berg, L., Danziger, W. L., Cohen, L. A., & Martin, R. L. (1982). A new clinical scale for the staging of dementia. *British Journal of Psychiatry, 140,* 566–572.

Hyer, L. (1995). Use of EMDR in a "dementing" PTSD survivor. *Clinical Gerontologist, 16,* 70–74.

Hyer, L. (1999). The effects of trauma: Dynamics and treatment of PTSD in the elderly. In M. Duffy (Ed.), *Handbook of counseling and psychotherapy with older adults* (pp. 539–560). New York: Wiley.

Hyer, L., & Brandsma, J. M. (1997). EMDR minus eye movements equals good psychotherapy. *Journal of Traumatic Stress, 10,* 515–522.

Hyer, L., Summers, M. N., Boyd, S., & Litaker, M. (1996). Assessment of older combat veterans with the Clinician-Administered PTSD Scale. *Journal of Traumatic Stress, 9,* 587–594.

Hyer, L., Swanson, G., Lefkowitz, R., Hillesland, D., Davis, H., & Woods, M. (1990). The application of the cognitive behavioral model to two older stressor groups. *Clinical Gerontologist, 9*(3–4), 145–190.

Judd, L. L., & Kunovac, J. L. (1998). Bipolar and unipolar depressive disorders in geriatric patients. *International Academy of Biomedical Drug Research, 13,* 1–10.

Kashner, T. M., Rodell, D. I., Ogden, S. R. et al. (1992). Outcomes and costs of two VA inpatient treatment programs for older alcoholic patients. *Hospital Community Psychiatry, 43,* 985–989.

Kasper, S., Lepine, J. P., Mendlewicz, J., Montgomery, S. A., & Rush, J. A. (1995). Efficacy, safety, and indications for tricyclic and newer antidepressants. *Depression, 2,* 127–137.

Katona, C. (2000). Managing depression and anxiety in the elderly patient. *European Neuropsychopharmacology, 10* (Suppl. 4), S427–S432.

Kaup, B., Ruskin, P., & Nyman, G. (1994). Significant life events and PTSD in elderly World War II veterans. *American Journal of Geriatric Psychiatry, 2,* 239–243.

Kawas, C. H. (1999). Inflammation, anti-inflammatory drugs and Alzheimer's disease. In R. Mayeaux & Y. Christen (Eds.), *Epidemiology of Alzheimer's disease: From gene to prevention* (pp. 65–72). New York: Springer-Verlag.

Klerman, G. L., Weissman, M. M., Rounsaville, B. J., & Chevron, E. S. (1984). *Interpersonal psychotherapy of depression*. New York: Basic Books.

Knight, B. (1986). *Psychotherapy with older adults*. Newbury Park, CA: Sage.

Kochanek, K. D., & Murphy, S. L. (1999). *Deaths: Final data for 1997*. National vital statistics report, 47(19). Hyattsville, MD: National Center for Health Statistics. DHHS Publication No. (PHS) 99–1120.

Kofoed, L. L., Tolson, R. L., Atkinson, R. M., et al (1987). Treatment compliance of older alcoholics: An elder-specific approach is superior to "mainstreaming." *Journal of Studies on Alcohol, 48*, 47–51.

Kolb, B., & Whishaw, I. Q. (1996). *Fundamentals of human neuropsychology* (4th ed.). New York: W. H. Freeman.

Laidlaw, K., Thompson, L. W., & Gallagher-Thompson, D. (2004). Comprehensive conceptualization of cognitive behaviour therapy for late life depression. *Behavioural & Cognitive Psychotherapy, 32*, 389–399.

Landreville, P., Laundry, J., Baillargeon, L., Guerette, A., & Matteau, E. (2001). Older adults' acceptance of psychological and pharmacological treatments for depression. *Journal of Gerontology: Psychological Sciences, 56B*(5), P285–P291.

Lauderdale, S. A., & Sheikh, J. I. (2003). Anxiety disorders in older adults. *Clinics in Geriatric Medicine, 19*(4), 721–741.

Lazarus, R. S., & Launier, R. (1978). Stress-related transactions between person and environment. In L. A. Pervin & M. Lewis (Eds.), *Perspectives in interactional psychology* (pp. 287–327). New York: Plenum.

Le Roux, H., Gatz, M., & Wetherell, J. L. (2005). Age at onset of generalized anxiety disorder in older adults. *American Journal of Geriatric Psychiatry, 13*, 23–30.

Lenze, E. J., Mulsant, B. H., Mohlman, J., Shear, M. K., Dew, M. A., Schulz, R., et al. (2005). Generalized anxiety disorders in late life: Lifetime course and comorbidity with major depressive disorder. *American Journal of Geriatric Psychiatry, 13*, 77–80.

Lerner, R. M. (1986). *Concepts and theories of human development* (2nd ed.). New York: Random House.

Levkoff, S. E., Chen, H., Fisher, J. E., & McIntyre, J. S. (Eds.). (2006). *Evidence-based behavioral health practices for older adults: A guide to implementation*. New York: Springer.

Lezak, M. D. (1995). *Neuropsychological assessment* (3rd ed.). New York: Oxford University Press.

Lichtenberg, P. A. (Ed.). (1996). *Handbook of assessment in clinical gerontology*. New York: Wiley.

Lindgren, C. L., Connelly, C. T., & Gaspar, H. L. (1999). Grief in spouse and children caregivers of dementia patients. *Western Journal of Nursing Research, 21*, 521–537.

Lipton, M. I., & Schaffer, W. R. (1988). Physical symptoms related to posttraumtic stress disorder (PTSD) in an aging population, *Military Medicine, 153*, 316–318.

Luis, C. A., Mittenberg, W., Gass, C. S., & Duara, R. (1999). Diffuse Lewy body disease: Clinical, pathological and neuropsychological review. *Neuropsychology Review, 9*(3), 137–150.

Maercker, A. (2002). Life-review technique in the treatment of PTSD in elderly patients: Rationale and three single case studies. *Journal of Clinical Geropsychology, 8*(3), 239–249.

Martenyi, F., Brown, E. B., Zhang, H., Prakah, A., & Koke, S. C. (2002). Fluoxetine versus placebo in posttraumatic stress disorder. *Journal of Clinical Psychiatry, 63*(3), 199–206.

Martin-Cook, K., Trimmer, C., Svetlik, D., & Weiner, M. F. (2000). Caregiver burden in Alzheimer's disease: Case studies. *American Journal of Alzheimer's Disease, 15*(1), 47–52.

Mattis, S. (1976). Mental Status examination for organic mental syndrome in the elderly patient. In L. Bellack & T. Karasu (Eds.), *Geriatric psychiatry* (pp. 77–120). New York: Grune & Stratton.

McFall, M. E., Smith, D. E., Mackay, P. W., & Tarver, D. J. (1990). Reliability and validity of the Mississippi scale for combat related PTSD. *Psychological Assessment, 2*, 114–121.

McFarlane, A. (1990). Posttraumatic stress disorder. *International Review of Psychiatry, 3*, 203–213.

McGivney, S. A., Mulvihill, M., & Taylor, B. (1994). Validating the GDS depression screen in the nursing home. *Journal of the American Geriatric Society, 42*, 490–492.

McIntoch, J. L., Santos, J. F., Hubbard, R. W., & Overholser, J. C. (1994). *Elder suicide research, theory and treatment*. Washington, D.C.: American Psychological Association.

McLeod, A. (1994). The reactivation of posttraumatic stress disorder in later life. *Australian and New Zealand Journal of Psychiatry, 28*, 625–634.

Miller, W. R., & Rollnick, S. (1991). *Motivational interviewing: Preparing people for change*. New York: Guilford.

Miller, W. R., & Rollnick, S. (2002). *Motivational interviewing: Preparing people for change* (2nd ed). New York: Guilford.

Molinari, V., & Williams, W. (1995). An analysis of aging World War II POWs with PTSD: Implications for practice and research. *Journal of Geriatric Psychiatry, 28*, 99–114.

Montgomery, S. A. (1998). Efficacy and safety of the selective serotonin reuptake inhibitors in treating depression in elderly patients. *International Clinical Psychopharmacology, 13*(Suppl. 5), S49–S54.

Montgomery, S. A., & Kasper, S. (1995). Comparison of compliance between serotonin reuptake inhibitors and tricyclic antidepressants: A meta-analysis. *International Clinical Psychopharmacology, 9*(Suppl. 4), 33–40.

Moore, A. A., Beck, J. C., Babor, T. F., Hays, R. D., & Reuben, D. B. (2002). Beyond alcoholism: Identifying older, at-risk drinkers in primary care. *Journal of Studies on Alcohol, 63*(3), 316–324.

Moos, R. M., Mertens, J. R., & Nrennan, P. L. (1993). Patterns of diagnosis and treatment among late-middle aged and older substance abuser patients. *Journal of Studies on Alcohol, 54*, 479–487.

Moscicki, E. K. (1995). Epidemiology of suicide. *International Psychogeriatrics, 7*, 137–148.

Mosimann, U. P., Schmitt, W., Greenberg, B. D., Kosel, M., Müri, R. M., Berkhoff, M., et al. (2004). Repetitive transcranial magnetic stimulation: A putative add-on treatment for major depression in elderly patients. *Psychiatry Research, 126*, 123–133.

Mui, A. C., Burnette, D., & Chen, L. M. (2001). Cross-cultural assessment of geriatric depression: A review of the CES-D and GDS. *Journal of Mental Health and Aging, 7*(1), 137–164.

National Institutes of Health, Consensus Development Conference. (1991). Consensus statement. *Diagnosis and treatment of depression in late life, 9*(3), 1–27.

Neal, L. A., Hill, N., Hughes, J., Middleton, A., & Busuttil, W. (1995). Convergent validity of measures of PTSD in an elderly population of former prisoners of war. *International Journal of Geriatric Psychiatry, 10,* 617–622.

Newmann, J. P., Engel, R. J., & Jensen, J. (1991a). Age differences in depressive symptom experiences. *Journal of Gerontology, 46*(5), P224–P235.

Newmann, J. P., Engel, R. J., & Jensen, J. (1991b). Changes in depressive symptom experiences among older women. *Psychology and Aging, 6*(2), 212–222.

Nordberg, A., & Swensson, A. L. (1998). Cholinesterase inhibitors in the treatment of Alzheimer's disease: A comparison of tolerability and pharmacology. *Drug Safety, 19,* 465–480.

O'Hara, R., Mumenthaler, M. S., & Yesavage, J. A. (2000). Update on Alzheimer's disease: Recent findings and treatments. *Western Journal of Medicine, 172,* 115–120.

Osgood, N. J. (1985). *Suicide in the elderly: A practitioner's guide to diagnosis and mental health intervention.* Richmond, VA: Aspen.

Oslin, D. W. (2004). Late-life alcoholism: Issues relevant to the geriatric psychiatrist. *American Journal of Geriatric Psychiatry, 12*(6), 571–583.

Oslin, D. W., Pettinati, H., & Volpicelli, J. R. (2005). Alcoholism treatment adherence: Older age predicts better adherence and drinking outcomes. *American Journal of Geriatric Psychiatry, 10*(6), 740–747.

Parmelee, P. A., Katz, I. R., & Lawton, M. P. (1989). Depression among institutionalized aged: Assessment and prevalence estimation. *Journal of Gerontology, 44,* M22–M29.

Pearson, J. L., Teri, L., Wagner, A., Truax, P., & Logsdon, R. (1993). The relationship of problem behaviors in dementia patients to the depression and burden of caregiving spouses. *American Journal of Alzheimer's Disease and Related Disorders Research, 8,* 15–22.

Perkins, B. R., & Rouanzoin, C. C. (2002). A critical evaluation of current views regarding eye movement desensitization and reprocessing (EMDR): Clarifying points of confusion. *Journal of Clinical Psychology, 58*(1), 77–97.

Peskind, E. R., Potkin, S. G., Pomara, N., Ott, B. R., Graham, S. M., Olin, J. T., et al. (2006). Memantine treatment in mild to moderate Alzheimer disease: A 24-week randomized, controlled trial. *American Journal of Geriatric Psychiatry, 14*(8), 704–715.

Petronis, A. (1999). Alzheimer's disease and Down syndrome: From meiosis to dementia. *Experimental Neurology, 158*(2):403–413.

Powers, D. V., Thompson, L., & Gallagher-Thompson, D. (2002). Depression in later life: Epidemiology, assessment, impact and treatment. In I. Gotlib & C. Hammen (Eds.), *The handbook of depression* (3rd ed.). New York: Guilford.

Radloff, L. (1977). A self-report depression scale for research in the general population. *Applied Psychological Measurement, 1,* 385–401.

Raj, B. A., & Sheehan, D. V. (1988). Medical evaluation of the anxious patient. *Psychiatric Annals, 18,* 176–181.

REACH II Investigators. (2006). Enhancing the quality of life of dementia caregivers from different ethnic or racial groups: A randomized, controlled trial. *Annals of Internal Medicine, 145,* 727–738.

Regier, D. A., Boyd, J. H., Burke, J. D., Rae, D. S., Myers, J. K., Kramer, M. et al. (1988). One-month prevalence of mental disorders in the United States: Based on five Epidemiologic Catchment Area sites. *Archives of General Psychiatry, 45,* 977–986.

Reisberg, B., Doody, R., Stoffler, A., Schmitt, F., Ferris, S., & Moebius H. J. (2003). A double-blind, placebo-controlled study of Memantine, an uncompetitive NMDA antagonist, in patients with advanced Alzheimer's Disease. *New England Journal of Medicine, 348,* 1333–1341.

Reynolds, C. F., Frank, E., Perel, J. M., Imber, S. D., Cornes, C., Morycz, R., et al. (1992). Combined pharmacotherapy and psychotherapy in the acute and continuation treatment with recurrent major depression: A preliminary report. *American Journal of Psychiatry, 149,* 1687–1692.

Rice, C., Longabaugh, R., Beattie, M., & Noel, N. (1993). Age-group differences in response to treatment for problematic alcohol use. *Addiction, 88,* 1369–1375.

Rice, P. L. (1999). *Stress and health* (3rd ed.). Pacific Grove, CA: Brooks/Cole.

Richman, J. (1999). Psychotherapy with the suicidal elderly: A family-oriented approach. In M. Duffy (Ed.), *Handbook of counseling and psychotherapy with older Adults* (pp. 650–661). New York: Wiley.

Riley, K. P., & Carr, M. (1989). Group psychotherapy with older adults: The value of an expressive approach. *Psychotherapy: Theory, Research, and Practice, 26,* 366–371.

Robinson, P. (1998). Behavioral health services in primary care: A new perspective for treating depression. *Clinical Psychology: Science and Practice, 51*(1), 77–93.

Rosen, W. G., Mohs, R. C., & Davis, K. L. (1984). A new rating scale for Alzheimer's disease. *American Journal of Psychiatry, 141,* 1356–1364.

Rowe, J. W., & Kahn, R. L. (1998). *Successful aging.* New York: Pantheon Books.

Salthouse, T. A. (1996). The processing-speed theory of adult age differences in cognition. *Psychological Review, 103,* 403–428.

Schoevers, R. A., Deeg, D. J. H., van Tilburg, W., & Beekman, A. T. F. (2005). Depression and generalized anxiety disorder co-occurrence and longitudinal patterns in elderly patients. *American Journal of Geriatric Psychiatry, 13,* 31–39.

Schonfeld, L., & Dupree, L. W. (1998). Relapse prevention approaches with the older problem drinker. *Southwest Journal on Aging, 14,* 43–50.

Schulz, R., O'Brien, A. T., Bookwala, J., & Fleissner, K. (1995). Psychiatric and physical morbidity effects of dementia caregiving: Prevalence, correlates, and causes. *Gerontologist, 35,* 771–791.

Scogin, F., Floyd, M., & Forde, J. (2000). Anxiety in older adults. In S. K. Whitbourne (Ed.), *Psychopathology in later adulthood* (pp. 117–140). New York: Wiley.

Scogin, F., Rickard, H. C., Keith, S., Wilson, J., & McElreath, L. (1992). Progressive and imaginal relaxation training for elderly persons with subjective anxiety. *Psychology and Aging, 7,* 419–424.

Sheikh, J. I., & Yesavage, J. A. (1986). Geriatric depression scale (GDS): Recent evidence and development of a shorter version. In T. L. Brink (Ed.), *Clinical gerontology: A guide to assessment and intervention* (pp. 165–173). Binghamton, NY: Haworth.

Siegel, J. S. (1999). Demographic introduction to racial/Hispanic elderly populations. In T. P. Miles (Ed.), *Full-color aging: Facts, goals, and recommendations for America's diverse elders* (pp. 1–19). Washington, D.C.: The Gerontological Society of America.

Simard, M., van Reekum, R., & Cohen, T. (2000). A review of the cognitive and behavioral symptoms in dementia with Lewy bodies. *Journal of Neuropsychiatry and Clinical Neuroscience, 12,* 425–450.

Sirvio, J. (1999). Strategies that support declining cholinergic neurotransmission in Alzheimer's disease patients. *Gerontology, 45,* 3–14.

Spiro, A., Schnurr, P. P., & Aldwin, C. M. (1994). Combat-related posttraumatic stress disorder symptoms in older men. *Psychology and Aging, 9*(1), 17–26.

Stanley, M. A., & Beck, J. G. (1998). Anxiety disorders. In M. Hersen & V. B. Van Hasselt (Eds.), *Handbook of Clinical Geropsychology* (pp. 217–238). New York: Plenum.

Stanley, M. A., Beck, J. G., & Glassco, J. D. (1996). Treatment of generalized anxiety in older adults: A preliminary comparison of cognitive-behavioral and supportive approaches. *Behavior Therapy, 27,* 565–581.

Stanley, M. A., Beck, J. G., & Zebb, B. J. (1996). Psychometric properties of four anxiety measures in older adults. *Behavior Research and Therapy, 34,* 827–838.

Steffens, D. C., & McQuoid, D. R. (2005). Impact of symptoms of generalized anxiety disorder on the course of late-life depression. *American Journal of Geriatric Psychiatry, 13,* 40–47.

Substance Abuse and Mental Health Services Administration (SAMHSA) (1998). *Substance abuse among older adults: Treatment improvement protocol (TIP) series #26.* Rockville, MD: U.S. Department of Health and Human Services.

Substance Abuse and Mental Health Services Administration (SAMHSA). (2004). *2004 National survey on drug use and health.* Rockville, MD: U.S. Department of Health and Human Services.

Tariot, P. N., Farlow, M. R., Grossberg, G. T., Graham, S. M., McDonald, S., & Gergel, I. (2004). Memantine treatment in patients with moderate to severe Alzheimer disease already receiving donepezil: A randomized controlled trial. *Journal of the American Medical Association, 291,* 317–324.

Teng, M. X., Stern, Y., Marder, K., Bell, K., Gurland, B., Lantigua, R., et al. (1998). The APOE-epsilon4 allele and the risk of Alzheimer's disease among African Americans, Whites, and Hispanics. *Journal of the American Medical Association, 279,* 751–755.

Teri, L. (1994). Behavioral treatment of depression in patients with dementia. *Alzheimer's disease and associated disorders, 8*(Suppl. 3), 66–74.

Teri, L. (1999). Training families to provide care: Effects on people with dementia. *International Journal of Geriatric Psychiatry, 14*(2), 110–116.

Teri, L., & Gallagher-Thompson, D. (1991). Cognitive-behavioral interventions for treatment of depression in Alzheimer's patients. *Gerontologist, 31,* 413–416.

Teri, L., Gibbons, L. E., McCurry, S. M., Logsdon, R. G., Buchner, D. M., Barlow, W. E., et al. (2003). Exercise plus behavioral management in patients with Alzheimer's disease: A randomized controlled trial. *Journal of the American Medical Association, 290*(15), 2015–2022.

Teri, L., & Logsdon, R. (1991). Identifying pleasant activities for Alzheimer's disease patients: The Pleasant Events Schedule-AD. *Gerontologist, 31,* 124–127.

Teri, L., Logsdon, R. G., Peskind, E., Raskind, M., Weiner, M. F., Tractenberg, R. E., et al. (2000). Treatment of agitation in AD: A randomized, placebo-controlled clinical trial. *Neurology, 55*(9), 1271–1278.

Teri, L., Logsdon, R. G., Uomoto, J., & McCurry, S. M. (1997). Behavioral treatment of depression in dementia patients: A controlled clinical trial. *Journal of Gerontology: Psychological Sciences, 52B*(4), P159–P166.

Teri, L., & McCurry, S. M. (1994). Psychosocial therapies. In C. E. Coffey & J. L. Cummings (Eds.), *The American Psychiatric Press textbook of geriatric neuropsychiatry* (pp. 662–682). Washington, D.C.: American Psychiatric Press.

Teri, L., & Reifler, B. V. (1987). Depression and dementia. In L. Carstensen & B. Edelstein (Eds.), *Handbook of clinical gerontology* (pp. 112–119). New York: Pergamon.

Teri, L., & Wagner, A. (1992). Alzheimer's disease and depression. *Journal of Consulting and Clinical Psychology, 3,* 379–391.

Thompson, C., & Thompson, G. (1999). Support for carers of people with Alzheimer's type dementia. *Cochrane Library, Issue 4.* Oxford: Update Software.

Thompson, L. W. (1996). Cognitive-behavioral therapy and treatment for late-life depression. *Journal of Clinical Psychiatry, 57*(Suppl. 5), 29–37.

Thompson, L. W., Coon, D., Gallagher-Thompson, D., Sommer, B., & Koin, D. (2001). Comparison of desipramine and cognitive/behavioral therapy in the treatment of elderly outpatients with mild to moderate depression. *American Journal of Geriatric Psychiatry, 9,* 225–240.

Thompson, L., Gallagher, D., & Breckenridge, J. S. (1987). Comparative effectiveness of psychotherapies for depressed elders. *Journal of Consulting and Clinical Psychology, 55,* 385–390.

Thompson, L., Gallagher-Thompson, D., & Dick, L. (1996). *Cognitive-behavioral therapy for late-life depression: A therapist manual.* Palo Alto, CA: Veterans Affairs Palo Alto Health Care System.

Thompson, L. W., Tang, P., Kaye, J., & Gallagher-Thompson, D. (2004). Bereavement and adjustment disorders in later life. In D. Blazer, D. Steffens, & E. Busse (Eds.), *Textbook of geriatric psychiatry* (3rd ed.). Washington, D.C.: American Psychiatric Press.

Tucker, P., Zaninelli, R., Yehuda, R., Ruggiero, L., Dillingham, K., & Pitts, C. D. (2001). Paroxetine in the treatment of chronic posttraumatic stress disorder: Results of a placebo-controlled, flexible-dosage trial. *Journal of Clinical Psychiatry, 62*(11), 860–868.

U.S. Administration on Aging. (2000). *A profile of older Americans.* Washington, D.C.: Author.

U.S. Administration on Aging. (2004). *A profile of older Americans.* Washington, D.C.: Author.

U.S. Department of Health and Human Services. (2000). *Progress report on Alzheimer's disease: Taking the next steps.* Rockville, MD: Author, Public Health Service, National Institutes of Health, National Institute on Aging.

U.S. Department of Health and Human Services. (2001). *Mental health: Culture, race, and ethnicity—A supplement to mental health: A report of the Surgeon General—Executive summary.* Rockville, MD: Author, Public Health Service, Office of the Surgeon General.

U.S. Department of Health and Human Services. (1999). *Mental health: A report of the surgeon general.* Rockville, MD: Author, Substance Abuse and Mental Health Services Administration, Center for Mental Health Services, National Institutes of Health, National Institute of Mental Health.

U.S. Department of Veterans Affairs. (1997). *Dementia identification and assessment: Guidelines for primary care practitioners.* Washington, D.C.: Author and the University Health System Consortium.

Van Zelst, W. H., De Beurs, E., Beekman, A. T. F., Deeg, D. J. H., & Van Dyck, R. (2003). Prevalence and risk factors of post-traumatic stress disorder in older adults. *Psychotherapy and Psychosomatics, 72,* 333–342.

Vedhara, K., Shanks, N., Anderson, S., & Lightman, S. (2000). The role of stressors and psychosocial variables in the stress process. A study of chronic caregiver stress. *Psychosomatic Medicine, 62*(3), 374–385.

Wagstaff, A. J., Cheer, S. M., Matheson, A. J., Ormrod, D., & Goa, K. L. (2002). Paroxetine: An update of its use in psychiatric disorders in adults, *Drugs, 62*(4), 655–703.

Watson, C. G. (1990). Psychometric PTSD measuring techniques: A review. *Psychological Assessment, 2,* 460–469.

Wechsler, H., Kuo, M., Lee, H., & Dowdall, G.W. (2000). Environmental correlates of underage alcohol use and related problems in college drinkers. *American Journal of Preventative Medicine, 19*(1), 24–29.

Weissman, M. M., Bruce, M. L., Leaf, P. J., Florio, L. P., & Holzer, C. (1991). Affective disorders. In L. N. Robins & D. A. Regier (Eds.), *Psychiatric disorders in America* (pp. 53–80). New York: Free Press.

Weitzman, E. A., & Wechsler, H. (2000). Alcohol use, abuse and related problems among children of problem drinkers: Findings from a national survey of college alcohol use. *Journal of Nervous & Mental Disease, 188*(3), 148–154.

Wetherell, J. L. (1998). Treatment of anxiety in older adults. *Psychotherapy, 35,* 444–458.

Wetherell, J. L. (2002). Behavior therapy for anxious older adults. *The Behavior Therapist, 25*(1), 16–17.

Wetherell, J. L., & Arean, P. A. (1997). Psychometric evaluation of the Beck Anxiety Inventory with older medical patients. *Psychological Assessment, 9,* 136–144.

Wetherell, J. L., Gatz, M., Craske, M. G. (2003). Treatment of generalized anxiety disorders in older adults. *Journal of Consulting and Clinical Psychology, 71*(1), 31–40.

Whitbourne, S. K. (2000). The normal aging process. In S. K. Whitbourne (Ed.), *Psychopathology in later adulthood* (pp. 27–60). New York: Wiley.

Wilkinson, D. G. (1999). The pharmacology of donepezil: A new treatment of Alzheimer's disease. *Expert Opinions in Pharmacotherapy, 1*(1), 121–135.

Wilson, J., Harel, Z., & Kahana, B. (1989). The day of infamy: The legacy of Pearl Harbor. In J. Wilson (Ed.), *Trauma, transformation, and healing* (pp. 129–156). New York: Brunner/Mazel.

Winblad, B., & Poritis, N. (1999). Memantine in severe dementia: Results of the 9M-Best Study (Benefit and efficacy in severely demented patients during treatment with memantine). *International Journal of Geriatric Psychiatry, 14,* 135–146.

Yesavage, J. A., Brink, T. L., Rose, T. L., Lum, O., Huang, V., Adey, M. B., & Leirer, V. O. (1983). Development and validation of a geriatric depression screening scale: A preliminary report. *Journal of Psychiatric Research, 17,* 37–49.

Zarit, S. H., & Haynie, D. A. (2000). Introduction to clinical issues. In S. K. Whitbourne (Ed.), *Psychopathology in later adulthood* (pp. 1–26). New York: Wiley.

Zarit, S. H., & Zarit, J. M. (1998). *Mental disorders in older adults: Fundamentals of assessment and treatment.* New York: Guilford.

Zeiss, A. M., & Steffen, A. (1996). Treatment issues with elderly clients. *Cognitive and Behavioral Practice, 3*(2), 371–390.

Index